Genetic Susceptibility to Infectious Diseases

Genetic Susceptibility to Infectious Diseases

Edited by
Richard A. Kaslow
Janet M. McNicholl
Adrian V.S. Hill

OXFORD
UNIVERSITY PRESS

2008

OXFORD
UNIVERSITY PRESS

Oxford University Press, Inc., publishes works that further
Oxford University's objective of excellence
in research, scholarship, and education.

Oxford   New York
Auckland   Cape Town   Dar es Salaam   Hong Kong   Karachi
Kuala Lumpur   Madrid   Melbourne   Mexico City   Nairobi
New Delhi   Shanghai   Taipei   Toronto

With offices in
Argentina   Austria   Brazil   Chile   Czech Republic   France   Greece
Guatemala   Hungary   Italy   Japan   Poland   Portugal   Singapore
South Korea   Switzerland   Thailand   Turkey   Ukraine   Vietnam

Published by Oxford University Press, Inc.
198 Madison Avenue, New York, New York 10016

www.oup.com

Oxford is a registered trademark of Oxford University Press

Library of Congress Cataloging-in-Publication Data
Kaslow, Richard A.
Genetic susceptibility to infectious diseases / Richard Kaslow, Janet
McNicholl, Adrian Hill.
   p.   cm.
Includes bibliographical references.
ISBN 978-0-19-517490-8
1. Communicable diseases—Genetic aspects.   2. Infection—Genetic aspects.
3. Disease susceptibility—Genetic aspects.   I. McNicholl, Janet.   II. Hill, Adrian.   III. Title.
[DNLM: 1. Communicable Diseases—genetics.   2. Genetic Predisposition
to Disease.   3. Variation (Genetics)—immunology. QZ 50 K19b 2007]
RC112.K27 2007
616.9042—dc22   2007008576

9 8 7 6 5 4 3 2 1
Printed in the United States of America
on acid-free paper

Preface

The twentieth century was filled with triumph in preventing and controlling infectious diseases. Much of that success was achieved through a combination of sanitation (simple alterations of the physical environment), antimicrobials (painstaking discovery and testing of compounds to inactivate or destroy etiologic agents), and immunization (elegant manipulation of the agents or their products to stimulate protective host immunity). Of the three approaches, only immunization depended on the genetically mediated host immune responses—and even then only indirectly and often imperceptibly. Numerous vaccines with impressive efficacies of 70–90% or higher—the most recent example being the remarkable human papillomavirus vaccine—were developed with little or no attention to the principles of human genetics. In short, throughout decades of progress, our meager knowledge of host genes and genetic variation was largely irrelevant to the many landmark victories.

During that same period, numerous assaults on infectious disease faltered, with grave consequences. The quarter-century-long explosion of HIV-1 infection, the resurgence of tuberculosis both with and without HIV/AIDS, the unshakable persistence of malaria, and biological threats such as anthrax continue to remind us of the inadequacy of previously effective strategies. Those "failures" as much as anything have refocused attention on the origins of infectious diseases in their full complexity. There has been increasing recognition that strategies for controlling these diseases will likely require insights at the deeper level of human and microbial genetics—a thorough understanding of the influences of host genetic variation on infection and immunity. The purpose of this volume is to organize existing knowledge of those influences into a foundation for future inquiry.

The book was conceived early in 2001 in the "pregenomic" era, a few months before the first draft sequence of the human genome was available and before the International HapMap Project was even designed. Beyond gathering in one place the information that a reader would otherwise be forced to excavate from many sites, this collection is intended to accomplish a secondary goal: to "cross-fertilize" the work of basic scientists, clinicians, and others who may be more familiar with genetics or infection but not both. It is thus meant to be a blend of the general and the specific—containing aspects of critical review, systematic progress report, clinical application, and prospectus.

In the gestational period between conception of the text and delivery of the manuscript to the publisher, many new candidate genes with probable influence on infection and immunity have surfaced, and previously quiescent or unrecognized infections of major public health consequence such as West Nile virus infection and corona virus–associated severe acute respiratory distress syndrome (SARS) have emerged. Meanwhile, revolutionary advances in the knowledge and technology of genetics have continued to sweep through every corner of the biomedical research enterprise. In the midst of such dynamic changes, we have tried to maintain as much currency as the constraints of space and time allowed.

To assist the diverse audience, we have divided the book into three parts that mirror that diversity in orientation and knowledge base. Part I describes the current methods for generating information about genetic variation in populations of humans and animals. Part II highlights families of genes whose variation is known or likely to contribute to susceptibility to human infectious disease, and part III covers the major infectious diseases on which the influences of host genetic variation are stronger or better established. Sections of individual chapters in parts II and III conform roughly to a general outline. General topic headings and the structure of certain tables correspond more closely across chapters; however, the inherent disparity in knowledge of each individual gene or disease limited further standardization.

We have made no attempt to catalogue every technique, gene, or disease with some connection to the title theme; that encyclopedic approach was beyond the scope of the endeavor. At the risk of diluting or omitting, we have tried to be rather more selective, to create an anthology with accessibility to readers in a broad set of disciplines. Chapters in part I provide more perspective than specifics. Including sections on such topics as bioinformatics tools and applications, the latest strategies for genomewide association studies, whole-genome sequencing or expression microarray analysis, proteomics, and alternative animal models might have added more specialized material of interest to some but are well reviewed elsewhere.

Part II covers 14 families of genes whose variation is known to contribute to differential susceptibility. The relevant polymorphisms of those selected range widely in the degree of certainty of their involvement and in their importance in terms of population frequency. For some gene families (e.g., those encoding certain complement components or immunoglobulin receptors), clinically significant variation is well established but relatively uncommon. Different chapters reflect varying perspectives among authors in accepting the validity or relevance of polymorphisms reported to alter immune function or disease susceptibility. For example, although experimental or epidemiologic studies of various inflammatory diseases have implicated the genes encoding MHC class I polypeptide–related sequence (MICA and MICB) and the Toll-like receptors (TLRs), the chapters on those gene clusters reflect considerable skepticism that published associations of infectious diseases with specific alleles represent effects that are functionally significant and independent of alleles in close linkage disequilibrium with unknown variants. Other chapters are more liberal in including reported relationships.

Part III reveals notable unevenness in current knowledge among the diseases of interest. Chapter 18 encompasses uncommon immune deficiencies due to derangements of immunoglobulin genes and others showing classic Mendelian inheritance. Subsequent chapters cover some diseases of major public health importance. Some other conditions of comparable impact on populations, such as dengue fever and human papillomavirus infection, are mentioned in the appropriate places in part II but not covered explicitly in their own right. For most of the disorders included, investigation of susceptibility due to genetic polymorphism has yielded relatively convincing evidence, but the diseases and the genes examined vary considerably in that regard. Malaria, HIV/AIDS, and tuberculosis show definitive relationships with variable gene content or allelic polymorphisms in numerous chromosomal regions. The work on malaria has been thorough enough to devote a separate chapter in part II to the profound impact of red blood cell genes and a chapter in part III to the disease itself.

Interest and information on genetic determinants of variable response to vaccines for preventing infections and to drugs for treating them are expanding. Aside from space limits, a simple reason explains our deliberate decision to include a chapter on the former but not the latter. Vaccines are biological products—in some cases actually replicating organisms—to which genetically mediated responses may well parallel responses to the naturally occurring pathogen. Accordingly, observations about variable vaccine response are quite likely to inform studies of infection and vice versa. On the other hand, anti-infective pharmaceuticals are transported and metabolized along pathways whose regulation, for the most part, involves a very different set of genes with more tenuous involvement in immunity or susceptibility.

Although we could not continue beyond a point to update the text with every new gene family, disease, or genotype–phenotype relationship to susceptibility whenever potentially relevant information appeared, two efforts have been made to maintain its currency during production. One effort resulted in an appendix containing a list of particularly informative Web sites among the many devoted to "postgenomic" activities. Compiling such a compendium was a challenge—one that is likely to grow as Web sites proliferate even further, but an exercise worth the effort because it will not be long before these and subsequent electronic sources will be providing rich and continuously timely information beyond the scope of this volume.

The other updating effort followed our decision to use current nomenclature and conventions of the U.S. National Center for Biotechnology Information (NCBI) as universally as possible. Names of genes are intended to follow official NCBI designations uniformly. Wherever possible, and with a few exceptions for those likely to be confusing in context, the NCBI gene symbol has been systematically substituted for the historical or more common abbreviation, often with a parenthetic reference to the older, familiar one. By convention, symbols that refer to a human gene rather than to its product or to its specific alleles are meant to be capitalized and italicized; a symbol for a human gene accompanied by one or more of its alleles is also usually capitalized but not italicized. Although the latter convention has not been widely adopted, we have tried for the most part to conform to it. For HLA genes and alleles, the more exacting nomenclature is explained in the text. Genes of nonhuman species may or may not be capitalized but are italicized.

As the mining of the human genome for susceptibility genes gathers pace, with greatly improved technologies and larger study populations, the relevance of this work to public health will expand. The number of susceptibility gene discoveries that have so far generated new intervention strategies is still small but likely to grow rapidly, particularly for the major killers that have proved most refractory to more traditional approaches. New susceptibility profiles will have application to risk assessment, to prioritization of individuals for prophylaxis, and to selection of alternative treatments. Equally important, pathways identified through the recognition of novel susceptibility genes have already suggested unexpected mechanisms with candidate molecular targets.

Research on genetic susceptibility to infectious diseases has often taken place at the interface between the science of evolutionary biology and the real world of treatment and prevention. The text summarizes the scientific discoveries of more than half a century in a series of stories about an ancient, ongoing struggle between host and pathogen. Victories on both sides of this coevolutionary contest between human and microbial life have forged remarkable patterns of polymorphism that remain with us—many probably persisting long after the pathogens responsible for driving the particular variation have ceased to colonize our species. However, the patterns in our DNA do not constitute mere "fossil record" of these encounters. Our genetic legacy continues to exert its force and, as in the past, will inevitably shape reemergent and newly recognized transmissible microorganisms into agents of future epidemics. The difference between the past and the future is that we have recently crossed a threshold into the promise of a postgenomic world. There we can envision far more powerful observational and experimental research that will accelerate the translation of discovery about human genetic susceptibility into effective measures of disease control. We hope that in some small way this text will equip each reader to contribute to that goal.

Acknowledgments

Every text is ultimately more than the sum of its published parts. This one represents the collective, organized wisdom of the authors and the product of continuous editorial exchange about content and form. However, other contributions were essential. At the earliest conceptual stages, three individuals with different orientations understood the theme of genetic susceptibility to infection and were of common mind as they envisioned something like this text. Jeffrey House, the Oxford University Press representative for many years; Emil Skamene, the eminent McGill University immunobiologist and physician; and Muin Khoury, the Centers for Disease Control and Prevention genetic epidemiologist and public health exponent, deserve our special gratitude for encouraging us to convert our shared vision into reality. Throughout the process that followed, we have relied on others behind the scenes to inspire, encourage, facilitate, tolerate, restrain, revive, and (still) love us for what we were trying to do. To them—our families, friends, colleagues—we owe our profound gratitude.

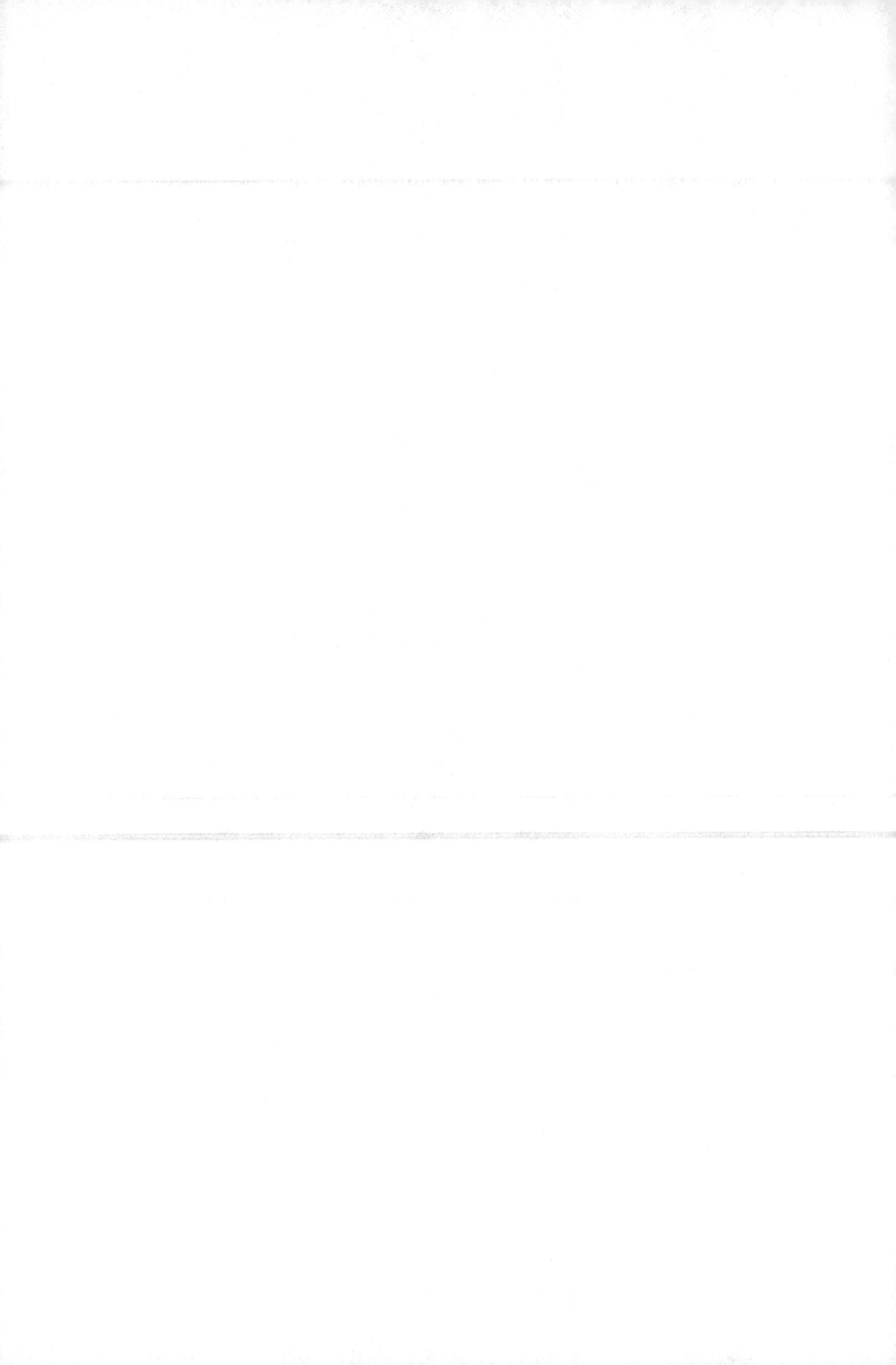

Contents

Contributors

Editors

Richard A. Kaslow, M.D., M.P.H.
Professor of Epidemiology, Medicine,
  Microbiology and Genetics
University of Alabama at Birmingham
220 Ryals Building
1665 University Blvd.
Birmingham, AL 35294-0022 USA
Tel: 205-975-8698
rkaslow@uab.edu

Janet M. McNicholl, M.D.
Medical Scientist and Section Chief, HIV/STD
  Laboratory
Thai MOPH-US CDC Collaboration,
Dept Med. Sciences, Bldg. 2
Ministry of Public Health
Tivanon Road, A. Muang
Nonthaburi, 11000, Thailand
or
U.S. postal address: CDC/HIV, Box 68
APO, AP, 96546
Tel: +66 (0)25915444
Fax: +66 (0)25800696
jkm7@cdc.gov
and
Assistant Professor, Department of Medicine
Emory University, Atlanta, GA, 30322 USA

Adrian V.S. Hill, D.M., F.Med.Sci.
Wellcome Trust Centre for Human Genetics
University of Oxford
Roosevelt Drive
Oxford OX3 7DN, UK
adrian.hill@well.ox.ac.uk

Authors

Chester A. Alper, M.D.
The CBR Institute for Biomedical
  Research
and
Department of Pediatrics
Harvard Medical School
800 Huntington Avenue
Boston, MA 02115 USA
Tel: 617-278-3333
alper@cbr.med.harvard.edu

Juan-Manuel Anaya
Cellular Biology and Immunogenetics
  Unit
Corporación para Investigaciones
  Biológicas
Cra. 72-A, No. 78-B-141
Medellín, Colombia
janaya@cib.org.co

Seiamak Bahram, M.D., Ph.D.
Laboratoire d'Immunogénétique Moléculaire
  Humaine
Centre de Recherche Immunologie et
  Hématologie
4 Rue Kirschleger
67085 Strasbourg Cedex, France
Tel : +33 0390243992
siamak@hemato-ulp.u-strasbg.fr

Charles R. M. Bangham, Sc.D., F.Med.Sci.
Department of Immunology
Imperial College, St Mary's Campus
London W2 1PG, UK
c.bangham@imperial.ac.uk

Terri H. Beaty, Ph.D.
Department of Epidemiology
Johns Hopkins University Bloomberg School
    of Public Health
615 N. Wolfe Street
Baltimore, MD 21205 USA
Tel: 410-955-6960
tbeaty@jhsph.edu

Richard Bellamy, M.D.
James Cook University Hospital
Marton Road
Middlesbrough TS4 3BW, UK
richard.bellamy@stees.nhs.uk

Bruce Beutler, M.D.
Department of Immunology
The Scripps Research Institute
10550 N. Torrey Pines Road
La Jolla, CA 92037 USA
Tel: 858-784-8610
bruce@scripps.edu

Jeremy M. Boss, Ph.D.
Professor
Department of Microbiology and Immunology
Emory University School of Medicine
Atlanta, GA 30322 USA
Tel: 404-727-5973
Fax: 404-727-1719
boss@microbio.emory.edu

Ellen Buschman, Ph.D.
The McGill University Centre for the Study
    of Host Resistance
1650 Cedar Avenue
Montreal, QC, Canada H3G 1A4[1]
Tel: 514-934-1934, ext. 42531
ellen.buschman@muhc.mcgill.ca

François Canonne-Hergaux Ph.D.
Chargé de Recherche INSERM
Institut de Chimie des Substances Naturelles
    (ICSN)
CNRS, Equipe 34

Bâtiment 27, Avenue de la Terrasse
91198 Gif-sur-Yvette Cedex France
Tel : +33 0169823081
Fax: +33 0169077247
fcanonne@icsn.cnrs-gif.fr

Mary Carrington, Ph.D.
Basic Research Program, Laboratory of Genomic
    Diversity
Science Applications International
    Corporation-Frederick, Inc.
National Cancer Institute
Building 560—FCRDC, 21-89
Frederick, MD 21702 USA
Tel: 301-846-1390
carringt@mail.ncifcrf.gov

Stephen J. Chanock, M.D.
Section on Genomic Variation
Pediatric Oncology Branch
National Cancer Institute
Advanced Technology Center
8717 Grovemont Circle
Bethesda, MD 20892-4605 USA
Tel: 301-435-7559
sc83a@nih.gov

Christophe Chevillard, Ph.D.
Inserm UMR399
Immunology and Genetics of Parasitic
    Diseases
Faculty of Medicine
Université de la Méditerranée
Marseille, France
Tel: +33 0491324524
Fax: +33 0491796063
christophe.chevillard@medecine.univ-mrs.fr

Graham Cooke, M.B., D.Phil.
Wellcome Trust Centre for Human
    Genetics
University of Oxford
Roosevelt Drive
Oxford OX3 7BN, UK

Keith D. Crawford, M.D., Ph.D.
The CBR Institute for Biomedical Research
and
Center for Molecular Orthopedics, Brigham
    and Women's Hospital

Department of Orthopedic Surgery
221 Longwood Avenue
Boston, MA 02115 USA
Tel: 617-732-8607
kdcrawford@partners.org

Jennifer A. Croker, Ph.D.
Division of Clinical Immunology and
    Rheumatology
Department of Medicine
Shelby Bldg. 172F
University of Alabama at Birmingham
Birmingham, AL 35294-2182 USA
Tel: 205-996-4478
Fax: 205-934-1564
Jennifer.Croker@ccc.uab.edu

Alain Dessein, Ph.D.
Inserm UMR399
Immunology and Genetics of Parasitic Diseases
Faculty of Medicine
Université de la Méditerranée
Marseille, France
alain.dessein@medecine.univ-mrs.fr

M. Tevfik Dorak, M.D., Ph.D.
Genomic Immunoepidemiology Laboratory
HUMIGEN, The Institute for Genetic
    Immunology
2439 Kuser Road
Hamilton, NJ 08690 USA
Tel: 609-570-1032
m.t.dorak@humigen.org

Priya Duggal, Ph.D., M.P.H.
Inherited Disease Research Branch
National Human Genome Research Institute
National Institutes of Health
333 Cassell Drive, Suite 1200
Baltimore, MD 21224 USA
Tel: 410-550-4621
pduggal@mail.nih.gov

Nasr Eldin Elwali, Ph.D.
Institute of Nuclear Medicine and
    Molecular Biology
University of Gezira
Wad Medani, Sudan
Tel: 249 511 466 40
Fax: 249 511 431 74
nasreldinelwali@yahoo.com

John R. Forbes, Ph.D.
Department of Biochemistry
Center for the Study of Host Resistance
Cancer Center
McGill University
3655 Sir William Osler Promenade
Montreal, QC, Canada, H3G 1Y6
Tel: 514-398-2489

Anny Fortin, Ph.D.
Emerillon Therapeutics
416 de Maisonneuve, West
Suite 1000
Montreal, QC, Canada H3A 1L2[2]
Tel: 514-985-0306, ext. 231
Anny.Fortin@emerillon.ca

Grant Gallagher, Ph.D.
Genetic Immunology Laboratory
HUMIGEN, the Institute for Genetic
    Immunology
2439 Kuser Road
Hamilton, NJ 08690 USA
G.Gallagher@Humigen.org

Philippe Gros, Ph.D.
Department of Biochemistry
McGill University
3655 Sir William Osler Promenade
Montreal, QC, Canada H3G 1Y6
Tel: 514-398-7291
philippe.gros@mcgill.ca

Margje H. Haverkamp, M.D.
Department of Infectious Diseases
Leiden University Medical Center
Leiden, The Netherlands
Tel: +31-71-5262613
and
NIAID, Room B3-4233
10 Center Drive, MSC 1684
Bethesda, MD 20892-1684 USA
Tel: 301-402-2087
mhaverkamp@niaid.nih.gov or
    m.h.haverkamp@lumc.nl

Stephen M. Holland, M.D.
Laboratory of Host Defenses
NIAID, Rm. 11N103
National Institutes of Health
10 Center Drive, MSC 1886

Bethesda, MD 20892-1886 USA
Tel: 301-402-7684
F: 301-402-4369
smh@nih.gov

Cynthia Horth, B.Sc.
Department of Biochemistry
Center for the Study of Host
    Resistance
Cancer Center
McGill University
3655 Sir William Osler Promenade
Montreal, QC, Canada H3G 1Y6
Tel: 514-398-2489

Tom W. J. Huizinga, M.D.
Department of Rheumatology, C1-41
Leiden University Medical Center
Albinusdreef 2
P.O. Box 9600
2300RC Leiden
The Netherlands
Tel: +31-71-5263598
Fax: +31-71-5266752

Robert M. Jacobson, M.D.
Mayo Vaccine Research Group
611 C Guggenheim Building
200 First Street SW
and
Department of Pediatric and Adolescent
    Medicine
Mayo Clinic College of Medicine
Rochester, MN 55905 USA
jacobson.robert@mayo.edu

Peter E. Jensen, M.D.
ARUP Professor and Chair
Department of Pathology
University of Utah
Emma Eccles Jones Medical Research Building
15 North Medical Drive East, Ste 1100
Salt Lake City, Utah 84112-5650 USA
Tel: 801-585-6217
Fax: 801-585-7376
peter.jensen@path.utah.edu

Robert P. Kimberly, M.D.
Division of Clinical Immunology and
    Rheumatology
Department of Medicine

Shelby Bldg. 172B
University of Alabama at Birmingham
Birmingham, AL 35294-2182 USA
Tel: 205-934-5306
Robert.Kimberly@ccc.uab.edu

Malak Kotb, Ph.D.
Veterans Affairs Medical Center, Research Service
Memphis, TN 38104 USA
and
The MidSouth Center for Biodefense and
    Security and
Departments of Surgery and Molecular Sciences
University of Tennessee Health Science Center
Memphis, TN 38163 USA
Tel: 901-448-7247
mkotb@utmem.edu

Dominic P. Kwiatkowski, F.R.C.P.
Wellcome Trust Centre for Human Genetics and
University Department of Paediatrics
Oxford University
Roosevelt Drive
Oxford OX3 7BN, UK
Tel: +44 (0)1865 287654
dominic@well.ox.ac.uk
and
Wellcome Trust Sanger Institute
Hinxton, Cambridge, CB10 1SA, UK

Gaia Luoni—Deceased
Wellcome Trust Centre for Human Genetics
Oxford University
Roosevelt Drive
Oxford OX3 7BN, UK

Jean-François Marquis, Ph.D.
Department of Biochemistry
Center for the Study of Host Resistance
Cancer Center
McGill University
3655 Sir William Osler Promenade
Montreal, QC, Canada, H3G 1Y6
Tel: 514-398-2489

Maureen P. Martin, Ph.D.
Basic Research Program, Laboratory
    of Genomic Diversity
Science Applications International
    Corporation-Frederick, Inc.

National Cancer Institute
Building 560, Room 21-46
Frederick, MD 21702 USA
Tel: 301-846-5318
martinm@ncifcrf.gov

Milton O. Moraes, Ph.D.
Functional Genomics and Genetic
    Epidemiology of Infectious Diseases
Leprosy Laboratory
Oswaldo Cruz Institute
FIOCRUZ
Av Brasil, 4365 Manguinhos
Rio de Janeiro RJ, Brazil 22441-140
Tel: 5521 25984467
Fax: 5521 22709997
mmoraes@fiocruz.br

Thomas R. O'Brien, M.D., M.P.H.
Senior Investigator
Division of Cancer Epidemiology and Genetics
National Cancer Institute
6120 Executive Blvd.
Room 8096
Rockville, MD 20852 USA
Tel: 301-435-4728
obrient@mail.nih.gov

Tom H. M. Ottenhoff, M.D., Ph.D.
Professor in Immunology
Head, Section Immunology and
    Immunogenetics of Bacterial Infectious
    Diseases
Dept. of Immunohematology & Blood
    Transfusion
and Dept. of Infectious Diseases
Leiden University Medical Center
Albinusdreef 2
2333 ZA Leiden
The Netherlands
Tel: +31-71-5265128 (main); 5263809 (direct)
Fax: +31-71-5265267
t.h.m.ottenhoff@lumc.nl

Inna G. Ovsyannikova, Ph.D.
Mayo Vaccine Research Group
611 C Guggenheim Building
200 First Street SW
Rochester, MN 55905 USA
Tel: 507-284-4968
ovsyannikova.inna@mayo.edu

Gregory A. Poland, M.D.
Mayo Clinic and Foundation
Director, Mayo Vaccine Research
    Group
and
Program in Translational Immunovirology
    and Biodefense
611 C Guggenheim Building
200 First Street SW
Rochester, MN 55905 USA
Tel: 507-284-4968
poland.gregory@mayo.edu

Harry W. Schroeder, M.D., Ph.D.
Division of Developmental and Clinical
    Immunology
Departments of Medicine and Microbiology
Shelby Bldg. 405
University of Alabama at Birmingham
Birmingham, AL 35294-2182 USA
Tel: 205-934-4769
hwsj@uab.edu

Emil Skamene, M.D., Ph.D.
The Research Institute of the McGill University
    Health Centre
Room A6.149
1650 Cedar Avenue
Montreal QC, H3G 1A4
Tel: 514-934-1934, ext. 42531
emil.skamene@muhc.mcgill.ca

Henry A. F. Stephens, Ph.D.
Centre for Nephrology & The Anthony Nolan
    Trust
Department of Medicine
Royal Free and University College Medical
    School
University College London
Royal Free Campus
Rowland Hill Street
London NW3 2PF, UK
Tel: +44 (0)2077 940500, ext. 5123 or 3447
h.stephens@ucl.ac.uk or
    Henry.Stephens@anthonynolan.org.uk

Jianming "James" Tang, Ph.D.
Department of Medicine
School of Medicine
and

Program in Epidemiology of Infection and
    Immunity
School of Public Health
University of Alabama at Birmingham
RPHB Room 624A
1665 University Blvd.
Birmingham, AL 35294-0022 USA
Tel: 205-975-8630
jtang@uab.edu

Mark R. Thursz, M.D., F.R.C.P.
Professor of Hepatology
Division of Medicine
Imperial College, St Mary's Campus
Norfolk Place
London W2 1PG, UK
Tel: + 44 (0) 2075 943851
m.thursz@imperial.ac.uk

David Weatherall, F.R.S.
Weatherall Institute of Molecular
    Medicine
University of Oxford
John Radcliffe Hospital
Headington
Oxford OX3 9DS, UK
T: +44 (0)1865 222360
david.weatherall@imm.ox.ac.uk

Robert A. Welch
Core Genotyping Facility
National Cancer Institute/SAIC
Advanced Technology Ctr, 143,
    MSC 4605
8717 Grovemont Circle

Gaithersburg, MD 20892-4605 USA
Tel: 301-435-7615
rw290r@nih.gov

Tania Mara Welzel, M.D., M.H.Sc.
Visiting Fellow
Division of Cancer Epidemiology and Genetics
National Cancer Institute
6120 Executive Blvd.
Rockville, MD 20852 USA
Tel: 301-435-4728

Meredith Yeager, Ph.D.
Core Genotyping Facility
National Cancer Institute/SAIC
Advanced Technology Center, 152B
8717 Grovemont Circle
Gaithersburg, MD 20892-4605 USA
Tel: 301-435-7613
YeagerM@mail.nih.gov

Leland J. Yee, Ph.D., M.P.H.
Assistant Professor
Department of Epidemiology
Graduate School of Public Health
and the Division of Infectious Diseases
Department of Medicine
School of Medicine
University of Pittsburgh
A511 Crabtree Hall
130 DeSoto Street
Pittsburgh, PA 15261 USA
YeeL@edc.pitt.edu
Tel: 412-624-5326

PART I

METHODS AND TOOLS

1

Genetic Epidemiology of Infectious Disease

Priya Duggal & Terri H. Beaty

Genetic epidemiology is a hybrid science that combines the tools of genetics and epidemiology to identify the role genes play in controlling susceptibility to complex diseases—diseases that have both genetic and environmental causes. Traditional medical genetics has focused primarily on single-gene traits and has successfully identified causal mutations controlling many phenotypes that follow the transmission patterns first outlined by Gregor Mendel. Mendelian diseases can be autosomal dominant, autosomal recessive, X-linked dominant, or X-linked recessive (with varying levels of incomplete penetrance possible) but are typically rare in the population (see glossary). Epidemiology, the methodologic science of public health, has conventionally focused on the study of more common diseases in an effort to identify factors that control the distribution of disease at the population level. The science of epidemiology evolved through the study of infectious diseases, and traditionally there has been little consideration of host genetic factors controlling susceptibility. During the last quarter of the twentieth century, however, genetic epidemiology emerged as a field that applies the principles of genetics to complex diseases, which generally cluster in families suggesting some genetic component but do not behave in a purely Mendelian fashion. Unlike the traditional single gene diseases, a complex disease is most likely to reflect effects of one or more genes (that may interact with each other) and the environment, and there is typically some degree of etiologic heterogeneity.

In many ways, an infectious disease epitomizes a complex disease because both genetic and environmental factors must play a role in susceptibility to and progression of such a disease. The genes of the host may determine susceptibility to infection, and risk or severity of disease after infection may be influenced by variable exposure to the infectious agent. The intricacy and redundancy of the human immune system provide many gene pathways that may be involved with susceptibility or resistance to infections, as well as the progression of disease. Although exposure to an environmental pathogen is obviously critical to risk, genes in the host can influence both risk of disease and severity. In this chapter, we describe study designs and analytical strategies that can be used to identify genetic factors in the host contributing to risk for infectious diseases. Although they may be important, issues of how genetic variability in the pathogen can influence risk are not addressed.

Defining the Phenotype

The first step in any genetic epidemiologic study is to evaluate the disease and correctly classify observable outcomes or phenotypes. Phenotypes can be classified as either qualitative or quantitative. A qualitative phenotype is a trait that can be categorized into two or more mutually exclusive groups (affected or unaffected; unaffected, mildly, or severely affected). For example, a person can be classified dichotomously as either having malaria or not having malaria, and the analysis would focus on predicting the probability of developing clinical symptoms of malaria, conditional on exposure to the parasite. Clearly, unexposed people would be unaffected, and hence infectious disease phenotypes always depend upon exposure. A quantitative phenotype, on the other hand, is a trait that exhibits continuous variation; each person has some measure of disease burden, from uninfected (zero burden) to heavily infected. In this situation, the trait being analyzed could be number of parasite eggs in a blood or stool sample. For each disease or a related phenotype, it is important to determine how to establish the phenotype and then identify the best study design and analytical model for the question at hand.

In general, the principles of genetic epidemiology involve a series of scientific questions aimed at determining whether or not a complex phenotype might be controlled by a genetic mechanism. This sequence includes (1) demonstrating there is significant familial aggregation of the disease or phenotype as a first step to documenting possible genetic control; (2) showing a genetic model can explain the data at hand better than a strictly nongenetic model; (3) providing evidence that a genetic marker or a chromosomal region is "linked" to an unobserved gene controlling the phenotype, which simultaneously provides strong evidence of genetic control and maps the causal gene to a particular region of the genome; and (4) testing for interaction between a causal gene and environmental risk factors or with other genes. This sequential approach to identifying a gene for a complex phenotype allows strong scientific inferences about causality. In general, family studies will be more informative about genetic mechanisms than will population-based studies of unrelated individuals. Thus, questions 1–3 are typically addressed by some form of family-based study design, but population-based studies or studies of unrelated individuals may be better for question 4. It is important to understand the underlying genetic principles when selecting the best study design or analytical approach to answer these four basic questions, and when each are appropriate to use for a truly complex phenotype, such as susceptibility to an infectious pathogen. In some situations, tests for interactions will be easier in population-based study designs, because exposure to the pathogen may not be universal. Conversely, if there is a true interaction between genes and environment, it will become vital to have a good understanding of the role of shared exposure to the pathogen to prevent these from being mistaken for effects of shared genes. This chapter outlines genetic epidemiologic study designs for both family and population studies, discusses their advantages and disadvantages, and specifically points out how they can be applied to the study of infectious diseases.

Family Studies

Familial Clustering/Aggregation of Risk

Phenotypes under genetic control typically cluster or aggregate in families, so the occurrence of one affected member signals a higher risk among other family members. This can be formally tested in a variety of settings, using data on the entire population or selected cohorts of individuals drawn from it, or using data from retrospective studies of families of cases and controls. The first step is to determine if there is any increased risk of disease for relatives of an affected proband (i.e., a case). If phenotype information on a set of cases and on their parents, siblings, or cousins is all available, familial clustering or aggregation of disease can be determined by simply comparing these classes of relatives to the general population. If there is an increased risk of disease among first-degree relatives (parents, full siblings, or offspring) of an individual with a disease, this suggests familial aggregation, whether it is genetic and/or environmental in nature. Some infectious diseases are more likely to aggregate in families because of intrafamilial spread of the infectious agent with or without an underlying genetic influence. Thus, it may be difficult to disentangle the genetic and environmental effects responsible for familial aggregation. The disease status of relatives can be collected through direct observation, reported status indirectly obtained from the index case/control, or population-based registries (if familial relationships can be identified). Of course, whenever the status of relatives is obtained indirectly, it would be desirable to validate this information in some manner to define the potential rate of misclassification. When relying on reported status of relatives obtained from the index person, there is also the potential for reporting bias because an affected informant (i.e., a case) might be more aware of the disease than would an unaffected informant (i.e., a control). In answering this preliminary question of familial clustering or aggregation, there is no need to genotype.

For qualitative traits, a retrospective case–control study comparing the risk of disease among first-degree relatives of index cases and controls is common. In a study of 243 Brazilian nuclear families that lived in an area endemic for visceral leishmaniasis, infection status was compared among family members (Cabello et al., 1995). In a simple χ^2 analysis, significant associations were found for parent–offspring and sibling–sibling pairs ($p < 0.001$), while no association was found between spouses. These results suggested a strong familial aggregation for infection by *Leishmania chagasi*.

Additionally, one can use individuals from an existing cohort in a nested case–control design. In a cohort study of 2- to 5-year-old children in Mirpur, Bangladesh, innate resistance to infection with *Entamoeba histolytica* was associated with the *absence* of serum anti-trophozoite IgG (Haque et al., 2002). Analysis of siblings of these index children showed almost a 5-fold increased risk of being positive for an anti-trophozoite IgG$^+$ antibody compared to siblings of anti-trophozoite IgG$^-$ index children (odds ratio [OR] = 4.8, 95% confidence interval [95% CI] = 2.34–9.90). This finding indicated familial aggregation of the anti-trophozoite antibody, which increased susceptibility to *E. histolytica* infection, suggesting genetic control of susceptibility.

For quantitative phenotypes, familial correlations can be estimated directly or by partitioning the observed variance and covariances among relatives using a variance components approach. This method provides an estimate of the heritability of the quantitative phenotype, which is defined as the ratio of the genetic variance to the total phenotypic variance in a population. Heritability serves as a measure of the relative importance of genetic factors without specifying the details of a model of inheritance. A study of 1,256 individuals comprising one extended pedigree of the indigenous Jirel population of Nepal was used to determine the genetic contribution to the helminth infection *Trichuris trichiura* by calculating the proportion of variation in the *T. trichiura* egg loads (from stool samples) that could be attributed to genetics and environmental factors (Williams-Blangero et al., 2002a). Familial correlations were determined for pairs of relatives including parent–offspring, siblings, grandparent–grandchild, uncle–niece/nephew, and so forth. This population was unique because the entire population was related in one way or another. Under a general linear model, where the observed phenotype (P) is viewed simply a sum of unobserved genes (G), unobserved household factors common to family members (C), and residual environmental factors (E), maximum likelihood methods were used to estimate separate components of variance that could be attributed to each of these distinct factors. Specifically, the total variance in egg counts was partitioned into

$$V_P = V_G + V_C + V_E$$

Assuming these components are uncorrelated and do not interact with one another, the covariance (or correlation) between any two relatives can also be expressed as the sum of an additive genetic component (V_G), a component due to shared household environment (V_C), and a residual term representing environments unique to the individual (V_E).

Under this general model, the phenotypic covariance between any two relatives can consequently be partitioned into the component parts listed above (i.e., V_G, V_C, and V_E). From these components, the heritability (h^2) or the proportion of variance attributable to additive genetic factors can be estimated as $h^2 = V_G/V_P$. It is important to understand that this heritability is a population-specific parameter so that, if either the genetic (V_G) or either environmental component (V_C or V_E) were altered, h^2 must also change. Therefore, direct comparisons of estimated heritability across populations should be made only after careful consideration of the similarity of the phenotype and its underlying causal factors. In the context of traits related to infectious diseases, the most likely variations across populations are in environmental factors reflecting severity of infection rather than in genetic factors in the host. The extreme case, of course, is the absence of the pathogen, which reduces the total variance to zero and makes it impossible to measure genetic heritability altogether.

To apply this variance-components approach to tests of linkage, the model is extended to include one additional term reflecting phenotypic variance attributable to sharing of marker alleles identical by descent (IBD). If this additional component accounts for a significant proportion of the phenotypic variance (or more specifically the covariance among relatives), it could reflect the existence of an unobserved gene controlling the quantitative phenotype tightly linked to the observed genetic marker. If such a quantitative trait locus (QTL) does not exist at or near a marker, patterns of allele sharing should always follow the prior probabilities shown in table 1.1. Spouses who are living together provide a measure of the effects of shared household environment since they are not expected to share any alleles IBD. Williams-Blangero et al. (2002a) determined that 28% of the variation in parasite burden could be attributable to genetic factors (this is the heritability of egg count), and only 4% of the variation in egg count arose from common household effects, suggesting a strong genetic component to susceptibility to *Trichuris* infection.

Defining Genetic Linkage

Linkage is the violation of Mendel's laws of independent assortment, which states that during meiosis alleles at different genes separate or "segregate" independently. If there is no linkage between two genes,

TABLE 1.1. Probability of different relative pairs sharing alleles identical by descent (IBD).

Relative Pairs	Probability of Sharing 0, 1, or 2 Alleles IBD (%)		
	0	1	2
Parent-offspring	0	100	0
Monozygotic twins	0	0	100
Dizygotic twins/Full sibs	25	50	25
Half sibs	50	50	0
Avuncular	50	50	0
First cousins	75	25	0
Grandparent-grandchild	50	50	0
Spouses	0	0	0

there will be 50% recombination of alleles during meiosis—this is independent assortment. If two genes are linked, however, the recombination fraction (θ) will be substantially reduced. Recombination results from an odd number of crossovers events between any two genes (two genetic markers or a single marker and a gene controlling a phenotype). If there is no recombination between the two loci (i.e., the alleles do not recombine during meiosis), they are considered completely linked. Thus, for unlinked genes, parental alleles at one gene are transmitted to offspring independently of alleles at another gene. Linkage becomes apparent when alleles at different genes cosegregate in a family or are passed together from generation to generation with little or no recombination. Linkage can be detected in genes syntenic (located on the same chromosome) and physically near one another by analyzing family data. Showing evidence for linkage between a known genetic marker and an unknown gene controlling risk for disease helps prove the causal gene exists at the same time it identifies the chromosomal region containing the putative gene.

Parametric Linkage Analysis

There are two major types of statistical methods to identify linkage: parametric and nonparametric. Parametric, or model-based, linkage analysis is the most powerful statistical method to test for linkage, but it requires prior knowledge of the true model of inheritance at the gene controlling the observed phenotype; that is, the allele frequency at the trait locus, the penetrance for each of its genotypes, and the transmission parameters are assumed to be known. These parameters need to be specified prior to the linkage analysis itself, even if the investigators simply guess. In a parametric linkage analysis, these parameters are used to compute a likelihood function that is a function of the key parameter of interest, the recombination fraction (θ). The null hypothesis of no linkage (i.e., $H_0:\theta = 0.5$) is formally tested by comparing the likelihood of the null hypothesis to this same likelihood function evaluated at the value of θ that best fits the observed data. This test statistic is called the log-odds or LOD score and is written as

$$LOD = -2[\ln L(\hat{\theta}) - \ln L(\theta = 0.5)]$$

Again, by convention, an LOD > 3.0 (odds 1,000:1 in favor of linkage) is taken as significant evidence of linkage when individual markers are considered (Ott, 1999). Parametric linkage analysis assumes the genetic model at the trait locus is known (e.g., autosomal dominant with some specified penetrance). Since the model of inheritance for the genetic marker is known, all focus falls on the recombination θ, the key parameter of interest. However, it is possible to use this LOD score method without knowing the genetic model, and many have adopted this strategy by simply assuming one or another model (perhaps with some allowance for nongenetic control of the phenotype) and testing for linkage. Since there is a relatively low risk of false positive signals for linkage, this may well be reasonable. When considering infectious diseases, however, there are more risks to simply assuming some specific model of inheritance because explicit consideration of exposure should be incorporated (unless exposure is truly universal, as for a holoendemic infection). This parametric linkage analysis method uses both phenotypic and genotypic information from all family members and can be used with one marker or with multiple markers in a defined chromosomal region.

While parametric linkage methods provide the most statistical power to map unobserved causal genes, there is a strict lower limit to the resolution of this linkage approach that depends on the number of informative matings (or meiotic events) that can be reconstructed from the observed data. Not all families will be informative for all markers, and although considering multiple markers improves the information level substantially, for small regions where few recombination events are expected (e.g., genetic distances representing 1–2% recombination) even dense marker maps in large numbers of families cannot provide adequate information to identify unknown genes.

Typically, parametric linkage analysis is used with qualitative phenotypes, but an important example of how a quantitative phenotype (egg count) can be used in a formal parametric linkage analysis arose from a study of *Schistosoma mansoni* infection in Brazil (Abel et al., 1991). A clinical survey of an entire Brazilian village population allowed Abel et al. (1991) to fit a single locus model for egg count burden. Later analysis of genetic markers in candidate genes and then a genomewide scan were successful in identifying a locus controlling burden of *S. mansoni* infection in these families (Marquet et al., 1996, 1999). Using the genetic model previously constructed from this entire endemically infected Brazilian population, parametric linkage analysis was performed on 142 individuals in 11 of the most informative families and yielded strong linkage evidence for a gene in region 5q31-q33 (two-point LOD score = 4.74). This example demonstrates the power of linkage analysis to identify unknown genes controlling parasite burden, but there are few other successful examples of using parametric linkage analysis for a quantitative phenotype.

Nonparametric Linkage Analysis

Nonparametric linkage analysis is a model-free approach where the genetic model is not specified ahead of time, and there is no effort to actually estimate the recombination fraction θ. Instead, the consequences of linkage become the focus of the statistical tests. In general, nonparametric linkage analysis methods use pairs (or sets) of relatives with the same phenotype and compare the distribution of alleles shared IBD to what would be expected under the null hypothesis of no linkage between the observed marker and an unobserved causal gene. These nonparametric approaches include affected sib-pair analysis, and their extensions to other pairs of affected relatives for qualitative phenotypes. The variance components approach mentioned above can also build upon tests for excess allele sharing at marker loci and can serve as a form of model-free test for linkage, although there are a number of assumptions made about the underlying biologic model.

Affected sib-pair methods are often used in studies of infectious diseases. Siddiqui et al. (2001) studied the qualitative trait leprosy in 245 independent affected sib pairs with paucibacillary leprosy from South India to search for genes influencing susceptibility. Evidence for linkage was found on chromosome 10p13 (maximum LOD score = 4.09, $p = 0.00002$). Mira et al. (2003) conducted another genomewide screen of 205 affected sib pairs from southern Vietnam with leprosy (both paucibacillary and multibacillary) and found evidence for linkage on chromosome 6q25 (maximum likelihood binomial LOD score = 4.31, $p = 0.000005$). These two reports raise the possibility that different genes control susceptibility to leprosy in two distinct populations, which is not unreasonable given the complexity of this disease.

The variance components linkage method described above was used to identify two regions of the genome that may contain genes controlling infection by roundworm *Ascaris lumbricoides*, an intestinal parasite, using a large Nepalese kindred (Williams-Blangero et al., 2002b). A single extended pedigree of 444 individuals provided 6,209 relative pairs that were included in a genomewide screen using the quantitative phenotype *Ascaris* egg counts. Significant evidence of linkage was identified on chromosome 13q32-q34 (LOD = 4.43, genomewide $p = 0.0009$) and chromosome 1p32 (LOD = 3.01, genomewide $p = 0.03$) for this helminth infection. Careful examination of the known genes in this region of chromosome 13, revealed a novel candidate gene (*TNFSF13B*), which controls B-cell activity and IgE levels and could well influence helminthic infection.

Genotyping for Linkage Studies

For genomewide linkage studies of either qualitative or quantitative phenotypes, both the phenotype and DNA of each individual are necessary. Every individual is genotyped for markers evenly spaced at 5–10 centimorgans (~1 cM = 1,000,000 base pairs) throughout the genome. The power of a linkage study comes from the polymorphic information content of markers (a function of marker allele frequency), as well as the size of the family and the relationships among individuals. Traditionally, evenly spaced microsatellite or short tandem repeat (STR) markers, short sequences of nucleotides (2–5bp) repeated in tandem, have been used for genomewide linkage analysis because the large number of alleles generates many informative matings. Biallelic single nucleotide polymorphisms (SNPs) are also being used for genomewide linkage analysis. Although SNPs are biallelic and individually do not contribute as much information as a multiallelic STR marker, they occur in greater density across the genome (10,000 SNPs in ~3 cM) and consequently provide better coverage of small chromosomal regions. Considering multiple SNP markers as haplotypes (combinations of alleles across multiple markers) can further increase the information content and may prove more powerful for case–control or other study designs.

Replication of Linkage Studies

Finally, it is important to replicate findings from linkage studies to confirm the existence of putative causal genes in separate samples of multiplex families. Although linkage provides very strong statistical evidence that a gene does exist, replication is notoriously difficult with complex phenotypes, and all infectious phenotypes must have a complex etiology. Significant differences in sample size, recruitment or ascertainment of individuals, diagnostic criteria, ethnicity, and statistical modeling across studies and across populations may result in a failure to replicate an initial finding, even if a true causal gene was identified in the first study (Suarez et al., 2000). Only through replication, however, can an initial finding be confirmed as biologically real. This is especially important in studies of the major infectious diseases such as malaria, which may reflect substantial selective pressure on human populations. In this context, the different histories of human populations and even different pathogenic agents may result in identifying distinct genes that control risk in different populations.

Association/Linkage Disequilibrium

Although linkage analysis, in its original form at least, has the advantage of having a well-defined and biologically meaningful null hypothesis, testing for association is a more general statistical approach where samples of individuals (either unrelated or sets of relatives) are compared to test for independence between genetic markers and observed phenotypes. The null hypothesis is complete independence between a qualitative phenotype (e.g., affected vs. unaffected) and allelic or genotypic classes, and the test statistic typically compares the frequency of a marker allele or genotype across different categories of individuals (e.g., cases and controls). For a quantitative phenotype, the statistical approach tests for a difference in the mean among different genotypes in a sample of unrelated individuals or an effect of observed genotype on the phenotypic variance/covariance among related individuals. Here, regression or analysis of variance (ANOVA) models can be used. In either situation, rejecting the null hypothesis of independence or no effect raises the possibility that the observed genetic marker controls or influences the phenotype, but the statistical test alone cannot discriminate between a *direct* and an *indirect* effect. A direct effect of a marker genotype implies the marker itself acts causally, perhaps as part of a complicated, causal pathway. If the marker genotype exerts a fixed effect on risk or the mean, it can be modeled as a covariate in a general multiple regression model. This is often called a "measured genotype" approach (Boerwinkle et al., 1986), and adjusting for allelic or genotypic effects can either increase the amount of variance explained by a predictive model for a quantitative phenotype or improve the ability to predict risk for a qualitative phenotype. In either situation, demonstrating a statistical association between the genetic marker and the phenotype documents part of the pathogenic pathway and may reflect direct genetic control.

A statistical association between a phenotype and a marker can also reflect an indirect effect of the marker, where the marker is linked to and in disequilibrium with some unobserved gene that controls the phenotype. Even if a marker has no direct effect on the phenotype, such an indirect relationship becomes very useful for mapping unobserved causal genes. Such an indirect association relies heavily on the concept of Hardy-Weinberg equilibrium (and its converse disequilibrium) commonly used in population genetics. For two alleles at one locus, Hardy-Weinberg equilibrium exists if genotypes occur as simple mathematical combinations of allele frequencies (see table 1.2, where the frequencies of homozygous AA genotypes is simply p^2, that for heterozygotes is simply $2pq$, etc.). There is a corresponding multilocus Hardy-Weinberg equilibrium expected if alleles at each of *two* loci combine independently, so that the haplotypes (combination of gametes) are a simple mathematical function of the individual alleles (see table 1.2, where homozygous AABB is simply p^2r^2). If alleles at two genes (two markers or a marker and an unobserved causal gene) are associated in the population, they are said to be in disequilibrium, because the principles of this two locus Hardy-Weinberg equilibrium no longer

hold. Although there are several possible causes for disequilibrium, a common cause is linkage disequilibrium (LD) where the two genes (A and B from table 1.2) are tightly linked and thus do not recombine at every meiosis. Even over many generations, there will be some degree of statistical association between alleles at nearby genes, and this will lead to higher than expected frequencies for some haplotypes and lower than expected for others. Figure 1.1 shows how a new mutation can arise next to an existing marker allele and thus will be in complete LD with those alleles initially. Over many generations, especially in expanding populations, this complete gametic association or complete LD will gradually decay, as recombination inevitably scrambles all allelic combinations and the population approaches full multilocus Hardy-Weinberg equilibrium. LD can be considered cosegregation of alleles at the population level.

The advantage of testing for association between markers and a phenotype (qualitative or quantitative) is that it allows samples of unrelated individuals to be used in the search for genes important in controlling risk for infectious diseases. Statistical tests alone can never discriminate between direct and indirect associations, nor do they necessarily prove that the observed disequilibrium reflects LD and is not the result of admixture of genetically distinct populations, selection, or genetic drift (all of which can produce disequilibrium). However, it opens up opportunities to use epidemiologic study designs and broader population samples to test for genes controlling risk for infectious disease. When studying infectious diseases, it becomes very

TABLE 1.2. Hardy-Weinberg equilibrium expected frequencies.

1 Locus			*2 Locus*				
Allele A with frequency p			Allele A with frequency p; a with frequency q				
Allele a with frequency q			Allele B with frequency r; b with frequency s				
Gametes			*Gametes*				
	A	a		AB	Ab	aB	ab
A	AA p^2	Aa pq	AB	AABB p^2r^2	AABb p^2rs	AaBB pqr^2	AaBb $pqrs$
			Ab	AABB p^2rs	AAbb p^2s^2	AaBb $pqrs$	Aabb pqs^2
a	Aa pq	aa q^2	aB	AaBB pqr^2	AaBb $pqrs$	aaBB q^2r^2	aaBb q^2rs
			ab	AaBb $pqrs$	Aabb pqs^2	*aaBb* q^2rs	aabb q^2s^2

a) ML1	DL	ML2		b) ML1	DL	ML2		c) ML1	DL	ML2
A	D	B		A	D	B		A	D	B
A	d	B		A	D	b		A	D	b
A	d	b		A	d	B		a	D	B
a	d	B		A	d	b		a	D	b
a	d	b		a	d	B		A	d	B
				a	d	b		A	d	b
								a	d	B
								a	d	b

Complete LD   **Moderate LD**   **No LD**

FIGURE 1.1. Alleles at two marker loci (ML1 = A/a and ML2 = B/b) and one disease locus (DL, D=disease, d=no disease). The recombination fraction between ML1 and DL is 0.01; the recombination fraction between ML2 and DL is 0.05. (a) When an initial mutation arises at the disease locus (D), it is in LD with alleles A and B. (b) After 20 generations, the LD begins to decay for ML2 due to the greater recombination fraction. The disease allele is now in moderate LD with ML1. After 1,000 generations, the LD has completely dissipated, the disease locus (D) occurs with each marker allele combination and there is Hardy-Weinberg equilibrium for all three genes.

important to use phenotypes from individuals (including their own exposure information) rather than a general phenotype assigned to the entire family, because not all members of a family may be equally exposed to the pathogenic agent. Family studies can be automatically more difficult if exposure varies with age, activity, household membership, and so on, because all such information must be collected on all family members.

Traditional epidemiologic methods (e.g., case–control designs) prescribe sampling unrelated individuals to determine the risk of disease attributable to a specific exposure variable (which could be a genetic marker). In a case–control study of susceptibility to *M. tuberculosis* in The Gambia, Bellamy et al. (1998) compared the frequency of two polymorphisms in the *NRAMP1* (*SLC11A1*) gene (located in intron 4 and the 3' untranslated region) among 410 adults with smear-positive pulmonary tuberculosis and 417 ethnically matched controls. Individuals heterozygous for both genetic variants had a 4-fold greater risk of tuberculosis than those without the polymorphisms (OR = 4.07, 95% CI = 1.86–9.12). Although this study design could not distinguish between susceptibility to infection and susceptibility to disease progression because tuberculosis was endemic in this population, it did suggest a gene that may play an important role in the development of clinical disease.

Family-Based Association Tests

The principles underlying case–control designs can also be applied to family-based designs by treating observed genotypes as paired observations (case and control alleles or genotypes). The original family-based test of association used trios of parents and an affected child to compare alleles or genotypes transmitted to the affected child as the "case" and alleles not transmitted as the "control" (Falk and Rubinstein, 1987; Rubinstein et al., 1981). Spielman et al. (1993) expanded this approach and developed the allelic transmission/disequilibrium test (TDT) as a formal test for linkage in the presence of disequilibrium, which tests a composite null hypothesis that there is no linkage *or* no LD between the observed genetic marker and an unobserved causal gene. Rejecting this null hypothesis constitutes evidence of both linkage *and* LD. However, for the allelic TDT to be valid and unbiased, genotype data on both parents are needed, although only heterozygous parents actually contribute to the test statistic. For many phenotypes with later ages of onset, it is difficult to obtain information on both parents, and modifications of this TDT have been developed that are essentially case–sib control designs. These include the sibship disequilibrium test (SDT; Horvath and Laird, 1998) and the sib-TDT (S-TDT; Spielman and Ewens, 1998). Sibling-based TDTs contrast marker data from an unaffected sibling (instead of the parents) to the genotype of the case, comparing genotypes transmitted to discordant siblings. The SDT is also a test for both linkage and LD, and the S-TDT is a test for linkage.

The TDT and S-TDT tests can also be used together to accommodate different types of trios or sib pairs available in more general pedigrees (Martin et al., 2000). However, in extended pedigrees where multiple family members are affected, this method is not a valid test of LD in the presence of linkage because genotypes of relatives are correlated, not independent. The pedigree disequilibrium test (Martin et al., 2000) and the family-based association test (FBAT) (Horvath et al., 2001) are better alternatives that can utilize information from most or all the family members to maximize statistical power. These statistical methods correct for the dependence among family members, so they are valid tests for linkage in the presence of LD (the original composite null hypothesis). The family-based tests of associations implemented in the FBAT package use both parents and siblings, can accommodate missing genotype data, and can consider qualitative or quantitative phenotypes. With qualitative phenotypes, a χ^2 statistic tests for strict adherence to Mendelian segregation of the marker that is independent of the observed phenotype under some prespecified model of inheritance (dominant or recessive). With quantitative or censored phenotypes, a similar goodness of fit χ^2 statistic is computed, but the fixed effect of marker genotype on the phenotypic mean becomes the center of focus.

For quantitative traits, several approaches that represent extensions of the ANOVA and regression models have been adapted to test for association or LD in family data, particularly sibship data (Abecasis et al., 2000, 2001; Fulker et al., 1999), conditional score tests (Rabinowitz, 1997; Schaid, 1996), and the use of offsets (Lunetta et al., 2000). Here the observed variance within and among families is contrasted to provide a test for LD under a random effects model. In studies of infectious diseases, many diseases can be easily classified into mutually exclusive categories (e.g., having the disease or not; having no infection, a mild infection, or a severe infection), and these can be analyzed under logistic regression models. However, available quantitative measurements including immune response levels (plasma viral load, delayed type hypersensitivity response) or degree of infection (number of diarrheal episodes, egg counts) may be more informative in identifying the effects of genes controlling susceptibility and disease severity.

A leprosy study of 197 Vietnamese case–parent trios yielded strong evidence for LD (or association) in the presence of linkage to a candidate region. The associated markers were in the region of the PARK2 and PACRG genes located on chromosome 6q25-26, a region previously mapped as a susceptibility locus for leprosy using multiplex families (Mira et al., 2003). Using the traditional TDT with no missing parental data, Mira et al. (2004) found evidence that two single nucleotide polymorphisms (SNPs) increased the risk of leprosy 5-fold for individuals who carried the high risk allele compared to those who had the alternate allele ($p = 0.0007$). Another family-based association study identified an association between tuberculosis and the 874A/T polymorphism in the interferon-γ gene (Rossouw et al., 2003). In a study of 131 South African case–parent trios, strong evidence for linkage and LD ($p = 0.0008$) with tuberculosis was seen among those carrying the interferon-γ 874A allele, whereas the T allele was overrepresented in controls. For both these studies, the cases and their parents and/or siblings were genotyped and the family-based association tests suggest these candidate genes control susceptibility to these infectious diseases.

Population Studies

Case–Control Study Design

For some infectious diseases, family studies become inappropriate because exposure to the pathogen is not uniform for all members of the family (e.g., sexually transmitted diseases). For these diseases, the usual genetic approach to measuring familial aggregation and then testing for linkage cannot be taken, and the focus shifts to identifying candidate genes that are associated with disease status using only unrelated individuals. For population-based case–control studies, it is necessary to recruit a representative sample of individuals with disease and a representative sample of at-risk (but unaffected) controls. If a particular high-risk allele is recognized or hypothesized from prior studies, a case–control design comparing individuals exposed (carrying the putative high-risk allele) to those unexposed among cases and controls may suffice. If no causal allele is known, several genetic markers within the gene can be typed, and haplotype analysis may identify the true high-risk allele or haplotype through tests for association among exposed cases and controls. A haplotype of several markers may well have greater statistical power to identify a causal gene, because it may uniquely identify the high-risk allele at the unobserved causal gene while individual markers show only weaker associations (Fallin et al., 2001). When the causal allele and a marker allele show no recombination, they will be inherited together (complete linkage), and this will likely result in strong LD in the population and measurable association in the exposed case–control sample at hand. In such situations, either individual markers or haplotypes should show distinctly different frequencies among exposed cases and controls. It is important to remember that when a pathogen is required for the disease, cases and controls should be at equal risk of this necessary exposure, and the gene may control risk conditional on exposure.

Case–Control Study Analysis

Traditional case–control methods can be used to compare a qualitative phenotype using a set of cases and unrelated controls in a simple contingency table comparing alleles or genotypes (Woolf, 1957). This presentation of data provides an easy way to calculate the OR, a ratio of the odds that cases carry the genotype to the odds that the controls carry the genotype. An $OR > 1$ indicates that individuals exposed to the genotype (carrying a variant allele or haplotype) are at an increased risk of disease compared to those who do not carry it; conversely, an $OR < 1$ indicates a negative association and can indicate that exposed individuals are protected from disease. This OR can also be modeled using logistic regression methods where the LOD is a linear function of several risk factors, so potential confounding variables and other covariates can be considered. Hobbs et al. (2002) presented a case–control study of 179 Tanzanian children that identified an apparent protective effect for symptomatic malaria among those carrying a polymorphic allele in the promoter region of the nitric oxide synthase (NOS2) gene (–1173C/T). The risk of symptomatic malaria was 88% lower in children carrying at least one copy of the 1173T allele (OR = 0.12, 95% CI = 0.03–0.48, $p = 0.0006$). Children carrying this T allele had increased fasting nitric oxide concentrations, suggesting this allele creates an actual functional effect in vivo.

ANOVA/Regression Methods

For a quantitative trait, ANOVA methods can also be used to compare individuals who carry an allele or haplotype to those who do not carry it. The ANOVA partitions the total variance in the observed phenotype (measured as the total sum of squares) into two main components: a within-group sum of squares and between-group sum of squares. Assuming the error terms (values beyond the fixed effects of observed covariates) are normally distributed, conventional least squares approaches use F-statistics to compare the variance between genotypic groups, allowing simple tests for genotypic effects. Simple and multiple linear regression approaches can also be used effectively in these situations. Whenever it is appropriate to conduct this kind of regression modeling on family data (i.e., when there is truly ubiquitous exposure to the pathogen), these regression models can be extended to consider dependence among relatives.

Time-to-Event/Longitudinal Cohort Studies

A case–control study can also be nested within a cohort study, where individuals are followed to observe the natural history of infection over time. As individuals develop infection or disease, they can be classified as cases and compared to those who have not yet developed infection/disease ("controls"). In these studies, the incidence of infection/disease can also be directly calculated based on the entire cohort. Additional analytical approaches, such as survival or relative hazards models, may also be used to see if a specific allele or genotype affects infection, disease progression, or overall survival. Time-to-event analysis has been used to assess the risk of HIV infection among serodiscordant heterosexual couples (Dorak et al., 2004). In a study of 125 initially serodiscordant partners with confirmed interpartner HIV transmission and 104 persistently discordant couples, the sharing of HLA-B alleles was associated with accelerated interpartner transmission (relative hazard = 2.23, 95% CI = 1.52–3.26). Survival analysis has been used extensively for HIV/AIDS to determine the effect of candidate genes on progression of HIV disease and overall survival. Using six cohorts of HIV seroincident and seroprevalent individuals ($n = 1,955$), the effect of a 32 base-pair deletion in the chemokine receptor CCR5 was evaluated (Dean et al., 1996). Despite repeated exposures, individuals homozygous for this 32 base-pair deletion were protected (at least via the *CCR5* pathway) from acquiring HIV infection. Individuals heterozygous for the deletion allele showed a delayed progression to AIDS compared with individuals who did not carry the deletion ($\chi^2 = 8.1$, $p = 0.0045$). The large sample size and the extensive longitudinal follow-up data from these six cohorts were critical to providing sufficient statistical power to detect this association with HIV disease progression.

Further Design Considerations

A critical aspect in the design of a case–control study is the proper sampling of controls. In studies of infectious diseases, controls should have the same exposure to the pathogen and therefore the same risk of developing infection as the cases. For some diseases, certain age groups or one gender may be at higher risk because of environmental exposures (access to drinking water, occupation, living conditions, etc.) or some other confounder. For example, the intestinal infection *Vibrio cholera* shows age-related attack rates especially where cholera is endemic (children 2–4 years old are at highest risk) versus areas with new infections (where all ages are at equal risk; Sack et al., 2004). Cholera infection is also seasonal, and as a result, the peak infection times or frequencies are not the same for all geographical regions. Understanding the natural history of infection is vital to developing the proper study design, so that cases and controls can be appropriately matched to ensure that they are similar in their exposure to the pathogen and other characteristics (i.e., age, gender) to minimize opportunities for spurious results.

A major source of confounding in studies of association is heterogeneity in ancestry (e.g., differences in genetic background; Deng et al., 2001; Heiman et al., 2004). A statistically significant association between a particular genetic marker and the phenotype of interest (e.g., infection or disease) may prove to be spurious if unrecognized subsets of a population differ in both their risk of infection and their allele frequencies at the marker locus. Population forces such as genetic drift or past selective pressures could produce different allele frequencies at any marker locus sufficient to create confounding. The distribution of the phenotype of interest may also differ across subsets of a population due to differences in allele frequencies at genes other than the marker being examined, different environmental factors, or some combination of both. Conventional case–control analysis ignoring the substructure of the whole

population could produce a statistical association even though the marker locus is neither a causal factor nor linked to a causal gene (Ewens and Spielman, 1995; Freedman et al., 2004; Heiman, et al., 2004). Confounding such as this has been described in various terms, including ethnic stratification or heterogeneity, background genetic heterogeneity, and latent class or population substructure. Whenever ancestral origins and the patterns of LD among affected cases and control subjects who represent the reference populations are uncertain, any newly detected statistical effect of a candidate gene without assurance of comparability in the genetic background of the population should be interpreted carefully.

To accommodate such genetic substructure or heterogeneity, alternative strategies have been proposed. One strategy is based on testing for substructure in the population of interest by estimating admixture (mixing of two or more genetically distinct populations; Satten et al., 2001; Allison and Neale, 2001). Another strategy involves using some form of "genomic control" wherein, in addition to markers in or near suspected candidate genes, a set of neutral markers distributed across the genome, capable of discriminating among subsets of different ancestries, is genotyped (Devlin et al., 2001; Pritchard and Rosenberg, 1999; Reiner et al., 2005). Practically speaking, using genomic controls usually means typing at least a number of SNP or microsatellite markers to help discriminate the subsets. Public databases including different ethnic groups are becoming more available, so selection of a set of genomic control markers for most ethnic groups will become simpler.

Additionally, it is important that any finding of a statistical association between a genetic marker be replicated in multiple populations to maximize the chance the association is not spurious. Replication and confirmation are also critical when multiple markers or genes are studied, as with all complex diseases. Multiple testing with many markers can result in false positives, especially when nominal *p*-values are relied on. Although current methods to control for multiple testing (i.e., the Bonferroni correction) are too stringent, any finding of association should still subscribe to a fairly rigorous analysis to confirm the statistical significance (e.g., empiric *p*-values obtained through simulation or permutation), and all findings, including those that may be nonsignificant, should be accurately reported. Finally, the lack of any statistically significant association may be the result of small sample sizes and an underpowered study. Negative findings should be analyzed to determine if the sample at hand provided enough power to detect a true association, given the observed marker allele frequency and/or the amount of LD within haplotypes. As with all epidemiologic analyses, the initial study design should specify the minimum sample size needed to have sufficient power to detect an association under various conditions.

Issues of study design go beyond how subjects are collected and phentoyped and include the issue of how many genes and markers are considered. Most studies to date have focused on one or a few "candidate genes" selected on the basis of current biologic knowledge. Markers are analyzed individually or together as haplotypes, either within a single gene or across several nearby genes in a chromosomal region. Even though candidate gene studies have substantial appeal (Tabor et al., 2002), they create problems of multiple testing based on markers that are not independent of one another. Therefore, not only are issues of multiple tests found in virtually any genetic study, but also the most appropriate way to minimize false positive and false negative results is not obvious. In addition to these issues of statistical error within a study, replication across studies of complex diseases remains elusive for both linkage and association tests. Because candidate gene studies are based on current knowledge, there is no guarantee that the list of candidates will include all causal genes, and genomewide approaches hold the promise of being unbiased in searching for causal genes. For linkage studies, genomewide screens with STR markers are practically guaranteed to locate a causal gene for any Mendelian disorder and have even proven somewhat successful for complex diseases. With technical improvements in SNP genotyping methods, genomewide association studies are now feasible (Klein et al., 2005; The Wellcome Trust Case Control Consortium, 2007; Diabetic Genetic Initiative, 2007; Scott et al., 2007). However, the sheer number of markers (100,000-650,000 SNPs) creates troublesome analytical problems in evaluating so many statistical tests and reliably defining rates of statistical error (Thomas et al., 2005). It is likely that genomewide association studies will become more widely used to identify genes controlling risk for infectious diseases in the near future. A genomewide case–control study of 1500 cases with tuberculosis and 1500 controls from The Gambia (The Wellcome Trust Case Control Consortium, 2007) and a genomewide family-based study of 1000 parent–child trios with severe malaria

from The Gambia (www.malariagen.net) are both currently underway. These studies hold the potential to identify completely new genes that may control susceptibility to infection or progression to clinical outcomes, but they require careful adherence to established epidemiologic principles such as case definition, sampling, and replication.

Summary

Genetic analyses of infectious disease can be critical to understanding the biologic and immunologic pathways of infection. However, infectious disease represents the epitome of complex diseases, because the pathogen is absolutely critical to risk. Appropriately designed studies may provide important insight into immunity and encourage the development of targeted treatments or more effective vaccines. As with any statistical genetic analysis, it is important that the study design be tailored for the disease (family- vs. population-based samples; tests of linkage vs. association) and issues of statistical power and sample size be addressed as early in the process as possible. Additionally, as with other studies, it is important that classification of disease status be accurate and stringent and that environmental exposure to the pathogen be somewhat uniform or at least consistent among diseased and nondiseased individuals, so that the underlying genetic risk of disease can be determined accurately. There are many opportunities for host genetic factors to play a major role in determining susceptibility and disease severity to infectious diseases. Our understanding of the natural history of these diseases will never be complete unless further efforts to identify key host factors are undertaken. In addition, building a better understanding of how host genes influence risk may advance important opportunities to control the burden of major infectious diseases.

References

Abecasis, G. R., Cardon, L. R., and Cookson, W. O. (2000) A general test of association for quantitative traits in nuclear families. *Am J Hum Genet.* 66:279–292.

Abecasis, G. R., Cookson, W. O., and Cardon, L. R. (2001) The power to detect linkage disequilibrium with quantitative traits in selected samples. *Am J Hum Genet.* 68:1463–1474.

Abel, L., Demenais, F., Prata, A., Souza, A. E., and Dessein, A. (1991) Evidence for the segregation of a major gene in human susceptibility/resistance to infection by Schistosoma mansoni. *Am J Hum Genet.* 48:959–970.

Allison, D. B., and Neale, M. C. (2001) Joint tests of linkage and association for quantitative traits. *Theoret Pop Biol.* 60:239–251.

Bellamy, R., Ruwende, C., Corrah, T., McAdam, K. P., Whittle, H. C., and Hill, A. V. (1998) Variations in the NRAMP1 gene and susceptibility to tuberculosis in West Africans. *N Engl J Med.* 338:640–644.

Boerwinkle, E., Chakraborty, R., and Sing, C. F. (1986) The use of measured genotype information in the analysis of quantitative phenotypes in man. I. Models and analytical methods. *Ann Hum Genet.* 50(pt 2):181–194.

Cabello, P. H., Lima, A. M., Azevedo, E. S., and Krieger, H. (1995) Familial aggregation of Leishmania chagasi infection in northeastern Brazil. *Am J Trop Med Hyg.* 52:364–365.

Dean, M., Carrington, M., Winkler, C., Huttley, G. A., Smith, M. W., Allikmets, R., Goedert, J. J., Buchbinder, S. P., Vittinghoff, E., Gomperts, E., Donfield, S., Vlahov, D., Kaslow, R., Saah, A., Rinaldo, C., Detels, R., and O'Brien, S. J. (1996) Genetic restriction of HIV-1 infection and progression to AIDS by a deletion allele of the CKR5 structural gene. Hemophilia Growth and Development Study, Multicenter AIDS Cohort Study, Multicenter Hemophilia Cohort Study, San Francisco City Cohort, ALIVE Study. *Science.* 273:1856–1862.

Deng, H. W., Chen, W. M., and Recker, R. R. (2001) Population admixture: detection by Hardy-Weinberg test and its quantitative effects on linkage-disequilibrium methods for localizing genes underlying complex traits. *Genetics.* 157:885–897.

Devlin, B., Roeder, K., and Wasserman L. (2001) Genomic control, a new approach to genetic-based association studies. *Theor Popul Biol.* 60(3):155–166.

Diabetes Genetics Initiative of Broad Institute of Harvard and MIT, Lund University, and Novartis Institutes of BioMedical Research, Saxena, R., Voight, B. F., Lyssenko, V., Burtt, N. P., de Bakker, P. I., Chen, H., Roix, J. J., Kathiresan, S., Hirschhorn, J. N., Daly, M. J., Hughes, T. E., Groop, L., Altshuler, D., Almgren, P., Florez, J. C., Meyer, J., Ardlie, K., Bengtsson Bostrom, K., Isomaa, B., Lettre, G., Lindblad, U., Lyon, H. N., Melander, O., Newton-Cheh, C., Nilsson, P., Orho-Melander, M., Rastam, L., Speliotes, E. K., Taskinen, M. R., Tuomi, T., Guiducci, C., Berglund, A., Carlson, J., Gianniny, L., Hackett, R., Hall, L., Holmkvist, J., Laurila, E., Sjogren, M., Sterner, M., Surti, A., Svensson, M., Svensson, M., Tewhey, R., Blumenstiel, B., Parkin, M., Defelice, M., Barry, R., Brodeur, W., Camarata, J., Chia, N., Fava, M., Gibbons, J., Handsaker, B., Healy, C., Nguyen, K., Gates, C., Sougnez, C., Gage, D., Nizzari, M., Gabriel, S. B., Chirn, G. W., Ma, Q., Parikh, H., Richardson, D., Ricke, D., and Purcell, S. (2007) Genome-wide association analysis identifies loci for type 2 diabetes and triglyceride levels. *Science.* 316(5829):1331–1336.

Dorak, M. T., Tang, J., Penman-Aguilar, A., Westfall, A. O., Zulu, I., Lobashevsky, E. S., Kancheya, N. G., Schaen, M. M., Allen, S. A., and Kaslow, R. A. (2004) Transmission of HIV-1 and HLA-B allele-sharing within serodiscordant heterosexual Zambian couples. *Lancet.* 363:2137–2139.

Ewens, W. J., and Spielman, R. S. (1995) The transmission/disequilibrium test: history, subdivision, and admixture. *Am J Hum Genet.* 2, 455–464.

Falk, C. T., and Rubinstein, P. (1987) Haplotype relative risks: an easy reliable way to construct a proper control sample for risk calculations. *Ann Hum Genet.* 51(pt 3):227–233.

Fallin, D., Cohen, A., Essioux, L., Chumakov, I., Blumenfeld, M., Cohen, D., and Schork, N. J. (2001) Genetic analysis of case/control data using estimated haplotype frequencies: application to APOE locus variation and Alzheimer's disease. *Genome Res.* 11: 143–151.

Freedman, M. L., Reich, D., Penney, K. L., McDonald, G. J., Mignault, A. A., Patterson, N., Gabriel, S. B., Topol, E. J., Smoller, J. W., Pato, C. N., Pato, M. T., Petryshen, T. L., Kolonel, L. N., Lander, E. S., Sklar, P., Henderson, B., Hirschhorn, J. N., and Altshuler, D. (2004) Assessing the impact of population stratification on genetic association studies. *Nat Genet.* 36:388–393.

Fulker, D. W., Cherny, S. S., Sham, P. C., and Hewitt, J. K. (1999) Combined linkage and association sib-pair analysis for quantitative traits. *Am J Hum Genet.* 64:259–267.

Haque, R., Duggal, P., Ali, I. M., Hossain, M. B., Mondal, D., Sack, R. B., Farr, B. M., Beaty, T. H., and Petri, W. A., Jr. (2002) Innate and acquired resistance to amebiasis in Bangladeshi children. *J Infect Dis.* 186:547–552.

Heiman G. A., Hodge S. E., Gorroochurn, P., Zhang J., and Greenberg, D. A. (2004) Effect of population stratification on case-control association studies. I. Elevation in false positive rates and comparison to confounding risk ratios (a simulation study). *Hum Hered.* 58:30–39.

Hobbs, M. R., Udhayakumar, V., Levesque, M. C., Booth, J., Roberts, J. M., Tkachuk, A. N., Pole, A., Coon, H., Kariuki, S., Nahlen, B. L., Mwaikambo,

E. D., Lal, A. L., Granger, D. L., Anstey, N. M., and Weinberg, J. B. (2002) A new NOS2 promoter polymorphism associated with increased nitric oxide production and protection from severe malaria in Tanzanian and Kenyan children. *Lancet.* 360:1468–1475.

Horvath, S., and Laird, N. M. (1998) A discordant-sibship test for disequilibrium and linkage: no need for parental data. *Am J Hum Genet.* 63:1886–1897.

Horvath, S., Xu, X., and Laird, N. M. (2001) The family based association test method: strategies for studying general genotype–phenotype associations. *Eur J Hum Genet.* 9:301–306.

Klein, R. J., Zeiss, C., Chew, E. Y., Tsai, J. Y., Sackler, R. S., Haynes, C., Henning, A. K., SanGiovanni, J. P., Mane, S. M., Mayne, S. T., Bracken, M. B., Ferris, F. L., Ott, J., Barnstable, C., and Hoh, J. (2005) Complement factor H polymorphism in age-related macular degeneration. *Science.* 308:385–389.

Lunetta, K. L., Faraone, S. V., Biederman, J., and Laird, N. M. (2000) Family-based tests of association and linkage that use unaffected sibs, covariates, and interactions. *Am J Hum Genet.* 66:605–614.

Marquet, S., Abel, L., Hillaire, D., and Dessein, A. (1999) Full results of the genome-wide scan which localises a locus controlling the intensity of infection by Schistosoma mansoni on chromosome 5q31-q33. *Eur J Hum Genet.* 7:88–97.

Marquet, S., Abel, L., Hillaire, D., Dessein, H., Kalil, J., Feingold, J., Weissenbach, J., and Dessein, A. J. (1996) Genetic localization of a locus controlling the intensity of infection by Schistosoma mansoni on chromosome 5q31-q33. *Nat Genet.* 14:181–184.

Martin, E. R., Monks, S. A., Warren, L. L., and Kaplan, N. L. (2000) A test for linkage and association in general pedigrees: the pedigree disequilibrium test. *Am J Hum Genet.* 67:146–154.

Mira, M. T., Alcais, A., Van Thuc, N., Thai, V. H., Huong, N. T., Ba, N. N., Verner, A., Hudson, T. J., Abel, L., and Schurr, E. (2003) Chromosome 6q25 is linked to susceptibility to leprosy in a Vietnamese population. *Nat Genet.* 33:412–415.

Mira, M. T., Alcais, A., Nguyen, V. T., Moraes, M. O., Di Flumeri, C., Vu, H. T., Mai, C. P., Nguyen, T. H., Nguyen, N. B., Pham, X. K., Sarno, E. N., Alter, A., Montepetit, A., Moraes, M. E., Morases, J. R., Dore, C., Gallant, C. J. Lepage, P., Verner, A., Van De Vosse, E., Hudson, T. J., Abel, L., and Schurr, E. (2004) Susceptibility to leprosy is associated with PARK2 and PACRG. *Nature.* 427(6975):636–640.

Ott, J. (1999) *Analysis of human genetic linkage.* Baltimore, MD: Johns Hopkins University Press.

Pritchard, J. K., and Rosenberg, N. A. (1999) Use of unlinked genetic markers to detect population stratification in association studies. *Am J Hum Genet.* 65:220–228.

Rabinowitz, D. (1997) A transmission disequilibrium test for quantitative trait loci. *Hum Hered.* 47:342–350.

Reiner, A. P., Ziv, E., Lind, D. L., Nievergelt, C. M., Schork, N. J., Cummings, S. R., Phong, A., Burchard, E. G., Harris, T. B., Psaty, B. M., and Kwok, P. Y. (2005) Population structure, admixture, and aging-related phenotypes in African American adults: the Cardiovascular Health Study. *Am J Hum Genet.* 76:463–477.

Rossouw, M., Nel, H. J., Cooke, G. S., van Helden, P. D., and Hoal, E. G. (2003) Association between tuberculosis and a polymorphic NFkappaB binding site in the interferon gamma gene. *Lancet.* 361:1871–1872.

Rubinstein, P., Ginsberg-Fellner, F., and Falk, C. (1981) Genetics of type I diabetes mellitus: a single, recessive predisposition gene mapping between HLA-B and GLO. With an appendix on the estimation of selection bias. *Am J Hum Genet.* 33:865–882.

Sack, D. A., Sack, R. B., Nair, G. B., and Siddique, A. K. (2004) Cholera. *Lancet.* 363:223–233.

Satten, G. A., Flanders, W. D., and Yang, Q. H. (2001) Accounting for unmeasured population substructure in case–control studies of genetic association using a novel latent-class model. *Am J Hum Genet.* 68:466–477.

Schaid, D. J. (1996) General score tests for associations of genetic markers with disease using cases and their parents. *Genet Epidemiol.* 13:423–449.

Scott, L. J., Mohlke, K. L., Bonnycastle, L. L., Willer, C. J., Duren, W. L., Erdos, M. R., Stringham, H. M., Chines, P. S., Jackson, A. U., Prokunina-Olsson, L., Ding, C. J., Swift, A. J., Narisu, N., Hu, T., Pruim, R., Xiao, R., Li, X. Y., Conneely, K. N., Riebow, N. L., Sprau, A. G., Tong, M., White, P. P., Hetric, K. N., Barnhart, M. W., Bark, C. W., Goldstein, J. L., Watkins, L., Xiang, F., Saramies, J., Buchanan, T. A., Watanabe, R. M., Valle, T. T., Kinnunen, L., Abecasis, G. R., Pugh, E. W., Doheny, K. F., Bergman, R. N., Tuomilheto, K., Collins, F. S., and Boehnke, M. (2007) A genome-wide association study of type 2 diabetes in Finns detects multiple susceptibility variants. *Science.* 316(5829):1341–1345.

Siddiqui, M. R., Meisner, S., Tosh, K., Balakrishnan, K., Ghei, S., Fisher, S. E., Golding, M., Shanker Narayan, N. P., Sitaraman, T., Sengupta, U., Pitchappan, R., and Hill, A. V. (2001) A major susceptibility locus for leprosy in India maps to chromosome 10p13. *Nat Genet.* 27:439–441.

Spielman, R. S., and Ewens, W. J. (1998) A sibship test for linkage in the presence of association: the sib transmission/disequilibrium test. *Am J Hum Genet.* 62:450–458.

Spielman, R. S., McGinnis, R. E., and Ewens, W. J. (1993) Transmission test for linkage disequilibrium: the insulin gene region and insulin-dependent diabetes mellitus (IDDM). *Am J Hum Genet.* 52:506–516.

Suarez, B. K., Lin, J., Witte, J. S., Conti, D. V., Resnick, M. I., Klein, E. A., Burmester, J. K., Vaske, D. A., Banerjee, T. K., and Catalona, W. J. (2000) Replication linkage study for prostate cancer susceptibility genes. *Prostate.* 45:106–114.

Tabor, H. K., Risch, N. J., Myers, R. M. (2002) Candidate-gene approaches for studying complex genetic traits: practical considerations. *Nat Rev Genet.* 3:391–397.

Thomas, D. C., Haile, R. W., and Duggan, D. (2005) Recent developments in genomewide association scans: a workshop summary and review. *Am J Hum Genet.* 77:337–345.

The Wellcome Trust Case Control Consortium. (2007) Genome-wide association study of 14,000 cases of seven common diseases and 3,000 shared controls. *Nature.* 447:661–678.

Williams-Blangero, S., McGarvey, S. T., Subedi, J., Wiest, P. M., Upadhayay, R. P., Rai, D. R., Jha, B., Olds, G. R., Guanling, W., and Blangero, J. (2002a) Genetic component to susceptibility to Trichuris trichiura: evidence from two Asian populations. *Genet Epidemiol.* 22:254–264.

Williams-Blangero, S., VandeBerg, J. L., Subedi, J., Aivaliotis, M. J., Rai, D. R., Upadhayay, R. P., Jha, B., and Blangero, J. (2002b) Genes on chromosomes 1 and 13 have significant effects on Ascaris infection. *Proc Natl Acad Sci USA.* 99:5533–5538.

Woolf, B. (1957) The log likelihood ratio test (the G-test); methods and tables for tests of heterogeneity in contingency tables. *Ann Hum Genet.* 21:397–409.

2

Laboratory Analysis of Genetic Variation

Meredith Yeager, Robert A. Welch, & Stephen J. Chanock

Recent technical and computational advances have dramatically accelerated the pace of laboratory analysis in the field of genetics. Historically, genotyping projects were small in scope and typically included analysis of a handful of single nucleotide polymorphisms (SNPs) in a candidate gene. The SNPs were often chosen because of known or putative function (e.g., in an amino acid–altering or promoter region) or on the basis of suggestive or corroborating laboratory data. However, in a matter of a few years, the horizon has changed dramatically; thousands of SNP markers can now be tested efficiently in large population-based studies.

Following the generation of a draft sequence of the human genome, annotation of genetic variation across the genome has reshaped the landscape for investigating the genetic basis of complex diseases (Risch and Merikangas, 1996; Risch, 2000). By definition, multiple genetic variants contribute to a complex disease, such as hypertension or cancer. Because it is now possible to assay thousands of genetic variants in a single sample with high precision, interest has shifted toward the examination of large sets of variants in studies designed to characterize germline variants. Already, it is possible to look "agnostically" at markers across the genome in genomewide association studies (GWAS), which can discover disease associations with novel regions of the genome, not all of which contain suitable candidate genes (Hunter et al., 2007a). For example, at least seven different regions of chromosome 8q24 have been associated with risk for prostate cancer (Yeager et al., 2007; Haiman et al. 2007; Gudmundsson et al. 2007; Carlson et al., 2004a). So far, GWAS have shown that confirmation studies are essential for verification, and particularly critical for markers that make relatively small contributions to a complex disease. Enhanced throughput capabilities permit rapid analysis of large sample sets, using smaller amounts of input DNA per assay. To support the investigation of complex diseases, formidable computation and informatic capacities are required to archive, manage and analyze the high-dimensional data sets.

Whole genome amplification (WGA) techniques can faithfully amplify nearly the entire genome, but there are regions that are not well represented and thus susceptible to genotype error (Dean et al., 2001; Hosono et al., 2003; Lasken and Egholm, 2003). Together, these developments have energized the field of molecular epidemiology and have established a foundation for discerning the contribution of genetics to human disease. Investigators no longer have to struggle with the arduous task of generating barely enough genetic markers to investigate the genetic contribution of a gene or set of genes. Instead, we face a more daunting challenge—how to handle the enormous amounts of data that can be routinely generated from increasingly smaller amounts of DNA.

Background

Germline variants that contribute to human disease can be divided into distinct categories based on the contribution of the variant to a well-defined phenotype. Classically, the penetrance of a variant is defined as the effect of the variant on a phenotype or outcome. Classic monogenic disorders, such as cystic fibrosis or classical hemophilia A (FVIII deficiency), are characterized by mutations in a single gene that have a highly predictable effect, or penetrance, resulting in disease. Even in these diseases, recent studies have shown that common genetic variants in other unlinked genes can modify the clinical course of the disease (Chanock and Foster, 1999; Taylor et al., 2001). For instance, several studies have shown that genetic variants in the mannose binding lectin gene, MBL2, can influence the severity of lung disease in patients with cystic fibrosis (Garred et al., 1999; Gabolde et al., 1999). In this regard, genetic modifiers can alter the risk for known complications or outcomes.

The availability of a large catalog of common and uncommon variants serves as the foundation for determining the contribution of many genes, albeit with small effects, or penetrance, to common and uncommon diseases (Botstein and Risch, 2003). According to the common disease–common variant hypothesis, ancestral genetic variants collectively contribute to the risk for common diseases, such as diabetes, hypertension, or mental illness. For the first two decades, the field was plagued by false positive reports, often owing to chance but also underpowered or improperly designed studies; reviews suggested that only a fraction of

reports were actually considered credible and reproducible (Lohmueller et al., 2003; see table 2.1).

The age of GWAS has ushered in a new era of discovery of regions and genes associated with common diseases, such as cancer, heart disease, and diabetes. Already, new loci have been discovered for breast and prostate cancer (Easton et al., 2007; Hunter et al., 2007b; Stacey et al., 2007; Haiman et al., 2007; Gudmundsson et al., 2007; Yeager et al., 2007), myocardial infarction (Helgadottir A. et al., 2007; McPherson et al., 2007), inflammatory bowel disease (Parkes et al., 2007) and diabetes (Saxena et al., 2007; Scott et al., 2007, Todd et al., 2007; Zeggini et al., 2007). In some diseases, at least 10 new regions have been established, but further studies are needed to fine-map the variants responsible for the biological effect. The success of GWAS has required analysis of over a thousand cases and controls with replication in larger data sets (Chanock et al., 2007). The combined analyses have generated very low p values for variants with estimated effects of 1.3 to 1.6 (Skol et al., 2006; Hunter et al., 2007a).

The capability of surveying thousands of well-chosen markers in whole-genome scans will certainly develop to the point of widespread application to a spectrum of diseases and outcomes, including pharmacogenomics (Carlson et al., 2004a). The ability to survey large sets of genetic variants has generated a series of new challenges, including the need for proper annotation of the human genome, an understanding of population genetics and evolution, the development of new tools to examine gene–gene and gene–environment interactions, and a framework for integrating this information into public and individual health.

TABLE 2.1. Replicated genetic association studies using a candidate gene approach.

Common Disease	Gene Symbol
Alzheimers disease	APOE-4
Deep venous thrombosis	FV-Leiden
Type 1 diabetes mellitus	INS (VNTR)
Type 2 diabetes mellitus	PPARG
Hemachromatosis	HFE
HIV infection and progression	CCR5
Severe RSV infection	IL4
Graves disease	CTL4A
Triglyceride levels	APOA
Lipid levels	LDL
Bladder cancer	NAT2
Gastric cancer	IL1

The most common type of variation in the human genome is the SNP, and advances in genotyping technologies have therefore concentrated on increasing the density of SNPs that can be analyzed at one time. Roughly 8–10 million SNPs occur with a minor allele frequency greater than 1% in at least one studied population (Kruglyak and Nickerson, 2001). The majority of SNPs, especially those of higher frequency (i.e., greater than 15–20%), are common to all human populations and are coveted for current approaches for SNP-based studies (Carlson et al., 2004b). An early survey found that 85% of more than 1.5 million SNPs were common to the three populations surveyed, while only a minority of high-frequency SNPs were private to a single population (Hinds et al., 2005). Because of historical bottlenecks associated with geographic isolation and evolutionary selection, the distribution of genetic diversity varies greatly across surveyed populations. The molecular evolution of human populations has resulted in a large number of common genetic variants, mainly SNPs with a minor allele frequency of greater than 10% (perhaps up to 5 million throughout the genome), which have been selected and maintained in populations (Clark et al., 2003; Hughes et al., 2005). Major differences in the allele frequencies of SNPs between populations reflect major differential and regional selective pressures, for example, infectious diseases such as malaria or tuberculosis, or environmental stresses such as temperature or diet (Hughes et al., 2005).

The recent success in employing the GWAS strategy has added a new dimension to the investigation of complex diseases. GWAS represent a discovery tool designed to identify new regions anywhere in the genome. This hypothesis-generating stage will be followed by effort to map and dissect the regions in search of the specific causal variants. In this regard, GWAS will direct some of the future selection of genes or regions for study in the genotype laboratory. At the same time, the candidate-gene approach, driven by biological or epidemiological observations as well as GWAS, will continue to be critical to explore the contribution of genetics to complex diseases. Moreover, it will continue to be productive to mine genetic databases and use comparative analysis strategies to identify regions for priority analysis. These strategies can include comparison of human populations or comparison of genome sequences from other species (Banerjee et al., 2002). In particular, the search for sequences shared between species represents a promising strategy for identifying common elements of potential functional importance. Conserved segments of sequence could represent preserved, functionally significant elements, especially regulatory regions (Banerjee et al., 2002).

Comparison of genetic sequences among human populations has yielded an unexpected finding: a greater density of common genetic variation in the human genome than previously appreciated (Cargill et al., 1999; Halushka et al., 1999; Schneider et al., 2003). Although common genetic variation represents less than 0.2% of the genome overall, SNPs are not inherited independently. Instead, SNPs are passed from one generation to the next on chromosomal segments (haplotypes), often within blocks (Reich et al., 2001; Gabriel et al., 2002). The observed patterns of LD between SNPs define haplotypes, which are very useful for mapping disease alleles. A relatively small number of SNPs can "tag" haplotypes that invariably contain certain others and thereby capture the most frequent and important variation in a region (Johnson et al., 2001, Carlson et al. 2004b). Quantitative methods have been developed to minimize the number of SNPs required to tag haplotypes (Stram et al., 2003a, 2003b; Carlson et al., 2004b). A number different programs and options are available for estimating haplotypes and tagging SNPs based on unphased genotype data generated in unrelated subjects (Salem et al., 2005).

The vast majority of SNPs are silent (i.e., they lack functional effect) but have been maintained on the backbone of an inherited block of DNA through generations. In contrast, a small subset of SNPs can alter the function or expression of a gene (Risch, 2000). These so-called "functional" SNPs are estimated to number between 50,000 and 250,000 (Chanock, 2001) and are of intense interest in disease association studies.

Advances in genomics have transformed the search for genetic contribution to disease susceptibility and outcome into a more systematic and comprehensive evaluation of genes. Since most SNPs are vestigial and appear to have no functional consequence, the challenge is to identify a set of informative SNPs, whether for scanning the genome or tagging a haplotype block in a candidate gene study. Laboratory analyses (e.g., in vitro or animal work) can certainly elucidate the basic mechanism or effect of a change in expression or function. The International HapMap Project represents a major milestone in establishing the patterns of common variation, which can differ substantially by population (International HapMap Consortium, 2003; Gabriel et al., 2002; Altshuler et al., 2005).

Choosing Genetic Variants for Study

Prior to the sequencing of the human genome, investigative strategies often depended on typing of signature repeat motifs (microsatellites). The generation of a draft sequence of the human genome led directly to efforts to annotate variation, resulting in a shift away from microsatellite analysis toward analysis of the more common SNP variants. Unlike microarray analysis, which examines the profile of all expressed mRNAs captured by an oligo dT primer, the analysis of a SNP is based on the ability to interrogate a single base change in a unique location in the genome. This can be accomplished either by direct sequence analysis or by using a genotyping assay that distinguishes between two bases. Current technologies require amplification of the flanking region using unique oligonucleotides. Recent estimates suggest that many regions of the genome have copy number variation (CNV; Redon et al., 2006). CNVs can vary in size and frequency in populations, resist easy detection, and can undermine the fidelity of bi-allelic SNP genotype assays. In fact, it has been estimated that perhaps one tenth of all genic regions have at least one paralog elsewhere in the genome; that is, a completely or nearly identical sequence has been duplicated on a different segment of the same chromosome or on a different chromosome (Bailey et al., 2002). Hence, great care must be exercised in designing SNP assays.

The primary public database is dbSNP (www.ncbi .nih.gov/SNP/), an international repository for SNPs (Marth et al., 2001). Currently, more than 8 million human SNPs have been deposited into dbSNP. However, these data are not all equally reliable. It is estimated that perhaps 15–20% of SNPs in dbSNP are monoallelic and represent sequence tracing errors. As several international efforts continue to verify SNPs, using different criteria, we can expect to see the number of new monoallelic entries decrease. Major international efforts, such as the SNP Consortium and the International HapMap Project, have deposited information on SNPs verified by a genotyping assay (International HapMap Consortium, 2003; Sachidanadam et al., 2001; Altshuler et al., 2005). Most of the SNPs from these programs, however, are not directly

resequenced but instead are optimized on one or more genotyping platforms. These strategies are biased toward high-frequency variants and do not characterize SNPs of lower frequency (<5%).

Several smaller scale programs have committed to resequencing genes in regions of interest for multiple individuals of different racial background to facilitate discovery of common SNPs (e.g., those with a minor allele frequency greater than 5%) and validate nominated SNPs of importance for molecular epidemiology studies (Schneider et al., 2003; Akey et al., 2004; Livingston et al., 2004; Packer et al., 2006). One strategy is to resequence across all introns and exons of the gene of interest (Akey et al., 2004; Livingston et al., 2004). This systematic coverage affords the optimal opportunity to characterize all common variation, the LD between them, and common haplotypes for each gene. An alternative approach has been to sequence in key genic regions, including exons, regulatory regions, and regions of high homology between mammals and humans; this approach emphasizes conserved function. For instance, the Breast and Prostate Cancer Cohort Consortium supported extensive resequencing in the 55 genes of the sex steroid hormone metabolism and insulin growth factor pathways and concurrently performed dense genotype analysis in reference samples to estimate the common haplotypes across each of the 55 genes (cgf.nci.nih.gov or www .uscnorris.com/mecgenetics/) (Hunter et al., 2005). Alternatively, the SNP500Cancer project (snp500 cancer.nci.nih.gov) linked sequence validation to optimization for genotype assays in four different populations, representing the four major self-described ethnic groups in the United States (Packer et al., 2006). Assay optimization is based on 100% concordance between sequence and genotype performance (see figure 2.1).

Although significant enthusiasm has been generated by the availability of a rapidly increasing set of common SNPs, choosing and designing a SNP assay may be less straightforward than it would appear. Because SNPs can vary by population, a thorough assessment of the sequence context (i.e., the sequence flanking the target SNP) is important for the design and performance of genotyping assays. A previously unknown SNP underlying a primer or probe can erroneously alter the performance of a SNP assay (see figure 2.1). Similarly, an adjacent SNP can prevent the design of a robust and reproducible assay. Additionally, because SNPs can vary by population, flanking

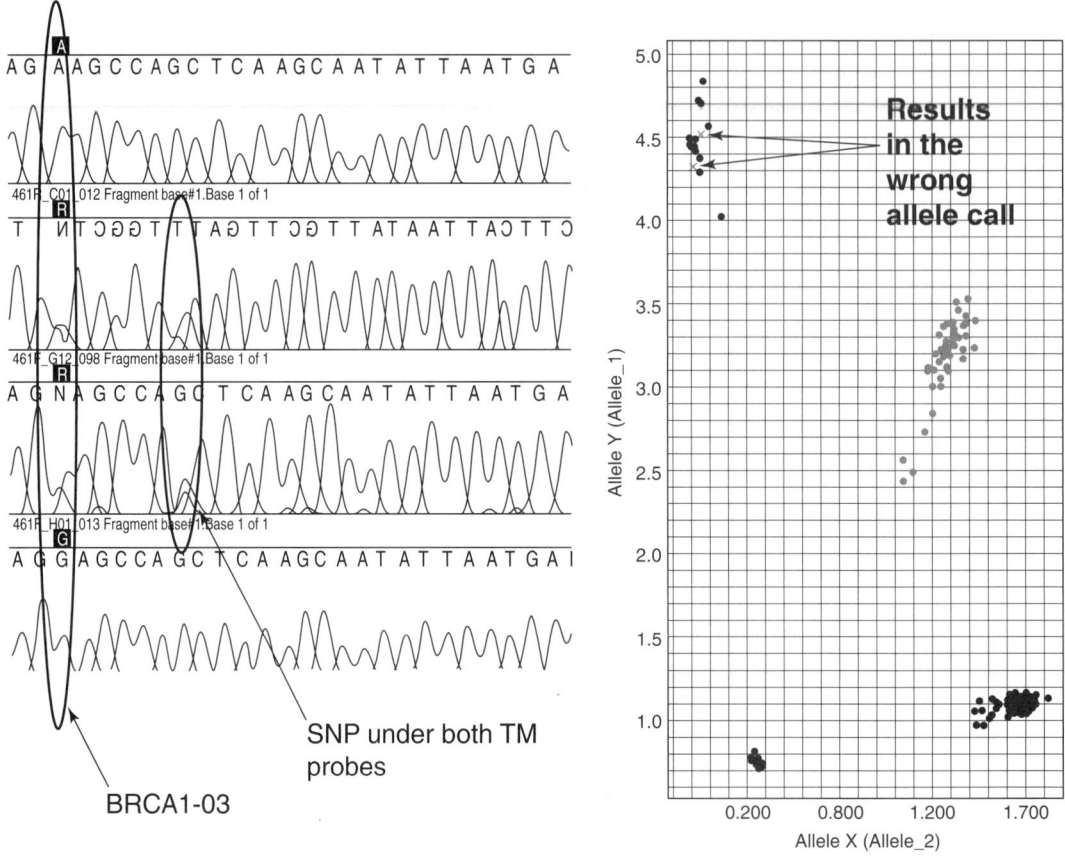

FIGURE 2.1. The problem of an unappreciated, neighboring SNP in the assay performance of the TaqMan assay system. All of the primers and probes are available for the optimized assay on the SNP500Cancer Web site (snp500cancer.nci.nih.gov; Packer et al., 2004).

sequences should be characterized in order to avoid these pitfalls. Furthermore, the population specificity of SNPs can vary—many SNPs observed in populations of African descent, known to be the most ancient, are not observed in other regions of the world (Tishkoff and Williams, 2002). Optimization of SNP assays is critical for minimizing genotyping error, which may be less than 0.4% as estimated by loss of a heterozygous marker (Sobel et al., 2002).

Because of the large number of SNPs, mining genomic databases can be a formidable task and requires extensive knowledge of the bioinformatic tools. The Web site, Genewindow (genewindow.nci.nih.gov), offers an example of a tool for gene-centric visualization of genetic variation across a locus (Staats et al., 2005). It facilitates navigation and selection of SNPs in preparation for genotyping analysis.

Genotype Platforms

The primary determinant of the choice of platform to be used for genotyping is the scope of the study. No single SNP detection technique is likely to meet all of the needs of any given study or laboratory. Design issues (e.g., guanine-cytosine [GC] content, neighboring SNPs) represent one challenge, while the presence of paralogous sequence is also a major obstacle. In fact, some regions are not amenable to unique amplification and thus cannot be assayed accurately (Bailey et al., 2002; Packer et al., 2006). SNP detection technologies can be applied in many different settings and circumstances, and selection of an appropriate one involves important considerations of cost, flexibility in the choice and substitution of SNP assays, commercial availability, and magnitude of assay throughput. In recent years, availability of alterative technologies and platforms has increased dramatically; these options have substantially lowered the price of genotyping and accelerated genotyping throughput. Indeed, these technical capabilities have surpassed statistical and other paradigms for analysis, in both their sheer size and complexity.

Options for genotyping technology span a wide spectrum—from single SNP detection to thousands of SNPs in one reaction (see table 2.2). With the nascent whole-genome scan technology, most investigators will probably focus on sets of SNPs, haplotypes, and genes in pursuit of the candidate gene approach in the short term (Taylor et al., 2001). Moreover, even as whole-genome scans become more common, it should be emphasized that the approach is designed to identify regions or loci that will still require the attention of the candidate gene approach, fine typing for haplotype assignment, and individual resequencing analysis. Earlier manual methods such as RFLP (restriction fragment length polymorphism) are increasingly obsolete; now only the exceptional variant is assayed with this or other laborious, error-prone techniques. Intermediate approaches include differential hybridization, primer extension, ligation reactions, and allele-specific probe cleavage (Kwok et al., 2003a; Kwok et al., 2003b).

To assay a small number of SNPs, many investigators have lately turned to fluorescence polarization detection technology (Kwok, 2002). This approach is based on a fluorescent molecule excited by plane-polarized light, resulting in an emitted polarized light detected by one of several types of sensors. Most commercial systems currently employ two-color technology, but efforts are under way to develop platforms with four or more colors. The TaqMan (Applied Biosystems, Foster City, Calif.) technology uses a single enzymatic step with universal reaction and thermocycling conditions, based on the principle of unique binding of a probe to the target sequence of interest followed by primer extension. Allelic discrimination is determined by selective annealing of exact matching probe and primer sequences, which in turn generate an allele-specific fluorescent signal. The reaction is capped by a modification of a nonfluorescent quencher with a Minor Grove Binder at the 3' end. (Kutyavin et al., 2000; Latif et al., 2001; de Kok et al., 2002). The TaqMan system can also be used for real-time PCR to estimate copy number or measure semi-quantitative differences. Another popular single-SNP genotyping assay is MGB Eclipse (Nanogen, Inc., San Diego, Calif.). This system is particularly suited for challenging regions, namely, those high in GC content or complicated by a nearby SNP that interferes with primer/probe design (Belousov et al., 2004). The latter system requires modified oligonucleotide probes that contain covalently attached duplex-stabilizing dihydrocyclopyrroloindole, which permits shorter probe sequences and improves mismatch discrimination. The Invader assay (Third Wave Technologies, Inc., Madison, Wisc.) is another option based on the cleavage of a specific structure formed by overlapping probes annealed to the DNA segment of interest (Hsu et al., 2001).

Several technologies are also available for analyzing between 5 and 50 SNPs at one time using a single sample. Optimization of these types of assays represents a significant challenge and requires effort to ensure high fidelity and throughput. Such "multiplexing" of assays offers the advantage of analyzing carefully selected SNPs, for instance, numerous SNPs tagging a region or locus; however, the flexibility to alter the assay composition is limited. One example is the SNPlex Genotyping System (Applied Biosystems), based on the oligonucleotide ligation/PCR assay with an additional probe for fluorescence detection (De la Vega et al., 2005). The genotype information is determined by ligation of the allele-specific oligonucleotide probes to the locus-specific oligonucleotide. An alternative technology uses chip-based MALDI-TOF (matrix-assisted laser desorption/ionization time-of-flight) mass spectrometry (Chiu et al., 2000). This technique is suited for smaller numbers of SNPs in a multiplex assay and is now widely used. It can be

TABLE 2.2. Spectrum of genotype platforms.

Intent	Type	SNPs per Day
Extreme genotyping: chips and beads	Whole genome	1,000,000
High throughput: smaller chips and bytes	Pathways and genes	250,000
Moderate throughput: probes and primers	Genes and haplotypes	100,000
Low throughput: RFLP	Gene or haplotype	500

RFLP, restriction fragment length polymorphism (gel-based analysis).

extended to embrace further applications such as analysis of mutations, the resequencing of amplicons with a known reference sequence, and the quantitative analysis of gene expression and allelic frequencies in complex DNA mixtures (Jurinke et al., 2004).

The next generation of SNP detection systems employs microarrays to capture even larger sets of SNPs. For instance, several groups have coupled allele-specific primer extension technology to microarray or membrane array platforms (Pastinen et al., 1997, 2000; Jobs et al., 2003).

New advances in technical capabilities are leading us into the age of high-density genotyping systems, also known as "extreme genotyping." New, high-density technologies are designed to genotype at least 500,000 and perhaps 1 million SNPs at once, using a small amount of DNA relative to the number of genotypes analyzed. The advantage of these technologies lies in analyzing an enormous set of genotypes. However, each of the technologies requires costly and extensive preparation of assays, particularly because thousands of data points are being generated in microliter amounts of specimen, and the bioinformatic challenges are formidable. Furthermore, there is little flexibility in choosing SNPs for inclusion in panels. The trade-off is between flexibility and cost. However, the success of GWAS has been the production of chips with representation of common genetic variation suitable for scanning the genome.

Several currently available commercial products have substantially increased the capabilities of SNP studies. Three are transportable but require extensive bioinformatic support and analytical capabilities. The Affymetrix (Santa Clara, Calif.) microchip system uses a simplification of the genome by restriction digest with one or more common restriction endonucleases. After the addition of universal adapting linkers, the reaction is globally amplified prior to fragmentation and labeling. SNP assays are analyzed on the microchip using an address system (Chee et al., 1996; Matsuzaki et al., 2004). The Illumina (San Diego, Calif.) system uses an allele-specific gap-fill process followed by ligation and amplification prior to readout on a bead-based capillary microarray or microchip system (Gunderson et al., 2004). The typing is performed with high multiplicity to ensure high performance. A fourth technology is provided by Perlegen Sciences (Mountain View, Calif.) on contract, but it cannot be transported to an external laboratory (Hinds et al., 2005). A PCR-based sample preparation promotes amplification across the genome.

High-density oligonucleotide arrays consisting of short DNA probes are synthesized on a glass surface and used to determine genotypes with great redundancy. Nearly one million SNPs have been sequenced by this technique, and the risk of encountering an unexpected neighboring SNP or other forms of interference with assay validity is very small.

Although the technical ingenuity of each platform is remarkable, a common feature of the detection process is the requirement of an amplification step, which undermines the accuracy of assessing CNV. Moreover, each of these technologies is challenged by SNPs that reside close together (within 60 or fewer nucleotides). Their capabilities do, however, represent a major step toward conducting whole-genome scans (Carlson et al., 2004a). Quality control is critical, and recommended procedures must be rigorously followed. Some investigators have already noted that, for each platform, a subset of the SNP assays do not perform well enough, due either to previously unappreciated neighboring SNPs or to local sequence peculiarities. The new high-density SNP platforms can also be applied to the study of loss of heterozygosity through somatic alterations, as often occurs in cancer. Techniques for detecting dense distribution of markers may also find useful application in studies of germline homozygosity in infectious diseases.

Additional approaches to high-density SNP analysis include, for example, a novel allele-specific primer elongation protocol using a DNA polymerase on oligonucleotide chips (Erdogan et al., 2001). With this platform, a set of oligonucleotide primers bearing the polymorphic sites on the 3′ end are covalently bound to glass slides. A set of single-stranded targets of genomic DNA containing each SNP is generated by an asymmetric PCR reaction or exonuclease treatment of phosphothioate-modified PCR products. DNA polymerase with Cy3-dUTP replacing dTTP is added, and the allele-specific extension of the immobilized primers takes place on a stretch of target DNA sequence.

Quality Control in the Laboratory

The success of a genotyping study begins with the efficient and meticulous handling of the samples. Close coordination between the laboratory performing the extraction and the biorepository storing the DNA samples is critical for enhancing the reliability of the study. Lapses in dilution of DNA following extraction, storage, and transport can undermine the integrity of the study, and optimal practice should not be taken for granted. Genomic DNA of questionable or poor quality often reduces completion rates and concordance between blind duplicates.

Many laboratories develop standard operating procedures for determining the quantity and quality of genomic DNA. Accurate assessment of the quantity of DNA can be interrogated by spectrophotometric measurement of DNA optical density, by PicoGreen (Turner BioSystems, Sunnyvale, Calif.) analysis or by real-time PCR analysis using a standardized TaqMan assay (Haque et al., 2003). Spectrophotometry and the PicoGreen assay measure total DNA present, regardless of source or quality, whereas a real-time PCR assay measures the total "amplifiable" human DNA. Establishing DNA quantity by real-time PCR is critical for DNA from buccal swabs, cytobrush samples, or other nonblood sources. Small differences between these techniques are important in assessing the amounts of single- and double-stranded DNA. Accurate quantification is critical for optimizing the genotyping results and minimizing the use of precious DNA samples (Haque et al., 2003). Further precautions can include additional analysis of all samples received, testing a forensic panel of 15 small tandem repeats and amelogenin, also known as the AmpF*l*STR Identifiler assay (Applied Biosystems). This analysis identifies contaminated samples as well as those on which the amplification step has failed. The individual profiles are also useful for ensuring that duplicate or replacement samples are identical and for resolving laboratory errors with plates or reagents.

The design of all molecular epidemiology studies should include undisclosed duplicates taken from the same sample, as well as replicates of different samples taken from the same individual. Genotype concordance among duplicates and replicates should exceed 98% for all assay systems. For the high density SNP chips, the concordance is higher, well above 99.5%. Errors in genotyping, mainly due to loss of one of the heterozygous alleles, occur in well below 1% of samples for commercial and academic platforms and techniques of highest quality. If standard operating procedures are followed closely, completion rates should be greater than 95% for most studies but may be slightly lower depending on the quality of genomic DNA. Completion rates below 90% should raise concern about technical or analytical deficiencies.

Whole-Genome Amplification (WGA)

Initially, PCR technology was used for genetic analysis at specific loci (Mullis et al., 1986), and early attempts to scale up the procedure with degenerate oligonucleotides proved to be inadequate. Intermediate milestones were accomplished by modifications of standard techniques (Cheung and Nelson, 1996). Advances in genomic technologies have evolved to permit the study of thousands of SNPs simultaneously from small quantities of DNA. While the amount of DNA required to conduct these analyses has diminished, new techniques can amplify the entire genome with excellent, but not perfect, fidelity. Improvements in the existing techniques to perform WGA have generated considerable enthusiasm but do not yet reproducibly amplify the entire genome nor recapture heavily degraded or damaged DNA (e.g., following electronic beam radiation used for protecting the U.S. mail system; Bergen et al., 2005a).

The optimization of new enzyme technologies has significantly improved WGA technology. The multiple displacement amplification approach utilizes a high-performance bacteriophage ϕ 29 DNA polymerase with degenerate hexamers (Dean et al., 2001, 2002; Pask et al., 2004). It has been applied to a spectrum of DNA sources, including whole blood, plasma, serum, dried blood, buccal cell swabs, cultured cells, and buffy coat cells. Under optimal conditions, the expected yield is approximately a 10,000-fold increase in genomic DNA, and allele loss has been estimated to be less than 1% or 2% (Dean et al., 2002; Hosono et al., 2003; Bergen et al., 2005b, 2005c). An alternative method utilizes OmniPlex (Rubicon Genomics, Ann Arbor, Mich.) libraries of 200–2,000 base-pair fragments created by random chemical cleavage of genomic DNA, followed by ligation of adaptor sequences to both ends and PCR amplification. It has been reported to faithfully amplify more than 99%, as measured by using whole-genome SNP linkage panels (Barker et al., 2004; Paez et al., 2004).

Several notable observations have emerged as more laboratories utilize WGA technologies. Specific loci might not amplify faithfully, and an allele may not be recognized. For instance, disproportional amplification in regions of high GC content and those near telomeres may result in the loss of one allele (Bergen et al., 2005b). This has significant implications for molecular epidemiology studies and should be monitored carefully for each study. Regardless of the genotype technology used, subtle but important differences in fidelity of amplification across regions and in success at genotyping may occur. It is also possible that WGA of water control specimens can generate a small, mono-allelic signal, which could be called positive during analysis. Thus, special care must be given to both the quality control analysis and the software programs for automating calls in high-throughput genotype analysis. Lastly, further studies are needed to determine the optimal amount and type of source genomic DNA to be amplified.

Further improvement of these techniques in the near future is expected to help identify specific genes or regions not amenable to reliable amplification and genotype analysis. Hopefully, public efforts along these lines will yield a valuable catalog of the more challenging regions of the genome.

Data Flow and Information Handling

The efficiency and effectiveness of a genotyping laboratory are based on the flow of information, from the preanalysis choice of markers through the analysis and presentation of the data to collaborators or for publication. Figure 2.2 shows a schematic view of the tasks involved. As the field has progressed and the number of genotypes performed on smaller quantities of DNA has rapidly expanded, the challenges of bioinformatics interpretation have increased substantially. Extensive resources are required for data storage, management, and archiving. Designated personnel are needed to manage the stream of information required to execute high-density genotyping and analyze the output.

Laboratories committed to high-throughput genotype analysis require a relational database for storing data to track and report study results. In turn, the relational database can link to a laboratory information management system (LIMS), which tracks data

through the entire flow of the laboratory. The specific features of the LIMS should be based on the needs and goals of the laboratory. Particular attention must be given to the details of laboratory workflow, often beginning in the biorepository through the provision of genotype reports (Henderson et al., 2005). The LIMS captures the movement of information into and out of the relational database, incorporating the results of experimental data, with linkage directly to *in silico* information, which includes the specific genomic coordinates and genotype assay. This systematic storage and linkage ensures the fidelity and accuracy of the genotype analysis. LIMS software should be subjected to rigorous quality-control and quality-assurance checks (Turner and Bolton, 2001). Select tasks, such as auto-reporting, reproducibility, throughput, and accuracy, are validated regularly to ensure high performance of stable data sets.

The relational database also houses information critical for quality control of specific assays. Standard data management techniques for quality control within a study and cross-validation (e.g., of the performance of technical platforms) with prior studies can ensure continued high-performance genotype analysis.

Conclusion

During the past decade, dramatic advances in genetic analyses have resulted in a major reorientation in the study of human genetic variation and disease. Instead of struggling with analysis on a handful of often individually typed genetic markers, we now face the daunting challenge of surveying thousands of markers per individual. Informative computational approaches are desperately needed to dissect the contribution of germline variation in human disease. The bottleneck has moved from the laboratory assay to the data analytic phase, where the major challenge now resides in

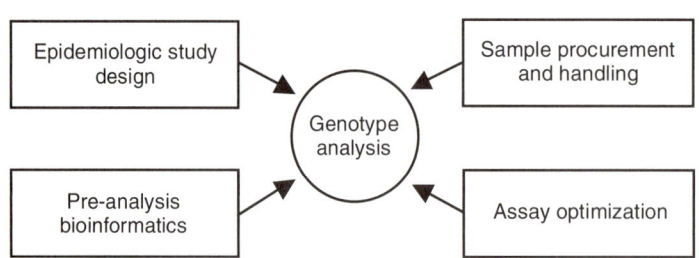

FIGURE 2.2. Schematic view of the tasks involved in high-throughput genotype analysis.

the mining of enormously dense data sets. Far greater effort must now focus on the search for meaningful effects of individual genotypes, haplotypes, and ultimately interactions between genetic markers. As the cost of genotyping drops, the temptation will be to analyze more markers. The next generation of technical platforms is expected to answer the call to increase the number of tested SNPs, but commercial and logistic constraints will likely yield sets of SNPs that are relatively few and fixed—less responsive to individual needs. Minor modification of a set of SNPs will exact a high cost, probably too high for most investigators to justify. Standardization across multiple studies could provide an unexpected advantage in the form of replication of results, but with the corresponding limit on discovery of the novel or unexpected.

The choice of study population and knowledge of the underlying structure of its genetic variants is critical for analysis, especially when investigating groups other than European or North American Caucasians. Information about the differences in patterns of linkage disequilibrium and haplotype structure is especially important when pursuing the candidate gene approach (Reich et al., 2001; Gabriel et al., 2002; Hinds et al., 2005).

For the near future, research into genetic susceptibility will continue to focus on SNP-based genotyping techniques, but within the next decade high-throughput sequence technology will likely become inexpensive enough to permit sequencing of the entire genome of an individual at a reasonable cost—the so-called "$1,000 genome" screen. At that point, it will be possible to examine both common and uncommon genetic variants, but the bioinformatic challenges will persist: to develop paradigms for interpreting the significance of rarer variants outside of families afflicted by a highly penetrant, severe disease phenotype (Pritchard, 2001). For now, however, an asymptotic limit, namely, the identification of rare variants in the absence of confirmation of their functional relevance, will remain the real challenge.

References

Akey JM, Eberle MA, Rieder MJ, Carlson CS, Shriver MD, Nickerson DA, Kruglyak L. 2004. Population history and natural selection shape patterns of genetic variation in 132 genes. *PLoS Biology*, 2, e286.

Altshuler D, Brooks LD, Chakravarti A, Collins FS, Daly MJ, Donnelly P; International HapMap Consortium. 2005. A haplotype map of the human genome. *Nature*, 437, 1299–1320.

Bailey JA, Gu Z, Clark RA, Reinert K, Samonte RV, Schwartz S, Adams MD, Myers EW, Li PW, Eichler EE. 2002. Recent segmental duplications in the human genome. *Science*, 297, 1003–1007.

Banerjee P, Bahlo M, Schwartz JR, Loots GG, Houston KA, Dubchak I, Speed TP, Rubin EM. 2002. SNPs in putative regulatory regions identified by human mouse comparative sequencing and transcription factor binding site data. *Mammalian Genome*, 13, 554–557.

Barker DL, Hansen MS, Faruqi AF, Giannola D, Irsula OR, Lasken RS, Latterich M, Makarov V, Oliphant A, Pinter JH, Shen R, et al. 2004. Two methods of whole-genome amplification enable accurate genotyping across a 2320-SNP linkage panel. *Genome Research*, 14, 901–907.

Belousov YS, Welch RA, Sander S, Mills A, Kulchenko A, Dempcy R, Afonina IA, Walburger DK, Glaser CL, Yadavalli S, Vermeulen NMJ, et al. 2004. Single nucleotide polymorphism genotyping by two colour melting curve analysis using the MGB Eclipse™ probe system in challenging sequence environment. *Human Genomics*, 1, 209–217.

Bergen AW, Qi Q, Haque K, Welch RA, Garcia-Closas M, Chanock S, Castle PE. 2005a. Effects of electron-beam irradiation on whole genome amplification. *Cancer Epidemiology Biomarkers and Prevention*, 14, 1016–1019.

Bergen AW, Haque KA, Qi Y, Beerman MB, Garcia-Closas M, Rothman N, Chanock SJ. 2005b. Comparison of: yield and genotyping performance of multiple displacement amplification and Omniplex™ whole genome amplified DNA generated from multiple DNA sources. *Human Mutation*, 26, 262–270.

Bergen AW, Qi Y, Haque KA, Welch RA, Chanock SJ. Effects of DNA mass on multiple displacement whole genome amplification and genotyping performance. 2005c. *BMC Biotechnology*, 5, 24.

Botstein D, Risch N. 2003. Discovering genotypes underlying human phenotypes: past successes for Mendelian disease, future approaches for complex disease. *Nature Genetics*, 33, 228–237.

Cargill M, Altshuler D, Ireland J, Sklar P, Ardlie K, Patil N, Shaw N, Lane CR, Lim EP, Kalyanaraman N, Nemesh J, et al. 1999. Characterization of single-nucleotide polymorphisms in coding regions of human genes. *Nature Genetics*, 22, 231–238.

Carlson CS, Eberle MA, Kruglyak L, Nickerson DA. 2004a. Mapping complex disease loci in whole-genome association studies. *Nature*, 429, 446–452.

Carlson CS, Eberle MA, Rieder MJ, Yi Q, Kruglyak L, Nickerson DA. 2004b. Selecting a maximally informative set of single-nucleotide polymorphisms for association analyses using linkage disequilibrium. *American Journal of Human Genetics*, 74, 106–120.

Chanock S. 2001. Candidate genes and single nucleotide polymorphisms (SNPs) in the study of human disease. *Disease Markers*, 17, 89–98.

Chanock SJ, Foster CB. 1999. SNPing away at innate immunity. *Journal of Clinical Investigations*, 104, 369–370.

Chanock SJ, Manolio T, Boehnke M, Boerwinckle E, Hunter DJ, Thomas G, Hirshhorn J, Abecasis G, et al. 2007. Replicating genotype-phenotype associations. *Nature*, 447, 655–660.

Chee M, Yang R, Hubbell E, Berno A, Huang XC, Stern D, Winkler J, Lockhart D, Morris MS, Fodor SP. 1996. Accessing genetic information with high-density DNA arrays. *Science*, 274, 610–614.

Cheung VG, Nelson SF. 1996. Whole genome amplification using a degenerate oligonucleotide primer allows hundreds of genotypes to be performed on less than one nanogram of genomic DNA. *Proceedings of the National Academy of Sciences of the United States of America*, 93, 14676–14679.

Chiu NH, Tang K, Yip P, Braun A, Koster H, Cantor CR. 2000. Mass spectrometry of single-stranded restriction fragments captured by an undigested complementary sequence. *Nucleic Acids Research*, 28, E31.

Clark AG, Nielsen R, Signorovitch J, Matise TC, Glanowski S, Heil J, Winn-Deen ES, Holden AL, Lai E. 2003. Linkage disequilibrium and inference of ancestral recombination in 538 single-nucleotide polymorphism clusters across the human genome. *American Journal of Human Genetics* 73, 285–300.

Dean FB, Nelson JR, Giesler TL, Lasken RS. 2001. Rapid amplification of plasmid and phage DNA using Phi 29 DNA polymerase and multiply-primed rolling circle amplification. *Genome Research*, 11, 1095–1099.

Dean FB, Hosono S, Fang L, Wu X, Faruqi AF, Bray-Ward P, Sun Z, Zong Q, Du Y, Du J, Driscoll M, et al. 2002. Comprehensive human genome amplification using multiple displacement amplification. *Proceedings of the National Academy of Sciences of the United States of America*, 99, 5261–5266.

de Kok JB, Wiegerinck ET, Giesendorf BA, Swinkels DW. 2002. Rapid genotyping of single nucleotide polymorphisms using novel minor groove binding DNA oligonucleotides (MGB probes). *Human Mutation*, 19, 554–559.

De la Vega FM, Lazaruk KD, Rhodes MD, Wenz MH. 2005. Assessment of two flexible and compatible SNP genotyping platforms: TaqMan SNP genotyping assays and the SNPlex genotyping system. *Mutation Research*, 573, 111–135.

Easton DF, Pooley KA, Dunning AM, Pharoah PD, Thompson D, Ballinger DG, et al. 2007. Genome-wide association study identifies novel breast cancer susceptibility loci. *Nature*, 447, 1087–1093

Erdogan F, Kirchner R, Mann W, Ropers HH, Nuber UA. 2001. Detection of mitochondrial single nucleotide polymorphisms using a primer elongation reaction on oligonucleotide microarrays. *Nucleic Acids Research*, 29, E36.

Gabolde M, Guilloud-Bataille M, Feingold J, et al. 1999. Association of variant alleles of mannose binding lectin with severity of pulmonary disease in cystic fibrosis: cohort study. *British Medical Journal*, 319, 1166–1167.

Gabriel SB, Schaffner SF, Nguyen H, Moore JM, Roy J, Blumenstiel B, Higgins J, DeFelice M, Lochner A, Faggart M, Liu-Cordero SN, et al. 2002. The structure of haplotype blocks in the human genome. *Science*, 296, 2225–2229.

Garred P, Pressler T, Madsen HO, et al. 1999. Association of mannose-binding lectin gene heterogeneity with severity of lung disease and survival in cystic fibrosis. *Journal of Clinical Investigation*, 104, 431–437.

Gudmundsson J, Sulem P, Manolescu A, Amundadottir LT, Gudbjartsson D, Helgason A, et al. 2007. Genome-wide association study identifies a second prostate cancer susceptibility variant at 8q24. *Nature Genetics*, 39, 631–637.

Gunderson KL, Kruglyak S, Graige MS, Garcia F, Kermani BG, Zhao C, Che D, Dickinson T, Wickham E, Bierle J, Doucet D, et al. 2004. Decoding randomly ordered DNA arrays. *Genome Research*, 14, 870–877.

Haiman CA, Patterson N, Freedman ML, Myers SR, Pike MC, Waliszewska A, et al. 2007. Multiple regions within 8q24 independently affect risk for prostate cancer. *Nature Genetics*, 39, 638–644.

Halushka MK, Fan JB, Bentley K, Hsie L, Shen N, Weder A, Cooper R, Lipshitz R, Chakravarti A. 1999. Patterns of single-nucleotide polymorphisms in candidate genes for blood-pressure homeostasis. *Nature Genetics*, 22, 239–247.

Haque KA, Pfeiffer RM, Beerman MB, Struewing JP, Chanock SJ, Bergen AW. 2003. Performance of high-throughput DNA quantification methods. *BMC Biotechnology*, 3, 20.

Helgadottir A, Thorleifsson G, Manolescu A, Gretarsdottir S, Blondal T, Jonasdottir A, et al. 2007. A common variant on chromosome 9p21 affects the risk of myocardial infarction. *Science*, 316, 1491–1493.

Henderson MK, Mohla C, Jacobs KB, Vaught JB. 2005. Challenges of scientific data management for large epidemiologic studies. *Cell Preservation Technology*, 3, 49–53.

Hinds DA, Stuve LL, Nilsen GB, Halperin E, Eskin E, Ballinger DG, Frazer KA, Cox DR. 2005. Whole-genome patterns of common DNA variation in three human populations. *Science*, 307, 1052–1053.

Hosono S, Faruqi AF, Dean FB, Du Y, Sun Z, Wu X, Du J, Kingsmore SF, Egholm M, Lasken RS. 2003. Unbiased whole-genome amplification directly from clinical samples. *Genome Research*, 13, 954–964.

Hunter DJ, Kraft P, Jacobs KB, Cox DG, Yeager M, Hankinson SE, et al. 2007. A genome-wide association study identifies alleles in FGFR2 associated with risk of sporadic postmenopausal breast cancer. *Nature Genetics*, 39, 870–874.

Hunter DJ, Riboli E, Haiman CA, Albanes D, Altshuler D, Chanock SJ, Haynes RB, Henderson BE, Kaaks R, Stram DO, Thomas G, et al.; National Cancer Institute Breast and Prostate Cancer Cohort Consortium. 2005. A candidate gene approach to searching for low-penetrance breast and prostate cancer genes. *Nature Reviews Cancer*, 5, 977–985.

Hunter DJ, Thomas G, Hoover R, Chanock SJ. 2007. Scanning the horizon: what is the future of genome-wide association studies in accelerating discoveries in cancer etiology and prevention? *Cancer Causes Control* 18, 479–484.

Hsu TM, Law SM, Duan S, Neri BP, Kwok PY. 2001. Genotyping single nucleotide polymorphisms by the invader assay with dual-color fluorescence polarization detection. *Clinical Chemistry*, 47, 1373–1377.

Hughes A, Packer B, Welch R, Bergen AW, Chanock SJ, Yeager M. 2005. Effects of natural selection on inter-population divergence at polymorphic sites in human protein-coding loci. *Genetics*, 170, 1181–1187.

International HapMap Consortium. 2003. The International HapMap Project. *Nature*, 426, 789–796.

Jobs M, Howell WM, Stromqvist L, Mayr T, Brookes AJ. 2003. DASH-2: flexible, low-cost, and high-throughput SNP genotyping by dynamic allele-specific hybridization on membrane arrays. *Genome Research*, 13, 916–924.

Johnson GC, Esposito L, Barratt BJ, Smith AN, Heward J, Di Genova G, Ueda H, Cordell HJ, Eaves IA, Dudbridge F, Twells RC, et al. 2001. Haplotype tagging for the identification of common disease genes. *Nature Genetics*, 29, 233–237.

Jurinke C, Oeth P, van den Boom D. 2004. MALDI-TOF mass spectrometry: a versatile tool for high-performance DNA analysis. *Molecular Biotechnology*, 26, 147–164.

Kruglyak L, Nickerson DA. 2001. The spice of life. *Nature Genetics*, 27, 234–235.

Kutyavin IV, Afonina IA, Mills A, Gorn, VV, Lukhtanov EA, Belousov ES, Singer MJ, Walburger DK, Lokhov SG, Gall AA, Dempcy R, et al. 2000. 3′-Minor groove binder-DNA probes increase sequence specificity at PCR extension temperatures. *Nucleic Acids Research*, 28, 655–661.

Kwok PY. 2002. SNP genotyping with fluorescence polarization detection. *Human Mutation*, 19, 315–323.

Kwok PY, Chen X. 2003a. Detection of single nucleotide polymorphisms. *Current Issues of Molecular Biology*, 5, 43–60.

Kwok PY, Duan S. 2003b. SNP discovery by direct DNA sequencing. *Methods of Molecular Biology*, 212, 71–84.

Lasken RS, Egholm M. 2003. Whole genome amplification: abundant supplies of DNA from precious samples or clinical specimens. *Trends in Biotechnology*, 21, 531–535.

Latif S, Bauer-Sardina I, Ranade K, Livak KJ, Kwok PY. 2001. Fluorescence polarization in homogeneous nucleic acid analysis II: 5′′-nuclease assay. *Genome Research*, 3, 436–40.

Livingston RJ, von Niederhausern A, Jegga AG, Crawford DC, Carlson CS, Rieder MJ, Gowrisankar S, Aronow BJ, Weiss RB, Nickerson DA. 2004. Pattern of sequence variation across 213 environmental response genes. *Genome Research*, 14, 1821–1831.

Lohmueller KE, Pearce CL, Pike M, Lander ES, Hirschhorn JN. 2003. Meta-analysis of genetic association studies supports a contribution of common variants to susceptibility to common disease. *Nature Genetics*, 33, 177–182.

Marth G, Yeh R, Minton M, Donaldson R, Li Q, Duan S, Davenport R, Miller RD, Kwok PY. 2001. Single-nucleotide polymorphisms in the public domain: how useful are they? *Nature Genetics*, 27, 371–372.

Matsuzaki H, Loi H, Dong S, Tsai YY, Fang J, Law J, Di X, Liu WM, Yang G, Liu G, Huang J, et al. 2004. Parallel genotyping of over 10,000 SNPs using a one-primer assay on a high-density oligonucleotide array. *Genome Research*, 14, 414–425.

McPherson R, Pertsemlidis A, Kavaslar N, Stewart A, Roberts R, Cox DR, et al. 2007. A common allele on chromosome 9 associated with coronary heart disease. *Science*, 316, 1488–1491.

Mullis K, Faloona F, Scharf S, Saiki R, Horn G, Erlich H. 1986. Specific enzymatic amplification of DNA in vitro: the polymerase chain reaction. *Cold Spring Harbor Symposium Quantitative Biology*, 51, 263–273.

Packer BR, Yeager M, Burdett L, Welch R, Beerman M, QI Y, Sicotte H, Staats B, Crenshaw A, et al. 2006.

SNP500Cancer: a public resource for sequence validation, assay development and frequency analysis for genetic variation in candidate genes. *Nucleic Acids Research*, 32, D617–D621.

Paez JG, Lin M, Beroukhim R, Lee JC, Zhao X, Richter DJ, Gabriel S, Herman P, Sasaki H, Altshuler D, Li C, et al. 2004. Genome coverage and sequence fidelity of phi29 polymerase-based multiple strand displacement whole genome amplification. *Nucleic Acids Research*, 32, e71.

Parkes M, Barrett JC, Prescott NJ, Tremelling M, Anderson CA, Fisher SA, et al. (2007). Sequence variants in the autophagy gene IRGM and multiple other replicating loci contribute to Crohn's disease susceptibility. *Nature Genetics*, 39, 830–832.

Pask R, Rance HE, Barratt BJ, Nutland S, Smyth DJ, Sebastian M, Twells RC, Smith A, Lam AC, Smink LJ, Walker NM, et al. 2004. Investigating the utility of combining phi29 whole genome amplification and highly multiplexed single nucleotide polymorphism BeadArray genotyping. *BMC Biotechnology*, 4, 15.

Pastinen T, Kurg A, Metspalu A, Peltonen L, Syvanen AC. 1997. Minisequencing: a specific tool for DNA analysis and diagnostics on oligonucleotide arrays. *Genome Research*, 7, 606–614.

Pastinen T, Raitio M, Lindroos K, Tainola P, Peltonen L, Syvanen AC. 2000. A system for specific, high-throughput genotyping by allele-specific primer extension on microarrays. *Genome Research*, 10, 1031–1042.

Pritchard JK. 2001. Are rare variants responsible for susceptibility to complex diseases? *American Journal of Human Genetics*, 69, 124–137.

Redon R, Ishikawa S, Fitch KR, Feuk L, Perry GH, Andrews TD, Fiegler H, Shapero MH et al. 2006. Global variation in copy number in the human genome. *Nature*. 444, 444–454.

Reich DE, Cargill M, Bolk S, Ireland J, Sabeti PC, Richter DJ, Lavery T, Kouyoumjian R, Farhadian SF, Ward R, Lander ES. 2001. Linkage disequilibrium in the human genome. *Nature*, 411, 199–204.

Risch NJ. 2000. Searching for genetic determinants in the new millennium. *Nature*, 405, 847–856.

Risch N, Merikangas K. 1996. The future of genetic studies of complex human diseases. *Science*, 273, 1516–1517.

Sachidanadam R, Weissman D, Schmidt SC, Kakol JM, Stein LD, Marth G, Sherry S, Mullikin JC, Mortimore BJ, Willey DJ, Hunt SE, et al. 2001. A map of human genome sequence variation containing 1.42 million single nucleotide polymorphisms. *Nature*, 409, 928–933.

Salem RM, Wessel J, Schork, NJ. 2005. A comprehensive literature review of haplotyping software and methods for use with unrelated individuals. *Human Genomics*, 2, 39–66.

Saxena R, Voight BF, Lyssenko V, Burtt NP, de Bakker PI, Chen H, et al. 2007. Genome-wide association analysis identifies loci for type 2 diabetes and triglyceride levels. *Science*, 316, 1331–1336.

Scott LJ, Mohlke KL, Bonnycastle LL, Willer CJ, Li Y, Duren WL, et al. 2007. A genome-wide association study of type 2 diabetes in Finns detects multiple susceptibility variants. *Science*, 316, 1341–1345.

Schneider JA, Pungliya MS, Choi JY, Jiang R, Sun XJ, Salisbury BA, Stephens JC. 2003. DNA variability of human genes. *Mechanisms of Ageing and Development*, 124, 17–25.

Skol AD, Scott LJ, Abecasis GR, Boehnke M. 2006. Joint analysis is more efficient than replication-based analysis for two-stage genome-wide association studies. *Nature Genetics*, 38, 209–213.

Sobel E, Papp JC, Lange K. 2002. Detection and integration of genotyping errors in statistical genetics. *American Journal of Human Genetics*, 70, 496–508.

Staats B, Qi L, Beerman M, Sicotte H, Burdett LA, Packer B, Chanock SJ, Yeager M. 2005. Genewindow: an interactive tool for visualization of genomic variation. *Nature Genetics*, 37, 109–110.

Stacey SN, Manolescu A, Sulem P, Rafnar T, Gudmundsson J, Gudjonsson SA, et al. 2007. Common variants on chromosomes 2q35 and 16q12 confer susceptibility to estrogen receptor-positive breast cancer. *Nature Genetics*, 39, 865–869.

Stram DO, Haiman CA, Hirschhorn JN, Altshuler D, Kolonel LN, Henderson BE, Pike MC. 2003a. Choosing haplotype-tagging SNPs based on unphased genotype data using a preliminary sample of unrelated subjects with an example from the Multiethnic Cohort Study. *Human Heredity*, 55, 27–36.

Stram DO, Leigh Pearce C, Bretsky P, Freedman M, Hirschhorn JN, Altshuler D, Kolonel LN, Henderson BE, Thomas DC. 2003b. Modeling and E-M estimation of haplotype-specific relative risks from genotype data for a case-control study of unrelated individuals. *Human Heredity*, 55, 179–190.

Taylor JG, Choi E, Foster CB, Chanock SJ. 2001. Using genetic variation to study human disease. *Trends in Molecular Medicine*, 7, 507–512.

Tishkoff AS, Williams SA. 2002. Genetic analysis of African populations: human evolution and complex disease. *Nature Review Genetics*, 3, 611–21.

Todd JA, Walker NM, Cooper JD, Smyth DJ, Downes K, Plagnol V, et al. 2007. Robustassociations of four new chromosome regions from genome-wide analyses of type 1 diabetes. *Nature Genetics*, 39, 857–864.

Turner E, Bolton J. 2001. Required steps for the validation of a laboratory information management system. *Quality Assurance*, 9, 217–224.

Yeager M, Orr N, Hayes RB, Jacobs KB, Kraft P, Wacholder S, et al. 2007. Genome-wide association study of prostate cancer identifies a second risk locus at 8q24. *Nature Genetics*, 39, 645–649.

Zeggini E, Weedon MN, Lindgren CM, Frayling TM, Elliott KS, Lango H, et al. 2007. Replication of genome-wide association signals in UK samples reveals risk loci for type 2 diabetes. *Science*, 316, 1336–1341.

3

Mouse Models for Genetic Susceptibility to Infection in Humans

Anny Fortin, Ellen Buschman, & Emil Skamene

Over the last several years, there has been a remarkable increase in the availability of new genomic strategies for analysis of complex traits in both human populations and mouse models. The advances in genome mapping, scanning, and analysis have been particularly valuable in the field of infectious diseases, leading to the cloning of a human gene for susceptibility to leprosy (Mira et al., 2003, 2004). In the mouse, the advent of genome scanning and new genetic strains has led to the identification of resistance/susceptibility loci for a large number of viral, bacterial, and eukaryotic pathogens.

In the mammalian host, genetic control of resistance to infection (encompassing both innate and acquired immune phases) is regarded as a complex phenotype. In order to identify genes influencing host response to infection, the infectious process can be strategically divided into four stages: exposure to the pathogen, establishment of infection, progression of infection to disease, and clinical manifestation of the disease. Within these stages, the most important points of possible genetic control are likely to act during the innate and acquired phases of immunity.

The mouse, in which single gene effects may have been either naturally segregated or experimentally isolated by breeding, is the model organism of choice to dissect the genetic components controlling host response to infection. This model organism is widely used because (1) the virulence status of the infectious agent, and the dose and route of infection, can be tightly controlled, thereby reducing microbial-induced variability; (2) large numbers of wild-type isolates and mutant stocks of mice are available in an inbred status; (3) informative segregating animals can be generated in large numbers for linkage mapping and positional cloning; (4) the sequence of the mouse genome provides a compendium of candidate genes for a particular region; (5) null alleles at candidate genes can be readily obtained by gene targeting; and (6) mutant variants of the gene can be reintroduced on a null background to analyze genotype/phenotype correlations.

Although mice are often privileged at the level of gene discovery, nonmouse models are also important in the study of infectious diseases, particularly when advancing to the clinical aspects. For example, for the development of efficacious vaccines against tuberculosis, it is necessary to use animals manifesting features of human tuberculosis. The rabbit model of tuberculosis is being employed to develop and test transmission-blocking vaccines because rabbits exhibit humanlike pulmonary tubercles and aerosol spread of the disease, features not seen in the mouse (Dannenberg et al., 2000). Similarly, a primate macaque model of tuberculosis is used to study vaccine efficacy (Capuano et al., 2003). Furthermore, characterization of the biochemical mechanism of identified genes and mutations often involves nonmouse models. Many aspects of the *Nramp1* gene, such as its transport function and evolutionary importance, were revealed through studies of nonmouse models in the chicken, sheep, and cow and model organisms such as *Escherichia coli* and yeast (Vidal, Gros, et al., 1995; Gruenheid and Gros, 2000). In addition, comparative genomic sequencing in model organisms has advanced considerably the detection of novel proteins and mechanisms involved in microbial pathogenicity. Comparative genome sequencing projects of *Entamoeba* and *Plasmodium* have detected new virulence and drug resistance proteins (Loftus et al., 2005; Marti et al., 2004). The combined information from all models is necessary for an understanding of the host–pathogen interplay.

Initial Mode of Inheritance Studies in Mouse Models

An initial analysis of inbred mouse strains for an infectious phenotype show whether the trait is continuous (quantitative) or discontinuous (qualitative). Should discontinuous phenotypes of either susceptibility or resistance appear among inbred strains, a single locus with two alternative alleles may be predicted to genetically control the trait (for reviews, see Malo and Skamene, 1994; Nadeau et al., 1995). The generation of informative crosses, in which the parental genetic effects are segregating, can subsequently be used to determine the mode of inheritance involved. The chromosomal location of the controlling gene can then be established through strain distribution pattern analysis in recombinant inbred strains of mice or by linkage studies in F_2 or backcross progeny, followed by

a positional cloning approach. The following sections describe examples for which this methodology was applied to identify loci and genes controlling mouse models of mycobacterial, bacterial, viral, and parasitic infections and briefly highlight how these discoveries have affected the study of these infections in humans.

Single Genes Controlling Host Resistance to Infection

The genetic control of the *in vivo* growth of small doses of *Mycobacterium bovis* BCG was shown to segregate as a single gene effect in inbred mouse strains, and genetic analyses using this model have led to the identification of *Nramp1*, the natural resistance-associated macrophage protein (Vidal et al., 1993). This gene, located on mouse chromosome 1 (Chr.1; formerly known as the *Bcg/Ity/Lsh* locus; currently named solute carrier family 11 member 1; *Slc11a1*), controls innate mouse susceptibility to BCG, *Mycobacterium lepraemurium*, *Mycobacterium avium*, *Salmonella typhimurium*, and *Leishmania donovani* (Govoni et al., 1996; Vidal et al., 1993, 1995a) and has no effect on the acquired immune response. Sequencing of *Nramp1* cDNA from 27 inbred strains of mice identified a G169D substitution within predicted TM4 of the Nramp1 protein in all susceptible strains but in none of the resistant strains (Malo et al., 1994).

The human homologue of *Nramp1*, formerly *NRAMP1* and now designated *SLC11A1*, has been cloned and mapped to chromosome 2q35 (Cellier et al., 1994). Several polymorphisms have been described in the human gene and were used to investigate the relevance of this gene to mycobacterium susceptibility in several human populations (see chapters 13 and 22). Linkage of *SLC11A1* to tuberculosis and leprosy has been demonstrated in some of these studies but not in others (reviewed in Bellamy, 2003). Overall, the different studies reported support a role of *SLC11A1* in the control of human mycobacterial infection but suggest a small contribution of this gene and the influence of other genes on overall disease susceptibility. In the mouse model of *M. tuberculosis*, *Nramp1* does not appear to affect the outcome of infection (Medina and North 1996a, 1998). Using survival time after intravenous or aerosol infection with *M. tuberculosis*, inbred mouse strains have been classified into either highly susceptible (CBA, C3H, DBA/2J, 129Svj) or highly resistant (C57Bl/6J, BALB/c) to infection

(Medina and North, 1998). Susceptibility in DBA/2J mice is characterized by progressive bacterial replication in the lung; extended neutrophil-dominated lung pathology, including large numbers of acid-fast bacilli and areas of necrosis; and early death (Medina and North, 1996b, 1998; Mitsos et al., 2000). Since *M. tuberculosis* is not a natural pathogen of rodents, it remains unclear whether infection of laboratory mice with this infectious agent represents a good model for human tuberculosis. Nevertheless, this model was successfully used to map several loci controlling various parameters of tuberculosis severity in mice (see below).

In another example of single gene effect identified in mouse models comes from the *Lps* locus, so named for the two alleles on Chr.4 denoting defective (Lps^d) and normal (Lps^n) responses to bacterial lipopolysaccharide (endotoxin), an abundant and essential component of the outer membrane of gram-negative bacteria. It was noted that Lps^d inbred strains of mice (C3H/He/J, C57BL/10ScCr, and C57BL/10ScN) had extremely high susceptibility to gram-negative *Salmonella typhimurium*, a natural pathogen of both mice and humans (Watson and Riblet, 1974; Roy and Malo, 2002). Positional cloning in informative crosses derived from Lps^d and Lps^n strains identified *Tlr4* (Toll-like receptor 4) as the *Lps* gene, which encodes the signaling component of the lipopolysaccharide receptor (Poltorak et al., 1998; Qureshi et al., 1996, 1999). In Lps^d mice, different mutations in the *Tlr4* gene render the signaling chain unable to sense the lipopolysaccharide component of *Salmonella*, and thus mice cannot contain the growth of the bacteria. The discovery of naturally occurring *Tlr4* mutations in mice has permitted functional and genetic characterization of the Toll-like receptor (TLR) molecules. In humans, 10 different TLR genes have been cloned to date (Zarember and Godowski, 2002), and research is ongoing to identify their ligands as well as accessory molecules that may aid the recognition process. The role of TLRs in the innate immune response in human diseases has been recently reviewed in this volume (see chapter 12) and elsewhere (Abreu and Arditi, 2004).

In a model of viral infection with murine cytomegalovirus (MCMV), the Cmv1 locus on Chr.6, originally identified in 1990, was associated with resistance and susceptibility to MCMV (Scalzo et al., 1990). Subsequently, the gene underlying Cmv1 was identified through positional cloning in C57BL/6 mouse strain as the *Ly49H* gene, encoding the Ly49H receptor protein in natural killer (NK) cells (Depatie et al., 1997; Lee et al., 2001a, 2001b). The Ly49H receptor mediates clearance of MCMV infection through direct recognition of an MCMV-encoded class I homologue (m157; see Lee et al., 2003). In resistant C57BL/6, it was proposed that Ly49H might have evolved as a countermeasure against virus-encoded MHC class I homologs, providing an overriding signal to the NK cell, and promoting the elimination of MCMV-infected cells. Additional studies involving the other MCMV-resistant strain Ma/My, which lacks Ly49H, led to the identification of a second NK cell mechanism in which resistance is mediated through a functional interaction between the receptor Ly49P and the MHC class I molecule H-2D^k (Desrosiers et al., 2005). The exact nature of the interaction remains to be defined, but it is plausible that ligation of the H-2D^k molecule depends on the presence of a MCMV-specific peptide.

Although no functional Ly49 family counterpart has been identified in humans, members of the killer-cell immunoglobulin-like receptor (KIR) family have been shown to act as virus-specific activating receptors on human leukocytes in a manner similar to Ly49 in mice. Indeed, genetic epidemiological studies have identified several combinations of KIR and MHC loci associated with disease outcome, including those reported for human *KIR2DL3* and *HLA-C* protection against hepatitis C (Khakoo et al., 2004), and human allelic forms *KIR3DS1/KIR3DL1* and *HLA-Bw4* activity delaying the progression of AIDS (Martin et al., 2002, 2007; see also in this volume chapters 7, 19, and 21). Finally, NK cells in general, and the Cmv1/Ly49 gene complex in particular, may play a more general role in host innate response to infections. Indeed, Hansen and colleagues have reported that different allelic combinations at this locus/complex affect susceptibility to cerebral malaria (CM), as caused by the protozoan *Plasmodium berghei* ANKA (Hansen et al., 2003). The authors concluded on a previously unsuspected general role of NK cells or NK T-cells in innate resistance against different pathogens (Hansen et al., 2005).

In mouse *Legionella* infection, a single locus on Chr.13, *Lgn1*, was shown (Yoshida et al., 1991) to control macrophage permissiveness to intracellular replication of *L. pneumophila* (Dietrich et al., 1995; Scharf et al., 1996; Beckers et al., 1997). The *Birc1e* or *Naip* gene on Chr.13 has been targeted as the most likely candidate for *Lgn1* (Beckers et al., 1995; Diez et al.,

2003). The Naip protein was originally shown to be an apoptosis inhibitor *in vitro* and *in vivo* (Liston et al., 1996; Xu et al., 1997). However, NAIP/BIRC proteins have recently been classified in the NACHT-LRR (NLR) protein family, a group of cytoplasmic proteins involved in intracellular recognition of microbial products (Chamaillard et al., 2003; Inohara and Nunez, 2003). Proteins in the NLR family are though to recognize conserved structures shared by many pathogens, notably through their so-called LRR (leucine-rich repeat) C-terminus domain, which is also found in TLRs. From this observation, it has been suggested that the innate immune system of vertebrates might use two sets of pathogen recognition molecules, one involved in "outside-in" signaling (TLRs) and one responsible for the "inside-in" signaling (NLRs) (Girardin et al., 2002).

The nature of the signal transduced by *Naip/Birc1e* in response to *Legionella* products is still unknown, but several scenarios including stimulation of Jun kinase, activation of the inflamasome (an intracellular complex that leads to the activation of proinflammatory caspases), or triggering of programmed cell death, have been recently reviewed in Fortier et al. (2005). In mouse *Bacillus anthracis* infection, the *Ltxs1* gene on Chr.11 controls macrophage susceptibility to anthrax lethal toxin (LT) *in vitro*. Mutations within the gene *Kif1c*, a kinesin-like motor protein, was proposed to account for the phenotypic function of *Ltxs1* (Watters et al., 2001). However, the exact mechanism linking LT to *Kif1c* remains unknown. The *Kif1c* gene is one of three linked loci on Chr.11 that control susceptibility of inbred mice to mortality following intravenous injection of LT (McAllister et al., 2003).

Complex Infectious Diseases and Mapping of Relevant QTLs: Malaria and More

Quantitative traits usually have a complex genetic component resulting from the combined effects of naturally occurring allelic variations at several genes with relatively major influences of the environment. A locus controlling a quantitative trait is commonly referred to as a quantitative trait locus (QTL). The ability to perform mapping of complex traits has improved greatly in recent years with the development of powerful tools such as recombinant congenic strains, advanced intercross lines, microarrays, and high-density genome scanning techniques. In fact, several recent

studies have employed the whole-genome scanning approach in the mouse in search of quantitative trait loci influencing the susceptibility to infection, and the first QTL for a mouse infectious disease was recently cloned for resistance to malaria (Min-Oo et al., 2003).

Plasmodium chabaudi is the parasite subspecies most commonly used to study malaria in mouse models. The pathophysiology associated with blood-stage infection of mice with *P. chabaudi* has many similarities to human malaria, which makes it a useful model to study the human disease (reviewed in Fortin et al., 2002). In fact, many of the blood-stage antigens expressed by *P. chabaudi* are similar to those of *P. falciparum*, and blood-stage parasites usually replicate in mature red cells, although reticulocytes can also be infected. Anemia is very severe, progresses rapidly, and is associated with postcrisis hyperreticulocytosis, erythrophagocytosis of infected and normal red cells, and enlarged spleens and liver. Renal damage is similar to that observed in humans and severe hypoglycemia may be observed. Infection of mice with *P. chabaudi* does not cause CM. However, a mouse model for CM has been developed using *P. berghei* ANKA as the infectious agent (Bagot et al., 2002; Nagayasu et al., 2002).

A whole-genome scan conducted in backcross and F_2 progeny derived from susceptible A/J and resistant C57BL/6J inbred strains identified a major locus on central Chr.8 controlling *P. chabaudi chabaudi* replication after intraperitoneal infection (Fortin et al., 1997). Independently, Foote et al. (1997) conducted similar linkage studies in (SJLXB6)F_2 and in (C3HXB6)F_2 female mice using an intravenous infection model with *P. chabaudi adami*. Two loci, termed *Char* (for *chabaudi resistance*), one on central Chr.8 (*Char2*) and the other on distal Chr.9 (*Char1*), were mapped and associated with parasite replication and/or survival to infection. Subsequently, linkage with the MHC locus (H-2) on Chr.17 was noted on the day following the peak of parasitemia in *P. chabaudi adami*–infected (C3HXB6)F_2 female animals (*Char3*; Burt et al., 1999). The *Char1* locus on Chr.9 was also associated to the control of blood parasitemia five days after infection with *P. yoelii* in a whole-genome scan using an informative backcross derived from susceptible NC/Jic and resistant 129/Sv parents (Ohno et al., 2001). Finally, linkage studies in F_2 mice derived from B6 and DBA/2 strains, respectively susceptible and resistant to experimental severe malaria induced by *P. berghei* ANKA, have mapped a major gene effect on the central portion of Chr.18, but additional suggestive linkage was also noted in the *Char2* region on Chr.8 (Nagayasu et al., 2002). Taken together, these studies demonstrated the importance of the *Char1* and *Char2* loci for regulation of blood stage parasite replication and survival from infection. These QTLs are of particular interest since they have been detected in different mouse strain combinations and using distinct species of *Plasmodium* parasites.

More examples of QTL mapping in mouse models of infections have been demonstrated in several recent genome scans studying various parameters of tuberculosis severity (Lavebratt et al., 1999; Mitsos et al., 2000, 2003; Kramnik et al., 2000). These analyses, conducted on mice of different genetic backgrounds, have identified several significant linkages, on chromosomes 1, 3, 5, 7, 9, 10, and 19. Interestingly, the location of the Chr.9 QTL, which influenced *M. tuberculosis*–triggered cachexia, exactly overlapped a QTL found in cutaneous leishmaniasis using lesion size as phenotype (Lavebratt et al., 1999; Roberts et al., 1997). The Chr.19 QTL (*Trl-4*) is also interesting because it seems to specifically regulate replication of *M. tuberculosis* in the lung after aerosol infection with small numbers of the pathogen (Mitsos et al., 2003). More important are the recent studies on the Chr.1 QTL (named *sst1*; Kramnik et al., 2000), for which a congenic mouse carrying the C57BL/6J-derived resistant *sst1* locus on the C3HeB/FeJ susceptible genetic background was used to refine the genetic interval. Using positional cloning and expression analysis of all the genes present in the interval, one isoform of the *Ifi75* gene, renamed *Ipr1* (intracellular pathogen resistance 1), was identified as underlying *sst1* (Pan et al., 2005). *Ipr1* is expressed in macrophages and the host cells in which *M. tuberculosis* replicates and appears to determine the type of death that macrophages will suffer following infection. Transgenic mice expressing full-length *Ipr1* cDNA on the susceptible C3HeB/FeJ background were shown to have an increased resistance to *M. tuberculosis in vivo*, and macrophages derived from these mice also showed strong resistance to *Listeria monocytogenes* infection *in vitro*, suggesting a general role for *Ipr1* in innate macrophage defenses against intracellular infections. In both cases, the resistance mechanism was linked to the fact that *Ipr1*-expressing macrophages control parasite multiplication by undergoing apoptosis (programmed cell death) rather than necrosis.

The closest homologue of the predicted Ipr1 protein in humans is SP110b, which localizes to a region of human Chr.2. Because polymorphisms in *SP110* have been associated with susceptibility to hepatitis C virus (Saito et al., 2004), this gene represented an attractive candidate for testing association with susceptibility to tuberculosis in human populations. Of four studies already reported (Tosh et al., 2006; Thye et al., 2006; Szeszko et al., 2007; Babb et al., 2007), only one detected an association of *SP110* with TB susceptibility (Tosh et al., 2006). Additional validation is needed to confirm a role of *SP110* in human susceptibility to tuberculosis. In cutaneous leishmaniasis, two independent studies have localized QTLs for a total of eight different chromosomal regions (Beebe et al., 1997; Roberts et al., 1997). In one study, parasites were injected into the footpad and footpad swelling was used as phenotype leading to the identification of six QTL linkages (Beebe et al., 1997). In the other study, parasites were injected intradermally and the size of the developing cutaneous lesion was used as phenotype leading to the localization of two QTLs (Roberts et al., 1997). Interestingly, there was no overlap in chromosomal regions identified in both studies, clearly demonstrating the importance of the phenotype for genetic analysis. The QTL approach has also been used to detect multiple gene control of variation in susceptibility to trypanosomiasis (Kemp et al., 1997) and toxoplasmosis (Johnson et al., 2002), as well as infection with the gastrointestinal nematode *Heligmosomoides polygyrus* (Menge et al., 2003).

Genes mapped in one species can be tested for their identity as QTL in another species. This strategy was used for the identification of *Tlr4* and *Nramp1* as QTL susceptibility genes for salmonellosis in chicken, genes that were originally identified in mice (Hu et al., 1997; Georges, 1997). In addition, QTLs identified in animal models can be used to directly determine whether the corresponding syntenic chromosomal regions in humans are associated with susceptibility to infection in different populations and in different areas of endemic disease worldwide.

Genetic Dissection of Infections with Newly Available Genetic Tools

The so-called recombinant congenic strains (RCS) strategy was pioneered by Demant and Hart (1986). The RCS are produced by limited backcrossing between two inbred strains and subsequent inbreeding by brother–sister mating. In this way, a series of strains is created, each of which carries a small fraction of the genome of one strain (donor strain) on the genetic background of a second strain (background strain). In RCS, unlinked genes contributing to a complex trait become separated and fixed in unique haplotype combinations in different strains and thus can be studied individually. Such genetic effects may be readily identified by examination of the strain distribution pattern of the RCS set for the phenotype of interest and can be further mapped by linkage analysis in F_2 crosses involving a specific RCS of interest (Demant and Hart, 1986).

Since an individual RCS may contain only one gene influencing a trait of interest, such strains can be used to breed recombinants in the region of interest and to further fine-map a given genetic interval. This approach was recently used in the 37-strain RCS panel constructed from A/J and C57Bl/6J mice (called the AcB/BcA RCS set) to clone the malaria susceptibility QTL on mouse Chr.3, termed *Char4* (Fortin et al., 2001a, 2001b). Characterization of this informative strain revealed that its resistance to malaria was associated with constitutive reticulocytosis and splenomegaly. As opposed to malaria resistance, the trait of constitutive reticulocytosis was shown to segregate as a monogenic trait. Genetic mapping using reticulocytosis as phenotypic marker showed that the *Char4* locus was also controlling this trait and allowed the positioning of the underlying gene more precisely. Subsequently, microarray analysis and sequencing of candidate genes identified a loss-of-function mutation in the pyruvate kinase gene (*Pklr*), which was specific to the informative strain. The *Pklr* mutation was shown to control the phenotype of constitutive reticulocytosis in a bimodal fashion while influencing the outcome of malaria infection in a more complex manner (Min-Oo et al., 2003). In humans, pyruvate kinase deficiency is the most common cause of hereditary nonspherocytic hemolytic anemia. A candidate approach can now test whether the high prevalence of this enzymatic deficiency was driven by natural selection against malaria infection.

Another series of RCS derived from BALB/c and STS/A mice was used to dissect the multigenic control of susceptibility to infection with *Leishmania major* (Lipoldova et al., 2000). In that study, different functional and pathological parameters of *L. major* infection were analyzed, and five QTL were mapped and linked with distinct phenotypes of host response. Another type of RCS panel, called interval-specific RCS

(IRCS), is selectively bred to carry various segments of specific chromosomes. An IRCS panel derived from DBA and BALB/c mice was recently used to map three QTL on Chr.11 controlling susceptibility *in vivo* to anthrax LT (McAllister et al., 2003).

Advanced intercross lines of mice are generated by producing an F_{11} generation between intercrossed nonsibling strains (Darvasi and Soller, 1995). This breeding scheme increases the likelihood of recombination between tightly linked genes. Such lines were recently used in *P. chabaudi* malaria to identify two QTLs (*Char5* and *Char6*) located on Chr.5, and controlling parasitemia in the A/J and C57Bl/6J strain combination (Hernandez-Valladares et al., 2004). The availability of chromosome substitution strains (CSS) derived from A/J and C57Bl/6J strains has been recently reported (Singer et al., 2004). These 22 CSS strains each carry a single chromosome from one strain on the genetic background of the other and may be useful in detecting more QTLs than can be found with other breeding panels.

Analysis of Gene Function in Mice

The ultimate aim of genetic studies of infectious diseases is the identification of molecular variants that modulate risk of infectious disease. In the mouse, the final proof of the identity of candidate genes can be established using transgenic animals expressing different forms of specific gene variants and by functional assays. Biological evidence should be consistent with the hypothesis that expression of allelic gene products can influence the underlying pathology of susceptibility.

Genetically engineered strains of mice are the major tool used to demonstrate directly the role of cloned genes. The *Nramp1* gene is such an example; through the use of transgenic animals, it was proven that a single G169D amino acid substitution caused susceptibility of certain inbred strains of mice to a large number of intracellular macrophage parasites (Govoni et al., 1996; Vidal et al., 1993, 1995b). The Nramp1 protein is a transmembrane protein that is expressed in the phagosomes of mature macrophages of resistant mice; susceptible mice do not express the Nramp1 protein (Vidal et al., 1996). It has been shown that Nramp1 can prevent phagosome acidification, possibly through depletion of the phagosome of divalent cations such as Fe; both functions are known to be required for microbial survival (Gruenheid et al., 1999; Hackam et al., 1998).

Recently, the availability of high-density oligonucleotide arrays for profiling of gene expression combined with QTL analysis in RCS has been explored as an approach to search for candidate susceptibility genes (Min-Oo et al., 2003). The strategy is to search for candidate susceptibility QTL according to both their location in the genome, as well as a tissue expression pattern consistent with expression of the studied phenotype. In the identification of the gene underlying the *Char4* locus, gene expression changes in spleen tissue were compared between informative RCS and the susceptible parental strain A/J (Min-Oo et al., 2003). This approach targeted differentially expressed genes specific to the informative RCS and was used to identify biochemical pathways and cell types underlying the presence of splenomegaly. It is likely that the RCS-microarray approach will be used frequently in the cloning of QTL.

An important consideration posed by the use of inbred strains of mice for genetic analysis is the low level of genetic variability in laboratory mice compared to that of human populations, limiting the number of genetic variants/mutations found in mice that may be relevant to humans. To circumvent this possible problem, wild mice, which have been subjected to different selective pressures compared to laboratory mice, can be used. Studies have used wild mice compared to laboratory mice to study resistance to worm infections (Derothe et al., 1997) and to murine leukemia viruses (Lyu and Kozak, 1996). In addition, the gene underlying resistance to West Nile virus infection, *flv1/Wnv*, was identified as being *Oasl1* using wild-derived mouse stocks (Mashimo et al., 2002). More than 146 new genetic loci have been mapped in wild-derived strains, thus providing an improved method of genome scanning for genetic loci (Elango et al., 1996).

Another important aspect is that the function of genes with major effects should be studied in the context of different genetic backgrounds (Erickson, 1996) to simulate the heterogeneity observed in human populations. Among the first models to study the effect of modifier genes was the creation of CFTR (Cystic fibrosis transmembrane conductance regulator) -deficient mice on different inbred backgrounds (Rozmahel et al., 1996). The results showed the existence of modifier genes that clearly changed the disease severity of the cystic fibrosis phenotype. Consequently, the role of genetic background is now considered an important factor in infectious models; for example, gene knockouts of interleukin-12 and nitric oxide synthase 2 have been bred onto different genetic backgrounds in the study of susceptibility to *M. tuberculosis* (Cooper et al., 1997; MacMicking et al., 1997). In addition, the use of double gene knockout mice strains is now established (Tourne et al., 1997; Weih et al., 1997). In a recent study, a loss-of-function mutation in *Icsbp/IRF8* (interferon consensus sequence-binding protein/interferon regulatory factor 8, $IRF8^{C294}$) encoding a transcription factor known to activate interferon-γ responsive genes (Tamura and Ozato, 2002), was shown to cause splenomegaly and myeloproliferation in the recombinant inbred strain BXH-2 (Turcotte et al., 2005). Interestingly, BXH-2 mice show increased susceptibility to infection with *M. bovis* BCG despite the presence of a "resistant" version of Nramp1 (G169). In this case, homozygosity at the mutant allele of IRF8 was shown to modify the level of resistance to mycobacterial infection conveyed by Nramp1, and this independently of their allelic combinations at *Nramp1*. It was concluded that IRF8 behaves as a true "genetic modifier" of the type of innate immunity imparted by *Nramp1*. This could take place through direct transcriptional regulation of Nramp1 expression (IRF8 binding sites have been found there) or through some indirect secondary mechanism. It will be interesting to analyze the effects of IRF8 loss-of-function on host defenses against other types of intracellular pathogens.

Finally, mouse strains carrying natural mutations, targeted gene knockouts, or transgenes are also used to investigate possible involvement of known immune pathways in response to infection by a given pathogen. The list of mouse strains mutated for key innate and adaptive immunity-related molecules is extensive and may be found on the Jackson Laboratories Web site (www.jax.org). These include cytokine-knockout mice (interferon-γ, interleukin-12), mice with gene deletions affecting innate immunity (TLR) and mice bearing natural mutations that affect lymphocyte function including SCID (severe combined immunodeficient) mice, beige mice, and nude mice. Such mutants, including nude mice, SCID mice, CD4$^+$ T-cell–depleted mice, and numerous cytokine knockout mice, have been used to investigate the effects of many mutations on susceptibility to mouse malaria (reviewed in Fortin et al. 2002; Ing et al., 2005).

Conclusion

Mouse models continue to provide important insight into the genetics of infectious diseases. Identification of genes in mouse models of infection may identify new defense mechanisms that could be directly targeted for therapeutic intervention in humans or can provide a conceptual framework to better comprehend infection processes, including entry points into cell biology, infectious pathogenesis, and molecular and cellular immunology.

References

Abreu, M.T., and Arditi, M. (2004) Innate immunity and toll-like receptors: clinical implications of basic science research. *J Pediatr.* **144**, 421–429.

Babb, C., Keet, E.H., van Helden, P.D., Hoal, E.G. (2007) SP110 polymorphisms are not associated with pulmonary tuberculosis in a South African population. *Hum Genet.* **121**, 521–522.

Bagot, S., Campino, S., Penha-Goncalves, C., Pied, S., Cazenave, P.A., and Holmberg, D. (2002) Identification of two cerebral malaria resistance loci using an inbred wild-derived mouse strain. *Proc Natl Acad Sci U S A.* **99**, 9919–9923.

Beckers, M.C., Ernst, E., Diez, E., Morissette, C., Gervais, F., Hunter, K., Housman, D., Yoshida, S., Skamene, E., and Gros, P. (1997) High-resolution linkage map of mouse chromosome 13 in the vicinity of the host resistance locus Lgn1. *Genomics.* **39**, 254–263.

Beckers, M.C., Yoshida, S.-I., Morgan, K., Skamene, E., and Gros, P. (1995) Natural resistance to infection with *Legionella pneumophila*: chromosomal localization of the *Lgn1* susceptibility gene. *Mamm Genome.* **6**, 540–545.

Beebe, A.M., Mauze, S., Schork, N.J., and Coffman, R.L. (1997) Serial backcross mapping of multiple loci associated with resistance to *Leishmania major* in mice. *Immunity.* **6**, 551–557.

Bellamy, R. (2003) Susceptibility to mycobacterial infections: the importance of host genetics. *Genes Immun.* **4**, 4–11.

Burt, R.A., Baldwin, T.M., Marshall, V.M., and Foote, S.J. (1999) Temporal expression of an H2-linked locus in host response to mouse malaria. *Immunogenetics.* **50**, 278–285.

Capuano, S.V., Croix, D.A., Pawar, S., Zinovik, A., Myers, A., Lin, P.L., Bissel, S., Fuhrman, C., Klein, E., and Flynn, J.L. (2003) Experimental *Myco-bacterium tuberculosis* infection of cynomolgus macaques closely resembles the various manifestations of human *M. tuberculosis* infection. *Infect Immun.* **71**, 5831–5844.

Cellier, M., Govoni, G., Vidal, S., Kwan, T., Groulx, N., Liu, J., Sanchez, F., Skamene, E., Schurr, E., and Gros, P. (1994) Human natural resistance-associated macrophage protein: cDNA cloning, chromosomal mapping, genomic organization, and tissue-specific expression. *J Exp Med.* **180**, 1741–1752.

Chamaillard, M., Girardin, S.E., Viala, J., and Philpott, D.J. (2003) Nods, Nalps and Naip: intracellular regulators of bacterial-induced inflammation. *Cell Microbiol.* **5**, 581–592.

Cooper, A.M., Magram, J., Ferrante, J., and Orme, I.M. (1997) Interleukin 12 (IL-12) is crucial to the development of protective immunity in mice intravenously infected with mycobacterium tuberculosis. *J Exp Med.* **186**, 39–45.

Dannenberg, A.M., Bishai, W.R., Parrish, N., Ruiz, R., Johnson, W., Zook, B.C., Boles, J.W., and Pitt, L.M. (2000) Efficacies of BCG and vole bacillus (*Mycobacterium microti*) vaccines in preventing clinically apparent pulmonary tuberculosis in rabbits: a preliminary report. *Vaccine.* **19**, 796–800.

Darvasi, A., and Soller, M. (1995) Advanced intercross lines, an experimental population for fine genetic mapping. *Genetics.* **141**, 1199–1207.

Demant, P., and Hart, A.A. (1986) Recombinant congenic strains—a new tool for analyzing genetic traits determined by more than one gene. *Immunogenetics.* **24**, 416–422.

Desrosiers, M.P., Kielczewska, A., Loredo-Osti, J.C., Adam, S.G., Makrigiannis, A.P., Lemieux, S., Pham, T., Lodoen, M.B., Morgan, K., Lanier, L.L., and Vidal, S.M. (2005) Epistasis between mouse Klra and major histocompatibility complex class I loci is associated with a new mechanism of natural killer cell-mediated innate resistance to cytomegalovirus infection. *Nat Genet.* **37**, 593–599.

Depatie, C., Muise, E., Lepage. P., Gros, P., and Vidal, S.M. (1997) High-resolution linkage map in the proximity of the host resistance locus Cmv1. *Genomics.* **39**, 154–163.

Derothe, J.M., Loubes, C., Orth, A., Renaud, F., and Moulia, C. (1997) Comparison between patterns of pinworm infection (*Aspiculuris tetraptera*) in wild and laboratory strains of mice, *Mus musculus*. *Int J Parasitol.* **27**, 645–651.

Dietrich, W.F., Damron, D.M., Isberg, R.R., Lander, E.S., and Swanson, M.S. (1995) *Lgn1*, a gene that determines susceptibility to *Legionella pneumophila*, maps to mouse chromosome 13. *Genomics.* **26**, 443–450.

Diez, E., Lee, S.H., Gauthier, S., Yaraghi, Z., Tremblay, M., Vidal, S., and Gros, P. (2003) *Birc1e* is the gene within the Lgn1 locus associated with resistance to *Legionella pneumophila. Nat Genet.* **33**, 55–60.

Elango, R., Riba, L., Housman, D., and Hunter, K. (1996) Generation and mapping of *Mus spretus* strain-specific markers for rapid genomic scanning. *Mamm. Genome.* **7**, 340–343.

Erickson, R.P. (1996) Mouse models of human genetic disease: which mouse is more like a man? *BioEssays.* **18**, 993–998.

Foote, S.J., Burt, R.A., Baldwin, T.M., Presente, A., Roberts, A.W., Laural, Y.L., Lew, A.M., and Marshall, V.M. (1997) Mouse loci for malaria-induced mortality and the control of parasitaemia. *Nat Genet.* **17**, 380–381.

Fortier, A., Diez, E., and Gros, P. (2005) Naip5/Birc1e and susceptibility to *Legionella pneumophila. Trends Microbiol.* **13**, 328–335.

Fortin, A., Belouchi, A., Tam, M.F., Cardon, L., Skamene, E., Stevenson, M.M., and Gros, P. (1997) Genetic control of blood parasitaemia in mouse malaria maps to chromosome 8. *Nat Genet.* **17**, 382–383.

Fortin, A., Cardon, L.R., Tam, M., Skamene, E., Stevenson, M.M., and Gros, P. (2001a) Identification of a new malaria susceptibility locus (Char4) in recombinant congenic strains of mice. *Proc Natl Acad Sci USA.* **98**, 10793–10798.

Fortin, A., Diez, E., Rochefort, D., Laroche, L., Malo, D., Rouleau, G.A., Gros, P., and Skamene, E. (2001b) Recombinant congenic strains derived from A/J and C57BL/6J: a tool for genetic dissection of complex traits. *Genomics.* **74**, 21–35.

Fortin, A., Stevenson, M.M., and Gros, P. (2002) Susceptibility to malaria as a complex trait: big pressure from a tiny creature. *Hum Mol Genet.* **11**, 2469–2478.

Georges, M. (1997) QTL mapping to QTL cloning: mice to the rescue. *Genome Res.* **7**, 665–667.

Girardin, S.E., Sansonetti, P.J., and Philpott, D.J. (2002) Intracellular vs extracellular recognition of pathogens—common concepts in mammals and flies. *Trends Microbiol.* **10**, 193–199.

Govoni, G., Vidal, S., Gauthier, S., Skamene, E., Malo, D., and Gros, P. (1996) The Bcg/Ity/Lsh locus: genetic transfer of resistance to infections in C57BL/6J mice transgenic for the *Nramp1 Gly169* allele. *Infect Immun.* **64**, 2923–2929.

Gruenheid, S., Canonne-Hergaux, F., Gauthier, S., Hackam, D.J., Grinstein, S., and Gros, P. (1999) The iron transport protein NRAMP2 is an integral membrane glycoprotein that colocalizes with transferrin in recycling endosomes. *J Exp Med.* **189**, 831–841.

Gruenheid, S., and Gros, P. (2000) Genetic susceptibility to intracellular infections: Nramp1, macrophage function and divalent cations transport. *Curr Opin Microbiol.* **3**, 43–48.

Hackam, D.J., Rotstein, O.D., Zhang, W., Gruenheid, S., Gros, P., and Grinstein, S. (1998) Host resistance to intracellular infection: mutation of natural resistance-associated macrophage protein 1 (Nramp1) impairs phagosomal acidification. *J Exp Med.* **188**, 351–364.

Hansen, D.S., Evans, K.J., D'Ombrain, M.C., Bernard, N.J., Sexton, A.C., Buckingham, L., Scalzo, A.A., and Schofield, L. (2005) The natural killer complex regulates severe malarial pathogenesis and influences acquired immune responses to *Plasmodium berghei* ANKA. *Infect Immun.* **73**, 2288–2297.

Hansen, D.S., Siomos, M.A., Buckingham, L., Scalzo, A.A., and Schofield, L. (2003) Regulation of murine cerebral malaria pathogenesis by CD1d-restricted NKT cells and the natural killer complex. *Immunity.* **18**, 391–402.

Hernandez-Valladares, M., Naessens, J., Gibson, J.P., Musoke, A.J., Nagda, S., Rihet, P., Ole-MoiYoi, O.K., and Iraqi, F.A. (2004) Confirmation and dissection of QTL controlling resistance to malaria in mice. *Mamm Genome.* **15**, 390–398.

Hu, J., Bumstead, N., Barrow, P., Sebastiani, G., Olien, L., Morgan, K., and Malo, D. (1997) Resistance to salmonellosis in the chicken is linked to NRAMP1 and TNC. *Genome Res.* **7**, 693–705.

Ing, R., Gros, P., and Stevenson, M.M. (2005) Interleukin-15 enhances innate and adaptive immune responses to blood-stage malaria infection in mice. *Infect Immun.* **73**, 3172–3177.

Inohara, N., and Nunez, G. (2003) NODs: intracellular proteins involved in inflammation and apoptosis. *Nat Rev Immunol.* **3**, 371–382.

Johnson, J., Suzuki, Y., Mack, D., Mui, E., Estes, R., David, C., Skamene, E., Forman, J., and McLeod, R. (2002) Genetic analysis of influences on survival following *Toxoplasma gondii* infection. *Int J Parasitol.* **32**, 179–185.

Kemp, S.J., Iraqi, F., Darvasi, A., Soller, M., and Teale, A.J. (1997) Localization of genes controlling resistance to trypanosomiasis in mice. *Nat Genet.* **16**, 194–196.

Khakoo, S.I., Thio, C.L., Martin, M.P., Brooks, C.R., Gao, X., Astemborski, J., Cheng, J., Goedert, J.J., Vlahov, D., Hilgartner, M., Cox, S., Little, A.M., Alexander, G.J., Cramp, M.E., O'Brien, S.J., Rosenberg, W.M., Thomas, D.L., and Carrington, M. (2004) HLA and NK cell inhibitory receptor genes in resolving hepatitis C virus infection. *Science.* **305**, 872–874.

Kramnik, I., Dietrich, W.F., Demant, P., and Bloom, B.R. (2000) Genetic control of resistance to experimental infection with virulent *Mycobacterium tuberculosis*. *Proc Natl Acad Sci USA*. **97**, 8560–8565.

Lavebratt, C., Apt, A., Nikonenko, B.V., Schalling, M., and Schurr, E. (1999) Severity of tuberculosis in mice is linked to distal chromosome 3 and proximal chromosome 9. *J Infect Dis*. **180**, 150–155.

Lee, S.H., Dimock, K., Gray, D.A., Beauchemin, N., Holmes, K.V., Belouchi, M., Realson, J., and Vidal, S.M. (2003) Maneuvering for advantage: the genetics of mouse susceptibility to virus infection. *Trends Genet*. **19**, 447–457.

Lee, S.H., Girard S., Macina, D., Busa, M., Zafer, A., Belouchi, A., Gros, P., and Vidal, S.M. (2001a) Susceptibility to mouse cytomegalovirus is associated with deletion of an activating natural killer cell receptor of the C-type lectin superfamily. *Nature Genet*. **28**, 42–45.

Lee, S.H., Gitas, J., Zafer, A., Lepage, P., Hudson, T.J., Belouchi, A., and Vidal, S.M. (2001b) Haplotype mapping indicates two independent origins for the Cmv1s susceptibility allele to cytomegalovirus infection and refines its localization within the Ly49 cluster. *Immunogenetics*. **53**, 501–505.

Lipoldova, M., Svobodova, M., Krulova, M., Havelkova, H., Badalova, J., Nohynkova, E., Holan, V., Hart, A.A., Volf, P., and Demant, P. (2000) Susceptibility to *Leishmania major* infection in mice: multiple loci and heterogeneity of immunopathological phenotypes. *Genes Immun*. **1**, 200–206.

Liston, P., Roy, N., Tamai, K., Lefebvre, C., Baird, S., Cherton-Horvat, G., Farahani, R., McLean, M., Ikeda, J.E., MacKenzie, A., and Korneluk, R.G. (1996) Suppression of apoptosis in mammalian cells by NAIP and a related family of IAP genes. *Nature*. **379**, 349–353.

Loftus, B., Anderson, I., Davies, R., Alsmark, U.C., Samuelson, J., Amedeo, P., Roncaglia, P., Berriman, M., Hirt, R.P., Mann, B.J., et al. (2005) The genome of the protist parasite Entamoeba histolytica. *Nature*. **433**, 865–868.

Lyu, M.S., and Kozak, C.A. (1996) Genetic basis for resistance to polytropic murine leukemia viruses in the wild mouse species *Mus castaneus*. *J Virol*. **70**, 830–833.

MacMicking, J.D., North, R.J., LaCourse, R., Mudgett, J.S., Shah, S.K., and Nathan, C.F. (1997) Identification of nitric oxide synthase as a protective locus against tuberculosis. *Proc Natl Acad Sci USA*. **94**, 5243–5248.

Malo, D., and Skamene, E. (1994) Genetic control of host resistance to infection. *Trends Genet*. **10**, 365–371.

Malo, D., Vogan, K., Vidal, S., Hu, J., Cellier, M., Schurr, E., Fuks, A., Bumstead, N., Morgan, K., and Gros, P. (1994) Haplotype mapping and sequence analysis of the mouse Nramp gene predict susceptibility to infection with intracellular parasites. *Genomics*. **23**, 51–61.

Marti, M., Good, R.T., Rug, M., Knuepfer, E., and Cowman, A.F. (2004) Targeting malaria virulence and remodeling proteins to the host erythrocyte. *Science*. **306**, 1930–1933.

Martin, M.P., Gao, X., Lee, J.H., Nelson, G.W., Detels, R., Goedert, J.J., Buchbinder, S., Hoots, K., Vlahov, D., Trowsdale, J., Wilson, M., O'Brien, S.J., and Carrington, M. (2002) Epistatic interaction between KIR3DS1 and HLA-B delays the progression to AIDS. *Nat Genet*. **31**, 429–434.

Martin M.P., Qi, Y., Gao, X., Yamada, E., Martin, J.N., Pereyra, F., Colombo, S., Brown, E.E., Shupert, W.L., Phair, J., Goedert, J.J., Buchbinder, S., Kirk, G.D., Telenti, A., Connors, M., O'Brien, S.J., Walker, B.D., Parham, P., Deeks, S.G., McVicar, D.W., and Carrington, M. (2007) Innate partnership of HLA-B and KIR3DL1 subtypes against HIV-1. *Nat Genet*. **39**, 733–40.

Mashimo, T., Lucas, M., Simon-Chazottes, D., Frenkiel, M.P., Montagutelli, X., Ceccaldi, P.E., Deubel, V., Guenet, J.L., and Despres, P. (2002) A nonsense mutation in the gene encoding 2″-5″-oligoadenylate synthetase/L1 isoform is associated with West Nile virus susceptibility in laboratory mice. *Proc Natl Acad Sci USA*. **99**, 11311–11316.

McAllister, R.D., Singh, Y., du Bois, W.D., Potter, M., Boehm, T., Meeker, N.D., Fillmore, P.D., Anderson, L.M., Poynter, M.E., and Teuscher, C. (2003) Susceptibility to anthrax lethal toxin is controlled by three linked quantitative trait loci. *Am J Pathol*. **163**, 1735–1741.

Medina, E., and North, R.J. (1996a) The Bcg gene (Nramp1) does not determine resistance of mice to virulent *Mycobacterium tuberculosis*. *Ann NY Acad Sci*. **797**, 257–259.

Medina, E., and North, R.J. (1996b) Evidence inconsistent with a role for the Bcg gene (Nramp1) in resistance of mice to infection with virulent *Mycobacterium tuberculosis*. *J Exp Med*. **183**, 1045–1051.

Medina, E., and North, R.J. (1998) Resistance ranking of some common inbred mouse strains to *Mycobacterium tuberculosis* and relationship to major histocompatibility complex haplotype and Nramp1 genotype. *Immunology*. **93**, 270–274.

Menge, D.M., Behnke, J.M., Lowe, A., Gibson, J.P., Iraqi, F.A., Baker, R.L., and Wakelin, D. (2003) Mapping of chromosomal regions influencing immunological responses to gastrointestinal nematode infections in mice. *Parasite Immunol.* **25**, 341–349.

Min-Oo, G., Fortin, A., Tam, M.F., Nantel, A., Stevenson, M.M., and Gros, P. (2003) Pyruvate kinase deficiency in mice protects against malaria. *Nat Genet.* **35**, 357–362.

Mira, M.T., Alcais, A., Van Thuc, N., Thai, V.H., Huong, N.T., Ba, N.N., Verner, A., Hudson, T.J., Abel, L., and Schurr, E. (2003) Chromosome 6q25 is linked to susceptibility to leprosy in a Vietnamese population. *Nat Genet.* **33**, 412–415.

Mira, M.T., Alcais, A., Nguyen, V.T., Moraes, M.O., Di Flumeri, C., Vu, H.T., Mai, C.P., Nguyen, T.H., Nguyen, N.B., Pham, X.K., Sarno, E.N., Alter, A., Montpetit, A., Moraes, M.E., Moraes, J.R., Dore, C., et al. (2004) Susceptibility to leprosy is associated with PARK2 and PACRG. *Nature.* **427**, 636–640.

Mitsos, L.M., Cardon, L.R., Fortin, A., Ryan, L., LaCourse, R., North, R.J., and Gros, P. (2000) Genetic control of susceptibility to infection with *Mycobacterium tuberculosis* in mice. *Genes Immun.* **1**, 467–477.

Mitsos, L.M., Cardon, L.R., Ryan, L., LaCourse, R., North, R.J., and Gros, P. (2003) Susceptibility to tuberculosis: a locus on mouse chromosome 19 (*Trl4*) regulates *Mycobacterium tuberculosis* replication in the lungs. *Proc Natl Acad Sci USA.* **100**, 6610–6615.

Nadeau, J.H., Arbuckle, L.D., and Skamene, E. (1995) Genetic dissection of inflammatory diseases. *J Inflamm.* **45**, 27–48.

Nagayasu, E., Nagakura, K., Akaki, M., Tamiya, G., Makino, S., Nakano, Y., Kimura, M., and Aikawa, M. (2002) Association of a determinant on mouse chromosome 18 with experimental severe *Plasmodium berghei* malaria. *Infect Immun.* **70**, 512–516.

Ohno, T., Ishih, A., Kohara, Y., Yonekawa, H., Terada, M., and Nishimura, M. (2001) Chromosomal mapping of the host resistance locus to rodent malaria (*Plasmodium yoelii*) infection in mice. *Immunogenetics.* **53**, 736–740.

Pan, H., Yan, B.S., Rojas, M., Shebzukhov, Y.V., Zhou, H., Kobzik, L., Higgins, D.E., Daly, M.J., Bloom, B.R., and Kramnik, I. (2005) Ipr1 gene mediates innate immunity to tuberculosis. *Nature.* **434**, 767–772.

Poltorak, A, He, X., Smirnova, I., Liu, M.Y., Huffel, C.V., Du, X., Birdwell, D., Alejos, E., Silva, M., Galanos, C., Freudenberg, M., Ricciardi-Castagnoli, P., Layton, B., and Beutler, B. (1998) Defective LPS signaling in C3 H/HeJ and C57BL/10ScCr mice: mutations in *Tlr4* gene. *Science.* 282, 2085–2088.

Qureshi, S.T., Lariviere, L., Leveque, G., Clermont, S., Moore, K.J., Gros, P., and Malo, D. (1999) Endotoxin-tolerant mice have mutations in Toll-like receptor 4 (*Tlr4*). *J Exp Med.* 189, 615–625

Qureshi, S.T., Larivière, L., Sebastiani, G., Clermont, S., Skamene, E., Gros, P., and Malo, D. (1996) A high-resolution map in the chromosomal region surrounding the *Lps* locus. *Genomics.* **31**, 283–294.

Roberts, L.J., Baldwin, T.M., Curtis, J.M., Handman, E., and Foote, S.J. (1997) Resistance to *Leishmania major* is linked to the H2 region on chromosome 17 and to chromosome 9. *J Exp Med.* **185**, 1705–1710.

Roy, M.F., and Malo, D. (2002) Regulation of host responses to *Salmonella* infection in mice. *Genes Immun.* **3**, 381–393.

Rozmahel, R., Wilschanski, M., Matin, A., Plyte, S., Oliver, M., Auerbach, W., Moore, A., Forstner, J., Durie, P., Nadeau, J., Bear, C., and Tsui, L.-C. (1996) Modulation of disease severity in cystic fibrosis transmembrane conductance regulator deficient mice by a secondary genetic factor. *Nat Genet.* **12**, 280–287.

Saito, T., Ji, G., Shinzawa, H., Okumoto, K., Hattori, E., Adachi, T., Takeda, T., Sugahara, K., Ito, J.I., Watanabe, H., Saito, K., Togashi, H., Ishii, K., Matsuura, T., Inageda, K., Muramatsu, M., and Kawata, S. (2004) Genetic variations in humans associated with differences in the course of hepatitis C. *Biochem Biophys Res Commun.* **317**, 335–341.

Scalzo, A.A., Fitzgerald, N.A., Simmons, A., La Vista, A.B., and Shellam, G.R. (1990) Cmv-1, a genetic locus that controls murine cytomegalovirus replication in the spleen. *J Exp Med.* **171**, 1469–1483.

Scharf, J.M., Damron, D., Frisella, A., Bruno, S., Beggs, A.H., Kunkel, L.M., and Dietrich, W.F. (1996) The mouse region syntenic for human spinal muscular atrophy lies within the Lgn1 critical interval and contains multiple copies of Naip exon 5. *Genomics.* **38**, 405–417.

Singer, J.B., Hill, A.E., Burrage, L.C., Olszens, K.R., Song, J., Justice, M., O'Brien, W.E., Conti, D.V., Witte, J.S., Lander, E.S., and Nadeau, J.H. (2004) Genetic dissection of complex traits with chromosome substitution strains of mice. *Science.* **304**, 445–448.

Szeszko, J.S., Healy, B., Stevens, H., Balabanova, Y., Drobniewski, F., Todd, J.A., and Nejentsev, S. (2007) Resequencing and association analysis of the SP110 gene in adult pulmonary tuberculosis. *Hum Genet.* **121**, 155–160.

Tamura, T., and Ozato, K. (2002) ICSBP/IRF-8: its regulatory roles in the development of myeloid cells. *J Interferon Cytokine Res.* **22**, 145–152.

Thye, T., Browne, E.N., Chinbuah, M.A., Gyapong, J., Osei, I., Owusu-Dabo, E., Niemann, S., Rusch-Gerdes, S., Horstmann, R.D., and Meyer, C.G. (2006) No associations of human pulmonary tuberculosis with Sp110 variants. *J Med Genet.* **43**, e32.

Tosh, K., Campbell, S.J., Fielding, K., Sillah, J., Bah, B., Gustafson, P., Manneh, K., Lisse, I., Sirugo, G., Bennett, S., Aaby, P., McAdam, K.P., Bah-Sow, O., Lienhardt, C., Kramnik, I., Hill, A.V. (2006) Variants in the SP110 gene are associated with genetic susceptibility to tuberculosis in West Africa. *Proc Natl Acad Sci USA.* **103**, 10364–10368.

Tourne, S., Miyazaki, T., Wolf, P., Ploegh, H., Benoist, C., and Mathis, D. (1997) Functionality of major histocompatibility complex class II molecules in mice doubly deficient for invariant chain and H-2M complexes. *Proc Natl Acad Sci USA.* **94**, 9255–9260.

Turcotte, K., Gauthier, S., Tuite, A., Mullick, A., Malo, D., and Gros, P. (2005) A mutation in the Icsbp1 gene causes susceptibility to infection and a chronic myeloid leukemia-like syndrome in BXH-2 mice. *J Exp Med.* **201**, 881–890.

Vidal, S., Gros, P., and Skamene, E. (1995) Natural resistance to infection with intracellular parasites: molecular genetics identifies *Nramp1* as the *Bcg/Ity/Lsh* locus. *J Leuk Biol.* **58**, 382–390.

Vidal, S. M., Malo, D., Vogan, K., Skamene, E., and Gros, P. (1993) Natural resistance to infection with intracellular parasites: isolation of a candidate for Bcg. *Cell.* **73**, 469–485.

Vidal, S.M., Pinner, E., Lepage, P., Gauthier, S., and Gros, P. (1996) Natural resistance to intracellular infections: *Nramp1* encodes a membrane phosphoglycoprotein absent in macrophages from susceptible (*Nramp1* D169) mouse strains. *J Immunol.* **157**, 3559–3568.

Vidal, S. M., Tremblay, M., Govoni, G., Gauthier, S., Sebastiani, G., Malo, D., Skamene, E., Olivier, M., Jothy, S., and Gros, P. (1995) The *Ity/Lsh/Bcg* locus: natural resistance to infection with intracellular parasites is abrogated by disruption of the *Nramp1* gene. *J Exp Med.* **182**, 655–666.

Watson, J., and Riblet, R. (1974) Genetic control of responses to bacterial lipopolysaccharides in mice. I. Evidence for a single gene that influences mitogenic and immunogenic responses to lipopolysaccharides. *J Exp Med.* **140**, 1147–1161.

Watters, J.W., Dewar, K., Lehoczky, J., Boyartchuk, V., and Dietrich, W.F. (2001) Kif1C, a kinesin-like motor protein, mediates mouse macrophage resistance to anthrax lethal factor. *Curr Biol.* **11**, 1503–1511.

Weih, F., Durham, S.K., Barton, D.S., Sha, W.C., Baltimore, D., and Bravo, R. (1997) p50-NF-kappaB complexes partially compensate for the absence of RelB: severely increased pathology in p50(–/–) relB(–/–) double-knockout mice. *J Exp Med.* **185**, 1359–1370.

Xu, D.G., Crocker, S.J., Doucet, J.P., St-Jean, M., Tamai, K., Hakim, A.M., Ikeda, J.E., Liston, P., Thompson, C.S., Korneluk, R.G., MacKenzie, A., and Robertson, G.S. (1997) Elevation of neuronal expression of NAIP reduces ischemic damage in the rat hippocampus. *Nat Med.* **3**, 997–1004.

Yoshida, S., Goto, Y., Miyamoto, H., Fujio, H., and Mizuguchi, Y. (1991) Association of Lps gene with natural resistance of mouse macrophages against Legionella pneumophila. *FEMS Microbiol Immunol.* **4**, 51–56.

Zarember, K.A., and Godowski, P.J. (2002) Tissue expression of human Toll-like receptors and differential regulation of Toll-like receptor mRNAs in leukocytes in response to microbes, their products, and cytokines. *J Immunol.* **168**, 554–561.

PART II

IMMUNE RESPONSE GENES AND INFECTION

4

MHC Class I and Related Genes

Henry A. F. Stephens

The Role of HLA Class I Molecules in Infection and Pathogenesis

Class I human leukocyte antigens (HLA) are highly polymorphic (see EBI/EMBL, 2007). A central issue in modern immunology is what forces have driven this variability. In the early 1990s, evidence emerged that one of the most common HLA class I molecules in African populations (HLA-B53) appeared to provide some degree of protection against severe life-threatening complications of malaria (Hill et al., 1991; see also chapter 24 in this volume). One implication of this work was that considerable microbial selective pressure has influenced HLA class I variability in different populations. However, much of the subsequent evidence for HLA class I associations with infectious diseases has come from the field of viral immunology. Here, the urgent need to develop vaccines against newly emerging infections such as HIV-1 (see chapter 19) has focused attention on how immune response genes determine initial infection and the subsequent course of disease after exposure to pathogens.

The human immune system has developed a variety of sophisticated mechanisms to identify and eliminate microbial pathogens. Playing a pivotal role in this strategy of seek and destroy are the HLA class I molecules, whose biological role is primarily to present at the cell surface foreign antigens, such as those produced endogenously in the cytosol of virally infected cells. The presence of HLA class I molecules, loaded with viral peptides, at the cell surface alerts both antigen-specific CD8[+] T cells of the adaptive immune response (Zinkernagel and Doherty, 1997) and natural killer (NK) cells that have the innate ability to spontaneously destroy infected cells (Trinchieri, 1989). Thus, HLA class I molecules are essential recognition elements of both the acquired and innate immune responses to infectious agents, particularly viruses.

An inevitable consequence of productive viral infection of human cells is the redirection of host biosynthetic processes to produce new viral proteins in the cytosol. For the virus, be it pathogenic or benign, this is an absolute requirement in order to render mature virions capable of further infection of other host cells. At the same time, viral proteins, like those of the host, are constantly being degraded and replaced within the cell. The degradation of viral proteins is performed by the host immune proteasomes, which are enzyme complexes or proteases composed of a variety of subunits, including the low-molecular-weight polypeptides LMP2 and LMP7 (Pamer and Cresswell, 1998). Short stretches of 8–12 amino acids derived from the virus are then diverted from the cytosol into the lumen of the endoplasmic reticulum (ER) via a pair of ATP-binding cassette host proteins called transporters associated with antigen processing (TAP-1 and TAP-2) (Koopman et al., 1997). Here, the viral peptides interact with the newly synthesized HLA class I molecules. The assembly of HLA class I molecules is largely dependent on stabilization by antigenic peptides of a complex of class I α- (heavy) chain with β2 microglobulin (light chain). Delivery of viral peptides to the HLA class I molecule is abetted by the ER chaperone proteins calnexin and calreticulin and further facilitated by tapasin, which forms a bridge between TAP and the assembling class I molecule. Once it is tightly complexed with viral antigen, the class I molecule can rapidly leave the ER and move via the Golgi apparatus to insert through the plasma membrane. There, the viral peptide is still held in the class I molecule but now located just inside the extracellular space. Thus, distinctive remnants of endogenously produced cellular pathogens held by transmembrane class I molecules can act as beacons, signaling to the CD8+ T and NK cell compartments of the immune response that a cell is infected.

The engagement of αβ T-cell receptors (TCRs) on T cells with viral peptides bound to HLA class I molecules is a key event in the generation of cytolytic responses to infections. The TCR–HLA–peptide complex is stabilized by the CD8 co-receptor, which facilitates the activation of cytotoxic T cells (CTLs). Signaling events mediated by the engaged TCR induce proliferation of CTLs, which release preformed granules of perforin and granzymes that lyse infected cells, and interferon-γ that down-regulates the synthesis of new virions. Activated CTLs also express Fas ligand (FasL), which can engage Fas on target cells and induce programmed cell death or apoptosis of the infected cell (Leonardo et al., 1999; Van Parijis and

Abbas, 1998). Thus, a formidable array of antiviral responses is induced in CTLs. However, up-regulation of FasL on CTLs exposes them to Fas, which is also expressed on CTLs, and to the possibility of self induced death. Hence, HLA-peptide signaling via the TCR not only activates CTLs to perform their prime function of recognizing and destroying infected cells but can also result in anergy or stunning of CTLs and may even induce apoptosis. For example, apoptotic stunning of memory CTL responses may occur in some individuals after secondary exposure to dengue virus (Mongkolsapaya et al., 2003). Nevertheless, the transport of viral peptides by HLA class I molecules to the cell surface provides the infected cell with a unique opportunity to control the expression of viral proteins through the HLA class I–restricted CTL pathway.

Not surprisingly, many adept viral pathogens have evolved a variety of mechanisms to avoid or interfere with this critical pathway of HLA class I–mediated CTL recognition and response to infection. Some can shut down the expression of HLA class I molecules and thus confound recognition of infected cells by CTLs. A variety of viruses, such as Epstein-Barr virus (EBV), human cytomegalovirus (CMV), herpes simplex virus (HSV), human papillomavirus (HPV), and human immunodeficiency virus (HIV-1), produce proteins that specifically down-regulate HLA class I protein expression. For example, EBV selectively down-regulates certain HLA class I gene products (Rickinson et al., 1992), CMV interferes with the stability of the class I heavy chain (Beersma et al., 1993; Park et al., 2004), and HSV produces a protein that binds to TAP and interferes with the transport of viral peptides into the ER (Hill et al., 1995). By contrast, proteins produced by HPV can bind directly to HLA class I molecules, confine them in the ER, and prevent their transport to the cell surface (Ashrafi et al., 2005). Similarly, the product of the HIV-1 Nef gene induces endocytosis and internalization of HLA class I molecules, thus preventing their transportation to the cell surface (Schwartz et al., 1996; Collins et al., 1998). However, the host countermeasure to this subversion of HLA class I–mediated immune recognition is a Nef fragment–specific CTL response (Mangasarian et al., 1999; Stephens, 2005). The host can also enlist NK cells, whose inhibitory killer immunoglobulin-like receptors (KIRs) and lectin-like receptors (e.g., NKG2) help monitor and destroy virus-infected cells with abnormally low levels of HLA class I expression (Moretta et al., 2004; Parham, 2005; see also chapter 7 in this volume).

Another strategy employed by relatively small RNA viruses such as HIV-1 is their highly defective replicative ability. As a result of an extreme propensity to mutate rapidly, HIV-1 replication generates immune-selected escape mutants producing peptides that no longer bind host HLA class I molecules or TCRs (Leslie et al., 2004) or that resist proteasome degradation (Yokomaku et al., 2004; Draenert et al., 2004). These evasive maneuvers currently appear to represent a major obstacle to the development of vaccines designed to elicit CTL-driven protective responses against HIV-1. This kind of strategic escape from immune recognition is by no means unique to RNA viruses, as evidenced by the loss of HLA class I recognition and CTL-driven responses to EBV in disparate populations (de Campos-Lima et al., 1994).

HLA Class I Molecular Structure

Structurally, HLA class I molecules are transmembrane glycoproteins composed of three extracellular α-chain domains (α1–α3) in complex with a β2 microglobulin, a transmembrane region, and a cytoplasmic tail (figure 4.1). The first crystallographic analysis of an HLA class I molecule in 1987 revealed a unique structure of antigenic peptides of specific length and composition held in a cleft formed by the α1 and α2 domains (Bjorkman et al., 1987a). The floor of the HLA class I cleft is composed of eight β-pleated strands surrounded by two flanking walls formed of α-helices (figure 4.2). From the seminal study (Bjorkman et al., 1987a) and many subsequent investigations, it is now well established that the amino acid side chains of antigens sit in specific pockets (named A–F) that form in the floor of the cleft, thus locking the peptide firmly into the class I molecule (figure 4.2). Most peptides are of a specific length (8–10 amino acids), with the amino-terminal (position 2) and carboxy-terminal (positions 8–10), respectively, engaged with the B and F pockets at either end of the cleft. Other antigenic peptide residues can interact directly with the secondary C, D, or E pockets. High-affinity hydrogen bonds between peptide residues and conserved tyrosine residues secure this interaction and prevent any exchange of bound peptides.

Individual class I molecules can bind a wide range of peptide sequences but also show specificity in the types of peptides bound. For any given peptide, not all pockets of the class I cleft are necessarily occupied by antigenic residues. Conversely, for any given HLA class I molecule, different pockets can be utilized to bind different antigens firmly (figure 4.3). Thus, the occupancy of pockets will vary between allelic variants

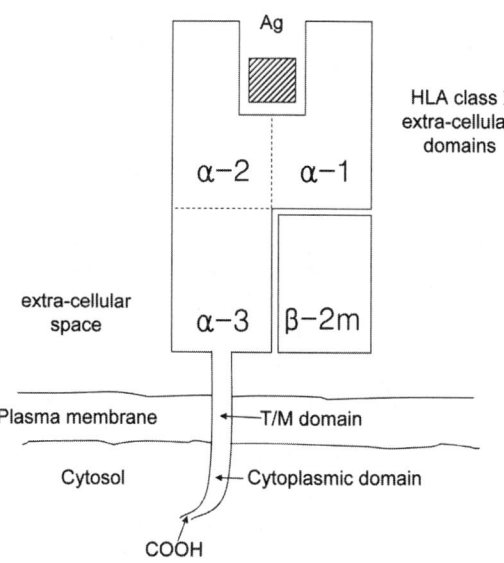

FIGURE 4.1. Orientation, configuration, and location of HLA class I α-chain protein domains with antigenic peptide (Ag) cargo, forming a heterodimer with β2 microglobulin.

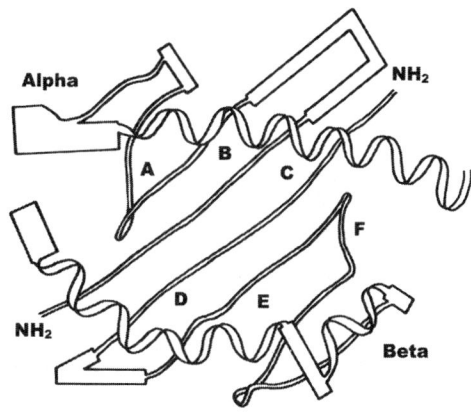

FIGURE 4.2. Three-dimensional structure of the HLA class I α1 and α2 protein domains forming an antigen-binding cleft, according to the model of Bjorkman et al. (1987a). The relative positions of the antigenic peptide-binding pockets (A–F) are as given. Two α-helices form the walls of the cleft, with β-pleated sheets forming the floor.

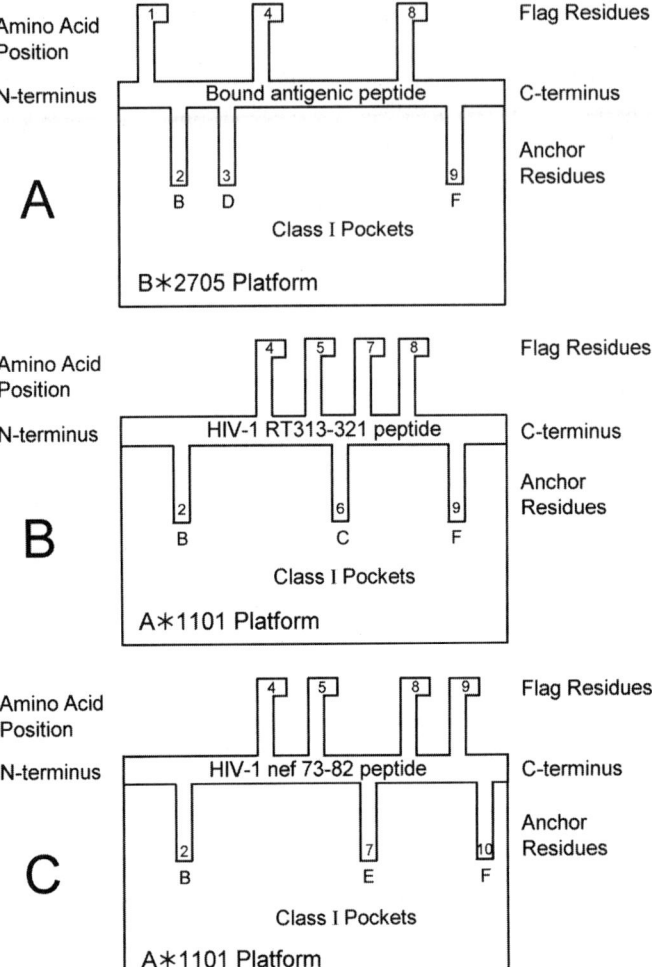

FIGURE 4.3. Antigenic anchor and flag positions vary between peptides and HLA class I molecules. (A) HLA-B*2705 platform showing the classic interaction of B, D, and F pockets with amino acid positions 2, 3, and 9 of an antigenic nonamer peptide (Madden et al., 1990), with positions 1, 4, and 8 acting as flag residues and interacting with the TCR (Bowness et al., 1994). (B and C) HLA-A*1101 platform varying in terms of pockets and antigenic anchor residues used, as well as flag residues presented to TCRs, depending on size and amino acid composition of two HIV-1–derived immunogenic peptides (Li and Bouvier, 2004).

of HLA class I molecules and the peptides they bind. Other antigenic peptide residues, called flag positions, are oriented away from the cleft and interact directly with the α- and β-chains of the TCR (Bjorkman et al., 1987b). These flag positions also vary between HLA class I molecules and the antigens they present (figure 4.3). Such flexibility in the size and specificity of peptide binding provides both permissiveness in the types of antigens presented by HLA class I molecules and the structural basis for genetic restriction of the immune response (Zinkernagel and Doherty, 1997).

HLA Class I Genes

The genes encoding HLA class I molecules are located within the major histocompatibility complex (MHC) on the short arm of chromosome 6, which is one of the most gene-dense regions of the human genome (MHC Sequencing Consortium, 1999; Horton et al., 2004). The extended MHC spans nearly 7.6 megabase pairs (Mb) and contains at least 421 gene loci, of which 252 (60%) are thought to be expressed. The remaining unexpressed loci are classified as pseudogenes, which are largely disabled remnants of evolution. The products of some 28% of the expressed loci are functionally involved in the immunity (Horton et al., 2004). This concentration of immune-response–related genes within a relatively small area of the human genome is likely to have evolved to enable coordinated expression of their functionally related and interacting products.

The MHC can be broadly categorized into three regions or clusters, designated classes I, II, and III. Six gene loci (*HLA-A, HLA-B, HLA-C, HLA-E, HLA-F,*

HLA-G) in the centromeric class I region encode functional class I α- or heavy chains (figure 4.4). *HLA-A, -B, -C* encode classical class I products, in the sense that they are ubiquitously expressed and recognized by CD8$^+$ CTLs (table 4.1). By contrast, the products of *HLA-E, -F,* and *-G* are considered nonclassical by virtue of their more restricted function and expression (table 4.1). The locus encoding the other component of all class I heterodimers, β2 microglobulin, does not reside on chromosome 6. On the other hand, both expressed *TAP1* and *TAP2* along with *PSMB9* and *PSMB8* (LMP2 and LMP7) gene loci reside within the MHC but are located in the telomeric class II region (figure 4.4).

HLA class I genes have the classic exon–intron configuration of eukaryote loci, with exons 2–4 encoding the three extracellular protein domains (α1–α3) of the mature protein (figure 4.5). The transcription and expression of classical class I genes occur in nearly all cell types and are regulated by a series of *cis-* and *trans-*acting elements. The majority of *cis-*acting control elements are noncoding nucleic acid promoter motifs located in the 5′ region flanking exon 1 (figure 4.5) (Gobin et al., 1999; Rousseau et al., 2004). These promoter motifs are highly conserved and drive the transcription of class I genes after interacting with *trans-*acting nuclear proteins. HLA class I inducers, such as interferon-γ and tumor necrosis factor-α, do not necessarily act directly on all *cis-*promoter motifs;

they may induce the intracellular production of other *trans-*acting proteins (Gobin et al., 1999).

HLA Class I Evolution, Polymorphism, Populations, and Disease

Each of the classical HLA class I loci is extremely polymorphic, encoding hundreds of alleles (table 4.2). *HLA-B* is the most polymorphic locus in the human genome; detection of nearly 900 molecularly defined alleles (EBI/EMBL, 2007) suggests that this locus is still undergoing rapid evolution. Profound selective microbial pressure is likely to be driving HLA class I allelic diversity by a variety of molecular processes, such as gene duplication and recombination, interallelic conversion, and retention of beneficial point mutations (Parham and Ohta, 1996; Prugnolle et al., 2005). At the population level, class I HLA loci show considerable differences in allele frequencies, both within and between different ethnic groups, be they African, Asian, or Caucasoid in origin (Cao et al., 2004; Chandanayingyong et al., 1997; Middleton et al., 2007). HLA class I allele frequencies in African populations tend to have the greatest range, perhaps related to a higher degree of local pathogen diversity and pressure on these populations (Prugnolle et al., 2005).

Another feature of HLA class I genes is the phenomenon of linkage disequilibrium, whereby certain

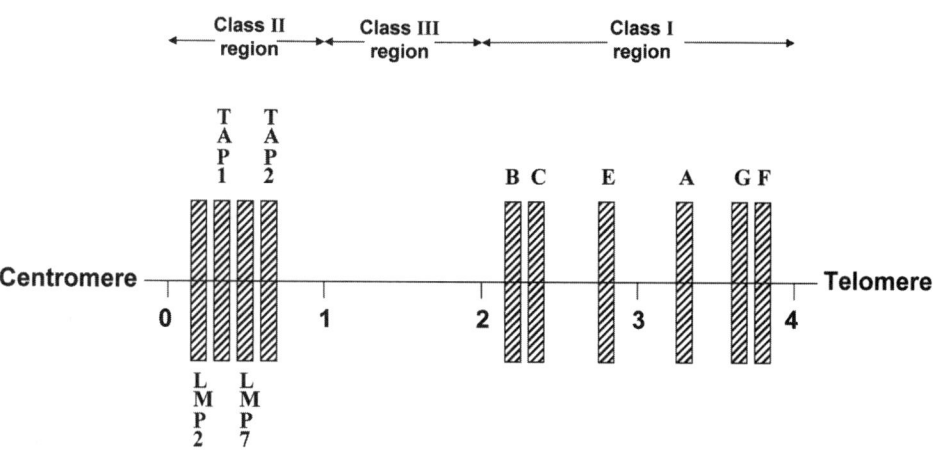

Relative position in mega bases

FIGURE 4.4. Relative and approximate locations of HLA class I, TAP (*TAP1* and *TAP2*), and LMP (*PSMB9* and *PSMB8*) gene loci (hatched boxes) in the human MHC on chromosome 6.

TABLE 4.1. Biological function and recognition of classical (HLA-A, -B, and -C) and nonclassical (HLA-E, -F, and -G) human class I molecules.

Human Class I Molecule	Cargo	Interacting Ligand/Receptor	Cell Type	Function
HLA-A	Peptide	TCR α/β, KIR3DL2, LILRB2 (ILT4/LIR2)	T + NK	Host defense
HLA-B	Peptide	TCR α/β, KIR3DL1, 3DL2, LILRB2 (ILT4/LIR2)	T + NK	Host defense
HLA-C	Peptide	TCR α/β, KIR2DL1, 2DL2, 2DL3, 2DS1, 2DS2, 2DS4	T + NK	Host defense, maternofetal tolerance, and trophoblast development
HLA-E	MHC class I leader peptide	CD94/NKG2-A, CD94/NKG2-B, CD94/NKG2-C, TCR α/β	NK + T	MHC class I expression
HLA-F	None	LILRB1 (ILT2/LIR1), LILRB2 (ILT4/LIR2)	NK + monocytes + dendritic cells	Maternofetal tolerance
HLA-G	Peptide	LILRB1 (ILT2/LIR-1), LILRB2 (ILT4/LIR2), KIR-2DL4	NK + monocytes	Maternofetal tolerance

The classical HLA-A and -B molecules are expressed by most cell types and are recognized by αβ TCRs, killer immunoglobulin-like receptors (KIRs; Hansasuta et al., 2004; Kollinberger et al., 2002), and leukocyte immunoglobulin-like receptors (LILRs). They are involved in host recognition of and defense against foreign proteins derived from microbial pathogens as well as transplanted and neoplastic cells. HLA-C molecules have a similar tissue distribution, are recognized by αβ TCRs and a variety of inhibiting and activating KIRs, and are involved in fetal trophoblast development as well as host defense (Parham, 2004; Hiby et al., 2004;). By contrast, HLA-E, -F, and -G have a more restricted tissue distribution. Each appears to be recognized by a different combination of receptors, including lectin-like NK receptors (CD94/NKG2), LILRs, and KIRs (Lepin et al., 2000; Ishitani et al., 2003). HLA-E is functionally involved in the control of MHC class I expression; HLA-F and -G regulate maternal-placental immune recognition, but both -E and -G may have functions related to host defense, as well. Earlier locus designations and nomenclature of LILR genes are given in parentheses.

combinations of alleles encoded at neighboring loci tend to form stable haplotypes that are inherited from one generation to another in a Mendelian fashion. Again, the composition and frequency of HLA haplotypes also vary considerably among different ethnic groups (Cao et al., 2004; Chandanayingyong et al., 1997; Middleton et al., 2007). Thus, class I alleles are recognized to be excellent markers of ethnicity. The

analysis of HLA class I genes has proved to be highly informative in anthropological studies, to the extent that class I allele and haplotype profiles show considerable parallelism with language diversification and other cultural and socioeconomic parameters that define ethnic groups (Cavalli-Sforza et al., 1988).

The extreme polymorphism of HLA class I genes also has a profound influence on the biological func-

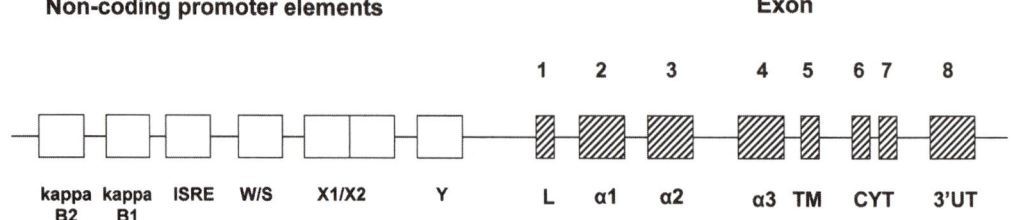

FIGURE 4.5. Exon–intron configuration of a gene encoding a classical HLA class I α or heavy chain (hatched boxes), together with 5' or upstream noncoding promoter motifs (open boxes). L = leader sequence; α1, α2, α3 are exons encoding the first three external protein domains; TM = transmembrane region; CYT = cytoplasmic tail; 3'UT = 3' untranslated region. For the *cis*-encoded promoter motifs (not drawn to scale), κB1 and κB2 = binding sites for NFκB1 and B2 transcription factors; ISRE = interferon-stimulated response element, which binds to interferon regulatory factor 1; W/S, X1/X2, and Y represent the different promoter boxes or conserved sequence motifs that are recognized by a variety of promoter-binding factors or proteins, such as RFX, BP, ATF, CREB, NF-Y, and CIITA (Gobin et al., 1999; Rousseau et al., 2004).

TABLE 4.2. Polymorphism of MHC encoded HLA class I and accessory molecules (June 2007).

Gene Name/Locus (NCBI)	Entrez Gene ID	Map Position	Number of Molecularly Defined Alleles	Number of Expressed Structural Variants	Number of Null (N) or Nonexpressers	Number of Low (L) Expressers	Number of Secreted (S) Expressers
HLA-A	3105	6p21.3	545	436	39	3	—
HLA-B	3106	6p21.3	894	766	31	1	1
HLA-C	3107	6p21.3	307	244	7	—	—
HLA-E	3133	6p21.3	8	3	—	—	—
HLA-F	3134	6p21.3	24	4	—	—	—
HLA-G	3135	6p21.3	23	6	1	—	—
TAP1	6890	6p21.3	7	5	1	—	—
TAP2	6891	6p21.3	4	4	—	—	—
TAPB (Tapasin)*	6892	6p21.3	2	2	—	—	—
PSMB9 (LMP-2)*	5698	6p21.3	2	2	—	—	—
PSMB8 (LMP-7)*	5696	6p21.3	4	4	—	—	—

Gene designations, Entrez gene IDs, and chromosomal location are as given in www.ncbi.nlm.nih.gov. LMP2 and LMP7 are now renamed as PSMB9 and PSMB8 respectively (see www.ncbi.nlm.nih.gov), which corresponds to proteasome (prosome, macropain) subunit, β-type (large multifunctional peptidase). HLA class I and TAP polymorphism are as given in EBI/EMBL (2007). *TAPBP (tapasin) and PSMB9 and PSMB8 (LMP2 and LMP7) polymorphism are shown according to Williams et al. (2000) and Lim et al. (1999), respectively.

tion of their products. Most polymorphism occurs in exons 2 and 3, particularly at codons for amino acids that form peptide-binding pockets (A–F) of the class I cleft, which in turn affects the binding and subsequent presentation of microbial peptides to antigen-specific T cells. Analysis of the protein sequence of antigenic peptides bound by different class I molecules has identified groups of HLA class I alleles (supertypes) with similar preferences for a pattern of peptide sequence or supermotifs that share a similar structure (Falk et al., 1991; Sidney et al., 1996; Sette and Sidney, 1999). Convergent evolution may have selected the current repertoire of HLA class I supertypes, because there is considerable overlap of the preferred supermotifs among alleles encoded by the same loci, among loci, and among different ethnic groups (Sette et al., 2003). Not surprisingly, current understanding of HLA class I binding preferences, in terms of the size and composition of their bound peptides, has begun to guide certain choices of target antigens in new vaccines.

The techniques used to type HLA molecules and their allelic variants have largely evolved in the field of human transplant immunology with its stringent requirements for matching compatible tissue types to reduce the risk of organ rejection, hence the "histocompatibility" component of the MHC acronym. The original serological HLA phenotyping methods utilized either sera from multiparous women who had developed antibodies to the HLA antigens of their biological partners or mixed lymphocyte culture proliferative assays. Once

HLA class I genes were cloned (Ploegh et al., 1980), Southern blot analysis of restriction-enzyme–digested genomic DNA with full-length HLA class I probes revealed good correlation between gross genomic profiles and serologically defined alleles. With the advent of PCR-based techniques came molecular methods involving PCR amplification of DNA coupled with sequence-specific oligonucleotide probes and sequence-specific primers or direct sequencing (Bunce et al., 1997).

The resulting profusion of molecularly defined alleles has benefited greatly from a rational internationally recognized nomenclature. The current scheme assigns each allele a unique identity consisting of the name of the class I locus followed by an asterisk and at least four digits. The first two digits designate the broad HLA type, roughly equivalent to the serologically defined antigen or serotype (allotype), and the third and fourth digits designate individual amino acid differences. For some alleles, fifth and sixth digits have been introduced to define noncoding, silent, or synonymous nucleotide base changes, and seventh and eighth digits refer to intronic, 5', or 3' polymorphism. Rarely, alleles are unexpressed or "null" (N), produced in low concentration (L), or secreted (S) (table 4.2).

A variety of molecular-based, high-resolution, and high-throughput HLA typing methods are available to test for class I allele, haplotype, and supertype associations with susceptibility and resistance to infectious diseases in different populations. Such studies are aimed at identifying immunogenetic factors that determine variability between individuals in their responses to infectious agents and vaccines. However, the interpretation of genetic associations in population studies can be complicated by a variety of factors (Cardon and Bell, 2001): size and ethnicity of the target populations, frequency and composition of the detected HLA alleles and haplotypes, degree of resolution of typing methods, and clinical or biological definitions of the disease outcomes under investigation. Larger cohorts of clinically well-characterized patients and controls (usually at least several hundred) are essential to provide adequate statistical power to detect HLA class I associations. The confounding effect of ethnic variation in association studies can be averted by careful consideration of the geography and environment of target populations, as well as their history, language, and culture. Thus, the gold standard for a meaningful HLA association with biologically relevant response is reproducibility in the same (intra-)ethnic group or detection of a similar relationship with an equivalent marker between different (inter-)ethnic groups.

Applications of this standard have probably been best illustrated by studies on HIV/AIDS (see chapter 19). The relatively recent zoonotic introduction and rapid spread of HIV-1 into human populations has revealed consistent associations between certain HLA class I alleles and haplotypes with either slow or rapid progression of AIDS in Africans and Caucasoids (Kaslow et al., 1996; Gao et al., 2001; Liu et al., 2003; Stephens, 2005; see also chapter 19). HIV-1–infected individuals who are fully heterozygous for HLA class I alleles have a clear advantage against developing AIDS, probably due to the increased range of immunodominant peptides presented to T cells in these individuals (Carrington et al., 1999; Tang et al., 1999). Several studies have recently demonstrated that as HIV-1 becomes established in exposed populations, it rapidly mutates to avoid CTL responses restricted by the major HLA class I alleles within those populations (Moore et al., 2002; Leslie et al., 2004 and 2005; Kiepiela et al., 2004). The virus is, in effect, being structurally remolded by immune responses restricted by HLA class I alleles. At the same time, some HLA class I alleles associated with fast progression to AIDS in highly exposed populations may eventually diminish in frequency (Kiepiela et al., 2004). Thus, we may now be observing real-time bidirectional natural selection or coevolution—rapid selective pressure by individual host HLA variants leading to viral mutation and immune escape, combined with slow selective pressure by HIV-

1 impinging on the most polymorphic human locus (*HLA-B*), leading to gradual realignment of population allele frequencies.

HLA class I allele, haplotype, and supertype profiles are also being carefully scrutinized in other chronic debilitating viral infections, such as those induced by human T-lymphotropic virus-1 and hepatitis B and C (see chapters 20 and 21). Although the evidence is not as conclusive for these infections as for HIV-1, HLA class I–driven CTL and NK responses are thought to play crucial roles in disease outcome (Jeffrey et al., 1999; Thio et al., 2002, 2003; Khakoo et al., 2004). An area of considerable public health concern, but more neglected, is that of acute and incapacitating viral infections. Two examples are dengue and severe acute respiratory syndrome (SARS), both of which have been associated with certain HLA class I alleles (Stephens et al., 2002; Ng et al., 2004). Dengue provides unique insight into HLA class I-driven T-cell memory and cross-reactivity with virus serotype responses, which can be both protective and in some cases detrimental to the host, particularly in those individuals who have been immunologically primed by previous exposure to different viral variants (Stephens et al., 2002).

Another illustration of complex involvement of HLA class I in infection is the intriguing role of HLA-B*27. It is a highly conserved class I molecule in Caucasian and some Asian populations where different variants occur in moderate to high frequency (Middleton et al., 2007). In certain populations, B*27 alleles may have conferred a selective advantage during evolution. Indeed, it facilitates vigorous CTL responses to many common pathogens such as influenza (Tussey et al., 1995), EBV (Brooks et al., 1993; Crotzer et al., 2000), and HIV-1 (Goulder et al., 1997). However, the downside of possessing HLA-B*27 is a propensity to develop reactive arthritis after enteric exposure to *Yersinia*, *Salmonella*, *Campylobacter*, and *Shigella* and after urogenital infection with *Chlamydia trachomatis* (Brewerton et al., 1973a). Probably the strongest interethnic HLA class I allele association with disease, albeit not of an established microbial origin, is that of HLA-B*27 and the spondyloarthropathies (Brewerton et al., 1973b; Lopez de Castro, 1998). For example, the relative risk of developing ankylosing spondylitis is some 20 times greater in Caucasoid individuals carrying a B*27 allele than in those without such an allele (Braun et al., 1998).

A variety of mechanisms have been proposed to account for the strong association between HLA-B*27 alleles and reactive arthritis or the spondyloarthropathies, such as reactivity to an arthritogenic peptide (Benjamin and Parham, 1990), prolonged B*27-restricted responses to persistent bacterial antigens in the affected joints (Keat et al., 1987; Rahman et al., 1992), abnormal splice variants generating a preponderance of soluble B27 molecules with an immunomodulatory capacity (Huang et al., 1997; Buelow et al., 1995), and molecular mimicry of B27 by bacterial pathogens (Schwimmbeck et al., 1987). Furthermore, B27 molecules display unique structural and functional features. The HLA*B2705 can load antigenic peptides without associating with TAP or tapasin (Peh et al., 1998). Unusual homodimeric forms of the α or heavy chain components of the B27 molecule without β2 microglobulin have been identified (Allen et al., 1999). The different structural forms of B27 vary in their ability to be recognized by leukocyte immunoglobulin-like receptors (LILRs), which are expressed on human NK cells (Allen et al., 2001). Similarly, recognition of B*2705 by the NK receptor KIR3DL1 is dependent on the antigenic peptide loaded into the HLA molecule (Stewart-Jones et al., 2005). B27 can also act like an HLA class II molecule and present antigenic peptides to CD4+ T cells (Roddis et al., 2004). Thus, a variety of structural features attributed to B27 may affect its biological functions and influence associations with infectious diseases.

At present there is little evidence that alleles or haplotypes of the nonclassical HLA class I genes *HLA-E*, *HLA-F*, and *HLA-G* are differentially related to the occurrence of infectious diseases. However, nasopharyngeal carcinoma, which is associated with EBV infection and certain classical HLA class I and II genes in Asian populations (Hildesheim et al., 2002), has also been associated with a homozygous HLA-E*0103 genotype in ethnic Thais (Hirankarn et al., 2004). There is evidence in Zimbabwean women that certain *HLA-E* and *HLA-G* alleles are associated with altered risk of acquiring heterosexual infections of HIV-1 (Matte et al., 2004; Lajoie et al., 2003). Similarly, the nonclassical MHC class I chain-related (MIC) genes that encode highly polymorphic stress-related molecules recognized by NK cells (see chapter 6) have been analyzed in a variety of infectious and autoimmune diseases. However, most MIC associations with disease appear to be secondary to linkage disequilibrium with primary disease-associated alleles at adjacent loci, particularly *HLA-B* (Stephens, 2002; see chapter 6). An area of some neglect is the epigenetic role HLA class I promoters (figure 4.5) and their transcription factors that drive HLA class I expression during infections. At the nucleotide level, there are several polymorphisms in and around the putative binding sites of transcription factors (EBI/EMBL, 2007), suggesting that natural selective pressures have generated this diversity, but at present HLA class I promoter associations with infection are unevaluated.

HLA Class I Accessory Genes

The *TAP1* and *TAP2*, *TAPBP* (tapasin), and *PSMB8* and *PSMB9* (LMP) genes have coevolved with the HLA class I loci to deliver peptides customized for particular class I alleles. However, these genes show limited polymorphism (table 4.2), they are not all in strong linkage disequilibrium with each other (Lim et al., 1999), and there is no apparent functional difference between allelic variants in peptide selection or transport (Obst et al., 1995; Daniel et al., 1997). Thus, early association studies of HIV-1 infection (Kaslow et al., 1996), most likely subject to analytic shortcomings, have not been widely replicated. In general, TAP and PSMB (LMP) polymorphisms are associated with infectious diseases either weakly (Cao et al., 2005) or not at all (Hohler et al., 1996). On the other hand, rare deficiencies in TAP genes resulting in down-regulation of HLA class I molecules have been associated with recurrent bacterial infections (Gadola et al., 2000). Defining a role for polymorphism of these genes in susceptibility to infections is further complicated by these genes being independently in linkage disequilibrium with HLA class II but not class I genes (Lim et al., 1999; Williams et al., 2000). Nevertheless, novel TAP polymorphisms have been detected in putative functional areas of the molecule, suggesting that selective pressures are maintaining these variations in different populations (Lajoie et al., 2003). In the future, suitably powered studies incorporating stratification for linkage disequilibrium with class II genes and population variability may resolve whether genes encoding TAP, tapasin, and LMP play a primary role in associations with infectious diseases.

HLA Class I Immunogenetics, Pharmocogenomics, Proteomics, and Vaccine Design

Accumulating information on the structure of HLA class I molecules and the influence of their allelic differences on the outcome of infectious diseases has led to various applications. For example, the synthesis of antigen-loaded HLA class I tetramers labeled with fluorescent tags has been extremely informative in real time flow cytometric analysis of the level and persistence of CTL responses to both acute and chronic viral infections (Ogg et al., 1998; McMichael and O'Callaghan, 1998). Prior to the development of HLA class I tetramer technology, monitoring of CTL responses was largely dependent on laborious limiting dilution cellular techniques, which probably grossly underestimated the strength and persistence of CTL responses, particularly during the acute viremic phase of infection. HLA class I tetramers are also helping to elucidate the antigen-specific nature of some NK-cell–mediated cell responses to HLA class I molecules presenting viral antigens, such as those derived from EBV (Hansasuta et al., 2004). Similarly, the development of transgenic animals expressing human HLA class I molecules such as B27 has enabled the production of animal models of human disease for testing novel therapeutic interventions (Hammer et al., 1990; Roddis et al., 2004). Furthermore, the reported association of hypersensitivity to an antiretroviral therapy agent in HIV/AIDS patients with HLA-B*57 and/or possibly another nearby linked gene disequilibrium, has extended the critical cross-fertilization between immunogenetics and pharmocogenomics to the realm of infectious diseases (Mallal et al., 2002; Martin et al., 2004).

Another development includes the numerous algorithms being used to analyze microbial genomic and proteomic studies in conjunction with host HLA class I profiles. These algorithms can predict the location, structure, and binding preferences of conserved immunogenic epitopes and supermotifs that are specific for HLA class I allele and supertype (Bond et al., 2001; Nussbaum et al., 2002; Sathiamurthy et al., 2003; Flower, 2003; Lund et al., 2004; Sylvester-Hvid et al., 2004). This approach holds considerable promise for vaccines designed to invoke protective CTL responses to various pathogens in disparate populations with variable HLA class I allele and supertype profiles. Publicly accessible international databases have collated pathogen proteomic data with the location of known CTL epitopes and their HLA class I restricting alleles (Nussbaum et al., 2002). As applied to HIV-1 (see www.hiv.lanl.gov), this approach has suggested that, despite the ability of virus to mutate and escape from CTL responses, certain highly conserved regions of viral proteins can act as hot spots of CTL recognition in diverse populations (Stephens, 2005). Thus, due consideration is now being paid to both microbial pathogen diversity and human HLA class I variability in the development of new immunological interventions designed to combat the major current and future threats from infectious diseases.

References

Allen, R.L., O'Callaghan, C.A., McMichael, A.J., & Bowness, P. (1999) Cutting edge: HLA-B27 can form a novel beta-2-microglobulin-free heavy chain homodimer structure. *Journal of Immunology* 162, 5045–5048.

Allen, R.L., Raine, T., Haude, A., Trowsdale, J., & Wilson, M.J. (2001) Cutting edge: Leukocyte receptor complex-encoded immunoregulatory receptors show differing specificity for alternative HLA-B27 structures. *Journal of Immunology* 167, 5543–5547.

Ashrafi, G.H., Haghshenas, M.R., Marchetti, B., O'Brien, P.M., & Campo, M.S. (2005) E5 protein of human papillomavirus type 16 selectively downregulates surface HLA class I. *International Journal of Cancer* 113, 276–283.

Beersma, M.F., Bijlmakers, M.J., & Ploegh, H.L. (1993) Human cytomegalovirus down-regulates HLA class I expression by reducing the stability of class I H chains. *Journal of Immunology* 151, 4455–4464.

Benjamin, R., & Parham, P. (1990) Guilt by association; HLA-B27 and ankylosing spondylitis. *Immunology Today* 11, 137–142.

Bjorkman, P.J., Sapper, M.A., Samraoui, B., Bennett, W.S., Strominger, J.L., & Wiley, D.C. (1987a) Structure of the human class I histocompatibility antigen HLA-A2. *Nature* 329, 526–512.

Bjorkman, P.J., Sapper, M.A., Samraoui, B., Bennett, W.S., Strominger, J.L., & Wiley, D.C. (1987b) The foreign antigen binding site and T cell recognition regions of class I histocompatibility antigens. *Nature* 329, 512–518.

Bond, K.B., Sriwanthana, B., Hodge, T.W., De Groot, A.S., Mastro, T.D., Young, N.L., Promadej, N., Altman, J.D., Limpakarnjanarat, K., & McNicholl, J.M. (2001) An HLA-directed molecular and bioinformatics approach identifies new HLA-A11 HIV-1 subtype E cytotoxic T lymphocyte epitopes in HIV-1-infected Thais. *AIDS Research and Human Retroviruses* 17, 703–717.

Bowness, P., Allen, R.L., & McMichael, A.J. (1994) Identification of T cell receptor recognition residues for a viral peptide presented by HLA B27. *European Journal of Immunology* 24, 2357–2363.

Braun, J., Bollow, M., Remlinger, G., Eggens, U., Rud-waleit, M., Distler, A., & Seiper, J. (1998) Prevalence of spondylarthopathies in HLA-B27 positive and negative blood donors. *Arthritis and Rheumatism* 41, 58–67.

Brewerton, D.A., Caffrey, M., Nicholls, A., Walters, D., Oates, J.K., & James, D.C. (1973a) Reiter's disease and HL-A 27. *Lancet* 2, 996–998.

Brewerton, D.A., Hart, F.D., Nicholls, A., Caffrey, M., James, D.C., & Sturrock, R.D. (1973b) Ankylosing spondylitis and HL-A 27. *Lancet* 1, 904–907.

Brooks, J.M., Murray, R.J., Thomas, W.A., Kurilla, M.G., & Rickinson, A.B. (1993) Different HLA-B27 subtypes present the same immunodominant Epstein-Barr virus peptide. *Journal of Experimental Medicine* 178, 879–887.

Buelow, R., Burlingham, W.J., & Clayberger, C. (1995) Immunomodulation by soluable HLA class I. *Transplantation* 59, 649–654.

Bunce, M., Young, N.T., & Welsh, K.I. (1997) Molecular HLA typing—the brave new world. *Transplantation* 64, 1505–1513.

Cao, K., Moormann, A.M., Lyke, K.E., Masaberg, C., Sumba, C., Doumbo, O.K., Koech, D., Lancaster, A., Nelson, M., Meyer, D., Single, R., Hartzman, R.J., Plowe, C.V., Kazura, J., Mann, D.L., Sztein, M.B., Thomson, G., & Fernandez-Vina, M.A. (2004) Differentiation between African populations is evidenced by the diversity of alleles and haplotypes of HLA class I loci. *Tissue Antigens* 63, 293–325.

Cao, B., Tian, X., Li, Y., Jiang, P., Ning, T., Xing, H., Zhao, Y., Zhang, C., Shi, X., Chen, D., Shen, Y., & Ke, Y. (2005) LMP7/TAP2 gene polymorphism and HPV infection in esophageal carcinoma patients from a high incidence area in China. *Carcinogenesis* 26, 1280–1284.

Cardon, L.R., & Bell, J.I. (2001) Association study designs for complex diseases. *Nature Reviews in Genetics* 2, 91–99.

Carrington, M., Nelson, G.W., Martin, M.P., Kissner, T., Vlahov, D., Goedert, J.J., Kaslow, R., Buchbinder, S., Hoots, K., & O'Brien, S.J. (1999) HLA and HIV-1: Heterozygote advantage and B*35-Cw*04 disadvantage. *Science* 283, 1748–1752.

Cavalli-Sforza, L.L., Piazza, A., Menozzi, M., & Mountain, J. (1988) Reconstruction of human evolution: Bringing together genetic, archeological, and linguistic data. *Proceedings of the National Academy of Sciences of the United States of America* 85, 6002–6006.

Chandanayingyong, D., Stephens, H.A.F., Klaythong, R., Sirkong, M., Udee, S., Longta, P., Chantangpol, R., Bejrachandra, S., & Runruang, E. (1997) HLA-A, -B, -DRB1, -DQA1 and -DQB1 polymorphism in Thais. *Human Immunology* 53, 174–182.

Collins, K.L., Chen, B.K., Kalams, S.A., Walker, B.D., & Baltimore, D. (1998) HIV-1 Nef protein protects infected primary cells against killing by cytotoxic T lymphocytes. *Nature* 391, 397–401.

Crotzer, V.L., Christian, R.E., Brooks, J.M., Shabanowitz, J., Settlage, R., Marto, J.A., White, F.M., Rickinson, A.B., Hunt, D.F., & Engelhard, V.H. (2000) Immunodominance among EBV-derived epitopes restricted by HLA-B27 does not correlate with epitope abundance in EBV-transformed B-lymphoblastoid cell lines. *Journal of Immunology* 164, 6120–6129.

Daniel, S., Caillat-Zucman, S., Hammer, J., Bach, J.F., & van Endert, P.M. (1997) Absence of functional relevance of human transporter associated with antigen processing polymorphism for peptide selection. *Journal of Immunology* 159, 2350–2357.

De Campos-Lima, P.O., Levitsky, V., Brooks, J., Lee S.P., Hu, L.F., Rickinson, A.B., & Masucci, M.G. (1994) T cell responses and virus evolution: Loss of HLA A11 restricted CTL responses in Epstein-Barr virus isolates from highly A11-positive populations by selective mutation of anchor residues. *Journal of Experimental Medicine* 179, 1297–1305.

Draenert, R., Le Gall, S., Pfafferott, K.J., Leslie, A.J., Chetty, P., Brander, C., Holmes, E.C., Chang, S.C., Feeney, M.E., Addo, M.M., Ruiz, L., Ramduth, D., Jueena, P., Altfield, M., Thomas, S., Tang, Y., Verrill, C.L., Dixon, C., Prado, J.G., Kiepiela, P., Martinez-Picado, J., Walker, B.D., & Goulder, P.J. (2004) Immune selection for altered antigen processing leads to cytotoxic T lymphocyte escape in chronic HIV-1 infection. *Journal of Experimental Medicine* 199, 905–915.

EBI/EMBL. (2007) IMGT/HLA Database, release 2.17.0. European Bioinformatics Institute/European Molecular Biology Laboratory. Available at www.ebi.ac.uk/imgt/hla/

Falk, K. Rotzschke, O., Stevanovic, S., Jung, G., & Rammensee, H-G. (1991) Allele-specific motifs revealed by sequencing of self-peptides. *Nature* 351, 290–296.

Flower, D.R. (2003) Towards in silico prediction of immunogenic epitopes. *Trends in Immunology* 24, 667–674.

Gadola, S.D., Moins-Teisserenc, H.T., Trowsdale, J., Gross, W.L., & Cerundolo, V. (2000) TAP deficiency syndrome. *Clinical and Experimental Immunlogy* 121, 173–178.

Gao, X., Nelson, G.W., Karacki, P., Martin, M.P., Phair, J., Kaslow, R., Goedert, J.J., Buchbinder, S., Hoots, K., Vlahov, D., O'Brien, S.J., & Carrington, M. (2001) Effect of a single amino acid change in MHC class I molecules on the rate of progression of AIDS. *New England Journal of Medicine* 344, 1668–1675.

Gobin, S.J.P., van Zutphen, M., Woltman, A.M., & van den Elsen, P.J. (1999) Transactivation of classical and nonclassical HLA class I genes through the IFN-stimulated immune response element. *Journal of Immunology* 163, 1428–1434.

Goulder, P.J.R., Phillips, R.E., Colbert, R.A., McAdam, S., Ogg, G., Nowak, M.A., Giangrande, P., Luzzi, G., Morgan, B., & Edwards, A. (1997) Late escape from an immunodominant cytotoxic T-lymphocyte response associated with progression to AIDS. *Nature Medicine* 3, 212–217.

Hammer, R.E., Maika, S.D., Richardson, J.A., Tang, J.P., & Taurog, J.D. (1990) Spontaneous inflammatory disease in transgenic rats expressing HLA-B27 and human beta 2m: An animal model of HLA-B27-associated human disorders. *Cell* 63, 1099–1122.

Hansasuta, P., Dong, T., Thananchai, H., Weckes, M., Willberg, C., Aledemir, H., Rowland-Jones, S., & Braud, V.M. (2004) Recognition of HLA-A3 and HLA-A11 by KIR3DL2 is peptide-specific. *European Journal of Immunology* 34, 1673–1679.

Hiby, S.E., Walker, J.J., O'Shaughnessy, K.M., Redman, C.W.G., Carrington, M., Trowsdale, J., & Moffett, A. (2004) Combinations of maternal KIR and fetal HLA-C genes influence the risk of preeclampsia and reproductive success. *Journal of Experimental Medicine* 200, 957–965.

Hildesheim, A., Apple, R.J., Chen, C.J., Wang, S.S., Cheng, Y.J., Klitz, W., Mack, S.J., Chen, I.H., Hsu, M.M., Yang, C.S., Brinton, L.A., Levine, P.H., & Erlich, H.A. (2002) Association of HLA class I and II alleles and extended haplotypes with nasopharyngeal carcinoma in Taiwan. *Journal of the National Cancer Institute* 94, 1780–1789.

Hill, A.V.S., Allsopp, C.E., Kwiatowski, D., Anstey, N.M., Twumansi, P., Rowe, P.A., Bennett, S., Brewster, S., McMichael, A.J., & Greenwood, B.M. (1991) Common west African HLA antigens are associated with protection from severe malaria. *Nature* 352, 595–600.

Hill, A., Jugovic, P., York, I., Russ, G., Bennink, J., Yewdell, J., Ploegh, H., & Johnson, D. (1995) Herpes simplex virus turns off the TAP to evade host immunity. *Nature* 375, 411–415.

Hirankarn, N., Kimkong, I., & Mutirangura, A. (2004) HLA-E polymophism in patients with nasopharyngeal carcinoma. *Tissue Antigens* 64, 588–592.

Hohler, T., Gerken, G., Schneider, P.M., Meyer zum Buschenfelde, K.H., & Rittner, C. (1996) Antigen-processing polymorphism in chronic hepatitis C infection. *Experimental and Clinical Immunogenetics* 13, 7–11.

Horton R., Wilming, L., Rand, V., Lovering, R.C., Bruford, E.A., Khodiyar, V.K., Lush, M.J., Povey, S., Talbot, C.C., Wright, M.W., Wain, H.M., Trowsdale, J., Ziegler, A., & Beck, S. (2004) Gene map of the extended human MHC. *Nature Reviews in Immunology* 5, 889–899.

Huang, F., Yamaguchi, A., Tsuchiya, N., Ikawa, T., Tamura, N., Virtala, M.M., Granfors, K., Yasaei, P., & Yu, D.T. (1997) Induction of alternative splicing of HLA-B27 by bacterial invasion. *Arthritis and Rheumatism* 40, 694–703.

Ishitani, A., Sageshima, N., Lee, N., Dorofeeva, N., Hatake, K., Marquadt, H., & Geraghty, D.E. (2003) Protein expression and peptide binding suggest unique and interacting functional roles for HLA-E, F, and G in maternal-placental immune recognition. *European Journal of Immunology* 171, 1376–1384.

Jeffrey, K.J., Ysuku, K., Hall, S.E., Matsumoto, W., Taylor, G.P., Procter, J., Bunce, M., Ogg, G.S., Welsh, K.I., Weber, J.N., Lloyd, A.L., Nowak, M.A., Nagai, M., Kodama, D., Izumo, S., Osame, M., & Bangham, C.R. (1999) HLA alleles determine human T-lymphotropic virus-1 (HTLV-1) proviral load and the risk of HTLV-1-associated myelopathy. *Proceedings of the National Academy of Sciences of the United States of America* 96, 3848–3853.

Kaslow, R.A., Carrington, M., Apple, R., Park, L., Munoz, A., Saah, A.J., Goedert, J.J., Winkler, C., O'Brien, S.J., Rinaldo, C., Detels, R., Blattner, W., Phair, J., Erlich, H., & Mann, D.L. (1996) Influence of combinations of human major histocompatibility complex genes on the course of HIV-1 infection. *Nature Medicine* 2, 405–411

Keat, A., Dixey, J., Sonnex, C., Thomas, B., Osborn, M., & Taylor-Robinson, D. (1987) Chlamydia trachomatis and reactive arthritis: The missing link. *Lancet* 1, 72–74.

Khakoo, S.I., Thio, C.L., Martin, M.P., Brooks, C.R., Gao, X., Astemborski, J., Cheng, J., Goedert, J.J., Vlahov, D., Hilgartner, M., Cox, S., Little, A.M., Alexander, G.J., Cramp, M.E., O'Brien, S.J., Rosenberg, W.M., Thomas, D.L., & Carrington, M. (2004) HLA and NK inhibitory receptor genes in resolving hepatitis C virus infection. *Science* 305, 872–874.

Kiepiela, P., Leslie, A.J., Honeyborne, I., Ramduth, D., Thobakgale, C., Chetty, S., Rathnavalu, P., Moore, C., Pjafferott, K.J., Hilton, L., Zimbwa, P., Moore, S., Allen T., Brander, C., Addo, M.M., Altfield, M., James, I., Mallal, S., Bunce, M., Barber, L.D., Szinger, J., Day, C., Klenerman, P., Mullins, J., Korber, B., Coovadia, H.M., Walker, B.D., & Goulder, P.J.R. (2004) Dominant influence of HLA-B in mediating the potential co-evolution of HIV and HLA. *Nature* 432, 769–774.

Kollinberger, S., Bird, L., Sun, M.Y., Retiere, C., Braud, V.M., McMichael, A., & Bowness, P. (2002) Cell surface expression and immune receptor recognition of HLA-B27 homodimers. *Arthritis and Rheumatism* 46, 2972–2982.

Koopman, J.O., Hammmerling, G.J., & Momburg, F. (1997) Generation, intracellular transport and loading of peptides associated with MHC class I molecules. *Current Opinions in Immunology* 9, 80–88.

Lajoie, J., Zijenah, L.S., Faucher, M-C., Ward, B.J., & Roger, M. (2003) Novel TAP-1 polymorphisms in indigenous Zimbabweans: Their potential implications on TAP function and in human diseases. *Human Immunology* 64, 823–829.

Lepin, E.J.M., Bastin, J.M., Allan, D.S.J., Roncador, G., Braud, V.M., Mason, D.Y., van der Merwe, A., McMichael, A.J., Bell, J.I., Powis, S.H., & O'Callaghan, C. (2000). Functional characterization of HLA-F tetramers to ILT2 and ILT4 receptors. *European Journal of Immunology* 30, 3552–3561.

Leonardo, M., Chan, K.M., Homung, F., McFarland, H., Siegel, R., Wang, J., & Zheng, L. (1999) Mature T lymphocyte apoptosis—immune regulation in a dynamic and unpredictable antigenic environment. *Annual Reviews in Immunology* 17, 221–253.

Leslie, A., Kavanagh, D., Honeyborne, I., Pfafferott, K., Edwards, C., Pillay, T., Hilton, L., Thobakgale, C., Ramduth, D., Draenert, R., Le Gall, S., Luzzi, G., Edwards, A., Brander, C., Sewell, A.K., Moore, S., Mullins, J., Moore, C., Mallal, S., Bhardwaj, N., Yusim, K., Phillips, R., Klenerman, P., Korber, B., Kiepiela, P., Walker, B., & Goulder, P. (2005) Transmission and accumulation of CTL escape variants drive negative associations between HIV polymorphisms and HLA. *Journal of Experimental Medicine* 201, 891–902.

Leslie, A.J., Pfafferott, K.J., Chetty, P., Draenert, R., Addo, M.M., Feeney, M., Tang, Y., Holmes, E.C., Allen, T., Prado, J.G., Altfield, M., Brander, C., Dixon, C., Ramduth, D., Jeena, P., Thomas, S.A., St John, A., Roach, T.A., Kupfer, B., Luzzi, G., Edwards, A., Taylor, G., Lyall, H., Tudor-Williams, G., Novelli, V., Martinez-Picado, J., Kiepiela, P., Walker, B.D., & Goulder, P.J. (2004) HIV evolution: CTL escape mutation and reversion after transmission. *Nature Medicine* 10, 282–289.

Li, L., & Bouvier, M. (2004) Structures of HLA-A1101 complexed with immunodominant nonamer and decamer HIV-1 epitopes clearly reveal the presence of a middle, secondary anchor residue. *Journal of Immunology* 172, 6175–6184.

Lim, J.K., Hunter, J., Fernandez-Vina, M., & Mann, D.L. (1999) Characterization of LMP polymorphism in homozygous typing cells and a random population. *Human Immunology* 60, 145–151.

Liu, C., Carrington, M., Kaslow, R.A., Gao, X., Rinaldo, C.R., Jacobson, L.P., Margolik, J.B., Phair, J., O'Brien, S.J., & Detels, R. (2003) Association of polymorphisms in HLA class I and transporter associated with antigen processing genes with resistance to HIV-1 infection. *Journal of Infectious Diseases* 187, 1404–1410.

Lopez de Castro, J. (1998) The pathogenic role of HLA-B27 in chronic arthritis. *Current Opinion in Immunology.* 10, 59–66.

Lund, O., Nielsen, M., Kesmir, C., Petersen, A.G., Lundegaard, C., Worning, P., Sylvester-Hvid, C., Lamberth, K., Roder, G., Justesen, S., Buus, S., & Brunak, S. (2004) Definition of supertypes for HLA molecules using clustering of specificity matrices. *Immunogenetics* 55, 797–810.

Madden, D.R., Gorga, J.C., Strominger, J.L., & Wiley, D.C. (1990) The structure of HLA B27 reveals nonamer self-peptides bound in an extended formation. *Nature* 353, 321–325.

Mallal, S., Nolan, D., Witt, C., Masel, G., Martin, A.M., Moore, C., Sayer, D., Castley, A., Mamotte, C., Maxwell, D., James, I., & Christiansen, F.T. (2002) Association between the presence of HLA-B*5701, HLA-DR7, and HLA-DQ3 and hypersensitivity to HIV-1 reverse-transcriptase inhibitor abacavir. *Lancet* 359, 727–732.

Mangasarian, A., Piguet, V., Wang, J.K., Chen, Y.L., & Trono, D. (1999) Nef-induced CD4 and major histocompatibility complex class I (MHC-1) downregulation are governed by distinct determinants: N-terminal alpha helix and proline repeat of *nef* selectively regulate MHC-1 trafficking. *Journal of Virology* 73, 1964–1973.

Martin, A.M., Nolan, D., Gaudieri, S., Almeida, C.A., Nolan, R., James, I., Carvalho, F., Phillips, E., Christiansen, F.T., Purcell, A.W., McCluskey, J., & Mallal, S. (2004) Predisposition to abacavir hypersensitivity conferred by HLA-B*5701 and a haplotypic Hsp70-Hom variant. *Proceedings of the National Academy of Sciences of the United States of America* 101, 4180–4185.

Matte, C., Lajoie, J., Lacaille, J., Zijenah, L.S., Ward, B.J., & Roger, M. (2004) Functionally active HLA-G polymorphisms are associated with the risk of heterosexual HIV-1 infection in African women. *AIDS* 18, 427–431.

McMichael, A.J., & O'Callaghan, C.A. (1998) A new look at T cells. *Journal of Experimental Medicine* 187, 1367–1371.

MHC Sequencing Consortium. (1999) Complete sequence and gene map of a human major histocompatibility complex. *Nature* 401, 921–923.

Middleton, D., Menchaca, L., Rood, H., & Komerofsky, R. 2007. Allele frequencies in worldwide populations: New allele frequency database. Available at www.allelefrequencies.net

Moore, C.B., John, M., James, I.R., Christiansen, F.T., Witt, C., & Mallal, S.A. (2002) Evidence of HIV-1 adaptation to HLA-restricted immune responses at a population level. *Science* 296, 1439–1443.

Mongkolsapaya, J., Dejinirattisai, W., Xu, X., Vasanwathana, S., Tangthawornchaikul, N., Chairunsri, A., Sawasdivorn, S., Duangchinda, T., Dong, T., Rowland-Jones, S., Yenchitsomanus, P.T., McMichael, A., Malasit, P., & Screaton, G. (2003) Original antigenic sin and apoptosis in the pathogenesis of dengue hemorrhagic fever. *Nature Medicine* 9, 921–927.

Moretta, L.O., Bottino, C., Pende, D., Vitale, M., Mingari, M.C., & Moretta, A. (2004) Different check points in human NK cell activation. *Trends in Immunology* 25, 670–676.

Ng, M.H.L., Lau, K-M., Li, L., Cheng, S-H., Chan, W.Y., Hui, P.K., Zee, B., Leung, C-H., & Sung, J.J.Y. (2004) Association of human-leukocyte-antigen class I (B*0703) and class II (DRB1*0301) genotypes with susceptibility and resistance to the development of severe acute respiratory syndrome. *Journal of Infectious Diseases* 190, 515–518.

Nussbaum, A.K., Kuttler, C., Tenzer, S.& Hansjorg, S. (2003) Using the world wide web for predicting CTL epitopes. *Current Opinion in Immunology* 15, 69–74.

Obst, R., Armandola, E.A., Nijenhuis, M., Momburg, F., & Hammerling, G.J. (1995) TAP polymorphism does not influence transport of peptide variants in mice and humans. *European Journal of Immunology* 25, 2170–2176.

Ogg, G.S., Jin, X., Bonhoeffer, S., Dunbar, P.R., Nowak, M.A., Monard, S., Segal, J.P., Cao, Y., Rowland-Jones, S.L., Cerundolo, V., Hurley, A., Markowitz, M., Ho, D.D., Nixon, D.F., & McMichael, A.J. (1998) Quantitation of HIV-1-specific cytotoxic T lymphocytes and plasma load of viral RNA. *Science* 279, 2103–2106.

Pamer, E., & Cresswell, P. (1998) Mechanisms of MHC class I-restricted antigen processing. *Annual Reviews in Immunology* 16, 323–358.

Parham, P. (2004) NK cells and trophoblasts: Partners in pregnancy. *Journal of Experimental Medicine* 200, 951–955.

Parham, P. (2005) MHC class I molecules and KIRS in human history, health and survival. *Nature Reviews in Immunology* 9, 201–214.

Parham, P., & Ohta, T. (1996) Population biology of antigen presentation by MHC class I molecules. *Science* 272, 67–74.

Park, B., Kim, Y., Shin, J., Lee, S., Cho, K., Fruh, K., & Ahn, K. (2004) Human cytomegalovirus inhibits tapasin-dependent peptide loading and optimization of the MHC class I peptide cargo for immune evasion. *Immunity* 20, 71–85.

Peh, C.A., Burrows, S.R., Barnden, M., Khanna, R., Cresswell, P., Moss, D.J., & McCluskey, J. (1998) HLA-B27 restricted antigen presentation in the absence of tapasin reveals polymorphism in mechanisms of HLA class I peptide loading. *Immunity* 8, 531–542.

Ploegh, H.L., Orr, H.T., & Strominger, J.L. (1980) Molecular cloning of a human histocompatibility antigen cDNA fragment. *Proceedings of the National Academy of Sciences of the United States of America* 77, 6081–6085.

Prugnolle, F., Manica, A., Charpentier, M., Guegan, J.F., Guernier, V., & Balloux, F. (2005) Pathogen-driven selection of worldwide HLA class I diversity. *Current Biology* 15, 1022–1027.

Rahman, M.U., Cheema, M.A., Schumacher, H.R., & Hudson, H.P. (1992) Molecular evidence for the presence of *Chlamydia* in the synovium of patients with Reiter's syndrome. *Arthritis and Rheumatism* 35, 521–529.

Rickinson, A.B., Murray, R.J., Brooks, J., Griffin, H., Moss, D.J., & Masucci, M.G. (1992) T cell recognition of Epstein-Barr virus associated lymphomas. *Cancer Surveys* 13, 53–80.

Roddis, M., Carter, R.W., Sun, M.Y., Weissensteiner, T., McMichael, A.J., Bowness, P., & Bodmer, H.C. (2004) Fully functional HLA-B27-restricted CD4(+) as well as CD8(+) T cell responses in TCR transgenic mice. *Journal of Immunology* 172, 155–161.

Rousseau, P., Masternak, K., Krawczyk, M., Reith, W., Dausset, J., Carosella, E.D., & Moreau, P. (2004) In vivo, RFX5 binds differently to the human leucocyte antigen-E, -F, and -G promoters and participates in HLA class I protein expression in a cell type-dependent manner. *Immunology* 111, 53–65.

Sathiamurthy, M., Hickman, H.D., Cavett, J.W., Zahoor, A., Prilliman, K., Metcalf, S., Fernandez Vina, M.A., & Hildebrand, W.H. (2003) Population of the HLA ligand database. *Tissue Antigens* 61, 12–19.

Schwartz, O., Marechal, V., LeGall, S., Lemmonier, F., & Heard, J.M. (1996) Endocytosis of major histocompatibility complex class I molecules is induced by the HIV-1 Nef protein. *Nature Medicine* 2, 338–342.

Schwimmbeck, P.L., Yu, D.T., & Oldstone, M.B. (1987) Autoantibodies to HLA-B27 in the sera of HLA B27 patients with ankylosing spondylitis and Reiter's syndrome. Molecular mimicry with *Klebsiella pneumoniae* as a potential mechanism of autoimmunity. *Journal of Experimental Medicine* 166, 173–181.

Sette, A., & Sidney, J. (1999) Nine major HLA class I supertypes account for the vast preponderance of HLA-A and -B polymorphism. *Immunogenetics* 50, 201–212.

Sette, A., Sidney, J., Livingston, B.D., Dzuris, J.L., Crimi, C., Walker, C.M., Southwood, S., Collins, E.J., & Hughes, A.I. (2003) Class I molecules with similar peptide-binding specificities are the result of both common ancestry and convergent evolution. *Immunogenetics* 54, 830–841.

Sidney, J., Grey, H.M., Kubo, R.T., & Sette, A. (1996) Practical, biochemical and evolutionary implications of the discovery of HLA class I supermotifs. *Immunology Today* 17, 261–266.

Stephens, H.A.F. (2002) MICA and MICB genes: Can the enigma of their polymorphism be resolved? *Trends in Immunology* 22, 378–385.

Stephens, H.A.F. (2005) HIV-1 diversity versus HLA class I polymorphism. *Trends in Immunology* 26, 41–47.

Stephens, H.A.F., Klaythong R., Sirikong, M., Vaughn, D.W., Green, S., Kalayanarooj, S., Endy, T.P., Libraty, D.H., Nisalak, A., Innis, B.L., Rothman, A.L., Ennis, F.A., & Chandanayingyong, D. (2002) HLA-A and B allele associations with secondary infections, correlate with disease severity and the infecting dengue virus serotype in ethnic Thais. *Tissue Antigens* 60, 309–318.

Stewart-Jones, G.B.E., di Gleria, K., Kollnberger, S., McMichael, A.J., Jones, E.Y., & Bowness, P. (2005) Crystal structures and KIR3DL1 recognition of three immunodominant viral peptides complexed to HLA-B*2705. *European Journal of Immunology* 35, 341–351.

Sylvester-Hvid, C., Nielsen, M., Lamberth, K., Justensen, S., Lundegaard, C., Worning, P., Thomadsen, H., Lund, O., Brunak, S., & Buus, S. (2004) SARS CTL vaccine candidates; HLA supertype-, genome-wide scanning and biochemical validation. *Tissue Antigens* 63, 395–400.

Tang, J., Costello, C., Keet, I.P., Rivers, C., Leblanc, S., Karita, E., Allen, S., & Kaslow, R.A. (1999) HLA class I homozygosity accelerates disease progression in HIV-1 infection. *AIDS Research and Human Retroviruses* 15, 317–324.

Thio, C.L., Gao, X., Goedert, J.J., Vlahov, D., Nelson, K.E., Hilgartner, M.W., O'Brien, S.J., Karacki, P., Astemborski, J., Carrington, M., & Thomas, D.L. (2002) HLA-Cw*04 and hepatitis C persistence. *Journal of Virology* 76, 4792–4797.

Thio, C.L., Thomas, D.L., Karacki, P., Gao, X., Marti, D., Kaslow, R.A., Goedert, J.J., Higartner, M.W., Strathdee, S.A., Duggal, P., O'Brien, S.J., Astemborski, J., & Carrington, M. (2003) Comprehensive analysis of class I and class II HLA antigens and chronic hepatitis B infection. *Journal of Virology* 77, 12083–12087.

Trinchieri, G. (1989) Biology of natural killer cells. *Advances in Immunology* 47, 187–376.

Tussey, L.G., Rowland-Jones, S., Zheng, T.S., Androlewicz, M.J., Cresswell, P., Frelinger, J.A., & McMichael, A.J. (1995) Different MHC class I alleles compete for presentation of overlapping viral epitopes. *Immunity* 3, 65–77.

Van Parijis, L., & Abbas, A.K. (1998) Homeostasis and self-tolerance in the immune system: Turning lymphocytes off. *Science* 280, 243–248.

Williams, A.P., Bevan, S., Bunce, M., Houlston, R., Welsh, K.I., & Elliott, T. (2000) Identification of novel *Tapasin* polymorphisms and linkage disequilibrium with MHC class I alleles. *Immunogenetics* 52, 9–11.

Yokomaku, Y., Miura, H., Tomiyama, H., Kawana-Tachikawa, A., Takiguchi, M., Kojima, A., Nagai, Y., Iwamoto, A., Matsuda, Z., & Ariyoshi, K. (2004) Impaired processing and presentation of cytotoxic-T-lymphocyte (CTL) epitopes are major escape mechanisms from CTL immune pressure in HIV-1 infection. *Journal of Virology* 78, 1324–1332.

Zinkernagel, R.M., & Doherty, P.C. (1997) The discovery of MHC restriction. *Immunology Today* 18, 14–17.

5

MHC Class II and Related Genes

Janet M. McNicholl, Peter E. Jensen, & Jeremy M. Boss

The MHC class II antigen-processing pathway plays a central role in the adaptive immune response to microbial pathogens as the mechanism through which ligands are generated for recognition by CD4$^+$ helper T cells. CD4$^+$ helper T cells are activated by recognition of short peptide antigens stably bound to MHC class II molecules expressed on the surface of specialized antigen-presenting cells (APC), such as dendritic cells. Activated CD4$^+$ T cells are required to generate high-affinity antibody responses through their capacity to interact with antigen-specific B cells to promote isotype switching, somatic mutation of immunoglobulin genes, and the generation of memory B cells. Through cytokine production and direct activation of dendritic cells, CD4$^+$ T cells also promote the induction of CD8$^+$ cytolytic T-cell responses. Moreover, helper T cells mediate delayed-type hypersensitivity effector mechanisms by recruiting and activating macrophages and other components of the innate immune system. By controlling antigen recognition by CD4$^+$ T cells, MHC class II proteins (e.g., the HLA-DR, -DP, and -DQ molecules), together with co-factor and accessory MHC molecules (e.g., HLA-DM and -DO and the invariant chain) and transcription factors (RFX and CIITA), have a profound impact on all the major effector mechanisms employed in adaptive immune responses.

MHC Genes and Alleles, Diversity, and Population Genetics

In humans, the genes encoding MHC class II α- and β-chains, including genes for HLA-DM and -DO, encompass almost 700,000 bp of DNA on chromosome 6p21.31 (MHC Sequencing Consortium, 1999) (figure 5.1, table 5.1). This region encodes more than 21 additional genes and more than 25 pseudogenes, making it one of the most gene-dense regions of the human genome (Mungall et al., 2003). MHC class II genes display tremendous allelic polymorphism. More than 790 alleles have been listed for the *DRA1* and

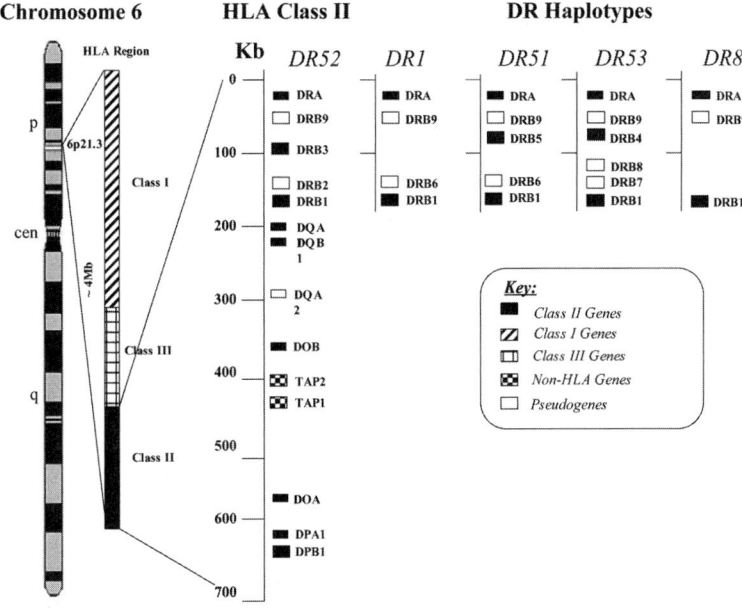

FIGURE 5.1. Organization of the MHC region on chromosome 6. Class I, II, and III regions are indicated. DR haplotypes comprising different combinations of genes and pseudogenes are indicated; serologic specificities are identified (top). Figure adapted from the MHC map at the NIH/NCBI db MHC Web site.

DRB1, DQA1 and *DQB1, DPA1* and *DPB1, DMA* and *DMB,* and *DOA* and *DOB* genes combined (table 5.1). Web sites such as the European Bioinformatics Institute (EBI) HLA Web site (www.ebi.ac.uk/imgt/hla) and others listed in table 5.1 provide updated lists, maps, sequence alignments, and additional allele and haplotype information. Loci for the accessory molecule, (Ii chain), the RFX components, and the CIITA occur on five different chromosomes outside the MHC.

The ability to express multiple MHC class II genes and alleles creates a system with great potential to present antigenic peptides. This enormous polymorphism among the alleles would seem to ensure that, within any relatively local subgroup of the human population, several individuals would be able to appropriately present an antigen from an epidemic/pandemic causing pathogen. Thus, this high degree of allelic polymorphism represents a way to ensure the survival of the species. In contrast, being diploid and expressing multiple genes and alleles are likely to benefit the individual, as well. Every individual has the potential to express multiple different allelic forms of MHC II molecules in various haplotypes (figure 5.1). However, the optimal number for effective immune function is not clear. If the expression of multiple MHC II alleles/haplotypes is beneficial, it might seem reasonable to assume that more variants would be better. On the other hand, the most advantageous number may be lower than expected, reflecting the dual role of MHC class II molecules. Because these molecules also function to select against self-reactive T cells, substantially greater diversity may lead to recognition of larger portions of self peptides, reduction in the T-lymphocyte repertoire and suppression of the critical antigen recognition function of MHC class II molecules.

Worldwide, substantial differences in frequencies of specific HLA alleles as well as in allelic and haplotypic diversity are observed from one population to another. Population diversity at the HLA loci is greatest in African populations (Olerup et al., 1991) and least in some isolated populations. Web sites such as www.allelefrequencies.net and others in table 5.1 can be used to examine MHC class II allelic differences by criteria such as geographic region, country, or race. The reasons for these differences include geographic isolation and population bottlenecks, natural selection, and environmental factors, including infectious

TABLE 5.1. Summary information on HLA class II and associated genes.

NCBI Gene ID	Common Name(s)	Entrez Gene ID (Locus Link)	Map Position[a]	Polymorphisms[b]	No. of Alleles[c]	mRNA (NM) No.
HLA-DRA	HLA-DR1; HGNC no. 4947	3122	6p21.3	≥ 83, mostly intronic or UTR; 6 coding	3	019111
HLA-DRB1[d]	HLA-DRB1, HLADRl1B; HGNC no. 4948	3123	6p21.3	≥ 1,042, mostly intronic, several nonsynonymous; 131 coding	429	002124
HLA-DQA1	CELIAC1, DQ-A1, HLA-QQA1; HGNC no. 4942	3117	1	≥ 722, mostly intronic or UTR, several nonsynonymous; 41 coding	32	002122
HLA-DQB1	CELIAC1, HLA-DQB1; HGNC no. 4944	3119	6p21.3	≥ 1,302, mostly intronic, some UTR; some coding;	69	002123
HLA-DPA1	HLA-DP1A, HLADP, HLASB; HGNC no. 4938	3113	6p21.3	≥ 125, mostly intronic and UTR; 14 coding	23	033554
HLA-DPB1	DPB1; HLA-DP1B, MHCDPB1; HGNC no. 4940	3115	6p21.3	≥ 378, mostly intronic or UTR, several nonsynonymous; 54 coding	121	002121
HLA-DMA	D6S222E, DMA, HLADM, RING6; HGNC no. 4934	3108	6p21.3	≥ 25, mostly intronic or UTR; 7 coding	4	006120
HLA-DMB	D6S221E, RING7; HGNC no. 4935	3109	6p21.3	≥ 40, mostly intronic or UTR; 6 coding	7	002118
HLA-DOA	HLA-DNA, HLA-DZA, HLADZ; HGNC no. 4936	3111	6p21.3	≥ 43, mostly intronic or UTR; 8 coding	12	002119
HLA-DOB	DOB; HGNC no. 4937	3112	6p21.3	≥ 15, mostly intronic or UTR; 14 coding	9	002120
CD74	Invariant chain, Ii, DHLAG, HLADG, Ia-γ, protein 41, HLA-DR-γ, Ia-associated invariant chain, MHC HLA-DR γ-chain, γ-chain of class II antigens	972	5q32	≥ 39, mostly intronic and UTR, some nonsynonymous; 3 coding		001025159

Gene	Description	Gene ID	Location	Polymorphisms	Entrez ID (last digits)
RFX5[e]	MHC class II regulatory factor RFX, enhancer factor C	5993	1q21	≥ 24, intronic, UTR and other regions; 9 coding	00449
RFXAP[e]	RFX DNA-binding complex 36 kDa subunit, RFX-associated protein	5994	13q14	≥ 21, intronic, UTR and other regions; some insertions and deletions; 3 coding	000538
RFXANK[e]	RFX-B, ANKRA1, DNA-binding protein RFXANK, ankyrin repeat-containing regulatory factor X-associated protein, regulatory factor X BLS group B	8625	19p12	≥ 16 including deletions (exons 4, 6), a transversion and others; 1 coding	003721
CIITA	MHC class II transactivator, MHC2TA	4261	16p13	≥ 18, mostly intronic and UTR (some nonsynonymous between amino acids 75 and 1057); 14 coding	000246

HGNC, Human Genome Organization (HUGO) Nomenclature Committee.

[a]To view a map of these genes at the NCBI Web site, use the Entrez gene ID as the last four digits of the search string. For example, to see a map of the HLA-DRA locus, use the following link: www.ncbi.nlm.nih.gov/mapview/map_search.cgi?direct=on&idtype=gene&id=3122. For other genes, use the same string and change the last four digits.

[b]Summary information only is provided here since new variants are frequently found. Single nucleotide polymorphism (SNP) counts are as of January 2006 in dpSNP (which includes short changes of several bases as well as single base changes). Not all reported SNPs have been validated. To access gene dbSNP data, a useful strategy is to go to www.ncbi.nlm.nih.gov/entrez, select the "Gene" database in the search field, and insert the gene name in the "for" field. When the gene information is retrieved, click on links, select "Gene view in dbSNP," and view the polymorphisms using the various "view rs (reference sequence number)" choices.

[c]The number of alleles is as of January 2006 from the EBI HLA Web site: www.ebi.ac.uk/imgt/hla/index.html. Allele frequencies are not listed for the accessory and co-factor genes since variants are rare. The NCBI dbMHC database (www.ncbi.nlm.nih.gov/projects/mhc) is synchronized with the IMGT/HLA database and has other useful information, including primer sequences and typing kits. Other useful Web sites are www.anthonynolan.org.uk/HIG/data.html, www.allelefrequencies.net, www.ashi-hla.org/, www.sanger.ac.uk/HGP/Chr6, www.hgmp.mrc.uk, and other linked Web sites.

[d]HLA-DRB1 information is listed. The total number of alleles for all DRB genes (DRB1–DRB9) is 511 in early 2006, including the following number at each locus other than DRB1: B2, 1; B3, 43; B4, 13; B5, 18; B6, 3; B7, 2; B8, 1; B9, 1.

[e]Proteins coded for by these three genes combine to form RFX.

diseases. Some evidence for pathogen-driven selection of certain MHC types has been provided by high frequencies of HLA class I and II alleles or haplotypes (e.g., HLA DRB1*1302-DQB1*0501) apparently associated with resistance to severe malaria in malaria-endemic regions of West Africa such as The Gambia (Hill et al., 1991; see also chapter 24).

Specific combinations of HLA class I, II, and III alleles are found more frequently than expected by chance alone. This phenomenon, known as linkage disequilibrium, has preserved large segments of the MHC as haplotypes of specific alleles inherited en bloc (see chapter 1). Although there is intense interest in the mechanisms of and reasons for linkage disequilibrium, it is generally accepted that combinations of alleles inherited in such linked segments provide some selection advantage to the host or population. The exceptional allelic diversity coupled with highly population-specific disequilibrium patterns must be taken into account in the design, sample size projection, and analysis of studies to identify HLA–disease associations. In analysis, the HLA data should be examined for Hardy-Weinberg equilibrium, and if possible, analyses should be performed at allelic, genotypic, and haplotypic levels. The large number of statistical tests performed on the many markers screened in a typical HLA study can easily generate false positive results and must be accounted for in interpreting the results, Multiplication of the calculated p-value for each separate statistical test by the number of tests performed (Bonferroni correction) is frequently considered too conservative. Alternative approaches (e.g., false discovery rate) are under investigation, but details are beyond the scope of this review. Replication of findings in one or more additional cohorts or using a different study design is essential. Weak associations will often fail to replicate (see chapters 1, 2, and 4).

Nomenclature and Typing Methods

Nomenclature used in HLA research has largely reflected the evolution of typing methods, from serologic to mixed lymphocyte culture (MLC) to present-day molecular methods, including sequencing. Standardized nomenclature now includes an official locus name composed of the letters of the historical serotype (e.g., DR), followed by a letter corresponding to the α- or β-chain gene (A or B). An asterisk signifies typing at the nucleic acid level and separates the name of the

gene from that of the allele, again broadly following the historical serotype designation (e.g., *01, *02, *03). The third and fourth digits indicate variation to the individual nonsynonymous nucleotide level (e.g., DRB1*0101, DRB1*0102, DRB1*0103). The relation between the older and new nomenclature is usually self-evident (e.g., DR1 corresponds to DRB1*01xx, and DR4 with DRB1*04xx). However, some serotype counterparts (e.g., DR2 and DR3) are not obvious: DR2 for DRB1*1501 and 1601 and DR3 for *1701 and *1801 (these are frequently termed "splits" of the serotype). The mixed lymphocyte culture (MLC)-based "Dw" specificities have also been renamed based on sequence data. Sequence-based typing may permit complete resolution to eight digits (e.g., DRB3*01010201). Polymorphisms at the fifth through eighth positions are noncoding or synonymous changes. New sequences are submitted to the EBI HLA sequence database for checking and assignment of an official name prior to publication. This prevents problems associated with renaming published sequences or use of multiple names for the same sequence. Nomenclature updates are published monthly, and the EBI Web site provides information on nomenclature and alleles. Additional publications include the proceedings from the meeting of the WHO Nomenclature Committee for Factors of the HLA System (held annually) and the International Histocompatibility Workshops (held every four years). Today, most HLA class II typing is performed with medium- (2–4 digit) to high- (>4 digit) resolution molecular typing methods, including sequencing. A wide assortment of methods and kits are available. The National Center for Biotechnology Information (NCBI) dbMHC database (www.ncbi.nlm.nih.gov/projects/mhc; see table 5.1) is a useful MHC typing resource listing kits, primers and other reagents.

Polymorphic MHC Class II Molecules (HLA-DR, -DQ, and -DP)

Gene Products in Infection and Pathogenesis

Molecular Structure and T-Cell Interaction

The HLA-DR, -DP, and -DQ MHC class II glycoproteins are composed of two noncovalently associated polymorphic transmembrane subunits, α (33 kDa) and β (29 kDa) (figures 5.2 and 5.3). Generally, the β-chain

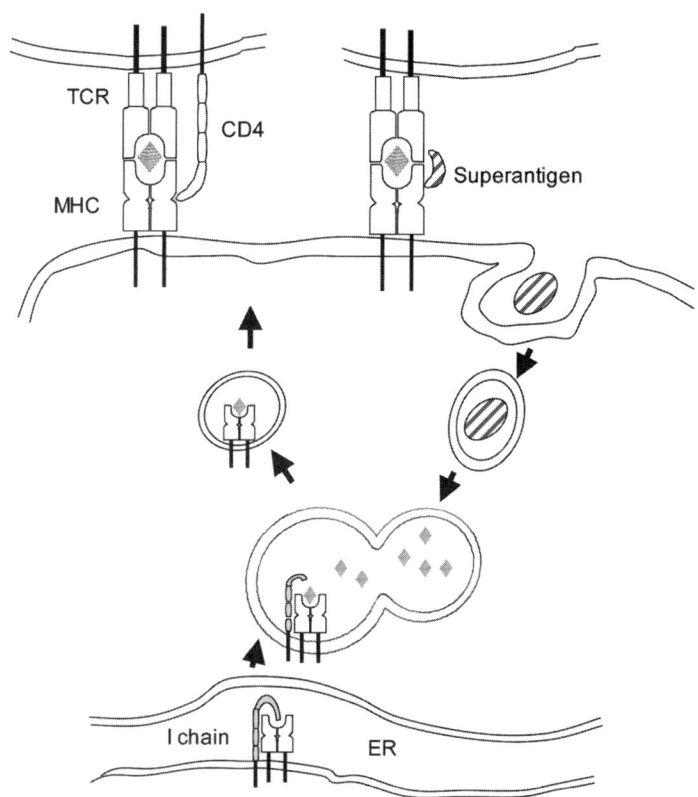

FIGURE 5.2. The HLA-class II pathway. HLA-class II molecules are synthesized in the endoplasmic reticulum (ER), where the invariant chain (Ii) blocks the peptide-binding site until the molecule transits to a compartment with processed antigen (peptide, diamond shape) where Ii is enzymatically removed and peptide is loaded. Loaded trimolecular complexes of peptide and class II heterodimer reach the cell surface where they can be recognized by T-cell receptors (TCRs) and stabilized with CD4 molecules. The interaction of superantigen with regions of TCR and MHC outside of the peptide binding site is also indicated.

is the most polymorphic of the two chains, and variability is found in the membrane-distal regions (encoded by exon 3) that fold to form the peptide-binding groove. During intracellular assembly, the proteins fold into dimers that are eventually expressed on the cell surface with bound peptide, where these trimolecular complexes are available for recognition by T-cell receptors (TCRs). The TCR variable regions (CDR3) bind to the MHC–peptide complex; docking occurs in such a way that CDR3 of the TCR overlaps the peptide, although several different configurations have been observed. The CD4 molecule on T cells binds to a relatively constant membrane-proximal part of the MHC, stabilizing it for TCR binding. After binding, signaling to the T cell (through the TCR) and to the APC (through the MHC) occurs (figure 5.2).

The ends of the MHC class II binding groove are "open," allowing binding of longer peptides (11 or more residues) than MHC class I molecules. The peptide-binding groove contains pockets that accommodate side chains of bound peptide antigen (Stern et al., 1994). The amino acids lining these pockets determine the peptide-binding motif of each MHC class

II molecule, giving it the capacity to bind peptides that share a common motif (Rammensee et al., 1999; Santori et al., 2002; Sathiamurthy et al., 2003). In HLA class II molecules, five pockets (1, 4, 6, 7, and 9, named after the peptide residues they bind), have been identified using crystallographic studies of a influenza hemagglutinin (HA) peptide-DRB*0101 complex (Stern et al., 1994). In the case of the DRB1*0401-restricted *Mycobacterium leprae* 18 kDa heat-shock protein T-cell epitope, ML38-50, a DRB1*0401-binding motif was identified that was predictable based on the characteristics of the five pockets of DRB1*0401 (McNicholl et al., 1995): a ring-structure amino acid (F) in pocket 1; an acidic, charged residue (E) in pocket 4 (where it interacts with the basic charged residue K at position 71 on the β-chain); and smaller residues in pockets 6, 7, and 9. The peptide extended beyond the binding site as predicted by the open ends. Interestingly, although the ML38-50 peptide is longer than the (HA) 307-319 peptide, it fits the MHC pockets in an almost identical register because a proline at position 8 allows it to kink out of the MHC-binding site (figure 5.3a,b). Lists of MHC-binding peptides and motif prediction programs,

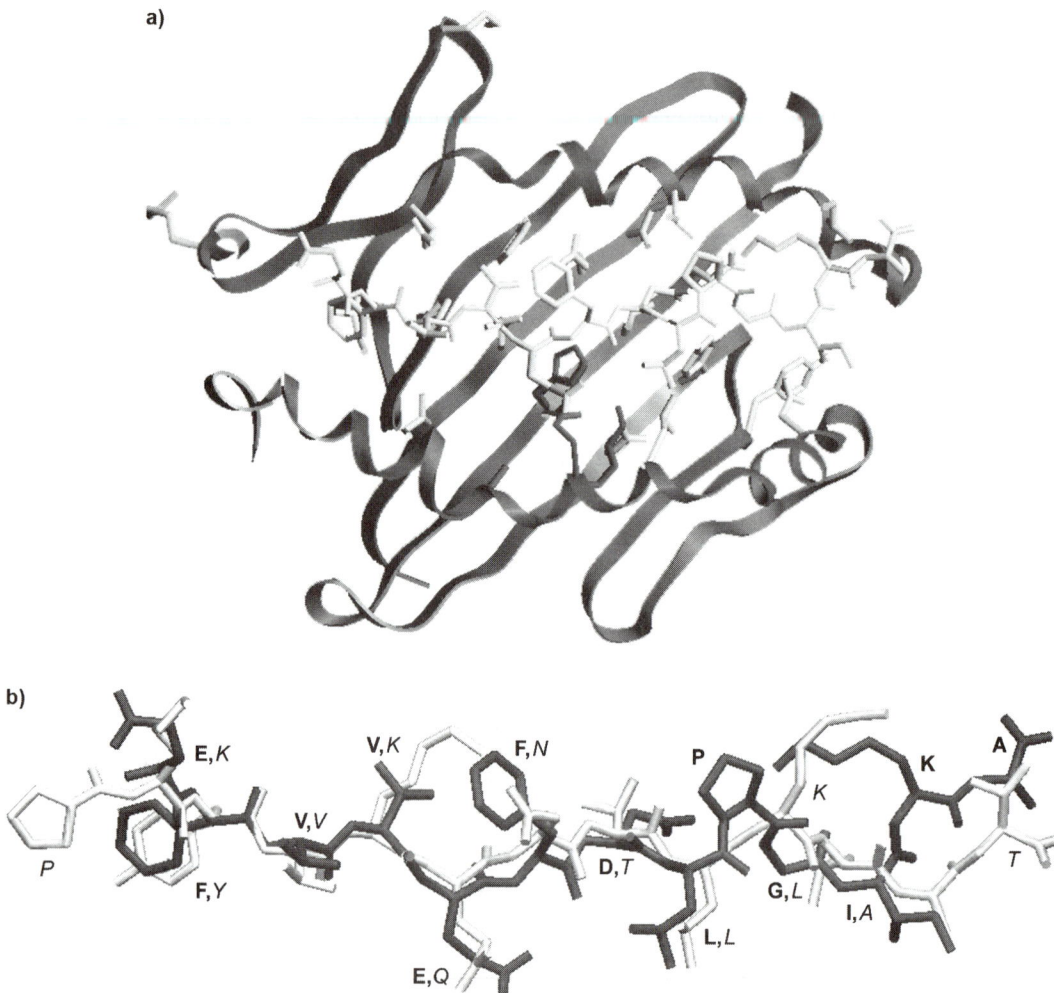

FIGURE 5.3. Views of peptide binding site and peptide. (a) Top view of a class II molecule (DRB1*0401) showing the bound 11-mer *M. leprae* heat-shock protein peptide ML38–50. The α-chain is indicated as the top ribbon; the β-chain as the bottom ribbon. ML38–50 amino acids are indicated in white, and interacting MHC amino acids in black. (b) Side views of ML-38–50 (dark gray bound to DRB1*0401) and the influenza hemagglutinin peptide, HA307–319 (light gray bound to DRB1*0101). Pocket binding residues for pockets 1, 4, 6, 7, and 9 are (in bold for ML38–50 and in regular italic font for HA307–319): **F**,*Y*; **E**, *Q*; **D**, *T*; **L**,*L*; **G**,*L*. Models are adapted from McNicholl et al., 1995.

based on MHC class II sequence and binding data, are available at several Web sites, including www.syfpeithi .de/, hiv-web.lanl.gov/content/index, and wehih.wehi .edu.au/mhcpep/.

MHC polymorphisms also have a major effect on the peripheral T-cell repertoire. During development, T cells undergo a rigorous selection process that removes T cells expressing TCRs with high affinity for self MHC–peptide complexes on APC in the thymus. In addition, developing T cells bearing TCRs with little or no affinity for self MHC–peptide complexes die from "neglect." This selection process produces a diverse repertoire of mature T cells that have some affinity for self MHC–peptide complexes, but not enough for activation of T cells to the point of generating an autoimmune pathologic response as they encounter self MHC–peptide complexes during recirculation through peripheral tissues (Goldrath and Bevan, 1999).

Thus, the T-cell repertoire is adapted to the MHC molecules expressed in the thymus of a given individual, and to the self peptides bound to these MHC molecules. Through this mechanism, MHC polymorphisms affect the repertoire of T cells that are available to respond to microbial pathogens.

In contrast to the almost ubiquitous expression of MHC class I molecules, MHC class II molecules and the co-factors that are required to promote peptide binding to these molecules are only constitutively expressed in dendritic cells, macrophages, B cells, and thymic epithelial cells, the so-called "professional" APCs. Expression of MHC class II molecules on other cells is tightly regulated by a variety of signals, including interferon-γ (IFN-γ; see below). In humans, HLA-DR variants are the most highly expressed class II molecules and likely contribute to the bulk of immune responses; however, many associations of infectious disease with HLA-DQ alleles have also been reported, and pathogen-derived DQ-restricted T-cell epitopes have been found.

Peptide Processing

The class II antigen processing and presentation pathway (figure 5.2) provides a mechanism to sample and display fragments of proteins that are present in the endosomal compartments of APC, which exhibit mechanisms for the uptake of components of microbial pathogens (Jensen et al., 1999). Protein antigens are internalized through a variety of mechanisms, including phagocytosis, receptor-mediated endocytosis, macropinocytosis, and fluid-phase endocytosis (Guermonprez et al., 2002). Internalized proteins progressively encounter more acidic and hydrolytic environment as they are transported from early endosomes to late endosomes and lysosomes. Most peptide complexes appear to be generated in lysosome-related compartments that are enriched for MHC class II molecules, termed MIIC. The mechanisms through which antigens are unfolded and cleaved into peptides remain an active area of investigation. An IFN-γ–inducible lysosomal thioreductase, GILT, has recently been discovered to catalyze the reduction of disulfide bonds, providing a key mechanism to facilitate the unfolding of disulfide-containing antigens (Arunachalam et al., 2000; Maric et al., 2001). For some antigens, exposure to the mildly acidic (~pH 5) environment in lysosomes can destabilize protein structure sufficiently to allow binding to MHC class II molecules without a requirement for proteolytic fragmentation (Jensen, 1993).

The open ends of the class II peptide binding groove impose little restriction on the length of the polypeptide that can be bound. The minimal requirement is that antigens unfold sufficiently to allow regions of the protein to structurally adapt to the peptide-binding groove. It is clear, however, that acidic endopeptidases play an important role in the processing of antigens to generate fragments available for binding to class II molecules. Several proteases have been shown to be important in the processing of model protein antigens (Manoury et al., 1998, 2002; Honey et al., 2002; Honey and Rudensky, 2003). It is likely that the key proteases differ depending on the particular APC type and the particular antigen in question. Nevertheless, this is an important area of investigation because there is no doubt that the cleavage specificity of endopeptidases involved in antigen processing has a major impact on the specific peptide epitopes that are made available for recognition by CD4[+] T cells.

Pathogen Interaction and Evasion

Given the critical role of HLA class II molecules in antigen presentation and T-cell recognition, it is not surprising that pathogens have evolved several mechanisms to harness these molecules for their own benefit. Virions of HIV-1, as they are newly generated and exit infected cells, acquire a coating of surface MHC class II and other host molecules that camouflage them to appear more like "self" (Guo and Hildreth, 1995; Lawn and Butera, 2000), and viral proteins such as Gag and Tat can alter levels of surface HLA-DR expression in infected cells (Nong et al., 1991; Kanazawa et al., 2000; Keppler et al., 2005). The Epstein-Barr virus (EBV) gp42 glycoprotein binds to HLA-DR, -DP, and -DQ molecules at a surface site on the molecule. This interaction plays a critical role in EBV infection of B lymphocytes, probably by facilitating membrane fusion (Haan and Longnecker, 2000; Mullen et al., 2002). Bacterial antigens known as superantigens (e.g., staphylococcal enterotoxin B) bind to relatively nonpolymorphic regions of HLA class II molecules and to TCRs (figure 5.2), activate multiple TCRs of different clonotypes in a non-peptide-specific way, and set in motion an immune response that can result in shock (see chapter 23). Recent studies indicate that there is some specificity to the interaction in that some superantigens such as streptococcal pyrogenic exotoxin may preferentially bind certain DR or DQ molecules (Norrby-Teglund et al., 2002; Llewelyn et al., 2004). A more peptide- and allele-specific mechanism by which pathogens may cause disease is through molecular mimicry. In this theory, pathogen-derived peptide presentation activates or expands T cells reactive for self-antigen–MHC complexes that are identical (or near identical) to the pathogen–peptide–MHC complex. In the case of an EBV protein, mimicry with a DRB1*1501-binding myelin-basic protein peptide has been implicated in the pathogenesis of multiple sclerosis (Lang et al., 2002), while mimicry between T-cell epitopes in self proteins and in the *Borrelia burgdorferi* outer surface protein has been implicated in the pathogenesis or severity of Lyme arthritis (Guerau-de-Arellano and Huber, 2002; Maier et al., 2000).

Gene Organization and Alleles

On chromosome 6p21, the loci for DP and DM are centromeric, for DQ more telomeric, and for DR most telomeric and closest to the class III region (figure 5.1). Class II genes have 5 exons: exon 1 codes for the leader peptide, exons 2 and 3 for the extracellular domains, and exons 4 and 5 for the transmembrane and cytoplasmic tails. With more than 500 alleles, *HLA-DRB1* is among the most polymorphic of the MHC class II genes, rivaled only by the *HLA-B* locus (for comparisons, see www.allelefrequencies.net). At the opposite extreme is DRA, with only three known alleles to date. Pseudogenes, often designated Ψ (or P in an official gene name) at the DRB (DRB 2-9) and other loci, do not generate expressed proteins. The combination of expressed β-chain genes and pseudogenes varies depending on the genetic haplotype of the individual (figure 5.1). Some genes and the lineages they identify were previously detected serologically (e.g., DR52 and -53). Pseudogenes are more common in individuals with fewer HLA-DRB genes. The occurrence of these pseudogenes and of the different copies of HLA-DRB genes in populations living today provides evidence that the MHC has undergone numerous evolutionary expansions/contractions.

Disease Associations

Studies of infectious disease associations with the HLA-DR, -DQ, and -DP loci span the entire range of human pathogens and cannot be fully reviewed in this chapter (see part III of this volume, and reviews in McNicholl and Cuenco, 1999; Segal and Hill, 2003). Here we emphasize some of the associations that illustrate accepted phenomena and concepts, recent and potentially novel findings, and some "orphan" areas not covered elsewhere in this text.

Studies of HLA associations with viruses that have been present in human populations for many generations have provided evidence for the phenomenon of heterozygote advantage (reviewed in Dean et al., 2002). In The Gambia, where 90% of adults are infected with hepatitis B virus before adulthood, homozygotes for DRB1 are less likely to clear hepatitis B infection and are at greater risk of becoming persistently infected and progressing to hepatocellular carcinoma (Almarri and Batchelor, 1994; Thursz et al., 1997). Since heterozygotes would be more likely to survive to reproductive age, they had a reproductive advantage. Presumably, greater diversity of HLA class II alleles in heterozygous individuals would reduce the ability of the virus to escape presentation to T cells. The observed heterozygous advantage was restricted to the HLA class II locus and was not observed for class I. Additional allelic association studies also found that DRB1*1301/2 (and other) alleles were associated with resistance to persistent infection, while DRB1*0301 and some other alleles conferred increased risk (Almarri and Batchelor, 1994; Thursz et al., 1995). It is interesting that the DRB1*0301 has also been associated with poor responses to hepatitis B vaccine (Alper et al., 1990) and with reduced risk or severity of hepatitis C infection (reviewed in Yee, 2004; see also chapter 21). These data suggest a key role for this allele in hepatitis, perhaps linked to antigen processing and presentation. Evidence for heterozygote advantage has also been found in studies of HIV-1 disease progression (e.g., Carrington et al., 1999; Tang et al., 1999). However, this has been observed only with class I and not with class II alleles. Studies of heterozygosity in human papillomavirus (HPV) infection and cervical cancer have not yet shown evidence for this phenomenon (Wang et al., 2002).

The hypothesis that HLA mismatch would reduce mother-to-child or person-to-person transmission of pathogens, perhaps by "rejection" of nonmatched cells infected with the pathogen, has been tested for HIV-1. Several studies provide evidence that mismatch at HLA class I and II loci, including the DRB3 locus, can reduce mother-to-child or heterosexual HIV-1 transmission (MacDonald et al., 1998; Lockett et al., 2001; Hader et al., 2002; Dorak et al., 2004). These observations, together with supporting data from non-human primate studies, have had implications for vaccine design, particularly in terms of choice of challenge stocks in animal studies modeling HIV-1 vaccine efficacy.

Studies of cancer have provided evidence that host gene–virus interactions lie in the causal pathway. Exposure to a HPV, particularly strain 16, in persons with HLA class II genotypes related to susceptibility, primarily HLA-DQB1*0301/2 alleles or the DRB1*1501-DQB1*0602, DQA1*0102-DQB1*0602, or DRB1*0401-DQB1*0301 haplotypes, may be associated with later development of cervical cancer, although these associations are not consistently found in all studies (reviewed in Hildesheim and Wang, 2002; Wu et al., 2006). In a recent study of HPV-16–associated cervical cancer in a Chinese population, where HLA-DQB1*0601 and 0602 were the most significantly associated alleles, analysis of shared polymorphic positions in associated versus nonassociated alleles suggested that presence of leucine at position 9 and aspartate at position 37 of the peptide-binding site were associated with risk of cervical cancer (Wu et al., 2006). These data provide a potential explanation for the association, related to antigen presentation, and may be relevant to understanding responses to the HPV vaccines licensed for the prevention of cervical cancer.

Interest in variable host susceptibility to newly emerging pathogens, such as hantavirus and severe acute respiratory syndrome (SARS), has led to studies of associations with HLA class II (and other genes). Interestingly, DRB1*03 positivity may be associated with increased risk for infection or poor outcome in SARS and hantavirus studies, respectively (Makela et al., 2002; Ng et al., 2004). These small initial studies need replication but, if confirmed, could have implications for epidemic control and vaccine design.

Few studies of genetic predisposition to infectious disease can carefully address quantitative aspects of pathogen exposure for two reasons. Disease is often identified after exposure has ended and would be difficult to quantify; moreover, the reference group (i.e., controls) usually consists of a convenience sample from a similar population rather than noncases known to have remained uninfected despite exposure. In a study of leptospirosis in triathletes where exposure to leptospire-contaminated water was quantifiable, HLA-DQ6 positivity in persons with documented exposure conferred the highest risk of infection, confirming a dose-related gene–environment interaction (Lingappa et al., 2004). The finding of an association with HLA-DQ6 but not with a specific DQ6 allele suggested a possible role for a superantigen-mediated pathogenesis. Whether this is unique to leptospirosis is not known. In the case of another spirochete, *Borrelia bugdorferi*, classical antigen presentation mechanisms are likely to influence Lyme disease risk and outcome. DRB1*01 and DRB1*04 alleles have been associated with Lyme disease susceptibility and chronic sequela; and T-cell epitopes restricted by these alleles have been identified in the outer surface protein of the spirochete.

HLA associations with mycobacterial disease (see also chapter 22) provide strong evidence that class II DR and DQ loci (particularly DRB1*15 and DQB1*06 alleles) influence disease risk or phenotype for *Mycobacterium tuberculosis* and *M. leprae*. Again, since many *M. tuberculosis* and *M. leprae* class II T-cell epitopes have been defined, it is likely that classical antigen presentation mechanisms are involved in pathogenesis. However, linkage disequilibrium between certain class II and class III alleles (e.g., at the tumor necrosis factor [TNF] locus) could implicate TNF-related mechanisms in these diseases. Polymorphisms in antigen-loading molecules such as DMA may also be relevant in mycobacterial disease pathogenesis, as observed in one study of disseminated *M. avium* complex (Naik et al., 2003; see also below).

With the exception of the superantigen-driven pathways of T-cell activation, most bacterial and viral infections appear to activate downstream events consistent with a T-helper-1 (Th-1) type cytokine profile. In contrast, in parasitic diseases, involvement or dominance of the Th-2 axis is frequently found, with eosinophilia, production of IgE and of cytokines such as interleukin-4. Despite these different downstream profiles, associations with HLA class II genes and mapping of class II–restricted epitopes indicate that classical antigen presentation is a key event in antigen recognition and pathogenesis for malaria, schistosome, and leishmania species (see chapters 24–26). If peptide-specific antigen presentation is central to infectious diseases that result in both Th-1- and Th-2-like immune responses, it is interesting to speculate what regulatory factors dictate the resultant cytokine helper type. Polymorphisms in other genes, particularly cytokine genes, or genes of natural immunity such as Toll-like receptors may be particularly important.

Accessory and Co-Factor MHC Molecules: Invariant Chain, DM, and DO

Invariant Chain (CD74, 5q32)

Gene Product in Infection and Pathogenesis

The MHC class II α- and β-chains initially assemble in the endoplasmic reticulum (ER) with the relatively nonpolymorphic chaperone protein, invariant chain (Ii) (figure 5.2). In the absence of bound peptide, "empty" αβ-heterodimers are inherently unstable. An important function of Ii is to stabilize newly synthesized class II molecules (Anderson and Miller, 1992). Ii contains an unstructured region encoded by exon 3 that fits into the class II binding groove in a manner that appears to analogous to that of the binding of peptide antigens (Ghosh et al., 1995). Other regions of Ii interact with class II molecules at sites outside of the peptide-binding groove, in essence forming a scaffolding that serves to position the exon 3-encoded segment in the peptide binding site (Thayer et al., 1999). Ii spontaneously assembles as a homotrimer that can interact with three class II αβ-heterodimers to form a nonameric oligomer (Roche et al., 1991). Ii is a type II membrane protein, and the cytoplasmic domain contains a di-leucine endosomal targeting and retention signal (Bakke and Dobberstein, 1990; Loss and Sant, 1993). Thus, a second function of Ii is to target class II molecules for localization in lysosome-related compartments. Ii is also believed to prevent class II molecules from binding peptides before they arrive in late endosomal compartments.

After transport of αβIi complexes to endosomes, Ii is degraded through a series of progressive proteolytic cleavage events, leaving only the fragment encoded by exon 3, termed class II–associated invariant chain peptide (CLIP), associated with the class II molecule. CLIP is protected from cleavage because it is largely buried in the class II peptide-binding groove. Several specific proteases have been identified that participate in proteolytic release of Ii in different cell types (Honey and Rudensky, 2003; Manoury et al., 2003). At this point, class II molecules are no longer tethered to endosomal targeting signals in the cytoplasmic domains of Ii, and they are free to travel to the cell surface. Thus, there is a short window of time within which CLIP must be released from the peptide-binding groove and replaced by antigenic peptides represented in the en-

dosomal compartment. The intrinsic affinity of class II molecules for the CLIP peptide differs widely depending on the allele. The CLIP sequence appears to have evolved such that it can bind to all class II molecules, but none too well (Thayer et al., 1999). If high binding affinity prevented easy release of CLIP from the peptide-binding groove in endosomes, the loading of peptide antigens would occur less efficiently or not at all (Doebele et al., 2003). It is interesting to consider the possibility that polymorphisms in class II molecules have been selected during evolution to avoid allelic products with high affinity for CLIP. In addition, alleles with especially low affinity for CLIP may be associated with increased risk for certain autoimmune diseases (Reed et al., 1997; Hausmann et al., 1999; Patil et al., 2001). Despite an apparent selection against class II molecules with high affinity for CLIP, the rate of spontaneous dissociation of this peptide from many class II molecules is too slow to allow effective sampling of peptides during the relatively short (<2 h) period of time that class II molecules reside in endosomal compartments prior to transport to the cell surface. A specialized co-factor, HLA-DM, catalyzes CLIP release and peptide exchange (see below).

Interesting interplays between Ii and pathogens have been observed. HIV-1 Nef up-regulates surface expression of Ii while at the same time down-regulating surface CD4 and MHC class I (Keppler et al., 2005) molecules. The role of this up-regulation in HIV-1 infection is not clear. On the other hand, herpes simplex virus-1 (HSV-1) infection appears to reduce Ii expression, and HSV-1 envelope glycoprotein B competes for HLA-DR binding to Ii (Neumann et al., 2003). These factors likely contribute to immune evasion. Recently, Ii has been noted to be highly expressed on gastric epithelial cells, where it appears to be able to bind *Helicobacter pylori* (Beswick et al., 2005).

Gene Organization and Sequence: Polymorphism and Populations

The Ii chain is encoded by a gene on chromosome 5q32. It has seven introns and three different mRNA transcripts have been described. Ii is relatively nonpolymorphic. However, in the coding region synonymous and nonsynonymous codon variants as well as others have been described (table 5.1). Few frequency data on these variants and no reports of their associations with infectious diseases have been published.

HLA-DM (6p21.3)

Gene Product in Infection and Pathogenesis

HLA-DM (DM) is a relatively nonpolymorphic trans-membrane heterodimer, composed of α- and β-chains and encoded in the class II region of the MHC (Cho et al., 1991; Kelly et al., 1991). It is selectively targeted to late endosomal compartment in APCs through a β-chain cytoplasmic domain targeting signal (Sanderson et al., 1994). It does not itself bind peptides, but instead plays a key role in the class II processing pathway through its capacity to catalyze CLIP dissociation and peptide exchange in other class II molecules (Sloan et al., 1995; Denzin and Cresswell, 1995; Sherman et al., 1995; Martin et al., 1996; Miyazaki et al., 1996; Fung-Leung et al., 1996). In the presence of DM, there is enhanced dissociation of preloaded peptide or class II binding to labeled peptides. At low concentrations of DM, the observed rate of peptide exchange is proportional to the DM concentration, and sub-stoichiometric concentrations of DM can catalyze peptide exchange in multiple class II molecules (Weber et al; 1996; Vogt et al., 1996). Thus, DM acts like an enzyme. However, there are unique features that differentiate DM from conventional enzymes. For example, DM has a relatively low turnover rate, and it does not catalyze the formation or breaking of covalent bonds. Under physiological conditions, DM may catalyze multiple rounds of peptide exchange, possibly favoring the most stable MHC–peptide complexes and thus editing the repertoire of peptides that are presented to CD4$^+$ T cells (Sloan et al., 1995; Weber et al., 1996; Kropshofer et al., 1996; van Ham et al., 1996; Katz et al., 1996; Raddrizzani et al., 1999; Nanda and Sant, 2000; Lovitch et al., 2003). In addition, DM has been shown to stabilize empty class II molecules, perhaps acting as a chaperone to prevent the denaturation of empty class II molecules as they await peptide loading in endosomal compartments (Denzin et al., 1996; Kropshofer et al., 1997; Kovats et al., 1998). During interaction with class II MHC–peptide complexes, DM appears to promote peptide exchange by stabilizing or inducing a conformational transition in which the peptide-binding groove is somehow "opened" and peptides are less tightly bound. The extent to which DM might have differential activity in catalyzing peptide exchange in different class II allelic products remains to be investigated.

Gene Organization and Sequence: Polymorphism and Populations

The two DM genes (A and B) are on chromosome 6p21.3 The DMA gene has five exons. The DMB gene has six exons and codes for a 26–28 kDa protein. The genes are relatively nonpolymorphic, but both contain some polymorphisms in coding regions, as well as in untranslated and intronic regions (table 5.1). Some of these polymorphisms have been investigated in relation to infectious disease susceptibility. In one study, presence or absence of HLA-DMA*0102 influenced the strength of an DRB1*1501 association with disseminated M. avium infection complex (Naik et al., 2003). This kind of interaction between antigen-loading and antigen-presenting molecules deserves further evaluation.

HLA-DO (6p21.3)

Gene Product in Infection and Pathogenesis

Another cofactor appears to be involved in the class II processing pathway. HLA-DO, like -DM, is also a relatively nonpolymorphic class II heterodimer, is composed of α- and β-chains and is encoded in the class II region of the MHC (Tonnelle et al., 1985; Wake and Flavell, 1985; Trowsdale and Kelly, 1985; Karlsson and Peterson, 1992). DO is an intracellular protein that localizes with DM in MIICs (Liljedahl et al., 1996; Denzin et al., 1997). There is no evidence that DO can bind peptides. Unlike other components of the class II processing pathway, DO (H2-O in mice) has been reported to be selectively expressed in B cells and thymic medullary epithelial cells, but not dendritic cells or macrophages. DO heterodimers are unstable in the absence of DM (H2-M in mice). In transfection experiments, DO is rapidly degraded through the ER quality-control mechanism unless it is co-expressed with DM (Liljedahl et al., 1996). Similarly, H2-O protein is absent in the B cells of H2-M–deficient mice (Liljedahl et al., 1998). Thus, DM acts as a chaperone for the intrinsically unstable DO heterodimer. DO forms a stable complex with DM in the ER, and DM/DO complexes are transported to MIIC, where they remain stably associated. In primary B cells, approximately 50% of DM molecules are bound to DO (Chen et al., 2002). A number of studies have demonstrated that DO is a negative regulator of DM function (Denzin et al., 1997; van

Ham et al., 1997; Liljedahl et al., 1998; Jensen, 1998; van Ham et al., 2000; Brocke et al., 2003). However, whether DO inhibits DM function or alternatively enhances peptide presentation remains controversial (Kropshofer et al., 1998).

Gene Organization and Sequence: Polymorphism and Populations

The DO proteins are coded for by the *DOA* and *DOB* genes on chromosome 6p21.3. These genes are relatively nonpolymorphic compared with others in class II but both coding and noncoding region polymorphisms have been investigated in relation to autoimmune diseases and leukemias. There are no published studies of DO associations with infectious diseases.

Regulation and Transcription of MHC Class II Genes: RFX, CIITA, and the Bare Lymphocyte Syndrome

HLA class II molecules and Ii genes are coordinately regulated. Their expression can be induced in numerous cell types following the exposure of those cells to cytokines, of which IFN-γ is the most potent (Collins et al., 1984). The expression of MHC II molecules on nonimmune cells may lead to the inappropriate activation of self-reactive T cells. Thus, tight regulation of this system is important. The expression of MHC class II DM and Ii genes is controlled by a common set of *cis*-acting elements, known as the W/Z, X1, X2, and Y boxes, which lie upstream of the promoters of each of these genes (reviewed in Boss and Jensen, 2003). The W-X-Y box elements are responsible for both the tissue-specific expression as well as IFN-γ induction. X and Y box elements can be found in all organisms encoding MHC class II genes, suggesting that the regulation of the gene system has coevolved with the genes themselves.

The RFX Complex: RFX-B/ANK (19p12), RFX-5 (1q21), and RFXAP (13q14)

Gene Product in Infection and Pathogenesis

While the X2 and Y box regulatory elements bind transcription factors common to many other genes (CREB and NF-Y, respectively), the X1 box binds RFX, a factor unique to this system (Hooft van Huijs-

duijnen et al., 1987; Reith et al., 1988; Mantovani et al., 1992; Moreno et al., 1999). RFX is a heterotrimer consisting of the subunits RFX-B (also called *RFXANK*), *RFX5*, and *RFXAP* (Steimle et al., 1995; Durand et al., 1997; Masternak et al., 1998; Nagarajan et al., 1999) (table 5.1). Mutation in any of the RFX subunit genes causes the inherited deficiency known as the bare lymphocyte syndrome (BLS), often considered a type of severe combined immunodeficiency (SCID). BLS patients do not express MHC II molecules (Griscelli et al., 1989; Elhasid and Etzioni, 1996; DeSandro et al., 1999), resulting in reduced numbers of CD4$^+$ T cells and the inability to mount CD4$^+$ T-cell responses. BLS patients succumb to a variety of opportunistic infections and often do not survive past childhood (for more information, see chapter 18). Interestingly *Chlamydia trachomatis* appears to be able to evade MHC-dependent T-cell recognition by synthesizing a protease-like factor that can degrade RFX5 (Zhong et al., 2001).

Gene Organization, Sequence, and Variation

Each of these proteins is coded for on different chromosomes (1, 13, and 19; table 5.1). Variations in these genes include single amino acid variations, insertions, deletions, transversions, and other polymorphisms. Most of the variants are rare, although some, such as those of RFX-B/ANK, have been mostly reported in North African patients. Other than those of the BLS-associated opportunistic infections, there are no published associations of any of the variants with other infectious diseases.

CIITA (16p13)

Gene Product in Infection and Pathogenesis

RFX, CREB, and NF-Y require the presence of another factor, the class II transactivator (CIITA), to activate transcription (Sloan and Boss, 1988; Reith et al., 1994; Louis-Plence et al., 1997, Steimle et al., 1993). Thus, mutations in *CIITA* also result in BLS, and together with the various RFX subunits define the four complementation groups of the disease (Hume and Lee, 1989). CIITA interacts with the scaffold of RFX, CREB, and NF-Y proteins and recruits chromatin remodeling complexes (Fontes et al., 1999; DeSandro et al., 2000; Masternak et al., 2000; Zhu et al., 2000; Beresford and Boss, 2001; Mudhasani and Fontes, 2002). The binding of CIITA to the X-Y scaffold is associated with specific modification to the local nucleosomal structure of MHC class II genes (Beresford and Boss, 2001; Gomez et al., 2005). CIITA is the only MHC II–specific factor that is regulated at the level of transcription. IFN-γ regulates CIITA, providing a direct mechanism by which MHC class II expression is controlled by IFN-γ (Steimle et al., 1994). Agents that down-modulate MHC II expression, such as transforming growth factor-β, also function by altering CIITA expression (Lee et al., 1997).

Targeting of CIITA appears to be a mechanism by which some pathogens evade host responses. Cytomegalovirus expresses proteins that target CIITA and prevent IFN-γ induction of MHC genes (Miller et al., 1998), HIV-1 Tat competes with CIITA for binding to a factor necessary for CIITA transcription (Kanazawa et al., 2000), and mycobacterial infections also influence CIITA expression (Wojciechowski et al., 1999; Pai et al., 2003).

Gene Organization, Sequence, and Polymorphisms

The *CIITA* gene is located on chromosome 16. Several variants have been reported (table 5.1), and there are four distinct promoters (Muhlethaler-Mottet et al., 1997), with cell-specific activity. Other than associations with the opportunistic infections typical of BLS patients, there are no published data on associations of *CIITA* polymorphisms with any specific infectious disease.

Animal Studies

MHC or MHC-like systems exist in vertebrates and even in nonvertebrates such as the lamprey, indicating the ancient role of such genes in host defense. Similarities in the *DRB1* locus of humans, apes, and other primates indicate divergence from ancestral genes millions of years ago but also allow for possibilities such as organ transplants across species. In some MHC–disease association studies in animals, the models closely resemble human disease (e.g., murine models of *Mycobacterium* and *Plasmodium* infections). However, primate models of certain diseases (e.g., HIV/AIDS) are far from perfect. Even in the best infectious disease models for MHC relationships, the alleles, the TCR responses and the presented epitopes differ from those in humans; these differences limit the ability to extrapolate to humans. Nevertheless, animal studies have been extremely useful for studies of almost every aspect of the MHC ranging from antigen processing and presentation to Ii chain function and regulators of transcription or translation. Web sites such as the one for the Jackson Laboratories (www.jax.org) list strains, including genetically engineered strains that are particularly suited to different questions about MHC effects.

Pharmacogenetics

The mapping of HLA class II (and class I) –restricted T-cell epitopes associated with responses to pathogens has led to the design of peptide-based vaccines for HIV-1 and other pathogens (reviewed in Sbai et al., 2001; Sette et al., 2002), some of which have reached preclinical or clinical trials. Common features of these vaccines include epitopes from conserved regions of the pathogen, epitopes with ability to bind broadly ("promiscuously") to many HLA class II alleles, and epitopes that can bind and be presented by HLA types prevalent in the population of interest. Development of reagents such as MHC multimers, with specific T-cell epitopes bound to DR or DQ molecules of interest, can be useful for monitoring responses to such vaccines, as well as responses to infections with pathogens of interest.

HLA class II genotypes have been shown to influence responses to several vaccines (Ovsyannikova et al., 2006a), cytokines, and drugs. HLA-associations with non-responsiveness to the hepatitis B and measles-mumps-rubella vaccines have been documented (Alper et al., 1990; Wang et al., 2004; Ovsyannikova et al., 2006b). Whether this is because of an inability to present certain epitopes or other aspects of antigen presentation or immune responsiveness is not clear. In the case of IFN-γ, hepatitis B–infected individuals with DRB1*07 appear to be low responders to the cytokine (Chu et al., 2005) whereas in hepatitis C infection, HLA-DR2 influences responses to IFN-γ (Almarri et al., 1998). Abacavir, an antiretroviral drug used in the treatment of HIV-1 infection, is associated with a hypersensitivity syndrome. In one study, individuals with a haplotype of European ancestry (HLA-B*5701-DR7-DQ3) were most likely to develop abacavir hypersensitivity, and presence of the ancestral haplotype had a positive predictive value of 100% for hypersensitivity (Mallal et al., 2002). Because B*5701 itself is equally predictive, it is not yet clear whether class II or other molecules encoded by genes in this haplotype contribute to the reaction.

Conclusions and Prospects/Needs

A complex and evolving interaction between the host HLA class II gene system and pathogen characterizes a number of responses to human infectious processes, vaccines, and antimicrobial agents. Future research will continue to translate this knowledge into better understanding of immune responses and design of new preventive and therapeutic measures.

Acknowledgments

Wanna Leelawiwat, Wanna Suwannaphan, and Baranee Balmongkol of the Thai Ministry of Public Health–U.S. CDC Collaboration, Nonthaburi, Thailand, provided assistance with tables, figures, and references and William Whitworth of Emory University, Atlanta, Georgia, USA, and Robert Linkins of the U.S. CDC, Atlanta, Georgia, USA, provided technical and editorial advice.

The findings and conclusions in this report are those of the authors and do not necessarily represent the views of the Centers for Disease Control and Prevention or the Agency for Toxic Substances and Disease Registry.

References

Almarri, A., Batchelor, J.R. (1994) HLA and hepatitis B infection. Lancet, 344(8931), 1194–1195.

Almarri, A., El Dwick, N., Al Kabi, S., Sleem, K., Rashed, A., Ritter, M.A., Batchelor, J.R. (1998) Interferon-alpha therapy in HCV hepatitis: HLA phenotype and cirrhosis are independent predictors of clinical outcome. Hum Immunol, 59(4), 239–242.

Alper, C.A., Kruskall, M.S., Marcus-Bagley, D., Craven, D.E., Katz, A.J., Brink, S.J., Dienstag, J.L., Awdeh, Z., Yunis, E.J. (1990) Genetic prediction of nonresponse to hepatitis B vaccine. N Engl J Med, 321(11), 708–712.

Anderson, M.S., Miller, J. (1992) Invariant chain can function as a chaperone protein for class II major histocompatibility complex molecules. Proc Natl Acad Sci USA, 89, 2282–2286.

Arunachalam, B., Phan, U.T., Geuze, H.J., Cresswell, P. (2000) Enzymatic reduction of disulfide bonds in lysosomes: characterization of a gamma-interferon-inducible lysosomal thiol reductase (GILT). Proc Natl Acad Sci USA, 97, 745–750.

Bakke, O., Dobberstein, B. (1990) MHC class II-associated invariant chain contains a sorting signal for endosomal compartments. Cell, 63, 707–716.

Beresford, G.W., Boss, J.M. (2001) CIITA coordinates multiple histone acetylation modifications at the HLA-DRA promoter. Nat Immunol, 2, 652–657.

Beswick, E.J., Bland, D.A., Suarez, G., Barrera, C.A., Fan, X., Reyes, V.E. (2005) Helicobacter pylori binds to CD74 on gastric epithelial cells and stimulates interleukin-8 production. Infect Immun, 73(5), 2736–2743.

Boss, J.M., Jensen, P.E. (2003) Transcriptional regulation of the MHC class II antigen presentation pathway. Curr Opin Immunol, 15, 105–111.

Brocke, P., Armandola, E., Garbi, N., Hammerling, G.J. (2003) Downmodulation of antigen presentation by H2-O in B cell lines and primary B lymphocytes. Eur J Immunol, 33, 411–421.

Carrington, M., Nelson, G.W., Martin, M.P., Kissner, T., Vlahov, D., Goedert, J.J., Kaslow, R., Buchbinder, S., Hoots, K., O'Brien, S.J. (1999) HLA and HIV-1: heterozygote advantage and B*35-Cw*04 disadvantage. Science, 283(5408), 1748–1752.

Chen, X., Laur, O., Kambayashi, T., Li, S., Bray, R.A., Weber, D.A., Karlsson, L., Jensen, P.E. (2002) Regulated expression of human histocompatibility leukocyte antigen (HLA)-DO during antigen-dependent and antigen-independent phases of B cell development. J Exp Med, 195, 1053–1062.

Cho, S.G., Attaya, M., Monaco, J.J. (1991) New class II-like genes in the murine MHC. Nature, 353, 573–576.

Chu, R.H., Ma, L.X., Wang, G., Shao, L.H. (2005) Influence of HLA-DRB1 alleles and HBV genotypes on interferon-alpha therapy for chronic hepatitis B. World J Gastroenterol, 11(30), 4753–4757.

Collins, T., Korman, A.J., Wake, C.T., Boss, J.M., Kappes, D.J., Fiers, W., Ault, K.A., Gimbrone, M.A., Jr., Strominger, J.L., Pober, J.S. (1984) Immune interferon activates multiple class II major histocompatibility complex genes and the associated invariant chain gene in human endothelial cells and dermal fibroblasts. Proc Natl Acad Sci USA, 81, 4917–4921.

Dean, M., Carrington, M., O'Brien, S.J. (2002) Balanced polymorphism selected by genetic versus infectious human disease. Annu Rev Genomics Hum Genet, 3, 263–292.

Denzin, L.K., Cresswell, P. (1995) HLA-DM induces CLIP dissociation from MHC class II alpha beta dimers and facilitates peptide loading. *Cell*, **82**, 155–165.

Denzin, L.K., Hammond, C., Cresswell, P. (1996) HLA-DM interactions with intermediates in HLA-DR maturation and a role for HLA-DM in stabilizing empty HLA-DR molecules. *J Exp Med*, **184**, 2153–2165.

Denzin, L.K., Sant'Angelo, D.B., Hammond, C., Surman, M.J., Cresswell, P. (1997) Negative regulation by HLA-DO of MHC class II-restricted antigen processing. *Science*, **278**, 106–109.

DeSandro, A., Nagarajan, U.M., Boss, J.M. (1999) The bare lymphocyte syndrome: molecular clues to the transcriptional regulation of major histocompatibility complex class II genes. *Am J Hum Genet*, **65**, 279–286.

DeSandro, A., Nagarajan, U.M., Boss, J.M. (2000) Associations and interactions among the bare lymphocyte syndrome factors. *Mol Cell Biol*, **20**, 6587–6599.

Doebele, R.C., Pashine, A., Liu, W., Zaller, D.M., Belmares, M., Busch, R., Mellins, E.D. (2003) Point mutations in or near the antigen-binding groove of HLA-DR3 implicate class II-associated invariant chain peptide affinity as a constraint on MHC class II polymorphism. *J Immunol*, **170**, 4683–4692.

Dorak, M.T., Tang, J., Penman-Aguilar, A., Westfall, A.O., Zulu, I., Lobashevsky, E.S., Kancheya, N.G., Schaen, M.M., Allen, S.A., Kaslow, R.A. (2004) Transmission of HIV-1 and HLA-B allele-sharing within serodiscordant heterosexual Zambian couples. *Lancet*, **363**(9427), 2137–2139.

Durand, B., Sperisen, P., Emery, P., Barras, E., Zufferey, M., Mach, B., Reith, W. (1997) RFXAP, a novel subunit of the RFX DNA binding complex, is mutated in MHC class II deficiency. *EMBO J*, **16**, 1045–1055.

Elhasid, R., Etzioni, A. (1996) Major histocompatibility complex class II deficiency: a clinical review. *Blood Rev*, **10**, 242–248.

Fontes, J.D., Kanazawa, S., Jean, D., Peterlin, B.M. (1999) Interactions between the class II transactivator and CREB binding protein increase transcription of major histocompatibility complex class II genes. *Mol Cell Biol*, **19**, 941–947.

Fung-Leung, W.P., Surh, C.D., Liljedahl, M., Pang, J., Leturcq, D., Peterson, P.A., Webb, S.R., Karlsson, L. (1996) Antigen presentation and T cell development in H2-M-deficient mice. *Science*, **271**, 1278–1281.

Ghosh, P., Amaya, M., Mellins, E., Wiley, D.C. (1995) The structure of an intermediate in class II MHC maturation: CLIP bound to HLA-DR3. *Nature*, **378**, 457–462.

Goldrath, A.W., Bevan, M.J. (1999) Selecting and maintaining a diverse T-cell repertoire. *Nature*, **402**, 255–262.

Gomez, J.A., Majumder, P., Nagarajan, U.M., Boss, J.M. (2005) X box-like sequences in the MHC class II region maintain regulatory function. *J Immunol*, **175**(2), 1030–1040.

Griscelli, C., Lisowska-Grospierre, B., Mach, B. (1989) Combined immunodeficiency with defective expression in MHC class II genes. *Immunodefic Rev*, **1**, 135–153.

Guerau-de-Arellano, M., Huber, B.T. (2002) Development of autoimmunity in Lyme arthritis. *Curr Opin Rheumatol*, **14**(4), 388–393.

Guermonprez, P., Valladeau, J., Zitvogel, L., Thery, C., Amigorena, S. (2002) Antigen presentation and T cell stimulation by dendritic cells. *Annu Rev Immunol*, **20**, 621–667.

Guo, M.M., Hildreth, J.E. (1995) HIV acquires functional adhesion receptors from host cells. *AIDS Res Hum Retroviruses*, **11**(9), 1007–1013.

Haan, K.M., Longnecker, R. (2000) Coreceptor restriction within the HLA-DQ locus for Epstein-Barr virus infection. *Proc Natl Acad Sci USA*, **97**(16), 9252–9257.

Hader, S.L., Hodge, T.W., Buchacz, K.A., Bray, R.A., Padian, N.S., Rausa, A., Slaviniski, S.A., Holmberg, S.D. (2002) Discordance at human leukocyte antigen-DRB3 and protection from human immunodeficiency virus type 1 transmission. *J Infect Dis*, **185**(12), 1729–1735.

Hausmann, D.H., Yu, B., Hausmann, S., Wucherpfennig, K.W. (1999) pH-dependent peptide binding properties of the type I diabetes-associated I-Ag7 molecule: rapid release of CLIP at an endosomal pH. *J Exp Med*, **189**, 1723–1734.

Hildesheim, A., Wang, S.S. (2002) Host and viral genetics and risk of cervical cancer: a review. *Virus Res*, **89**(2), 229–240.

Hill, A.V., Allsopp, C.E., Kwiatkowski, D., Anstey, N.M., Twumasi, P., Rowe, P.A., Bennett, S., Brewster, D., McMichael, A.J., Greenwood, B.M. (1991) Common west African HLA antigens are associated with protection from severe malaria. *Nature*, **352**, 595–600. Honey, K., Nakagawa, T., Peters, C., Rudensky, A. (2002) Cathepsin L regulates CD4+ T cell selection independently of its effect on invariant chain: a role in the generation of positively selecting peptide ligands. *J Exp Med*, **195**, 1349–1358.

Honey, K., Rudensky, A.Y. (2003) Lysosomal cysteine proteases regulate antigen presentation. *Nat Rev Immunol*, **3**, 472–482.

Hooft van Huijsduijnen, R.A., Bollekens, J., Dorn, A., Benoist, C., Mathis, D. (1987) Properties of a CCAAT box-binding protein. *Nucl Acids Res*, **15**, 7265–7282.

Hume, C.R., Lee, J.S. (1989) Congenital immunodeficiencies associated with absence of HLA class II antigens on lymphocytes result from distinct mutations in trans-acting factors. *Hum Immunol*, **26**, 288–309.

Jensen, P.E. (1993) Acidification and disulfide reduction can be sufficient to allow intact proteins to bind class II MHC. *J Immunol*, **150**, 3347–3356.

Jensen, P.E. (1998) Antigen processing: HLA-DO—a hitchhiking inhibitor of HLA-DM. *Curr Biol*, **8**, 128–131.

Jensen, P.E., Weber, D.A., Thayer, W.P., Chen, X., Dao, C.T. (1999) HLA-DM and the MHC class II antigen presentation pathway. *Immunol Res*, **20**, 195–205.

Kanazawa, S., Okamoto, T., Peterlin, B.M. (2000) Tat competes with CIITA for the binding to P-TEFb and blocks the expression of MHC class II genes in HIV infection. *Immunity*, **12**(1), 61–70.

Karlsson, L., Peterson, P.A. (1992) The alpha chain gene of H-2O has an unexpected location in the major histocompatibility complex. *J Exp Med*, **176**, 477–483.

Katz, J.F., Stebbins, C., Appella, E., Sant, A.J. (1996) Invariant chain and DM edit self-peptide presentation by major histocompatibility complex (MHC) class II molecules. *J Exp Med*, **184**, 1747–1753.

Kelly, A.P., Monaco, J.J., Cho, S.G., Trowsdale, J. (1991) A new human HLA class II-related locus, DM. *Nature*, **353**, 571–573.

Keppler, O.T., Tibroni, N., Venzke, S., Rauch, S., Fackler, O.T. (2005) Modulation of specific surface receptors and activation sensitization in primary resting CD4+ T lymphocytes by the Nef protein of HIV-1. *J Leukoc Biol*, **79**(3), 616–627.

Kovats, S., Grubin, C.E., Eastman, S., deRoos, P., Dongre, A., Van Kaer, L., Rudensky, A.Y. (1998) Invariant chain-independent function of H-2M in the formation of endogenous peptide-major histocompatibility complex class II complexes in vivo. *J Exp Med*, **187**, 245–251.

Kropshofer, H., Arndt, S.O., Moldenhauer, G., Hammerling, G.J., Vogt, A.B. (1997) HLA-DM acts as a molecular chaperone and rescues empty HLA-DR molecules at lysosomal pH. *Immunity*, **6**, 293–302.

Kropshofer, H., Vogt, A.B., Moldenhauer, G., Hammer, J., Blum, J.S., Hammerling, G.J. (1996) Editing of the HLA-DR-peptide repertoire by HLA-DM. *EMBO J*, **15**, 6144–6154.

Kropshofer, H., Vogt, A.B., Thery, C., Armandola, E.A., Li, B.C., Moldenhauer, G., Amigorena, S., Hammerling, G.J. (1998) A role for HLA-DO as a cochaperone of HLA-DM in peptide loading of MHC class II molecules. *EMBO J*, **17**, 2971–2981.

Lang, H.L.E., Jacobsen, H., Ikemizu, S., Andersson, C., Harlos, K., Madsen, L., Hjorth, P., Sondergaard, L., Svejgaard, A., Wucherpfennig, K., Stuart, D.I., Bell, J.I., Jones, E.Y., Fugger, L. (2002) A functional and structural basis for TCR cross-reactivity in multiple sclerosis. *Nat Immunol*, **3**, 940–943.

Lawn, S.D., Butera, S.T. (2000) Incorporation of HLA-DR into the envelope of human immunodeficiency virus type 1 in vivo: correlation with stage of disease and presence of opportunistic infection. *J Virol*, **74**(21), 10256–10259.

Lee, Y.-J., Han, Y., Lu, H.-T., Nguyen, V., Qin, H., Howe, P.H., Hocevar, B.A., Boss, J.M., Ransohoff, R.M., Benveniste, E.N. (1997) TGF-beta suppresses IFN-gamma induction of class II MHC gene expression by inhibiting class II transactivator mRNA expression. *J Immunol*, **158**, 2065–2075.

Liljedahl, M., Kuwana, T., Fung-Leung, W.P., Jackson, M.R., Peterson, P.A., Karlsson, L. (1996) HLA-DO is a lysosomal resident which requires association with HLA-DM for efficient intracellular transport. *EMBO J*, **15**, 4817–4824.

Liljedahl, M., Winqvist, O., Surh, C.D., Wong, P., Ngo, K., Teyton, L., Peterson, P.A., Brunmark, A., Rudensky, A.Y., Fung-Leung, W.P., Karlsson, L. (1998) Altered antigen presentation in mice lacking H2-O. *Immunity*, **8**, 233–243.

Lingappa, J., Kuffner, T., Tappero, J., Whitworth, W., Mize, A., Kaiser, R., McNicholl, J. (2004) HLA-DQ6 and ingestion of contaminated water: possible gene-environment interaction in an outbreak of Leptospirosis. *Genes Immun*, **5**(3), 197–202.

Llewelyn, M., Sriskandan, S., Peakman, M., Ambrozak, D.R., Douek, D.C., Kwok, W.W., Cohen, J., Altmann, D.M. (2004) HLA class II polymorphisms determine responses to bacterial superantigens. *J Immunol*, **172**(3), 1719–1726.

Lockett, S.F., Robertson, J.R., Brettle, R.P., Yap, P.L., Middleton, D., Leigh Brown, A.J. (2001) Mismatched human leukocyte antigen alleles protect against heterosexual HIV transmission. *J Acquir Immune Defic Syndr*, **27**, 277–280.

Loss, G.E., Jr., Sant, A.J. (1993) Invariant chain retains MHC class II molecules in the endocytic pathway. *J Immunol*, **150**, 3187–3197.

Louis-Plence, P., Moreno, C.S., Boss, J.M. (1997) Formation of a regulatory factor X/X2 box-binding protein/nuclear factor-Y multiprotein complex on the conserved regulatory regions of HLA class II genes. *J Immunol*, **159**, 3899–3909.

Lovitch, S.B., Petzold, S.J., Unanue, E.R. (2003) Cutting edge: H-2DM is responsible for the large differences in presentation among peptides selected by I-Ak during antigen processing. *J Immunol*, **171**, 2183–2186.

MacDonald, K.S., Embree, J., Njenga, S., Nagelkerke, N.J., Ngatia, I., Mohammed, Z., Barber, B.H.,

Ndinya-Achola, J., Bwayo, J., Plummer, F.A. (1998) Mother-child class I HLA concordance increases perinatal human immunodeficiency virus type 1 transmission. *J Infect Dis*, 177, 551–556.

Maier, B., Molinger, M., Cope, A.P., Fugger, L., Schneider-Mergener, J., Sonderstrup, G., Kamradt, T., Kramer, A. (2000) Multiple cross-reactive self-ligands for *Borrelia burgdorferi*-specific HLA-DR4-restricted T cells. *Eur J Immunol*, 30(2), 448–457.

Makela, S., Mustonen, J., Ala-Houhala, I., Hurme, M., Partanen, J., Vapalahti, O., Vaheri, A., Pasternack, A. (2002) Human leukocyte antigen-B8-DR3 is a more important risk factor for severe Puumala hantavirus infection than the tumor necrosis factor-alpha(-308) G/A polymorphism. *J Infect Dis*, 186(6), 843–846.

Mallal, S., Nolan, D., Witt, C., Masel, G., Martin, A.M., Moore, C., Sayer, D., Castley, A., Mamotte, C., Maxwell, D., James, I., Christiansen, F.T. (2002) Association between presence of HLA-B*5701, HLA-DR7, and HLA-DQ3 and hypersensitivity to HIV-1 reverse-transcriptase inhibitor abacavir. *Lancet*, 359(9308), 727–732.

Manoury, B., Hewitt, E.W., Morrice, N., Dando, P.M., Barrett, A.J., Watts, C. (1998) An asparaginyl endopeptidase processes a microbial antigen for class II MHC presentation. *Nature*, 396, 695–699.

Manoury, B., Mazzeo, D., Fugger, L., Viner, N., Ponsford, M., Streeter, H., Mazza, G., Wraith, D.C., Watts, C., Antoniou, A.N., Blackwood, S.L., Hewitt, E.W., Morrice, N., Dando, P.M., Barrett, A.J. (2002) Destructive processing by asparagine endopeptidase limits presentation of a dominant T cell epitope in MBP. *Nat Immunol*, 3, 169–174.

Manoury, B., Mazzeo, D., Li, D.N., Billson, J., Loak, K., Benaroch, P., Watts, C., Fugger, L., Viner, N., Ponsford, M., Streeter, H., Mazza, G., Wraith, D.C., Antoniou, A.N., Blackwood, S.L., Hewitt, E.W., Morrice, N., Dando, P.M., Barrett, A.J. (2003) Asparagine endopeptidase can initiate the removal of the MHC class II invariant chain chaperone. *Immunity*, 18, 489–498.

Mantovani, R., Pessara, U., Tronche, F., Li, X.Y., Knapp, A.M., Pasquali, J.-L., Benoist, C., Mathis, D. (1992) Monoclonal antibodies to NF-Y define its function in MHC class II and albumin gene transcription. *EMBO J*, 11, 3315–3322.

Maric, M., Arunachalam, B., Phan, U.T., Dong, C., Garrett, W.S., Cannon, K.S., Alfonso, C., Karlsson, L., Flavell, R.A., Cresswell, P. (2001) Defective antigen processing in GILT-free mice. *Science*, 294, 1361–1365.

Martin, W.D., Hicks, G.G., Mendiratta, S.K., Leva, H.I., Ruley, H.E., Van Kaer, L. (1996) H2-M mutant mice are defective in the peptide loading of class II molecules, antigen presentation, and T cell repertoire selection. *Cell*, 84, 543–550.

Masternak, K., Barras, E., Zufferey, M., Conrad, B., Corthals, G., Aebersold, R., Sanchez, J.-C., Hochstrasser, D.F., Mach, B., Reith, W. (1998) A gene encoding a novel RFX-associated transactivator is mutated in the majority of MHC class II deficiency patients. *Nat Genet*, 20, 273–277.

Masternak, K., Muhlethaler-Mottet, A., Villard, J., Zufferey, M., Steimle, V., Reith, W. (2000) CIITA is a transcriptional coactivator that is recruited to MHC class II promoters by multiple synergistic interactions with an enhanceosome complex. *Genes Devel*, 14, 1156–1166.

McNicholl, J.M., Cuenco, K.T. (1999) Host genes and infectious diseases: HIV, other pathogens and a public health perspective. *Am J Prev Med*, 16(2), 131–154.

McNicholl, J.M., Whitworth, W.C., Oftung, F., Fu, X., Shinnick, T., Jensen, P.E., Simon, M., Wohlhueter, R.M., Karr, R.W. (1995) Structural requirements of peptide and MHC for DR(alpha, beta 1*0401)-restricted T cell antigen recognition. *J Immunol*, 155, 1951–1963.

MHC Sequencing Consortium. (1999) Complete sequence and gene map of a human major histocompatibility complex. *Nature*, 401, 921–923.

Miller, D.M., Rahill, B., Durbin, J.E., Lairmore, M., Boss, J.M., Sedmak, D.D. (1998) Human cytomegalovirus inhibits major histocompatibility complex class II expression by disruption of the Jak/Stat pathway. *J Exp Med*, 187, 675–683.

Miyazaki, T., Wolf, P., Tourne, S., Waltzinger, C., Dierich, A., Barois, N., Ploegh, H., Benoist, C., Mathis, D. (1996) Mice lacking H2-M complexes, enigmatic elements of the MHC class II peptide-loading pathway. *Cell*, 84, 531–541.

Moreno, C.S., Beresford, G.W., Louis-Plence, P., Morris, A.C., Boss, J.M. (1999) CREB regulates MHC class II expression in a CIITA-dependent manner. *Immunity*, 10, 143–151.

Mudhasani, R., Fontes, J.D. (2002) The class II transactivator requires brahma-related gene 1 to activate transcription of major histocompatibility complex class II genes. *Mol Cell Biol*, 22, 5019–5026.

Muhlethaler-Mottet, A., Otten, L.A., Steimle, V., Mach, B. (1997) Expression of MHC class II molecules in different cellular and functional compartments is controlled by differential usage of multiple promoters of the transactivator CIITA. *EMBO J*, 16, 2851–2860.

Mullen, M.M., Haan, K.M., Longnecker, R., Jardetzky, T.S. (2002) Structure of the Epstein-Barr virus gp42 protein bound to the MHC class II receptor HLA-DR1. *Mol Cell*, 9(2), 375–385.

Mungall, A.J., Palmer, S.A., Sims, S.K., Edwards, C.A., Ashurst, J.L., Wilming, L., et al. (2003) The DNA sequence and analysis of human chromosome 6. *Nature*, **425**, 805–811.

Nagarajan, U.M., Louis-Plence, P., DeSandro, A., Nilsen, R., Bushey, A., Boss, J.M. (1999) RFX-B is the gene responsible for the most common cause of the bare lymphocyte syndrome, an MHC class II immunodeficiency. *Immunity*, **10**, 153–162.

Naik, E., LeBlanc, S., Tang, J., Jacobson, L.P., Kaslow, R.A. (2003) The complexity of HLA class II (DRB1, DQB1, DM) associations with disseminated Mycobacterium avium complex infection among HIV-1-seropositive whites. *J Acquir Immune Defic Syndr*, **33**(2), 140–145.

Nanda, N.K., Sant, A.J. (2000) DM determines the cryptic and immunodominant fate of T cell epitopes. *J Exp Med*, **192**, 781–788.

Neumann, J., Eis-Hubinger, A.M., Koch, N. (2003) Herpes simplex virus type 1 targets the MHC class II processing pathway for immune evasion. *J Immunol*, **171**(6), 3075–3083.

Newman, M.J., Livingston, B., McKinney, D.M., Chesnut, R.W., Sette, A. (2002) T-lymphocyte epitope identification and their use in vaccine development for HIV-1. *Front Biosci*, **7**, d1503–1515.

Ng, M.H., Lau, K.M., Li, L., Cheng, S.H., Chan, W.Y., Hui, P.K., Zee, B., Leung, C.B., Sung, J.J. (2004) Association of human-leukocyte-antigen class I (B*0703) and class II (DRB1*0301) genotypes with susceptibility and resistance to the development of severe acute respiratory syndrome. *J Infect Dis*, **190**(3), 515–518.

Nong, Y., Kandil, O., Tobin, E.H., Rose, R.M., Remold, H.G. (1991) The HIV core protein p24 inhibits interferon-gamma-induced increase of HLA-DR and cytochrome b heavy chain mRNA levels in the human monocyte-like cell line THP1. *Cell Immunol*, **132**(1), 10–16.

Norrby-Teglund, A., Nepom, G.T., Kotb, M. (2002) Differential presentation of group A streptococcal superantigens by HLA class II DQ and DR alleles. *Eur J Immunol*, **32**(9), 2570–2577.

Olerup, O., Troye-Blomberg, M., Schreuder, G.M.T., Riley, E.M. (1991) HLA-DR and -DQ gene polymorphism in West Africans is twice as extensive as in North European Caucasians: evolutionary implications. *Proc Natl Acad Sci USA*, **88**, 8480–8484.

Ovsyannikova, I.G., Dhiman, N., Jacobson, R.M., Poland, G.A. (2006a) Human leukocyte antigen polymorphisms: variable humoral immune responses to viral vaccines. *Expert Rev Vaccines*, **5**(1), 33–43.

Ovsyannikova, I.G., Pankratz, V.S., Vierkant, R.A., Jacobson, R.M., Poland, G.A. (2006b) Human leukocyte antigen haplotypes in the genetic control of immune response to measles-mumps-rubella vaccine. *J Infect Dis*, **193**(5), 655–663.

Pai, R.K., Convery, M., Hamilton, T.A., Boom, W.H., Harding, C.V. (2003) Inhibition of IFN-gamma-induced class II transactivator expression by a 19-kDa lipoprotein from Mycobacterium tuberculosis: a potential mechanism for immune evasion. *J Immunol*, **171**, 175–184.

Patil, N.S., Pashine, A., Belmares, M.P., Liu, W., Kaneshiro, B., Rabinowitz, J., McConnell, H., Mellins, E.D. (2001) Rheumatoid arthritis (RA)-associated HLA-DR alleles form less stable complexes with class II-associated invariant chain peptide than non-RA-associated HLA-DR alleles. *J Immunol*, **167**, 7157–7168.

Raddrizzani, L., Bono, E., Vogt, A.B., Kropshofer, H., Gallazzi, F., Sturniolo, T., Hammerling, G.J., Sinigaglia, F., Hammer, J. (1999) Identification of destabilizing residues in HLA class II-selected bacteriophage display libraries edited by HLA-DM. *Eur J Immunol*, **29**, 660–668.

Rammensee, H., Bachmann, J., Emmerich, N.P., Bachor, O.A., Stevanovic, S., Rammensee, H.G., Friede, T., Stevanoviic, S. (1999) SYFPEITHI: database for MHC ligands and peptide motifs. *Immunogenetics*, **50**, 213–219.

Reed, A.M., Collins, E.J., Shock, L.P., Klapper, D.G., Frelinger, J.A. (1997) Diminished class II-associated Ii peptide binding to the juvenile dermatomyositis HLA-DQ alpha 1*0501/DQ beta 1*0301 molecule. *J Immunol*, **159**, 6260–6265.

Reith, W., Satola, S., Herreo-Sanchez, C., Amaldi, I., Lisowska-Grospierre, B., Griscelli, C., Hadam, M.R., Mach, B. (1988) Congenital immunodeficiency with a regulatory defect in MHC class II gene expression lacks a specific HLA-DR promoter binding protein, RF-X. *Cell*, **53**, 897–906.

Reith, W., Siegrist, C.A., Durand, B., Barras, E., Mach, B. (1994) Function of major histocompatibility complex class II promoters requires cooperative binding between factors RFX and NF-Y. *Proc Natl Acad Sci USA*, **91**, 554–558.

Roche, P.A., Marks, M.S., Cresswell, P. (1991) Formation of a nine-subunit complex by HLA class II glycoproteins and the invariant chain. *Nature*, **354**, 392–394.

Sanderson, F., Kleijmeer, M.J., Kelly, A., Verwoerd, D., Tulp, A., Neefjes, J.J., Geuze, H.J., Trowsdale, J. (1994) Accumulation of HLA-DM, a regulator of antigen presentation, in MHC class II compartments. *Science*, **266**, 1566–1569.

Santori, F.R., Brown, S.M., Vukmanovic, S. (2002) Genomics-based identification of self-ligands with

T cell receptor-specific biological activity. *Immunol Rev*, **190**, 146–160.

Sathiamurthy, M., Hickman, H.D., Cavett, J.W., Zahoor, A., Prilliman, K., Metcalf, S., Fernandez Vina, M., Hildebrand, W.H. (2003) Population of the HLA ligand database. *Tissue Antigens*, **61**, 12–19.

Sbai, H., Mehta, A., DeGroot, A.S. (2001) Use of T cell epitopes for vaccine development. *Curr Drug Targets Infect Disord*, **1**(3), 303–313.

Segal, S., Hill, A.V. (2003) Genetic susceptibility to infectious disease. *Trends Microbiol*, **11**(9), 445–448.

Sette, A., Newman, M., Livingston, B., McKinney, D., Sidney, J., Ishioka, G., Tangri, S., Alexander, J., Fikes, J., Chesnut, R. (2002) Optimizing vaccine design for cellular processing, MHC binding and TCR recognition.*Tissue Antigens*. **59**, 443–451.

Sherman, M.A., Weber, D.A., Jensen, P.E. (1995) DM enhances peptide binding to class II MHC by release of invariant chain-derived peptide. *Immunity*, **3**(2), 197–205.

Sloan, J.H., Boss, J.M. (1988) Conserved upstream sequences of human class II major histocompatibility genes enhance expression of class II genes in wild-type but not mutant B-cell lines. *Proc Natl Acad Sci USA*, **85**, 8186–8190.

Sloan, V.S., Cameron, P., Porter, G., Gammon, M., Amaya, M., Mellins, E., Zaller, D.M. (1995) Mediation by HLA-DM of dissociation of peptides from HLA-DR. *Nature*, **375**, 802–806.

Steimle, V., Durand, B., Emmanuele, B., Zufferey, M., Hadam, M.R., Mach, B., Reith, W. (1995) A novel DNA-binding regulatory factor is mutated in primary MHC class II deficiency (bare lymphocyte syndrome). *Genes Devel*, **9**, 1021–1032.

Steimle, V., Otten, L.A., Zufferey, M., Mach, B. (1993) Complementation cloning of an MHC class II transactivator mutated in hereditary MHC class II deficiency (or bare lymphocyte syndrome). *Cell*, **75**, 135–146.

Steimle, V., Siegrist, C.-A., Mottet, A., Lisowska-Grospierre, B., Mach, B. (1994) Regulation of MHC class II expression by interferon-gamma mediated by the transactivator gene CIITA. *Science*, **265**, 106–108.

Stern, L.J., Brown, J.H., Jardetzky, T.S., Gorga, J.C., Urban, R.G., Strominger, J.L., Wiley, D.C. (1994) Crystal structure of the human class II MHC protein HLA-DR1 complexed with an influenza virus peptide. *Nature*, **368**, 215–221.

Tang, J., Costello, C., Keet, I.P.M., Rivers, C., LeBlanc, S., Karita, E., Allen, S. Kaslow, R.A. (1999) HLA class I homozygosity accelerates disease progression in human immunodeficiency virus type 1 infection. *AIDS Res Hum Retrovir*, **15**, 317–324.

Thayer, W.P., Ignatowicz, L., Weber, D.A., Jensen, P.E. (1999) Class II-associated invariant chain peptide-independent binding of invariant chain to class II MHC molecules. *J Immunol*, **162**, 1502–1509.

Thursz, M.R., Kwiatkowski, D., Allsopp, C.E., Greenwood, B.M., Thomas, H.C., Hill, A.V. (1995) Association between an MHC class II allele and clearance of hepatitis B virus in the Gambia. *N Engl J Med*, **332**, 1065.

Thursz, M.R., Thomas, H.C., Greenwood, B.M., Hill, A.V.S. (1997) Heterozygote advantage for HLA class-II type in hepatitis B virus infection. *Nature Genet*, **17**, 11–12.

Tonnelle, C., DeMars, R., Long, E.O. (1985) DO beta: a new beta chain gene in HLA-D with a distinct regulation of expression. *EMBO J*, **4**, 2839–2847.

Trowsdale, J., Kelly, A. (1985) The human HLA class II alpha chain gene DZ alpha is distinct from genes in the DP, DQ and DR subregions. *EMBO J*, **4**, 2231–2237.

van Ham, S.M., Gruneberg, U., Malcherek, G., Broker, I., Melms, A., Trowsdale, J. (1996) Human histocompatibility leukocyte antigen (HLA)-DM edits peptides presented by HLA-DR according to their ligand binding motifs. *J Exp Med*, **184**, 2019–2024.

van Ham, S.M., Tjin, E.P., Lillemeier, B.F., Gruneberg, U., van Meijgaarden, K.E., Pastoors, L., Verwoerd, D., Tulp, A., Canas, B., Rahman, D., Ottenhoff, T.H., Pappin, D.J., Trowsdale, J., Neefjes, J. (1997) HLA-DO is a negative modulator of HLA-DM-mediated MHC class II peptide loading. *Curr Biol*, **7**, 950–957.

van Ham, M., van Lith, M., Lillemeier, B., Tjin, E., Gruneberg, U., Rahman, D., Pastoors, L., van Meijgaarden, K., Roucard, C., Trowsdale, J., Ottenhoff, T., Pappin, D., Neefjes, J. (2000) Modulation of the major histocompatibility complex class II-associated peptide repertoire by human histocompatibility leukocyte antigen (HLA)-DO. *J Exp Med*, **191**, 1127–1136.

Vogt, A.B., Kropshofer, H., Moldenhauer, G., Hammerling, G.J. (1996) Kinetic analysis of peptide loading onto HLA-DR molecules mediated by HLA-DM. *Proc Natl Acad Sci U S A*, **93**, 9724–9729.

Wake, C.T., Flavell, R.A. (1985) Multiple mechanisms regulate the expression of murine immune response genes. *Cell*, **42**, 623–628.

Wang, S.S., Hildesheim, A., Gao, X., Schiffman, M., Herrero, R., Bratti, M.C., Sherman, M.E., Barnes, W.A., Greenberg, M.D., McGowan, L., Mortel, R., Schwartz, P.E., Zaino, R.J., Glass, A.G., Burk, R.D., Karacki, P., Carrington, M. (2002) Human leukocyte antigen class I alleles and cervical neoplasia: no heterozygote advantage. *Cancer Epidemiol Biomarkers Prev*, 11(4), 419–420.

Weber, D.A., Evavold, B.D., Jensen, P.E. (1996) Enhanced dissociation of HLA-DR-bound peptides in the presence of HLA-DM. *Science*, 274, 618–620.

Wojciechowski, W., DeSanctis, J., Skamene, E., Radzioch, D. (1999) Attenuation of MHC class II expression in macrophages infected with Mycobacterium bovis bacillus Calmette-Guerin involves class II transactivator and depends on the *Nramp1* gene. *J Immunol*, 163, 2688–2696.

Wu, Y., Chen, Y., Li, L., Cao, Y., Liu, Z., Liu, B., et al. (2006) Polymorphic amino acids at codons 9 and 37 of HLA-DQB1 alleles may confer susceptibility to cervical cancer among Chinese women. *Int J Cancer*, 118, 3006–3011.

Yee, L.J. (2004) Host genetic determinants in hepatitis C virus infection. *Genes Immun*, 5(4), 237–245.

Zhong, G., Fan, P., Ji, H., Dong, F, Huang, Y. (2001) Identification of a chlamydial protease-like activity factor responsible for the degradation of host transcription factors. *J Exp Med*, 193, 935–942.

Zhu, X.S., Linhoff, M.W., Li, G., Chin, K.C., Maity, S.N., Ting, J.P. (2000) Transcriptional scaffold: CIITA interacts with NF-Y, RFX, and CREB to cause stereospecific regulation of the class II major histocompatibility complex promoter. *Mol Cell Biol*, 20, 6051–6061.

6

MHC Class I Polypeptide-Related Sequence A and B (MICA and MICB) Genes

Seiamak Bahram

The prime relevance of the so-called classical MHC class I genes in fighting infectious diseases is established beyond doubt (Segal and Hill 2003). These highly polymorphic, ubiquitously expressed, β2-microglobulin linked molecules (*HLA-A,-B* and *-C* in man, *H2-K1, -D1,* and *-L* in mouse) present short, endogenously produced peptide antigens (derived from degradation of intracellular proteins, including viruses and certain bacteria) to the αβ T-cell receptor (TCR) of CD8[+] cytotoxic T lymphocytes (CTLs) (Bjorkman and Parham 1990). These CTLs consequently eliminate the infected cells and, in case of most infections, thereby stop further microbial diffusion. The hallmark of these classical MHC class I genes is their staggering number of alleles (see chapter 4). This diversity is most important at the population level, conferring on the species a capacity to resist an epidemic/pandemic, because there are likely certain group of individuals that harbor particular disease-resistant combinations of these HLA alleles (Robinson et al. 2003). This high level of diversity within these classical HLA molecules contrasts with the signifi-

cantly lower number of alleles identified for the so-called nonclassical MHC I genes (*HLA-E, -F,* and *-G* in humans and *H-2QTM* in mice): 5 for *HLA-E,* 2 for *HLA-F* and 15 for *HLA-G* (Radosavljevic and Bahram 2003). Again, this makes sense because these molecules either do not interact with peptides or interact with only a restricted set of them and hence do not need a large allelic repertoire for this purpose.

Beside these "conventional" class I genes, a number of other MHC I genes have been identified. For most, these are located outside the MHC (chromosome 6p21.3 in man) and are involved in a variety of physiological functions, often with no obvious link with the immune system. However, one gene family, MIC (MHC class I chain related), identified about a decade ago, is of interest here not only because of its function in immunity but also for its unexpected level of polymorphism (Bahram 2000; Bahram et al. 1994). In this chapter I provide an overall view of the structure and function of MIC with special emphasis on diversity as related to defense against infections.

Pathophysiology

The two functional MIC gene products, MICA and MICB, are single-chain glycoproteins that do not interact with the TCR; instead, they bind to NKG2D, an activating C-type lectin-like molecule expressed on the majority of human T ($\gamma\delta$ and CD8$^+$ $\alpha\beta$) and natural killer (NK) cells. MIC molecules share this faculty with RAET1 (ULBP) molecules, an apparently dissimilar gene family located on the opposite end of chromosome 6 (6q24.2-25.3) (Radosavljevic et al. 2002). Upon engagement, the NKG2D homodimer recruits mainly (in humans) the DAP10 signaling molecule, which ultimately leads to the triggering of the cellular cytotoxic arsenal leading to the elimination of the distressed cell. It seems that the stress signal is defined somewhat by the cell-surface expression of MIC molecules, which is in turn stress dependant. Other than the experimental artifact of heat shock, MIC genes have been shown to be induced following infection, tumor development, and other types of cellular stress (Bahram and Spies 1996; Das et al. 2001; Groh et al. 1996, 2001).

Genomics

There are seven MIC genes within the 1.8 Mb human MHC class I region. These are interspersed between the HLA loci. *MICA* and *MICB* are centromeric—47 and 130 kb, respectively—to *HLA-B*, *MICC* is 70 kb telomeric to *HLA-E*; *MICD* 28 kb centromeric to *HLA-A*; *MICE* and *MICG* 18 and 85.5 kb centromeric to *HLA-F*; and *MICF* 24 kb centromeric to *HLA-G*

(Shiina et al. 2001). Within these seven loci, only *MICA* and *MICB* harbor an intact open reading frame and give rise to functional glycoproteins. They are rather large genes of approximately 12 kb, compared to 3.5 kb for a typical HLA gene. Despite this length difference, their overall genomic structures is similar to those of all class I genes, where extracellular domains are encoded by distinct exons. *MICC*, *MICD*, *MICE*, *MICF*, and *MICG* are pseudogenes (Bahram 2000).

Genetics

Using the criteria mentioned above to try to classify HLA genes as classical or nonclassical, MIC genes defy easy categorization: Because they do not present peptides, they could be dubbed nonclassical, whereas given their significant level of polymorphism, they could be called classical. For the purposes of this discussion, these molecules are assigned to the large group of nonconventional MHC I, along with other genes such as *RAET1* and *CD1*.

MICA

MICA (table 6.1) is quite polymorphic—56 alleles have been documented to date (Fodil et al. 1996, 1999; Robinson et al. 2003). (Sequence alignments of the MIC alleles officially assigned to date may be found at www.ebi.ac.uk/imgt/hla/align.html.) *MICA* alleles are notable for several features, which also apply to *MICB* alleles (see below): (1) no clear hypervariable site, such as those seen in antigen presenting class I molecules,

TABLE 6.1. *MICA* and *MICB* gene summary.

Gene ID (NCBI)	Common Name(s)	Entrez Gene No. (Locus Link)	Map Position	Notes on Important SNPs, Indels, Truncations (Region, Reference Sequence [rs] Number)	References
MICA	MHC class I polypeptide-related sequence A MHC class I chain-related gene A	4276	6p21.3	Triplet repeat polymorphism in the transmembrane region with a common dysfunctional allele; extensive other polymorphisms	Mizuki et al. (1997) Suemizu et al. (2002)
MICB	MHC class I polypeptide-related sequence B MHC class I chain-related gene B	4277	6p21.3	Many variants, with one, MICB010, encoding a premature termination codon	Ando et al. (1997b)

can be readily identified; (2) all three extracellular domains are more or less equally polymorphic, again in contrast to classical molecules where the mainly structural α3 domain shows very little diversity; and (3) a large number of alleles are defined by reshuffling of an initial set of polymorphic sites. Along with these general characteristics, several unique features of MICA deserve attention.

During the genomic sequencing of the MICA locus, an unforeseen polymorphism was uncovered within the transmembrane exon (Mizuki et al. 1997). This fifth exon was shown to harbor a polymorphic short tandem repeat (STR) composed of a variable number of GCT repeats encoding 4, 5, 6, 9, and 10 alanine (A) residues (Mizuki et al. 1997; Perez-Rodriguez et al. 2000). Additionally, alleles carrying the 5.1 STR, which is defined by a nucleotide insertion (GCT → GGCT) in the 5 STR, encode truncated glycoproteins due to a premature stop codon (resulting from frame shift mutation) within this transmembrane segment (Mizuki et al. 1997). These 5.1-carrying alleles thus encode a glycoprotein lacking the cytoplasmic tail, which eventually does reach the plasma membrane albeit at an apparently nonphysiological location in polarized cells (Suemizu et al. 2002). It was therefore interesting to address the functional consequences of the absence of the MICA cytoplasmic tail, especially given the fact that the MICA008/5.1 allele carrying this variant is the most frequent MICA allele in several analyzed populations. Previous data have hinted at an elective expression of MICA within the intestinal epithelium where the molecule is capable of engaging the numerous intraepithelial lymphocytes (IELs) expressing the activatory NKG2D receptor; it was therefore important to study the fate of the MICA008/5.1 within this physiological niche (Groh et al. 1996; Hue et al. 2004). Transfection studies in polarized epithelial cell lines (reminiscent of the human gut) have unequivocally demonstrated improper targeting and expression of this particular allele. Subsequent site-directed mutagenesis, combined with transfection and confocal laser microscopy analysis, led to the identification of a dihydrophobic sequence (Leu-Val; residues 344–345) within the cytoplasmic tail responsible for the subcellular (basolateral) targeting of the molecule (Suemizu et al. 2002). Given the presence of IELs within intercellular spaces of enterocytes, it is tempting to consider that the presence of 008/5.1 allele at homozygosity will preclude the surveillance exerted by IELs against pathological (infected, malignant) enterocytes or other epi-

thelial cells. Finally, another MICA allele, MICA010, has also been reported to be unable to reach the cell surface, due to a single, R6P change, at the start of the α1 domain (Li et al. 2000). However, it is possible that in homozygous MICA008/5.1 or MICA010 individuals, the adjacent MICB gene product will supplant the dysfunctional MICA.

Another interesting MICA variant was identified by Kimura and colleagues while sequencing MICA in a cohort of HLA homozygous cell lines. Two alleles, MICA*017 and MICA*015, harbor a guanine deletion at the end of their fourth exon (α3 domain), which engenders a translational frame shift resulting in a premature stop codon at the start of the sixth exon, encoding the cytoplasmic tail (Obuchi et al. 2001). The transmembrane segments of these two alleles, initially thought to carry alanine repeats (GCT$_9$), carry instead a long leucine-rich hydrophobic region and terminate at the second position in the cytoplasmic domain. The functional behavior of these alleles has not yet been investigated.

Given the very short distance separating MICA from the highly polymorphic HLA-B, a strong degree of linkage disequilibrium was expected, for example, association of MICA008/5.1 (the latter MICA allele is found within the conserved haplotype HLA-A*0101-B*0801-DRB1*0301) with HLA-B*0702 and B*0801, MICA011/6 with HLA-B*1402, and MICA007/4 with HLA-B*27052 (Fodil et al. 1999). Exceptions exist, however; for example, the most common MICA allele, MICA008/5.1 is variously linked to HLA-B*0702, HLA-B*0801, HLA-B*1302, HLA-B*4001, HLA-B*4402, and HLA-B*4701. A growing number of reports have shown evidence of varying degrees of linkage or association between several MICA alleles and diseases. These include gastrointestinal disorders, such as Crohn's disease and ulcerative colitis (Glas et al. 2001; Orchard et al. 2001; Ding et al. 2005); primary sclerosing cholangitis (Norris et al. 2001; Wiencke et al. 2001); type I diabetes (Sanjeevi et al. 2002); systemic lupus erythematosis (Gambelunghe et al. 2005); rheumatoid arthritis (Martinez et al. 2001); psoriasis (Choi et al. 2000; Gonzalez et al. 2001); psoriatic arthritis (Gonzalez et al. 2002); Kawasaki disease (Huang et al. 2000); various neoplasia, for example, oral squamous cell carcinoma (Chung-Ji et al. 2002) and cervical cancer (Ghaderi et al. 2001); Addison's disease (Gambelunghe et al. 1999); familial Mediterranean fever (Touitou et al. 2001); and Behçet disease (Mizuki et al. 1997, 1999). Deciphering the part due to linkage disequilibrium with classical

HLA alleles or a primary contribution of MIC to disease etiology may remain an unachievable task as it has been for HLA alleles per se. However, the contribution of MIC diversity to the definition of HLA haplotypes may facilitate our final understanding of the genetic contribution of this critical segment of the genome to susceptibility to more than 100 diseases, some of which of major public health concern. Although the fact that infectious agents are supposed to play a (decisive) role—as a triggering device—in the pathogenesis of several if not most autoimmune diseases, thorough analysis of MIC diversity in susceptibility/resistance to infectious diseases per se is still lacking despite some initial endeavors regarding hepatitis B and C infections (Karacki et al. 2004; Lopez-Vazquez et al. 2004) and coxsackie B virus (Gupta et al. 2003). Despite this scarcity of data at present, a thorough investigation of MIC association with various infectious diseases might be worthwhile given the functional implication of MIC/NKG2D interactions in destroying infected cells.

MICB

The seemingly less rich *MICB* (table 6.1) diversity appears to be the result of a lesser effort in that sense. At present, at least 24 *MICB* alleles have been officially registered (Ando et al. 1997b; Pellet et al. 1997). The most interesting aspect of *MICB* diversity is the existence of two null alleles. The first one was initially reported by Ando et al. (1997a). This allele, MICB010 (also called MICB0107N), carries a stop codon within the α2 domain. Interestingly, this allele is invariably linked to a 100-kb genomic deletion, including the more telomeric *MICA* gene, carried thus far only on the HLA-B*4801 haplotype, prevalent in Southeast Asia and South America (Komatsu-Wakui et al. 1999, 2001; Aida et al. 2002). A fraction of these HLA-B*4801 chromosomes are *MICA–MICB* compound knockouts. Present estimates from a limited number of cases suggest that slightly more than half of the HLAB*4801 haplotypes are MIC null. Given the 3.2% frequency of the HLA-B*4801 in Japan, a 0.1024% homozygote rate is expected. So far, and based on a very limited number of cases, 62.5% (5 of 8) of these haplotypes carry the MIC null configuration. Hence, given the current size of the Japanese population, more than 80,000 individuals in Japan alone carry this haplotype at homozygosity. Because the first examined MIC gene knockout (*MICA-MICB^{-}/$^{-}$*) individuals were blood donors, "MIC deficiency" apparently does not engender any

overt clinical symptoms, in contrast to the mild to severe immune deficiencies consequent to the lack of MHC I or II molecules. These homozygous individuals (*MICA MICB^{-}/$^{-}$*) are therefore crucial in dissecting the *in vivo* role of MIC genes notably in defense against infections. The second report of a tentative *MICB* null allele is that of MICB-H018N, where a frame shift mutation leads to a stop codon within this time the first extracellular (α1) domain and hence leads very likely to a rapidly degraded gene product (Schroeder et al. 2004).

Conclusion

Like classical MHC class I molecules, MIC genes are involved in defense against infection, albeit via a distinct molecular and cellular pathway. The diversity of MIC genes is therefore of central value in this respect. However, the amount of available data is considerably less than that at hand for antigen-presenting MHC molecules. The challenge will be to perform the molecular typing of MIC genes in parallel with those of closely linked HLA loci in order to collectively grasp the extent of involvement of MHC diversity in our ability to fight infection and to be able eventually to segregate the fraction supported by HLA and MIC genes.

References

Aida, K., Russomando, G., Kikuchi, M., Candia, N., Franco, L., Almiron, M., Ubalee, R., and Hirayama, K.: High frequency of MIC null haplotype (HLA-B48-MICA-del-MICB*0107 N) in the Angaite Amerindian community in Paraguay. *Immunogenetics* 54: 439–41, 2002.

Ando, H., Mizuki, N., Ohno, S., Tabbara, K.F., Taguchi, S., Yamazaki, M., Miyata, Y., Wakisaka, K., and Inoko, H.: Identification of a novel HLA-B allele (B*4202) in a Saudi Arabian family with Behcet's disease. *Tissue Antigens* 49: 526–28, 1997a.

Ando, H., Mizuki, N., Ota, M., Yamazaki, M., Ohno, S., Goto, K., Miyata, Y., Wakisaka, K., Bahram, S., and Inoko, H.: Allelic variants of the human MHC class I chain-related B gene (MICB). *Immunogenetics* 46: 499–508, 1997b.

Bahram, S.: MIC genes: from genetics to biology. *Adv Immunol* 76: 1–60, 2000.

Bahram, S., Bresnahan, M., Geraghty, D.E., and Spies, T.: A second lineage of mammalian major histocompatibility complex class I genes [see comments]. *Proc Natl Acad Sci USA* 91: 6259–63, 1994.

Bahram, S., and Spies, T.: Nucleotide sequence of a human MHC class I MICB cDNA. *Immunogenetics* 43: 230–33, 1996.

Bjorkman, P.J., and Parham, P.: Structure, function, and diversity of class I major histocompatibility complex molecules. *Annu Rev Biochem* 59: 253–88, 1990.

Choi, H.B., Han, H., Youn, J.I., Kim, T.Y., and Kim, T.G.: MICA 5.1 allele is a susceptibility marker for psoriasis in the Korean population. *Tissue Antigens* 56: 548–50, 2000.

Chung-Ji, L., Yann-Jinn, L., Hsin-Fu, L., Ching-Wen, D., Che-Shoa, C., Yi-Shing, L., and Kuo-Wei, C.: The increase in the frequency of MICA gene A6 allele in oral squamous cell carcinoma. *J Oral Pathol Med* 31: 323–28, 2002.

Das, H., Groh, V., Kuijl, C., Sugita, M., Morita, C.T., Spies, T., and Bukowski, J.F.: MICA engagement by human vgamma2vdelta2 T cells enhances their antigen-dependent effector function. *Immunity* 15: 83–93, 2001.

Ding Y., Xia B., Lu M., Zhang Y., Li J., Ye M., Luo H., Yu J., Zhang X., and Tan J.: MHC class I chain-related gene A-A5.1 allele is associated with ulcerative colitis in Chinese population. *Clin Exp Immunol.* 142: 193–98, 2005.

Fodil, N., Laloux, L., Wanner, V., Pellet, P., Hauptmann, G., Mizuki, N., Inoko, H., Spies, T., Theodorou, I., and Bahram, S.: Allelic repertoire of the human MHC class I MICA gene. *Immunogenetics* 44: 351–57, 1996.

Fodil, N., Pellet, P., Laloux, L., Hauptmann, G., Theodorou, I., and Bahram, S.: MICA haplotypic diversity. *Immunogenetics* 49: 557–60, 1999.

Gambelunghe, G., Falorni, A., Ghaderi, M., Laureti, S., Tortoioli, C., Santeusanio, F., Brunetti, P., and Sanjeevi, C.B.: Microsatellite polymorphism of the MHC class I chain-related (MIC-A and MIC-B) genes marks the risk for autoimmune Addison's disease. *J Clin Endocrinol Metab* 84: 3701–07, 1999.

Gambelunghe, G., Gerli, R., Bocci, E.B., Del Sindaco, P., Ghaderi, M., Sanjeevi, C.B., Bistoni, O., Bini, V., and Falorni, A.: Contribution of MHC class I chain-related A (MICA) gene polymorphism to genetic susceptibility for systemic lupus erythematosus. *Rheumatology* 44: 287–92, 2005.

Ghaderi, M., Nikitina Zake, L., Wallin, K., Wiklund, F., Hallmans, G., Lenner, P., Dillner, J., and Sanjeevi, C.B.: Tumor necrosis factor A and MHC class I chain related gene A (MIC-A) polymorphisms in Swedish patients with cervical cancer. *Hum Immunol* 62: 1153–58, 2001.

Glas, J., Martin, K., Brunnler, G., Kopp, R., Folwaczny, C., Weiss, E.H., and Albert, E.D.: MICA, MICB and C1_4_1 polymorphism in Crohn's disease and ulcerative colitis. *Tissue Antigens* 58: 243–49, 2001.

Gonzalez, S., Brautbar, C., Martinez-Borra, J., Lopez-Vazquez, A., Segal, R., Blanco-Gelaz, M.A., Enk, C.D., Safriman, C., and Lopez-Larrea, C.: Polymorphism in MICA rather than HLA-B/C genes is associated with psoriatic arthritis in the Jewish population. *Hum Immunol* 62: 632–38, 2001.

Gonzalez, S., Martinez-Borra, J., Lopez-Vazquez, A., Garcia-Fernandez, S., Torre-Alonso, J.C., and Lopez-Larrea, C.: MICA rather than MICB, TNFA, or HLA-DRB1 is associated with susceptibility to psoriatic arthritis. *J Rheumatol* 29: 973–78, 2002.

Groh, V., Bahram, S., Bauer, S., Herman, A., Beauchamp, M., and Spies, T.: Cell stress-regulated human major histocompatibility complex class I gene expressed in gastrointestinal epithelium. *Proc Natl Acad Sci USA* 93: 12445–50, 1996.

Groh, V., Rhinehart, R., Randolph-Habecker, J., Topp, M.S., Riddell, S.R., and Spies, T.: Costimulation of CD8alphabeta T cells by NKG2D via engagement by MIC induced on virus-infected cells. *Nat Immunol* 2: 255–60, 2001.

Gupta, M., Nikitina-Zake, L., Landin-Olsson, M., Kockum, I., and Sanjeevi, C.B.: Coxsackie virus B antibodies are increased in HLA DR3-MICA5.1 positive type 1 diabetes patients in the Linkoping region of Sweden. *Hum Immunol* 64: 874–79, 2003.

Huang, Y., Lee, Y.J., Chen, M.R., Hsu, C.H., Lin, S.P., Sung, T.C., Chang, S.C., and Chang, J.G.: Polymorphism of transmembrane region of MICA gene and Kawasaki disease. *Exp Clin Immunogenet* 17: 130–37, 2000.

Hue, S., Mention, J.J., Monteiro, R.C., Zhang, S., Cellier, C., Schmitz, J., Verkarre, V., Fodil, N., Bahram, S., Cerf-Bensussan, N., and Caillat-Zucman, S.: A direct role for NKG2D/MICA interaction in villous atrophy during celiac disease. *Immunity* 21: 367–77, 2004.

Karacki, P.S., Gao, X., Thio, C.L., Thomas, D.L., Goedert, J.J., Vlahov, D., Kaslow, R.A., Strathdee, S., Hilgartner, M.W., O'Brien, S.J., and Carrington, M.: MICA and recovery from hepatitis C virus and hepatitis B virus infections. *Genes Immun* 5: 261–66, 2004.

Komatsu-Wakui, M., Tokunaga, K., Ishikawa, Y., Kashiwase, K., Moriyama, S., Tsuchiya, N., Ando, H., Shiina, T., Geraghty, D.E., Inoko, H., and Juji, T.: MIC-A polymorphism in Japanese and a MIC-A-MIC-B null haplotype. *Immunogenetics* 49: 620–28, 1999.

Komatsu-Wakui, M., Tokunaga, K., Ishikawa, Y., Leelayuwat, C., Kashiwase, K., Tanaka, H., Moriyama, S., Nakajima, F., Park, M.H., Jia, G.J., Chimge, N.O., Sideltseva, E.W., and Juji, T.: Wide distribution of the MICA-MICB null haplotype in East Asians. *Tissue Antigens* 57: 1–8, 2001.

Li, Z., Groh, V., Strong, R.K., and Spies, T.: A single amino acid substitution causes loss of expression of a MICA allele. *Immunogenetics* 51: 246–48, 2000.

Lopez-Vazquez, A., Rodrigo, L., Mina-Blanco, A., Martinez-Borra, J., Fuentes, D., Rodriguez, M., Perez, R., Gonzalez, S., and Lopez-Larrea, C.: Extended human leukocyte antigen haplotype EH18.1 influences progression to hepatocellular carcinoma in patients with hepatitis C virus infection. *J Infect Dis* 189: 957–63, 2004.

Martinez, A., Fernandez-Arquero, M., Balsa, A., Rubio, A., Alves, H., Pascual-Salcedo, D., Martin-Mola, E., and de la Concha, E.G.: Primary association of a MICA allele with protection against rheumatoid arthritis. *Arthritis Rheum* 44: 1261–65, 2001.

Mizuki, N., Ota, M., Katsuyama, Y., Yabuki, K., Ando, H., Goto, K., Nakamura, S., Bahram, S., Ohno, S., and Inoko, H.: Association analysis between the MIC-A and HLA-B alleles in Japanese patients with Behcet's disease. *Arthritis Rheum* 42: 1961–6, 1999.

Mizuki, N., Ota, M., Kimura, M., Ohno, S., Ando, H., Katsuyama, Y., Yamazaki, M., Watanabe, K., Goto, K., Nakamura, S., Bahram, S., and Inoko, H.: Triplet repeat polymorphism in the transmembrane region of the MICA gene: a strong association of six GCT repetitions with Behcet disease. *Proc Natl Acad Sci USA* 94: 1298–303, 1997.

Norris, S., Kondeatis, E., Collins, R., Satsangi, J., Clare, M., Chapman, R., Stephens, H., Harrison, P., Vaughan, R., and Donaldson, P.: Mapping MHC-encoded susceptibility and resistance in primary sclerosing cholangitis: the role of MICA polymorphism. *Gastroenterology* 120: 1475–82, 2001.

Obuchi, N., Takahashi, M., Nouchi, T., Satoh, M., Arimura, T., Ueda, K., Akai, J., Ota, M., Naruse, T., Inoko, H., Numano, F., and Kimura, A.: Identification of MICA alleles with a long Leu-repeat in the transmembrane region and no cytoplasmic tail due to a frameshift-deletion in exon 4. *Tissue Antigens* 57: 520–35, 2001.

Orchard, T.R., Dhar, A., Simmons, J.D., Vaughan, R., Welsh, K.I., and Jewell, D.P.: MHC class I chain-like gene A (MICA) and its associations with inflammatory bowel disease and peripheral arthropathy. *Clin Exp Immunol* 126: 437–40, 2001.

Pellet, P., Renaud, M., Fodil, N., Laloux, L., Inoko, H., Hauptmann, G., Debre, P., Bahram, S., and Theodorou, I.: Allelic repertoire of the human MICB gene. *Immunogenetics* 46: 434–36, 1997.

Perez-Rodriguez, M., Corell, A., Arguello, J.R., Cox, S.T., McWhinnie, A., Marsh, S.G.E., and Madrigal, J.A.: A new MICA allele with ten alanine residues in the exon 5 microsatellite. *Tissue Antigens* 55: 162 65, 2000.

Radosavljevic, M., and Bahram, S.: In vivo immunogenetics: from MIC to RAET1 loci. *Immunogenetics* 55: 1–9, 2003.

Radosavljevic, M., Cuillerier, B., Wilson, M.J., Clement, O., Wicker, S., Gilfillan, S., Beck, S., Trowsdale, J., and Bahram, S.: A cluster of ten novel MHC class I related genes on human chromosome 6q24.2-q25.3. *Genomics* 79: 114–23, 2002.

Robinson, J., Waller, M.J., Parham, P., de Groot, N., Bontrop, R., Kennedy, L.J., Stoehr, P., and Marsh, S.G.: IMGT/HLA and IMGT/MHC: sequence databases for the study of the major histocompatibility complex. *Nucleic Acids Res* 31: 311–14, 2003.

Sanjeevi, C.B., Gambelunghe, G., Falorni, A., Shtauvere-Brameus, A., and Kanungo, A.: Genetics of latent autoimmune diabetes in adults. *Ann NY Acad Sci* 958: 107–11, 2002.

Schroeder, M., Elsner, H.A., Kim, T.D., and Blaszyk, R.: Eight novel MICB alleles, including a null allele, identified in gastric MALT lymphoma patients. *Tissue Antigens* 64: 276–80, 2004.

Segal, S., and Hill, A.V.: Genetic susceptibility to infectious disease. *Trends Microbiol* 11: 445–48, 2003.

Shiina, T., Asako, A., Suto, Y., Kasai, F., Shigenari, A., Takishima, N., Kikkawa, E., Iwata, K., Kuwano, Y., Kitamura, Y., Matsuzawa, Y., Sano, K., Nogami, M., Kawata, H., Li, S., Fukuzumi, Y., Yamazaki, M., Tashiro, H., Tamiya, G., Kohda, A., Okumura, K., Ikemura, T., Soeda, E., Mizuki, N., Kimura, M., Bahram, S., and Inoko, H.: Genomic anatomy of a premier major histocompatibility complex paralogous region on human chromosome 1q21-q22. *Genome Res* 11: 789–802, 2001.

Suemizu, H., Radosavljevic, M., Kimura, M., Sadahiro, S., Yoshimura, S., Bahram, S., and Inoko, H.: A basolateral sorting motif in the MICA cytoplasmic tail. *Proc Natl Acad Sci USA* 99: 2971–76, 2002.

Touitou, I., Picot, M.C., Domingo, C., Notarnicola, C., Cattan, D., Demaille, J., and Kone-Paut, I.: The MICA region determines the first modifier locus in familial Mediterranean fever. *Arthritis Rheum* 44: 163–69, 2001.

Wiencke, K., Spurkland, A., Schrumpf, E., and Boberg, K.M.: Primary sclerosing cholangitis is associated to an extended B8-DR3 haplotype including particular MICA and MICB alleles. *Hepatology* 34: 625–30, 2001.

7

Killer Immunoglobulin-Like Receptor and Related Genes

Maureen P. Martin, M. Tevfik Dorak, & Mary Carrington

Natural killer (NK) cells are an important component of the innate immune system; they participate in early responses against infected or transformed cells by production of cytokines and direct cytotoxicity (Bancroft 1993; Biron et al. 1999; Cooper et al. 2001; French and Yokoyama 2003; Robertson and Ritz 1990; Trinchieri 1989). The importance of NK cells in antiviral immunity is evidenced by the report of an NK-cell–deficient individual with otherwise normal B and T cells who suffered from recurrent herpesvirus infections (Biron et al. 1989). Other studies have also implicated NK cells in the pathogenesis of viral infections, including cytomegalovirus (CMV), Epstein-Barr virus, herpes simplex virus (HSV), hepatitis B, hepatitis C (HCV), and HIV-1, as well as a variety of intracellular bacteria and protozoan parasites (reviewed in Bancroft 1993; Biron et al. 1999; See et al. 1997). Thus, it is clear that NK cells, key components of the innate immune system, are essential in limiting pathogens during the early phases of a primary infection before the adaptive immune system is able to respond.

The mechanisms that regulate the function of NK cells have only recently begun to be understood (Biassoni et al. 2001; Cerwenka and Lanier 2001; Diefenbach and Raulet 2001), but little is still known about how NK cells recognize virally infected cells. Quiescent NK cells can be activated either by soluble mediators such as cytokines or by direct cell–cell contact. A large number of inhibitory and activating NK cell receptors that bind to ligands on target cells mediate the specificity and strength of cell–cell contact leading up to cytotoxicity (Moretta et al. 2002; Moretta and Moretta 2004), with a prominent role being played by inhibitory receptors that interact with major histocompatibility complex (MHC) class I molecules. The original hypothesis proposed that these receptors protect normal cells from attack while rendering cells with altered levels of MHC class I expression susceptible to NK cell lysis, a concept termed the "missing self

TABLE 7.1. Characteristics of NK cell receptor families.

NK Receptor Family	Protein Structure	Genetic Complex	Ligands
KIR	Ig superfamily	LRC	HLA-A, Bw, Cw
ILT/LIR/LILR	Ig superfamily	LRC	HLA class Ia (-G)
CD94/NKG2 (KLR)	C-type lectin-like	NKC	HLA class Ib (-E)
NKG2D (KLRK)	C-type lectin-like	NKC	MIC and MHC class I-like
NCR	Ig superfamily	Various, including MHC, LRC	Viral hemagglutinins and others

hypothesis" (Ljunggren and Karre 1990). The current model, on the other hand, proposes that NK cell cytotoxicity is instead controlled by the equilibrium between activating and inhibitory signals (Lanier 2005). Thus, NK cells not only target cells that lack MHC class I, but also those that overexpress ligands for activating receptors. Consequently, for example, when multiple activating receptors are engaged, the signal might be sufficiently potent to overcome inhibition. The main types of class I specific receptors used by human NK cells are the killer immunoglobulin-like receptors (KIRs) and the CD94/NKG2 heterodimer group belonging to the killer cell lectin-like receptor (KLR) family (Lanier 1998; Long 1999; Lopez-Botet et al. 2000; Moretta et al. 1996; table 7.1). NK receptors usually recognize missing self (MHC), induced self (stress signals), or modified self (stress signals) proteins as their ligands (Long and Rajagopalan 2002). The inhibitory members of the KIR family are indirectly responsible for activation. In the absence of inhibitory signals from missing self MHC molecules, they screen HLA-E expression as a marker for overall MHC class I expression. The same interaction may be interfered by modified self (heat-shock protein 60) as a stress signal to induce NK cell activation. A unique member of the KLR family, KLRK or NKG2D, recognizes a variety of stress-induced self molecules from inflamed, infected, or transformed cells (Raulet 2003).

The KIR family belongs to the immunoglobulin (Ig) superfamily of receptors and consists of a group of regulatory molecules that are expressed on NK cells and a subset of T cells. They were first identified by their ability to impart some specificity to NK cell cytolysis (Harel-Bellan et al. 1986; Moretta et al. 1990). Thus far, only HLA class I molecules have been identified as ligands for KIRs. Through the interaction of inhibitory KIR with HLA class I, healthy cells are protected from spontaneous destruction by NK cell–mediated cytolysis. Other KIR isotypes stimulate the activity of NK cells. Thus, KIRs play a significant role in the control of the immune response.

Gene Product in Infection

To date, 16 KIR genes have been identified of which two are pseudogenes (table 7.2). The naming of KIR is based primarily on their protein structure (Marsh et al. 2003). There are four major subdivisions based on two features: the number of extracellular Ig domains (2D or 3D) and length of the cytoplasmic tail (L or S; see figure 7.1).

KIRs with long cytoplasmic tails are inhibitory by virtue of the immunoreceptor tyrosine-based inhibition motifs (ITIMs) present in their cytoplasmic domains. One exception to this is KIR2DL4 which is unique in that in addition to the single ITIM in the cytoplasmic tail, it also possesses a charged arginine residue in the transmembrane domain. This allows it to associate with the accessory molecule FcεRI-γ, which possesses an immunoreceptor tyrosine-based activation motif (ITAM; Kikuchi-Maki et al. 2005). Engagement of 2DL4 thus results in activation despite the inhibitory potential conferred by the ITIM in its cytoplasmic tail. Short-tailed KIRs transmit activating signals through their interaction with the adaptor molecule DAP-12 (DNAX activation protein of 12 kDa; this molecule is also known as killer cell activating receptor-associated protein, KARAP), which contains ITAMs (Lanier et al. 1998; Olcese et al. 1997). DAP-12 is also a member of the immunoglobulin superfamily and is encoded at the centromeric end of the leukocyte receptor complex (LRC).

TABLE 7.2. KIR genes identified to date.

Symbol	Aliases	Gene ID	Location
KIR2DL1	NKAT1, p58.1, CD158a	3802	19q13.4
KIR2DL2[a]	NKAT6, CD158b1, p58.2	3803	19q13.4
KIR2DL3[a]	NKAT2, NKAT2a, NKAT2b, CD158b2, p58.2	3804	19q13.4
KIR2DL4[b]	KIR103, CD158d	3805	19q13.4
KIR2DL5A	KIR2DL5.1, CD158f	57292	19q13.4
KIR2DL5B	KIR2DL5.2, KIR2DL5.3, KIR2DL5.4, KIR2DLX	553128	19q13.4
KIR2DS1	CD158h, p50.1	3806	19q13.4
KIR2DS2	NKAT5, CD158j, p50.2	3807	19q13.4
KIR2DS3	NKAT7	3808	19q13.4
KIR2DS4	NKAT8, CD158i, KIR1D	3809	19q13.4
KIR2DS5	NKAT9, CD158g	3810	19q13.4
KIR3DL1[a]	NKAT3, CD158e1, p70	3811	19q13.4
KIR3DL2[b]	NKAT4, NKAT4a, NKAT4b, CD158k	3812	19q13.4
KIR3DL3[b]	KIRC1, KIR3DL7, KIR44, CD158z	115653	19q13.4
KIR3DS1[a]	NKAT10, CD158e2	(3811)[b]	19q13.4
KIR2DP1	KIRZ, KIRY, KIR15, KIR2DL6	554300	19q13.4
KIR3DP1[b]	KIRX, KIR2DS6, KIR3DS2P, CD158c	548594	19q13.4

Modified from Human Genome Organization (HUGO) Nomenclature Committee's KIR Gene Family Nomenclature Web site (www.gene.ucl.ac.uk/nomenclature/genefamily/kir.html), European Molecular Biology Laboratory/European Bioinformatics Institute's IPD KIR Sequence Database (www.ebi.ac.uk/ipd/kir/loci.html), and National Center for Biotechnology Information's Entrez-Gene (www.ncbi.nlm.nih.gov/sites/entrez).

[a] Alleles of a single locus

[b] Framework (anchor) genes present on all KIR haplotypes

Pathogenesis

HLA molecules precipitate in adaptive aspects of anti-pathogen defense by presenting peptide fragments to immune effector cells (Bjorkman et al. 1987; Zinkernagel and Doherty 1974). Cytotoxic T lymphocytes (CTLs) interact with the HLA class I peptide complex on target cells via the T-cell receptor (TCR), which instigates cytolytic activity if the peptide is considered foreign. HLA class I expression can be down-regulated in virally infected or transformed cells, rendering the cells resistant to cytolysis by CTLs but lowering the threshold for attack by NK cells or T cells by relieving them of inhibitory signals. In addition, the presence of activating receptors might allow for recognition of cells expressing the appropriate ligands. Although neither the ligand nor the direct mode of action of many NK receptors is known, it is widely accepted that normal cells are protected from spontaneous killing when they express an appropriate ligand for an inhibitory receptor on the cytotoxic cell (NK or CTL). NK cells need to discriminate between healthy and infected or transformed cells, corresponding with the observed phenotypic dominance of KIR-mediated inhibition over activation (Biassoni et al. 1997; Sivori et al. 1997; Vales-Gomez et al. 1998a; Watzl et al. 2000b). However, NK cell tolerance mechanisms are not completely understood. The previous dogma assumed that each NK cell had at least one inhibitory receptor specific for self MHC class I (the "at least one" model) that accounted for self-tolerance (Raulet et al. 1997; Valiante et al. 1997b). However, in view of the stochastic expression of KIR, this model seems unlikely. Furthermore, studies of NK cells from MHC class I-deficient mice indicate that the absence of ligands for inhibitory receptors does not leave the mice with autoreactive NK cells (Liao et al. 1991). Two models have recently been proposed to explain this self-tolerance in mice. The so-called "disarming" model proposes that NK cells that do not express inhibitory receptors for self-MHC are chronically stimulated and consequently become anergic (Fernandez et al. 2005). The alternative model proposes that inhibitory receptors for self-MHC play an active role in the functional maturation of NK cells. Thus, NK cells that possess inhibitory receptors that recognize self-MHC become functionally competent or "licensed," whereas those that do not are functionally incompetent or "unlicensed" (Kim et al. 2005). Whether or not human NK cell activity is regulated in a similar manner remains to be determined. The ligands for several of the inhibitory KIR molecules are subsets of HLA class I molecules, as shown by assays measuring binding of inhibitory KIR to specific HLA molecules and inhibition of NK-mediated cytolysis of target cells bearing those HLA allotypes (Long and Rajagopalan 2000; Sawicki et al. 2001; Vilches and Parham 2002).

Dimorphisms in the HLA-Cw α1 domain that are characterized by Ser77/Asn80 and Asn77/Lys80 define serologically distinct allotypes of HLA-Cw (Cw group

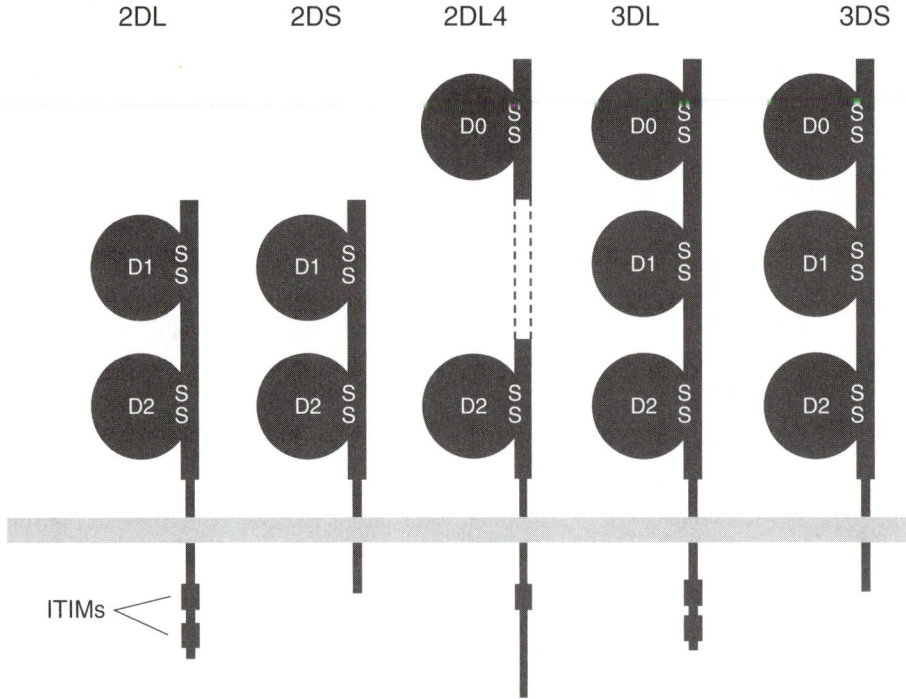

FIGURE 7.1. General protein structure of the KIR family. From Protein Reviews on the Web: KIR (www.ncbi.nlm.nih.gov/). D0 is the first Ig domain in KIR3D, D1 and D2 and first and second Ig domains in *KIR2D* and are closely related in amino acid sequence to the second and third Ig domains in *KIR3D*. Long cytoplasmic tails carry two ITIMs (immunoreceptor tyrosine-based inhibition motifs); while short cytoplasmic tails are truncated before the first ITIM and are connected to a transmembrane region which includes a lysine residue.

1 and group 2, respectively). The inhibitory KIR2DL1 interacts with group 2 allotypes, while 2DL2 and 2DL3 interact with group 1 allotypes (Biassoni et al. 1995; Colonna et al. 1992; Winter and Long 1997). Similarly, the inhibitory KIR3DL1 interacts with HLA-B allotypes that contain Bw4 (Cella et al. 1994; Gumperz et al. 1995), a serologically defined motif. KIR3DL2 interacts with HLA-A3 and HLA-A11 (Dohring et al. 1996b; Pende et al. 1996), and KIR2DL4 recognizes the non-classical class I molecule HLA-G (Ponte et al. 1999; Rajagopalan et al. 2006; Rajagopalan and Long 1999). The ligands for the activating KIR2DS3 and KIR2DS5 and the inhibitory KIR2DL5 and 3DL3 have not been identified. The activating KIR2DS1 and KIR2DS2 demonstrate weak binding to Cw group 2 and 1 allotypes, respectively (Moretta et al. 1995; Vales-Gomez et al. 1998a), but their high affinity ligands have not been identified. The distinct binding affinities of activating compared to inhibitory KIR may also

contribute to the dominance of inhibition. For example, *KIR2DL2* has a higher affinity than *KIR2DS2* for HLA-Cw3 due to a single amino acid substitution (Boyington et al. 2001).

The importance of NK cell receptors in defense against viral infections can be inferred from the complex mechanisms used by viruses to evade immune recognition (Tortorella et al. 2000). Several viruses down-regulate the expression of MHC class I molecules, thus diminishing TCR-mediated activation of CTLs (Tortorella et al. 2000) but also reducing the engagement of NK cell inhibitory receptors, thus rendering the infected cells more susceptible to NK cell lysis. However, expression of HLA-C and HLA-E, which less effectively stimulate antigen-specific CTL but are recognized by inhibitory KIR and CD94/NKG2A, respectively, may be unaffected (Cohen et al. 1999; Coscoy and Ganem 2000; Gewurz et al. 2001; Ishido et al. 2000). The HIV Nef protein (Cohen et al. 1999) and

Kaposi sarcoma herpesvirus K5 protein (Ishido et al. 2000), for example, selectively down-regulate HLA-A and HLA-B while preserving HLA-C and HLA-E expression. Alternatively, HLA-E may be up-regulated by the human CMV UL40 protein, which contains a sequence identical to the leader sequence of HLA-C presented by HLA-E (Tomasec et al. 2000; Ulbrecht et al. 2000). Herpesviruses also encode MHC class I-like molecules such as m144 that bind to inhibitory receptors (Cretney et al. 1999; Farrell et al. 1997). The mouse CMV protein m157 exhibits structural but not sequence homology to MHC class I molecules and binds the Ly49I inhibitory receptor and the Ly49H activating receptor in mice (Arase et al. 2002; Smith et al. 2002).

NK cells become activated when inhibition is removed, so activation must involve stimulatory receptors (Karre et al. 1986). Based on assays measuring target cell killing, stimulatory KIRs can mediate NK cell activity through recognition of HLA ligands (Moretta et al. 1995), however, they bind with very weak affinity if at all to their putative HLA ligands. Thus, the identity of their high-affinity physiologic ligands remains in question. Candidate ligands include non-MHC molecules, such as foreign or microbial antigens expressed on infected cells, normal cell-surface proteins that are aberrantly expressed, stress-induced proteins, and complexes of pathogen-derived peptides bound to MHC class I molecules. The mouse CMV m157 gene product was shown to bind the mouse activating NK cell receptor Ly49H, an interaction that leads to NK cell killing of the infected targets (Arase et al. 2002; Brown et al. 2001; Daniels et al. 2001; Lee et al. 2001; Smith et al. 2002; Vivier and Biron 2002). Although they lack sequence homology, the mouse Ly49 and human KIR families are considered to be functionally equivalent (Hanke et al. 1999). Ly49H recognition of m157 provides strong support for the possibility that non-HLA molecules can behave as ligands for activating KIR.

Although some interactions with KIR have been shown to be independent of peptide (Mandelboim et al. 1996), several studies also indicated that specificity depends on the presented peptide (Hansasuta et al. 2004; Kim et al. 1997; Maenaka et al. 1999a; Malnati et al. 1995; Peruzzi et al. 1996; Rajagopalan and Long 1997; Winter et al. 1998). Peptide-dependent protection of killing by NK cells has been observed (Malnati et al. 1995; Zappacosta et al. 1997). It has been suggested that inhibiting and activating receptors specific for the same HLA may respond differentially depending on bound peptides (Mandelboim et al. 1997;

Young et al. 1998). Peptide recognition could provide KIR with one further means for mediating pathogen-specific immunity.

Comparisons of KIR sequences and haplotypes within and across species indicate that the KIR gene family is evolving rapidly, perhaps in response to species-specific pathogens (Grendell et al. 2001; Guethlein et al. 2002; Guethlein et al. 2007; Khakoo et al. 2000; Rajalingam et al. 2001; Sambrook et al. 2005). It was initially thought that KIR were only present in higher primates, although KIR-like sequences have been found recently in lower primates (Hershberger et al. 2001; Mager et al. 2001), ungulates (McQueen et al. 2002), and other mammals (Hoelsbrekken et al. 2003; Sambrook et al. 2006a; Volz et al. 2001).

Extensive phylogenetic analysis among primates (Rajalingam et al. 2004; Sambrook et al. 2005) has revealed five lineages of KIR genes that originated from the recently identified ancestral lineage of KIR3DL0 genes present in all primate species (Sambrook et al. 2006b). Besides KIR3DL0, KIR2DL4 orthologs have also been maintained in all primate species tested. KIR2DL5, KIR3DL3, and KIR2DS4 have also been conserved to some extent, but all other genes appear to have evolved in a species-specific manner. Identical receptor specificity for MHC-Cw molecules has also been observed in human and chimpanzees, and the two species are xenocompatible in that KIR from chimpanzee can functionally recognize some human MHC class I molecules and vice versa (Khakoo et al. 2000).

It has been suggested that MHC class I and KIR are coevolving (Arase and Lanier 2002; Gumperz et al. 1995; Khakoo et al. 2000). Evidence for the coevolutionary process is illustrated by the observation that orangutans have KIR2D genes that are predicted to encode receptors that specify only the Cw1 epitope (asparagine at position 80) of MHC-Cw molecules, which correlates with the observation that allotypes with the Cw2 epitope (lysine at position 80) are missing in this species (Guethlein et al. 2002). Additional selective pressures may also act directly on the KIR loci during early phases of infection by selecting for variants that enhance innate immune responsiveness, potentially increasing the rate of evolution at a speed surpassing that at the HLA class I loci (Khakoo et al. 2000; Martin et al. 2000). In agreement with this hypothesis, all functional HLA class I genes have chimpanzee orthologues (Adams et al. 2000), but there are only three human–chimpanzee KIR orthologues (Khakoo et al. 2000; Martin et al. 2000).

Gene Organization and Sequence

The KIR locus contains a family of polymorphic and highly homologous genes that maps to chromosome 19q13.4 within the leukocyte receptor complex (LRC). The LRC also encodes other related members of the Ig superfamily, including the leukocyte immunoglobulin-like receptor family (LILR) and the leukocyte-associated immunoglobulin-like receptor (LAIR) family. KIR genes are tandemly arrayed over about 100–200 kb (Carrington and Norman 2003; Trowsdale 2001), with the remarkable feature that gene content varies among haplotypes (Uhrberg et al. 1997). The KIR genes show extensive sequence similarity to one another reflecting their origin from an ancestral gene. Indeed, the recently described *KIR3DL0*, which is distinct from all other KIRs, seems to represent the prototypic sequence from which all other KIRs were derived (Sambrook et al. 2006b).

There are four framework genes *KIR3DL3*, *KIR2DL4*, *KIR3DL2*, and *KIR3DP1* that are present on nearly all haplotypes. However, the regions between these genes have undergone multiple gene duplication and deletion events that have resulted in diverse KIR haplotypes having between 6 and 14 expressed KIR genes. *KIR2DL2* and *2DL3* were originally thought to be two distinct genes but data derived from segregation analysis indicate that they actually segregate as alleles of the same locus. The same is also true for the inhibitory *KIR3DL1* and the activating *KIR3DS1*. Almost all haplotypes contain either *KIR2DL2* or *KIR2DL3* and either *KIR3DL1* or *KIR3DS1*; thus they can also be considered as additional framework genes.

The order of the KIR genes along the chromosome has been determined for two distinct haplotypes, providing a framework for their genomic order (Wende et al. 1999, 2000; Wilson et al. 2000). The 10–16 kb-long genes are each oriented in the same direction and separated by about 2 kb; an exception is *KIR2DL4*, which is flanked by an additional 12-kb of sequence. Linkage disequilibrium (LD) studies between pairs of KIR genes have revealed a pattern of strong LD for pairs of genes located centromeric and pairs located telomeric of the central framework gene *KIR2DL4* (Shilling et al. 2002). Although significant in many instances, weaker disequilibrium patterns have been observed between pairs of genes located in opposite halves of the complex. In general, however, patterns of LD that have been observed to date appear to correspond quite well with physical distance between genes.

Exon–Intron Structure of the KIR Genes

Organization of the exon–intron structure of the various KIR genes is fairly consistent with the following basic arrangement: The signal sequence is encoded by the first two exons, each Ig domain (D_0, D_1, and D_2, starting from the N-terminus) corresponds to a single exon (exons 3–5, respectively), the linker and transmembrane regions are each encoded by a single exon (exons 6 and 7), and the cytoplasmic domain is encoded by exons 8 and 9 (figure 7.1) (Trowsdale et al. 2001; Wilson et al. 1997, 2000). The genomic organization of the so-called type 1 two-domain genes: *KIR2DL1*, both *2DL2* and *2DL3*, and all *2DS* genes (Vilches and Parham 2002) is identical to those encoding KIR3D molecules. However, exon 3 is a pseudoexon in these two-domain KIR genes, which often remains in-frame but is eventually spliced out, possibly due to a 3 base-pair deletion (Vilches and Parham 2002). The protein products of type 1 two-domain KIR are therefore missing the D_0 domain (Vilches et al. 2000b). The type 2 two-domain KIRs, which include *KIR2DL4*, *KIR2DL5A*, and *KIR2DL5B* (Vilches and Parham 2002), are characterized by the complete absence of exon 4 (Selvakumar et al. 1997), and therefore their protein product lacks the D_1 domain. The *KIR3DL3* gene closely resembles the other 3D genes, except that it is missing exon 6. The two KIR pseudogenes *KIR2DP1* and *KIR3DP1* have similar exon–intron structures to expressed KIR genes. *KIR2DP1* is closely related to *2DL2/3* and *2DL1* (>97% homology at the nucleotide level) and contains two pseudoexons, 3 and 4. Pseudoexon 3 of *2DP1* contains the same 3 base-pair deletion as the type 1 two-domain KIR genes, and an additional single base-pair deletion in pseudoexon 4 which results in a frame shift that introduces a premature stop codon. *KIR3DP1* is severely truncated, and alternate forms of the gene are differentiated by a 1.5-kb deletion, which removes exon 2 (Wilson et al. 2000).

Polymorphisms and Populations

The high sequence similarity of the KIR genes likely facilitates the occurrence of non-allelic homologous recombination (NAHR) (Carrington and Cullen 2004; Lupski 1998). Indeed, the propensity for NAHR likely explains the expansion and contraction of the KIR complex and the variation in gene content of KIR

Haplotype A

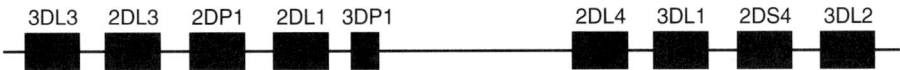

Haplotype B

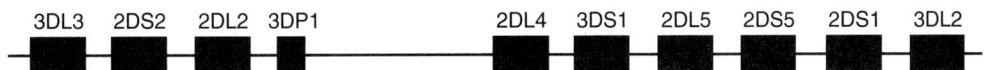

FIGURE 7.2.   Gene order of KIR haplotypes A and B. The genes are organized in a head-to-tail fashion, and each gene is roughly 10–16 kb in length with a sequence of about 2 kb separating each pair of genes, except for a 14-kb stretch of unique sequence upstream of 2DL4. The KIR genes 3DL3, 2DL4, and 3DL2 are framework genes and are present on both haplotypes. These haplotypes are two random examples of many possible haplotype configurations.

haplotypes (Martin et al. 2003; Williams et al. 2003; Wilson et al. 2000). Variation at the KIR gene complex is a function of both variability in the number and types of genes present on any given haplotype and allelic polymorphism within several KIR genes (Selvakumar et al. 1997; Shilling et al. 2002; Uhrberg et al. 1997). Well more than 400 KIR sequences have been deposited into either EMBL GenBank, or the IPD nucleotide sequence databases.

The number of putatively expressed KIR genes present on a single haplotype ranges from about 7 to 12, depending primarily on the presence or absence of activating KIR loci (Uhrberg et al. 1997; Wilson et al. 2000; Witt et al. 1999). Based on gene content, the haplotypes have been divided into two primary groups, termed A and B, which were originally differentiated by the presence of a 24-kb HindIII fragment on Southern blot analysis (Uhrberg et al. 1997). Haplotype A has a uniform gene content composed of nine loci: 2DL1, 2DL3, 2DL4, 2DS4, 3DL1, 3DL2, 3DL3, 2DP1, and 3DP1. Haplotype B, on the other hand, contains various combinations of KIR genes. Perhaps the most functionally relevant distinction between haplotypes A and B is the number of activating receptors present. Haplotype A contains only two activating KIR genes, *KIR2DS4* and *KIR2DL4*, whereas haplotype B contains various combinations of activating 2D and 3D genes. Furthermore, the *KIR2DS4* gene has a null allele with a population frequency of about 84% (allele frequency of 60%) (Maxwell et al. 2002). Similarly, some alleles of *KIR2DL4* encode a molecule that is not expressed on the cell surface, but rather is secreted due to the splicing out of the transmembrane region (Goodridge et al. 2007). Thus, some individuals are homozygous for an A haplotype from which no activating KIR is expressed (Hsu et al. 2002).

Several studies in families and unrelated individuals indicate that there is a great deal of haplotypic diversity across distinct populations (Cook et al. 2003; Crum et al. 2000; Denis et al. 2005; Frassati et al. 2006; Gendzekhadze et al. 2006; Jiang et al. 2005; Middleton et al. 2007; Norman et al. 2001; Rajalingam et al. 2001a; Rajalingam et al. 2002; Toneva et al. 2001; Velickovic et al. 2006; Whang et al. 2005; Witt et al. 1999; Yawata et al. 2002a; Yawata et al. 2002b). The frequencies of haplotypes A and B are roughly equal in Caucasian populations, but in Japanese, Han Chinese, and Koreans, the A haplotype is more frequent (~75%), in stark contrast to the Australian Aborigines with an approximate frequency of 13% for the A haplotype. Based on segregation analysis, more than 40 different B haplotypes have been described (Khakoo and Carrington 2006) and this number is likely to increase as more populations are genotyped.

Expansion and contraction of the KIR region appear to have occurred due in part to unequal crossing over and in some cases has resulted in the generation of KIR haplotypes that have two (or more) copies of a gene on a single haplotype, the rearrangement of gene order, and the generation of hybrid molecules, further expanding diversity (Gomez-Lozano et al. 2005; Martin et al. 2003; Williams et al. 2003).

Allelic Variability

Allelic variation of KIRs creates a further level of diversity such that it is extremely unlikely that any two individuals will be 100% identical (Shilling et al. 2002b). Thus far, the number of alleles per locus ranges from 3–54 (Robinson et al. 2005). Variation tends to occur throughout all regions of the gene, unlike the pattern observed in HLA class I and II genes, where nucleotide variation is restricted primarily to one or two exons (Hughes 2002). Moreover, many of the amino acid residues that vary among KIR allotypes are found in the extracellular domains, suggesting selection of polymorphisms that might alter their interaction with ligands or other molecules (Fan et al. 2001; Gardiner et al. 2001; Snyder et al. 1999).

KIR3DL1 and KIR3DL2, which encode molecules that bind certain allotypes of HLA-B and–A respectively, are quite polymorphic (Gardiner et al. 2001). Polymorphisms in the KIR3DL1 gene appear to have phenotypic consequences as determined by staining with the 3DL1-specific monoclonal antibody (mAb) DX9. Allotypes with high, low, and no binding have been observed and expression levels correlate with variation at specific amino acid residues of the 3DL1 molecule (Gardiner et al. 2001; Pando et al. 2003). Recently, it was also shown that NK cell inhibitory capacity of individual KIR3DL1 allotypes is closely linked to their expression levels on NK cells and to the percent of cells expressing these molecules within the NK cell population of a given individual (Carr et al. 2005; Yawata et al. 2006). Allelic variation also appears to affect the affinity for ligand (Carr et al. 2005; Yawata et al. 2006), where the high expressing allotypes that have been tested show higher affinity for Bw4 allotypes with isoleucine at position 80 (Bw4–80I) than they do for allotypes with threonine at position 80 (Bw4–80T), leading to greater inhibition through Bw4–80I recognition.

Promoter Region Variability

The promoter regions of most KIR genes share >90% sequence similarity (Valiante et al. 1997a) which suggests that they may be controlled by similar mechanisms. The promoter regions of KIR3DL3 and KIR2DL4, however, are more divergent (89% and 69% sequence similarity, respectively) (Trompeter et al. 2005; van Bergen et al. 2005). Differences in promoter regions of these framework loci may account for the relatively low expression of KIR3DL3 (Trundley et al. 2006) and, alternatively, the expression of KIR2DL4 in virtually 100% of NK cell clones, a characteristic unique to KIR2DL4 (Valiante et al. 1997a). Measurements of KIR2DL5A mRNA in NK cells indicate that it is expressed, whereas KIR2DL5B is not (Vilches et al. 2000a) and this correlates with a mutation in a putative AML1 transcription factor site in the promoter region, a variant that is also present in the pseudogene KIR3DP1.

KIRs are clonally expressed in a variegated fashion on NK cells (Ciccone et al. 1992; Moretta et al. 1990; Wagtmann et al. 1995) and the control of clonal expression is one of the most intriguing aspects of NK cell genetics. Recent studies have suggested epigenetic mechanisms to explain the regulation of clonal KIR expression (Chan et al. 2003; Gomez-Lozano et al. 2007; Santourlidis et al. 2002). One such mechanism is DNA hypomethylation in the 5′ region of the gene that was shown to correlate with silencing of KIR transcription in a stochastic fashion. DNA methylation also appears to maintain the stability of the KIR repertoire in NK cell clones (Chan et al. 2005; Santourlidis et al. 2002), and the silencing of KIR3DL3 in a subpopulation of NK cells (Trundley et al. 2006). More recently, an interesting mechanism to explain the stochastic expression of Ly49 was described in the mouse (Saleh et al. 2004). This mechanism is based on the presence of bidirectional promoters that behave as probabilistic switches. The KIR proximal promoter region has also recently been shown to possess bi-directional transcriptional activity (Davies et al. 2007).

Population Studies of Infectious Diseases

Because KIR genes, haplotypes, and allelic polymorphisms have only recently been characterized, few studies to date have addressed genetic associations of KIR with specific diseases. Given the receptor–ligand relationship between certain combinations of KIR and HLA class I molecules, early investigations hypothesized interactions, including synergistic relationships, between these two systems of polymorphic loci that may ultimately regulate NK cell–mediated immunity against infectious pathogens. Such epistatic interaction has been shown in two successive population studies of HIV-1 infection (Martin et al. 2002; Martin et al. 2007; see also chapter 19 in this volume). In those analyses, the combinations of either KIR3DS1 and KIR3DL1 which are alleles of the same locus, with certain HLA-B Bw4 alleles that encode molecules with isoleucine at position 80, Bw4-80I resulted in delayed progression to AIDS after HIV-1 infection. Neither of the two KIR allelic forms by itself was associated with slower disease progression, and homozygosity for *KIR3DS1* in the absence of Bw4–80I was significantly associated with more rapid progression to AIDS. The more recent of these studies also documented further variability of NK receptor expression based on allelic differences of *KIR3DL1*. The models proposed to account for the distinctive effects of the products of these two KIR genes in conjunction with their HLA-B ligands reflect complex host-virus interplay along with context-specific competition between NK activation and inhibition that will be the focus of much future investigation.

The effects of HLA class I and KIR have also been studied in a large study of HCV infection that enrolled 352 individuals with HCV clearance and 685 matched persistently infected individuals (Khakoo et al. 2004). The genes encoding the inhibitory NK cell receptor KIR2DL3 and its HLA-C1 ligand, which transmit relatively weak inhibitory signals, enhanced resolution of HCV infection. The protection was observed only among individuals presumably receiving low-dose HCV inocula, suggesting that the difference in the ability of distinct KIR-HLA genotypes to regulate NK cell activity is great enough to alter the outcome when faced with low-dose but not high-dose infection (Khakoo et al. 2004).

The results of these studies on HIV-1 and HCV infection are consistent with the experimental evidence for specific interaction between KIR and HLA molecules. Although these findings await biologic and epidemiologic confirmation, they emphasize the possibility that HLA associations with some diseases may actually stem from such molecular interaction on NK or T cells.

Gazit et al. (2004) described a patient with recurrent infections, mainly due to CMV. The patient, whose entire NK cell population expressed KIR2DL1, had symptoms almost identical to those seen in patients with NK cell deficiency. This case highlights the importance of inhibitory NK cell interactions in antiviral immunity and suggests that diminished inhibitory responses confer protection against infection, while increased inhibition may lead to susceptibility to infection. A recent report also showed an association of KIR and the course of HSV-1 infection (Estefania et al. 2007). The authors provide preliminary evidence suggesting that *KIR2DL2* and *KIR2DS2*, which are in strong LD, predispose to symptomatic HSV-1 infection and favor the frequently recurring forms of the disease perhaps by hindering an effective cellular response to the virus.

Conclusion and Prospects

KIR genes have been associated with several disease processes, primarily through their interaction with polymorphic HLA class I molecules. The importance of NK cells for early defense against infection suggests that human KIR genotype diversity reflects the cumulative impact of many successive selective encounters between different pathogens and the machinery of the human NK cell response (Parham 2004; Yawata et al. 2002a). In addition to demonstrating associations with infectious diseases, population studies have also suggested that selection acts on KIR. The KIR haplotype composition and allele frequency distributions are consistent with the influence of balancing selection. The high interpopulation heterogeneity measure a for the LRC-encoded leukocyte immunoglobulin-like receptor A3 (*LILRA3*) is an illustration of pathogen-driven disruptive selection (Norman et al. 2004). These observations, coupled with further delineation of the diversity at the KIR gene complex and development of efficient typing systems, will surely foster disease association studies as plentiful, varied, and ultimately enlightening as those that focused HLA loci. To achieve the ultimate aim of such association studies, predicting the relative risk and protection, researchers should aim to fulfill sound principles of epidemiologic investigation, including careful definition of phenotypes and adequate power (Dahlman et al. 2002). Future work will also focus on identification of ligands, especially for the NK cell receptors other than KIR, and the precise role of individual receptors especially in bridging the innate and adaptive immunity.

References

Adams, E.J., Cooper, S., Thomson, G., & Parham, P. (2000) Common chimpanzees have greater diversity than humans at two of the three highly polymorphic MHC class I genes. *Immunogenetics*, 51, 410–424.

Andre, P., Biassoni, R., Colonna, M., Cosman, D., Lanier, L.L., Long, E.O., Lopez-Botet, M., Moretta, A., Moretta, L., Parham, P., Trowsdale, J., Vivier, E.,

Wagtmann, N., & Wilson, M.J. (2001) New nomenclature for MHC receptors. *Nature Immunology*, **2**, 661.

Arase, H., & Lanier, L.L. (2002) Virus-driven evolution of natural killer cell receptors. *Microbes and Infection*, **4**, 1505–1512.

Arase, H., Mocarski, E.S., Campbell, A.E., Hill, A.B., & Lanier, L.L. (2002) Direct recognition of cytomegalovirus by activating and inhibitory NK cell receptors. *Science*, **296**, 1323–1326.

Bancroft, G.J. (1993) The role of natural killer cells in innate resistance to infection. *Current Opinion in Immunology*, **5**, 503–510.

Biassoni, R., Cantoni, C., Pende, D., Sivori, S., Parolini, S., Vitale, M., Bottino, C., & Moretta, A. (2001) Human natural killer cell receptors and co-receptors. *Immunological Reviews*, **181**, 203–214.

Biassoni, R., Falco, M., Cambiaggi, A., Costa, P., Verdiani, S., Pende, D., Conte, R., Di Donato, C., Parham, P., & Moretta, L. (1995) Amino acid substitutions can influence the natural killer (NK)-mediated recognition of HLA-C molecules. Role of serine-77 and lysine-80 in the target cell protection from lysis mediated by "group 2" or "group 1" NK clones. *Journal of Experimental Medicine*, **182**, 605–609.

Biassoni, R., Pessino, A., Malaspina, A., Cantoni, C., Bottino, C., Sivori, S., Moretta, L., & Moretta, A. (1997) Role of amino acid position 70 in the binding affinity of p50.1 and p58.1 receptors for HLA-Cw4 molecules. *European Journal of Immunology*, **27**, 3095–3099.

Biron, C.A., Byron, K.S., & Sullivan, J.L. (1989) Severe herpesvirus infections in an adolescent without natural killer cells. *New England Journal of Medicine*, **320**, 1731–1735.

Biron, C.A., Nguyen, K.B., Pien, G.C., Cousens, L.P., & Salazar-Mather, T.P. (1999) Natural killer cells in antiviral defense: function and regulation by innate cytokines. *Annual Review of Immunology*, **17**, 189–220.

Bjorkman, P.J., Saper, M.A., Samraoui, B., Bennett, W.S., Strominger, J.L., & Wiley, D.C. (1987) The foreign antigen binding site and T cell recognition regions of class I histocompatibility antigens. *Nature*, **329**, 512–518.

Blery, M., Olcese, L., & Vivier, E. (2000) Early signaling via inhibitory and activating NK receptors. *Human Immunology*, **61**, 51–64.

Boyington, J.C., Brooks, A.G., & Sun, P.D. (2001) Structure of killer cell immunoglobulin-like receptors and their recognition of the class I MHC molecules. *Immunological Reviews*, **181**, 66–78.

Boyington, J.C., Motyka, S.A., Schuck, P., Brooks, A.G., & Sun, P.D. (2000) Crystal structure of an NK cell immunoglobulin-like receptor in complex with its class I MHC ligand. *Nature*, **405**, 537–543.

Brown, M.G., Dokun, A.O., Heusel, J.W., Smith, H.R., Beckman, D.L., Blattenberger, E.A., Dubbelde, C.E., Stone, L.R., Scalzo, A.A., & Yokoyama, W.M. (2001) Vital involvement of a natural killer cell activation receptor in resistance to viral infection. *Science*, **292**, 934–937.

Bruhns, P., Marchetti, P., Fridman, W.H., Vivier, E., & Daeron, M. (1999) Differential roles of N- and C-terminal immunoreceptor tyrosine-based inhibition motifs during inhibition of cell activation by killer cell inhibitory receptors. *Journal of Immunology*, **162**, 3168–3175.

Brumbaugh, K.M., Binstadt, B.A., Billadeau, D.D., Schoon, R.A., Dick, C.J., Ten, R.M., & Leibson, P.J. (1997) Functional role for Syk tyrosine kinase in natural killer cell-mediated natural cytotoxicity. *Journal of Experimental Medicine*, **186**, 1965–1974.

Burshtyn, D.N., Scharenberg, A.M., Wagtmann, N., Rajagopalan, S., Berrada, K., Yi, T., Kinet, J.P., & Long, E.O. (1996) Recruitment of tyrosine phosphatase HCP by the killer cell inhibitor receptor. *Immunity*, **4**, 77–85.

Carlin, L.M., Eleme, K., McCann, F.E., & Davis, D.M. (2001) Intercellular transfer and supramolecular organization of human leukocyte antigen C at inhibitory natural killer cell immune synapses. *Journal of Experimental Medicine*, **194**, 1507–1517.

Carr, W. H., Pando, M. J., & Parham, P. (2005) KIR3DL1 polymorphisms that affect NK cell inhibition by HLA-Bw4 ligand. *Journal of Immunology*, **175**, 5222–5229.

Carrington, M., & Cullen, M. (2004) Justified chauvinism: Advances in defining meiotic recombination through sperm typing. *Trends in Genetics*, **20**, 196–205.

Carrington, M., & Norman, P.J. (2003) *The KIR gene cluster*. Vol. 2003. Bethesda, MD: U.S. National Library of Medicine, National Center for Biotechnology Information. Available from www.ncbi.nlm .nih.gov/entrez/query.fcgi?db=Books

Cella, M., Longo, A., Ferrara, G.B., Strominger, J.L., & Colonna, M. (1994) NK3-specific natural killer cells are selectively inhibited by Bw4-positive HLA alleles with isoleucine 80. *Journal of Experimental Medicine*, **180**, 1235–1242.

Cerwenka, A., & Lanier, L.L. (2001) Ligands for natural killer cell receptors: redundancy or specificity. *Immunological Reviews*, **181**, 158–169.

Chan, H. W., Kurago, Z. B., Stewart, C. A., Wilson, M. J., Martin, M. P., Mace, B. E., Carrington, M., Trowsdale, J., & Lutz, C.T. (2003) DNA methylation maintains allele-specific KIR gene expression in human natural killer cells. *Journal of Experimental Medicine*, **197**, 245–255.

Chan, H.W., Miller, J.S., Moore, M.B., & Lutz, C.T. (2005) Epigenetic control of highly homologous killer Ig-like receptor gene alleles. *Journal of Immunology*, **175**, 5966–5974.

Ciccone, E., Pende, D., Viale, O., Di Donato, C., Tripodi, G., Orengo, A. M., Guardiola, J., Moretta, A., & Moretta, L. (1992) Evidence of a natural killer (NK) cell repertoire for (allo) antigen recognition: definition of five distinct NK-determined allospecificities in humans. *Journal of Experimental Medicine*, **175**, 709–718.

Cohen, G.B., Gandhi, R.T., Davis, D.M., Mandelboim, O., Chen, B.K., Strominger, J.L., & Baltimore, D. (1999) The selective downregulation of class I major histocompatibility complex proteins by HIV-1 protects HIV-infected cells from NK cells. *Immunity*, **10**, 661–671.

Colonna, M., & Samaridis, J. (1995) Cloning of immunoglobulin-superfamily members associated with HLA-C and HLA-B recognition by human natural killer cells. *Science*, **268**, 405–408.

Colonna, M., Spies, T., Strominger, J.L., Ciccone, E., Moretta, A., Moretta, L., Pende, D., & Viale, O. (1992) Alloantigen recognition by two human natural killer cell clones is associated with HLA-C or a closely linked gene. *Proceedings of the National Academy of Sciences of the United States of America*, **89**, 7983–7985.

Cook, M.A., Moss, P.A., & Briggs, D.C. (2003) The distribution of 13 killer-cell immunoglobulin-like receptor loci in UK blood donors from three ethnic groups. *European Journal of Immunogenetics*, **30**, 213–221.

Cooper, M.A., Fehniger, T.A., & Caligiuri, M.A. (2001) The biology of human natural killer-cell subsets. *Trends in Immunology*, **22**, 633–640.

Coscoy, L., & Ganem, D. (2000) Kaposi's sarcoma-associated herpesvirus encodes two proteins that block cell surface display of MHC class I chains by enhancing their endocytosis. *Proceedings of the National Academy of Sciences of the United States of America*, **97**, 8051–8056.

Cretney, E., Degli-Esposti, M.A., Densley, E.H., Farrell, H.E., Davis-Poynter, N.J., & Smyth, M.J. (1999) m144, a murine cytomegalovirus (MCMV)-encoded major histocompatibility complex class I homologue, confers tumor resistance to natural killer cell-mediated rejection. *Journal of Experimental Medicine*, **190**, 435–444.

Crum, K.A., Logue, S.E., Curran, M.D., & Middleton, D. (2000) Development of a PCR-SSOP approach capable of defining the natural killer cell inhibitory receptor (KIR) gene sequence repertoires. *Tissue Antigens*, **56**, 313–326.

Dahlman, I., Eaves, I.A., Kosoy, R., Morrison, V.A., Heward, J., Gough, S.C., Allahabadia, A., Franklyn, J.A., Tuomilehto, J., Tuomilehto-Wolf, E., Cucca, F., Guja, C., Ionescu-Tirgoviste, C., Stevens, H., Carr, P., Nutland, S., McKinney, P., Shield, J.P., Wang, W., Cordell, H.J., Walker, N., Todd, J.A., & Concannon, P. (2002) Parameters for reliable results in genetic association studies in common disease. *Nature Genetics*, **30**, 149–150.

D'Andrea, A., Chang, C., Franz-Bacon, K., McClanahan, T., Phillips, J.H., & Lanier, L.L. (1995) Molecular cloning of NKB1. A natural killer cell receptor for HLA-B allotypes. *Journal of Immunology*, **155**, 2306–2310.

Daniels, K.A., Devora, G., Lai, W.C., O'Donnell, C.L., Bennett, M., & Welsh, R.M. (2001) Murine cytomegalovirus is regulated by a discrete subset of natural killer cells reactive with monoclonal antibody to Ly49H. *Journal of Experimental Medicine*, **194**, 29–44.

Davies, G.E., Locke, S.M., Wright, P.W., Li, H., Hanson, R.J., Miller, J.S., & Anderson, S.K. (2007) Identification of bidirectional promoters in the human KIR genes. *Genes and Immunity*, **8**, 245–253.

Davis, D.M., Chiu, I., Fassett, M., Cohen, G.B., Mandelboim, O., & Strominger, J.L. (1999) The human natural killer cell immune synapse. *Proceedings of the National Academy of Sciences of the United States of America*, **96**, 15062–15067.

Denis, L., Sivula, J., Gourraud, P.A., Kerdudou, N., Chout, R., Ricard, C., Moisan, J.P., Gagne, K., Partanen, J., & Bignon, J.D. (2005) Genetic diversity of KIR natural killer cell markers in populations from France, Guadeloupe, Finland, Senegal and Reunion. *Tissue Antigens*, **66**, 267–276.

Diefenbach, A., & Raulet, D.H. (2001) Strategies for target cell recognition by natural killer cells. *Immunological Reviews*, **181**, 170–184.

Dohring, C., Samaridis, J., & Colonna, M. (1996a) Alternatively spliced forms of human killer inhibitory receptors. *Immunogenetics*, **44**, 227–230.

Dohring, C., Scheidegger, D., Samaridis, J., Cella, M., & Colonna, M. (1996b) A human killer inhibitory receptor specific for HLA-A1. *Journal of Immunology*, **156**, 3098–3101.

Estefania, E., Gomez-Lozano, N., Portero, F., de Pablo, R., Solis, R., Sepulveda, S., Vaquero, M., Gonzalez,

M.A., Suarez, E., Roustan, G., & Vilches, C. (2007) Influence of KIR gene diversity on the course of HSV-1 infection: resistance to the disease is associated with the absence of KIR2DL2 and KIR2DS2. *Tissue Antigens*, **70**, 34–41.

Fan, Q.R., Long, E.O., & Wiley, D.C. (2001) Crystal structure of the human natural killer cell inhibitory receptor KIR2DL1–HLA-Cw4 complex. *Nature Immunology*, **2**, 452–460.

Farrell, H.E., Vally, H., Lynch, D.M., Fleming, P., Shellam, G.R., Scalzo, A.A., & Davis-Poynter, N.J. (1997) Inhibition of natural killer cells by a cytomegalovirus MHC class I homologue in vivo. *Nature*, **386**, 510–514.

Fassett, M.S., Davis, D.M., Valter, M.M., Cohen, G.B., & Strominger, J.L. (2001) Signaling at the inhibitory natural killer cell immune synapse regulates lipid raft polarization but not class I MHC clustering. *Proceedings of the National Academy of Sciences of the United States of America*, **98**, 14547–14552.

Fernandez, N.C., Treiner, E., Vance, R.E., Jamieson, A.M., Lemieux, S., & Raulet, D.H. (2005) A subset of natural killer cells achieves self-tolerance without expressing inhibitory receptors specific for self-MHC molecules. *Blood*, **105**, 4416–4423.

Frassati, C., Touinssi, M., Picard, C., Segura, M., Galicher, V., Papa, K., Gagne, K., Vivier, E., Degioanni, A., Boetsch, G., Mercier, P., Vely, F., de Micco, P., Reviron, D., & Chiaroni, J. (2006) Distribution of killer-cell immunoglobulin-like receptor (KIR) in Comoros and Southeast France. *Tissue Antigens*, **67**, 356–367.

French, A.R., & Yokoyama, W.M. (2003) Natural killer cells and viral infections. *Current Opinion in Immunology*, **15**, 45–51.

Fry, A.M., Lanier, L.L., & Weiss, A. (1996) Phosphotyrosines in the killer cell inhibitory receptor motif of NKB1 are required for negative signaling and for association with protein tyrosine phosphatase 1C. *Journal of Experimental Medicine*, **184**, 295–300.

Gardiner, C.M., Guethlein, L.A., Shilling, H.G., Pando, M., Carr, W.H., Rajalingam, R., Vilches, C., & Parham, P. (2001) Different NK cell surface phenotypes defined by the DX9 antibody are due to KIR3DL1 gene polymorphism. *Journal of Immunology*, **166**, 2992–3001.

Gazit, R., Garty, B.Z., Monselise, Y., Hoffer, V., Finkelstein, Y., Markel, G., Katz, G., Hanna, J., Achdout, H., Gruda, R., Gonen-Gross, T., & Mandelboim, O. (2004) Expression of KIR2DL1 on the entire NK cell population: a possible novel immunodeficiency syndrome. *Blood*, **103**, 1965–1966.

Gendzekhadze, K., Norman, P.J., Abi-Rached, L., Layrisse, Z., & Parham, P. (2006) High KIR diversity in Amerindians is maintained using few gene-content haplotypes. *Immunogenetics*, **58**, 474–480.

Gewurz, B.E., Wang, E.W., Tortorella, D., Schust, D.J., & Ploegh, H.L. (2001) Human cytomegalovirus US2 endoplasmic reticulum-lumenal domain dictates association with major histocompatibility complex class I in a locus-specific manner. *Journal of Virology*, **75**, 5197–5204.

Gomez-Lozano, N., Gardiner, C.M., Parham, P., & Vilches, C. (2002) Some human KIR haplotypes contain two KIR2DL5 genes: KIR2DL5A and KIR2DL5B. *Immunogenetics*, **54**, 314–319.

Gomez-Lozano, N., Trompeter, H.I., de Pablo, R., Estefania, E., Uhrberg, M., & Vilches, C. (2007) Epigenetic silencing of potentially functional KIR2DL5 alleles: Implications for the acquisition of KIR repertoires by NK cells. *European Journal of Immunology*, **37**, 1954–1965.

Goodridge, J.P., Lathbury, L.J., Steiner, N.K., Shulse, C.N., Pullikotil, P., Seidah, N.G., Hurley, C.K., Christiansen, F.T., & Witt, C.S. (2007) Three common alleles of KIR2DL4 (CD158d) encode constitutively expressed, inducible and secreted receptors in NK cells. *European Journal of Immunology*, **37**, 199–211.

Grendell, R.L., Hughes, A.L., & Golos, T.G. (2001) Cloning of rhesus monkey killer-cell Ig-like receptors (KIRs) from early pregnancy decidua. *Tissue Antigens*, **58**, 329–334.

Guethlein, L.A., Flodin, L.R., Adams, E.J., & Parham, P. (2002) NK cell receptors of the orangutan (Pongo pygmaeus): a pivotal species for tracking the coevolution of killer cell Ig-like receptors with MHC- C. *Journal of Immunology*, **169**, 220–229.

Guethlein, L.A., Older Aguilar, A.M., Abi-Rached, L., & Parham, P. (2007) Evolution of Killer Cell Ig-Like Receptor (KIR) Genes: Definition of an Orangutan KIR Haplotype Reveals Expansion of Lineage III KIR Associated with the Emergence of MHC-C. *Journal of Immunology*, **179**, 491–504.

Gumperz, J.E., Litwin, V., Phillips, J.H., Lanier, L.L., & Parham, P. (1995) The Bw4 public epitope of HLA-B molecules confers reactivity with natural killer cell clones that express NKB1, a putative HLA receptor. *Journal of Experimental Medicine*, **181**, 1133–1144.

Hanke, T., Takizawa, H., McMahon, C.W., Busch, D.H., Pamer, E.G., Miller, J.D., Altman, J.D., Liu, Y., Cado, D., Lemonnier, F.A., Bjorkman, P.J., & Raulet, D.H. (1999) Direct assessment of MHC class I binding by seven Ly49 inhibitory NK cell receptors. *Immunity*, **11**, 67–77.

Hansasuta, P., Dong, T., Thananchai, H., Weekes, M., Willberg, C., Aldemir, H., Rowland-Jones, S., & Braud, V.M. (2004) Recognition of HLA-A3 and

HLA-A11 by *KIR3DL2* is peptide-specific. *European Journal of Immunology*, **34**, 1673–1679.

Harel-Bellan, A., Quillet, A., Marchiol, C., DeMars, R., Tursz, T., & Fradelizi, D. (1986) Natural killer susceptibility of human cells may be regulated by genes in the HLA region on chromosome 6. *Proceedings of the National Academy of Sciences of the United States of America*, **83**, 5688–5692.

Hershberger, K.L., Shyam, R., Miura, A., & Letvin, N.L. (2001) Diversity of the killer cell Ig-like receptors of rhesus monkeys. *Journal of Immunology*, **166**, 4380–4390.

Hoelsbrekken, S.E., Nylenna, O., Saether, P.C., Slettedal, I.O., Ryan, J.C., Fossum, S., & Dissen, E. (2003) Cutting edge: molecular cloning of a killer cell Ig-like receptor in the mouse and rat. *Journal of Immunology*, **170**, 2259–2263.

Horton, R., Wilming, L., Rand, V., Lovering, R.C., Bruford, E.A., Khodiyar, V.K., Lush, M.J., Povey, S., Talbot, C.C., Jr., Wright, M.W., Wain, H.M., Trowsdale, J., Ziegler, A., & Beck, S. (2004) Gene map of the extended human MHC. *Nature Reviews. Genetics*, **5**, 889–899.

Hsu, K.C., Chida, S., Dupont, B., & Geraghty, D.E. (2002) The killer cell immunoglobulin-like receptor (KIR) genomic region: gene-order, haplotypes and allelic polymorphism. *Immunological Reviews*, **190**, 40–52.

Hughes, A.L. (2002) Natural selection and the diversification of vertebrate immune effectors. *Immunological Reviews*, **190**, 161–168.

Ishido, S., Wang, C., Lee, B.S., Cohen, G.B., & Jung, J.U. (2000) Downregulation of major histocompatibility complex class I molecules by Kaposi's sarcoma-associated herpesvirus K3 and K5 proteins. *Journal of Virology*, **74**, 5300–5309.

Jiang, K., Zhu, F.M., Lv, Q.F., & Yan, L.X. (2005) Distribution of killer cell immunoglobulin-like receptor genes in the Chinese Han population. *Tissue Antigens*, **65**, 556–563.

Karre, K., Ljunggren, H.G., Piontek, G., & Kiessling, R. (1986) Selective rejection of H-2-deficient lymphoma variants suggests alternative immune defence strategy. *Nature*, **319**, 675–678.

Khakoo, S. I. & Carrington, M. (2006) KIR and disease: A model system or system of models? *Immunological Reviews*, **214**, 186–201.

Khakoo, S.I., Geller, R., Shin, S., Jenkins, J.A., & Parham, P. (2002) The D0 domain of KIR3D acts as a major histocompatibility complex class I binding enhancer. *Journal of Experimental Medicine*, **196**, 911–921.

Khakoo, S.I., Rajalingam, R., Shum, B.P., Weidenbach, K., Flodin, L., Muir, D.G., Canavez, F., Cooper, S.L., Valiante, N.M., Lanier, L.L. & Parham, P. (2000) Rapid evolution of NK cell receptor systems demonstrated by comparison of chimpanzees and humans. *Immunity*, **12**, 687–698.

Khakoo, S.I., Thio, C., Martin, M., Brooks, C., Gao, X., Astemborski, J., Cheng, J., Goedert, J., Vlahov, D., Hilgartner, M., Cox, S., Little, A., Alexander, G., Cramp, M., O'Brien, S., Rosenberg, W., Thomas, D. & Carrington, M. (2004) HLA and NK cell inhibitory receptor genes in resolving hepatitis C virus infection. *Science*, **305**, 872–874.

Kikuchi-Maki, A., Catina, T.L., & Campbell, K.S. (2005) Cutting edge: KIR2DL4 transduces signals into human NK cells through association with the Fc receptor gamma protein. *Journal of Immunology*, **174**, 3859–3863.

Kim, J., Chwae, Y.J., Kim, M.Y., Choi, I.H., Park, J.H., & Kim, S.J. (1997) Molecular basis of HLA-C recognition by p58 natural killer cell inhibitory receptors. *Journal of Immunology*, **159**, 3875–3882.

Kim, S., Poursine-Laurent, J., Truscott, S.M., Lybarger, L., Song, Y.J., Yang, L., French, A.R., Sunwoo, J.B., Lemieux, S., Hansen, T.H., & Yokoyama, W.M. (2005) Licensing of natural killer cells by host major histocompatibility complex class I molecules. *Nature*, **436**, 709–713.

Lanier, L.L. (1998) NK cell receptors. *Annual Review of Immunology*, **16**, 359–393.

Lanier, L.L. (2005) NK cell recognition. *Annual Review of Immunology*, **23**, 225–274.

Lanier, L.L., Corliss, B.C., Wu, J., Leong, C., & Phillips, J.H. (1998) Immunoreceptor DAP12 bearing a tyrosine-based activation motif is involved in activating NK cells. *Nature*, **391**, 703–707.

Lee, S.H., Girard, S., Macina, D., Busa, M., Zafer, A., Belouchi, A., Gros, P., & Vidal, S.M. (2001) Susceptibility to mouse cytomegalovirus is associated with deletion of an activating natural killer cell receptor of the C-type lectin superfamily. *Nature Genetics*, **28**, 42–45.

Leibson, P.J. (1997) Signal transduction during natural killer cell activation: inside the mind of a killer. *Immunity*, **6**, 655–661.

Liao, N.S., Bix, M., Zijlstra, M., Jaenisch, R., and Raulet, D. (1991) MHC class I deficiency: susceptibility to natural killer (NK) cells and impaired NK activity. *Science*, **253**, 199–202.

Ljunggren, H.G., & Karre, K. (1990) In search of the "missing self": MHC molecules and NK cell recognition. *Immunology Today*, **11**, 237–244.

Long, E.O. (1999) Regulation of immune responses through inhibitory receptors. *Annual Review of Immunology*, **17**, 875–904.

Long, E.O., & Rajagopalan, S. (2000) HLA class I recognition by killer cell Ig-like receptors. *Seminars in Immunology*, **12**, 101–108.

Long, E.O., & Rajagopalan, S. (2002) Stress signals activate natural killer cells. *Journal of Experimental Medicine*, **196**, 1399–1402.

Lopez-Botet, M., Llano, M., Navarro, F., & Bellon, T. (2000) NK cell recognition of non-classical HLA class I molecules. *Seminars in Immunology*, **12**, 109–119.

Lupski, J.R. (1998) Charcot-Marie-Tooth disease: lessons in genetic mechanisms. *Molecular Medicine*, **4**, 3–11.

Maenaka, K., Juji, T., Nakayama, T., Wyer, J.R., Gao, G.F., Maenaka, T., Zaccai, N.R., Kikuchi, A., Yabe, T., Tokunaga, K., Tadokoro, K., Stuart, D.I., Jones, E.Y., & van der Merwe, P.A. (1999a) Killer cell immunoglobulin receptors and T cell receptors bind peptide-major histocompatibility complex class I with distinct thermodynamic and kinetic properties. *Journal of Biological Chemistry*, **274**, 28329–28334.

Maenaka, K., Juji, T., Stuart, D.I., & Jones, E.Y. (1999b) Crystal structure of the human p58 killer cell inhibitory receptor (*KIR2DL3*) specific for HLA-Cw3-related MHC class I. *Structure*, **7**, 391–398.

Mager, D.L., McQueen, K.L., Wee, V., & Freeman, J.D. (2001) Evolution of natural killer cell receptors: co-existence of functional Ly49 and KIR genes in baboons. *Current Biology*, **11**, 626–630.

Malnati, M.S., Peruzzi, M., Parker, K.C., Biddison, W.E., Ciccone, E., Moretta, A., & Long, E.O. (1995) Peptide specificity in the recognition of MHC class I by natural killer cell clones. *Science*, **267**, 1016–1018.

Mandelboim, O., Reyburn, H.T., Vales-Gomez, M., Pazmany, L., Colonna, M., Borsellino, G., & Strominger, J.L. (1996) Protection from lysis by natural killer cells of group 1 and 2 specificity is mediated by residue 80 in human histocompatibility leukocyte antigen C alleles and also occurs with empty major histocompatibility complex molecules. *Journal of Experimental Medicine*, **184**, 913–922.

Mandelboim, O., Wilson, S.B., Vales-Gomez, M., Reyburn, H.T., & Strominger, J.L. (1997) Self and viral peptides can initiate lysis by autologous natural killer cells. *Proceedings of the National Academy of Sciences of the United States of America*, **94**, 4604–4609.

Marsh, S.G., Parham, P., Dupont, B., Geraghty, D.E., Trowsdale, J., Middleton, D., Vilches, C., Carrington, M., Witt, C., Guethlein, L.A., Shilling, H., Garcia, C.A., Hsu, K.C., & Wain, H. (2003) Killer-cell immunoglobulin-like receptor (KIR) nomenclature report, 2002. *Tissue Antigens*, **62**, 79–86.

Martin, A.M., Freitas, E.M., Witt, C.S., & Christiansen, F.T. (2000) The genomic organization and evolution of the natural killer immunoglobulin-like receptor (KIR) gene cluster. *Immunogenetics*, **51**, 268–280.

Martin, M.P., Bashirova, A., Traherne, J., Trowsdale, J., & Carrington, M. (2003) Cutting edge: expansion of the KIR locus by unequal crossing over. *Journal of Immunology*, **171**, 2192–2195.

Martin, M.P., Gao, X., Lee, J.H., Nelson, G.W., Detels, R., Goedert, J.J., Buchbinder, S., Hoots, K., Vlahov, D., Trowsdale, J., Wilson, M., O'Brien, S.J., & Carrington, M. (2002) Epistatic interaction between *KIR3DS1* and HLA-B delays the progression to AIDS. *Nature Genetics*, **31**, 429–434.

Martin, M.P., Gao, X., Yamada, E., Martin, J.N., Pereyra, F., Colombo, S., Brown, E.E., Shupert, W.L., Phair, J., Goedert, J.J., Buchbinder, S., Kirk, G.D., Telenti, A., Connors, M., O'Brien, S.J., Walker, B.D., Parham, P., Deeks, S.G., McVicar, D.W., Carrington, M. (2007) Innate partnership of HLA-B and *KIR3DL1* subtypes against HIV-1. *Nat Genet*, **39**, 733–740.

Maxwell, L.D., Wallace, A., Middleton, D., & Curran, M.D. (2002) A common KIR2DS4 deletion variant in the human that predicts a soluble KIR molecule analogous to the KIR1D molecule observed in the rhesus monkey. *Tissue Antigens*, **60**, 254–258.

McQueen, K.L., Wilhelm, B.T., Harden, K.D., & Mager, D.L. (2002) Evolution of NK receptors: a single Ly49 and multiple KIR genes in the cow. *European Journal of Immunology*, **32**, 810–817.

Middleton, D., Meenagh, A., & Gourraud, P. A. (2007) KIR haplotype content at the allele level in 77 Northern Irish families. *Immunogenetics*, **59**, 145–158.

Moretta, A., Bottino, C., Pende, D., Tripodi, G., Tambussi, G., Viale, O., Orengo, A., Barbaresi, M., Merli, A., & Ciccone, E. (1990) Identification of four subsets of human CD3-CD16+ natural killer (NK) cells by the expression of clonally distributed functional surface molecules: correlation between subset assignment of NK clones and ability to mediate specific alloantigen recognition. *Journal of Experimental Medicine*, **172**, 1589–1598.

Moretta, A., Bottino, C., Vitale, M., Pende, D., Biassoni, R., Mingari, M.C., & Moretta, L. (1996) Receptors for HLA class-I molecules in human natural killer cells. *Annual Review of Immunology*, **14**, 619–648.

Moretta, A., Sivori, S., Vitale, M., Pende, D., Morelli, L., Augugliaro, R., Bottino, C. & Moretta, L. (1995) Existence of both inhibitory (p58) and activatory (p50) receptors for HLA-C molecules in human natural killer cells. *Journal of Experimental Medicine*, **182**, 875–884.

Moretta, A., Tambussi, G., Bottino, C., Tripodi, G., Merli, A., Ciccone, E., Pantaleo, G. & Moretta, L. (1990) A novel surface antigen expressed by a subset of human CD3- CD16+ natural killer cells. Role in cell activation and regulation of cytolytic function. *Journal of Experimental Medicine*, **171**, 695–714.

Moretta, L., Bottino, C., Pende, D., Mingari, M.C., Biassoni, R., & Moretta, A. (2002) Human natural killer cells: their origin, receptors and function. *European Journal of Immunology*, **32**, 1205–1211.

Moretta, L. & Moretta, A. (2004) Unravelling natural killer cell function: triggering and inhibitory human NK receptors. *EMBO Journal*, **23**, 255–259.

Norman, P.J., Carrington, C.V., Byng, M., Maxwell, L.D., Curran, M.D., Stephens, H.A., Chandanayingyong, D., Verity, D.H., Hameed, K., Ramdath, D.D., & Vaughan, R.W. (2002) Natural killer cell immunoglobulin-like receptor (KIR) locus profiles in African and South Asian populations. *Genes and Immunity*, **3**, 86–95.

Norman, P.J., Cook, M.A., Carey, B.S., Carrington, C.V., Verity, D.H., Hameed, K., Ramdath, D.D., Chandanayingyong, D., Leppert, M., Stephens, H.A., & Vaughan, R.W. (2004) SNP haplotypes and allele frequencies show evidence for disruptive and balancing selection in the human leukocyte receptor complex. *Immunogenetics*, **56**, 225–237.

Norman, P.J., Stephens, H.A., Verity, D.H., Chandanayingyong, D. & Vaughan, R.W. (2001) Distribution of natural killer cell immunoglobulin-like receptor sequences in three ethnic groups. *Immunogenetics*, **52**, 195–205.

Olcese, L., Cambiaggi, A., Semenzato, G., Bottino, C., Moretta, A., & Vivier, E. (1997) Human killer cell activatory receptors for MHC class I molecules are included in a multimeric complex expressed by natural killer cells. *Journal of Immunology*, **158**, 5083–5086.

Pando, M.J., Gardiner, C.M., Gleimer, M., McQueen, K.L., & Parham, P. (2003) The protein made from a common allele of *KIR3DL1* (3DL1*004) is poorly expressed at cell surfaces due to substitution at positions 86 in Ig domain 0 and 182 in Ig domain 1. *Journal of Immunology*, **171**, 6640–6649.

Parham, P. (2004) Killer cell immunoglobulin-like receptor diversity: balancing signals in the natural killer cell response. *Immunology Letters*, **92**, 11–13.

Pende, D., Biassoni, R., Cantoni, C., Verdiani, S., Falco, M., di Donato, C., Accame, L., Bottino, C., Moretta, A., & Moretta, L. (1996) The natural killer cell receptor specific for HLA-A allotypes: a novel member of the p58/p70 family of inhibitory receptors that is characterized by three immunoglobulin-like domains and is expressed as a 140-kD disulphide-linked dimer. *Journal of Experimental Medicine*, **184**, 505–518.

Peruzzi, M., Wagtmann, N., & Long, E.O. (1996) A p70 killer cell inhibitory receptor specific for several HLA-B allotypes discriminates among peptides bound to HLA-B*2705. *Journal of Experimental Medicine*, **184**, 1585–1590.

Ponte, M., Cantoni, C., Biassoni, R., Tradori-Cappai, A., Bentivoglio, G., Vitale, C., Bertone, S., Moretta, A.,

Moretta, L., & Mingari, M.C. (1999) Inhibitory receptors sensing HLA-G1 molecules in pregnancy: decidua-associated natural killer cells express LIR-1 and CD94/NKG2A and acquire p49, an HLA-G1-specific receptor. *Proceedings of the National Academy of Sciences of the United States of America*, **96**, 5674–5679.

Rajagopalan, S., Bryceson, Y.T., Kuppusamy, S.P., Geraghty, D.E., van der Meer, A., Joosten, I., & Long, E.O. (2006) Activation of NK cells by an endocytosed receptor for soluble HLA-G. *PLoS Biology*, **4**, e9.

Rajagopalan, S., & Long, E.O. (1997) The direct binding of a p58 killer cell inhibitory receptor to human histocompatibility leukocyte antigen (HLA)-Cw4 exhibits peptide selectivity. *Journal of Experimental Medicine*, **185**, 1523–1528.

Rajagopalan, S., & Long, E.O. (1999) A human histocompatibility leukocyte antigen (HLA)-G-specific receptor expressed on all natural killer cells. *Journal of Experimental Medicine*, **189**, 1093–1100.

Rajalingam, R., Gardiner, C.M., Canavez, F., Vilches, C., & Parham, P. (2001a) Identification of seventeen novel KIR variants: fourteen of them from two non-Caucasian donors. *Tissue Antigens*, **57**, 22–31.

Rajalingam, R., Hong, M., Adams, E.J., Shum, B.P., Guethlein, L.A., & Parham, P. (2001b) Short KIR haplotypes in pygmy chimpanzee (Bonobo) resemble the conserved framework of diverse human KIR haplotypes. *Journal of Experimental Medicine*, **193**, 135–146.

Rajalingam, R., Krausa, P., Shilling, H.G., Stein, J.B., Balamurugan, A., McGinnis, M.D., Cheng, N.W., Mehra, N.K., & Parham, P. (2002) Distinctive KIR and HLA diversity in a panel of north Indian Hindus. *Immunogenetics*, **53**, 1009–1019.

Rajalingam, R., Parham, P., & Abi-Rached, L. (2004) Domain shuffling has been the main mechanism forming new hominoid killer cell Ig-like receptors. *Journal of Immunology*, **172**, 356–369.

Raulet, D.H. (2003) Roles of the NKG2D immunoreceptor and its ligands. *Nat Rev Immunol*, **3**, 781–790.

Raulet, D.H., Held, W., Correa, I., Dorfman, J.R., Wu, M.F., & Corral, L. (1997) Specificity, tolerance and developmental regulation of natural killer cells defined by expression of class I-specific Ly49 receptors. *Immunological Reviews*, **155**, 41–52.

Robertson, M.J., & Ritz, J. (1990) Biology and clinical relevance of human natural killer cells. *Blood*, **76**, 2421–2438.

Robinson, J., Waller, M.J., Stoehr, P., & Marsh, S.G. (2005) IPD—the Immuno Polymorphism Database. *Nucleic Acids Research*, **33**, D523–526.

Rojo, S., Wagtmann, N., & Long, E.O. (1997) Binding of a soluble p70 killer cell inhibitory receptor to HLA-B*5101: requirement for all three p70 immunoglobulin domains. *European Journal of Immunology*, 27, 568–571.

Saleh, A., Davies, G.E., Pascal, V., Wright, P.W., Hodge, D.L., Cho, E.H., Lockett, S.J., Abshari, M., & Anderson, S.K. (2004) Identification of probabilistic transcriptional switches in the Ly49 gene cluster: A eukaryotic mechanism for selective gene activation. *Immunity*, 21, 55–66.

Sambrook, J.G., Bashirova, A., Palmer, S., Sims, S., Trowsdale, J., Abi-Rached, L., Parham, P., Carrington, M., & Beck, S. (2005) Single haplotype analysis demonstrates rapid evolution of the killer immunoglobulin-like receptor (KIR) loci in primates. *Genome Research*, 15, 25–35.

Sambrook, J.G., Sehra, H., Coggill, P., Humphray, S., Palmer, S., Sims, S., Takamatsu, H. H., Wileman, T., Archibald, A.L., & Beck, S. (2006a) Identification of a single killer immunoglobulin-like receptor (KIR) gene in the porcine leukocyte receptor complex on chromosome 6q. *Immunogenetics*, 58, 481–486.

Sambrook, J.G., Bashirova, A., Andersen, H., Piatak, M., Vernikos, G.S., Coggill, P., Lifson, J.D., Carrington, M., & Beck, S. (2006b) Identification of the ancestral killer immunoglobulin-like receptor gene in primates. *BMC Genomics*, 7, 209.

Santourlidis, S., Trompeter, H.I., Weinhold, S., Eisermann, B., Meyer, K.L., Wernet, P., & Uhrberg, M. (2002) Crucial role of DNA methylation in determination of clonally distributed killer cell Ig-like receptor expression patterns in NK cells. *Journal of Immunology*, 169, 4253–4261.

Sawicki, M.W., Dimasi, N., Natarajan, K., Wang, J., Margulies, D.H., & Mariuzza, R.A. (2001) Structural basis of MHC class I recognition by natural killer cell receptors. *Immunological Reviews*, 181, 52–65.

See, D.M., Khemka, P., Sahl, L., Bui, T., & Tilles, J.G. (1997) The role of natural killer cells in viral infections. *Scandinavian Journal of Immunology*, 46, 217–224.

Selvakumar, A., Steffens, U., & Dupont, B. (1997) Polymorphism and domain variability of human killer cell inhibitory receptors. *Immunological Reviews*, 155, 183–196.

Shilling, H.G., Lienert-Weidenbach, K., Valiante, N.M., Uhrberg, M., & Parham, P. (1998) Evidence for recombination as a mechanism for KIR diversification. *Immunogenetics*, 48, 413–416.

Shilling, H.G., Guethlein, L.A., Cheng, N.W., Gardiner, C.M., Rodriguez, R., Tyan, D. & Parham, P. (2002a) Allelic polymorphism synergizes with variable gene content to individualize human KIR genotype. *Journal of Immunology*, 168, 2307–2315.

Shilling, H.G., Young, N., Guethlein, L.A., Cheng, N.W., Gardiner, C.M., Tyan, D., & Parham, P. (2002b) Genetic control of human NK cell repertoire. *Journal of Immunology*, 169, 239–247.

Sivori, S., Vitale, M., Morelli, L., Sanseverino, L., Augugliaro, R., Bottino, C., Moretta, L., & Moretta, A. (1997) p46, a novel natural killer cell-specific surface molecule that mediates cell activation. *Journal of Experimental Medicine*, 186, 1129–1136.

Smith, H.R., Heusel, J.W., Mehta, I.K., Kim, S., Dorner, B.G., Naidenko, O.V., Iizuka, K., Furukawa, H., Beckman, D.L., Pingel, J.T., Scalzo, A.A., Fremont, D.H., & Yokoyama, W.M. (2002) Recognition of a virus-encoded ligand by a natural killer cell activation receptor. *Proceedings of the National Academy of Sciences of the United States of America*, 99, 8826–8831.

Snyder, G.A., Brooks, A.G., & Sun, P.D. (1999) Crystal structure of the HLA-Cw3 allotype-specific killer cell inhibitory receptor KIR2DL2. *Proceedings of the National Academy of Sciences of the United States of America*, 96, 3864–3869.

Spaggiari, G.M., Contini, P., Carosio, R., Arvigo, M., Ghio, M., Oddone, D., Dondero, A., Zocchi, M.R., Puppo, F., Indiveri, F., & Poggi, A. (2002) Soluble HLA class I molecules induce natural killer cell apoptosis through the engagement of CD8: evidence for a negative regulation exerted by members of the inhibitory receptor superfamily. *Blood*, 99, 1706–1714.

Tabiasco, J., Espinosa, E., Hudrisier, D., Joly, E., Fournie, J.J., & Vercellone, A. (2002) Active trans-synaptic capture of membrane fragments by natural killer cells. *European Journal of Immunology*, 32, 1502–1508.

Tomasec, P., Braud, V.M., Rickards, C., Powell, M.B., McSharry, B.P., Gadola, S., Cerundolo, V., Borysiewicz, L.K., McMichael, A.J., & Wilkinson, G.W. (2000) Surface expression of HLA-E, an inhibitor of natural killer cells, enhanced by human cytomegalovirus gpUL40. *Science*, 287, 1031.

Toneva, M., Lepage, V., Lafay, G., Dulphy, N., Busson, M., Lester, S., Vu-Trien, A., Michaylova, A., Naumova, E., McCluskey, J., & Charron, D. (2001) Genomic diversity of natural killer cell receptor genes in three populations. *Tissue Antigens*, 57, 358–362.

Tortorella, D., Gewurz, B.E., Furman, M.H., Schust, D.J., & Ploegh, H.L. (2000) Viral subversion of the immune system. *Annual Review of Immunology*, 18, 861–926.

Trinchieri, G. (1989) Biology of natural killer cells. *Advances in Immunology*, 47, 187–376.

Trompeter, H. I., Gomez-Lozano, N., Santourlidis, S., Eisermann, B., Wernet, P., Vilches, C., & Uhrberg, M. (2005) Three structurally and functionally divergent kinds of promoters regulate expression of clonally distributed killer cell Ig-like receptors (KIR), of *KIR2DL4*, and of *KIR3DL3*. *Journal of Immunology*, 174, 4135–4143.

Trowsdale, J. (2001) Genetic and functional relationships between MHC and NK receptor genes. *Immunity*, 15, 363–374.

Trowsdale, J., Barten, R., Haude, A., Stewart, C.A., Beck, S., & Wilson, M.J. (2001) The genomic context of natural killer receptor extended gene families. *Immunological Reviews*, 181, 20–38.

Trundley, A.E., Hiby, S.E., Chang, C., Sharkey, A.M., Santourlidis, S., Uhrberg, M., Trowsdale, J., & Moffett, A. (2006) Molecular characterization of *KIR3DL3*. *Immunogenetics*, 57, 904–916.

Uhrberg, M., Parham, P. & Wernet, P. (2002) Definition of gene content for nine common group B haplotypes of the Caucasoid population: KIR haplotypes contain between seven and eleven KIR genes. *Immunogenetics*, 54, 221–229.

Uhrberg, M., Valiante, N.M., Shum, B.P., Shilling, H.G., Lienert-Weidenbach, K., Corliss, B., Tyan, D., Lanier, L.L., & Parham, P. (1997) Human diversity in killer cell inhibitory receptor genes. *Immunity*, 7, 753–763.

Ulbrecht, M., Martinozzi, S., Grzeschik, M., Hengel, H., Ellwart, J.W., Pla, M., & Weiss, E.H. (2000) Cutting edge: the human cytomegalovirus UL40 gene product contains a ligand for HLA-E and prevents NK cell-mediated lysis. *Journal of Immunology*, 164, 5019–5022.

Vales-Gomez, M., Reyburn, H.T., Erskine, R.A., & Strominger, J. (1998a) Differential binding to HLA-C of p50-activating and p58-inhibitory natural killer cell receptors. *Proceedings of the National Academy of Sciences of the United States of America*, 95, 14326–14331.

Vales-Gomez, M., Reyburn, H.T., Mandelboim, M., & Strominger, J.L. (1998b) Kinetics of interaction of HLA-C ligands with natural killer cell inhibitory receptors. *Immunity*, 9, 337–344.

Valiante, N.M., Lienert, K., Shilling, H.G., Smits, B.J., & Parham, P. (1997a) Killer cell receptors: keeping pace with MHC class I evolution. *Immunological Reviews*, 155, 155–164.

Valiante, N.M., Uhrberg, M., Shilling, H.G., Lienert-Weidenbach, K., Arnett, K.L., D'Andrea, A., Phillips, J.H., Lanier, L.L., & Parham, P. (1997b) Functionally and structurally distinct NK cell receptors for repertoires in the peripheral blood of two human donors. *Immunity*, 7, 739–751.

van Bergen, J., Stewart, C.A., van den Elsen, P.J., & Trowsdale, J. (2005) Structural and functional differences between the promoters of independently expressed killer cell Ig-like receptors. *European Journal of Immunology*, 35, 2191–2199.

Velickovic, M., Velickovic, Z., & Dunckley, H. (2006) Diversity of killer cell immunoglobulin-like receptor genes in Pacific Islands populations. *Immunogenetics*, 58, 523–532.

Vilches, C., Gardiner, C.M., & Parham, P. (2000a) Gene structure and promoter variation of expressed and nonexpressed variants of the *KIR2DL5* gene. *Journal of Immunology*, 165, 6416–6421.

Vilches, C., Pando, M.J., & Parham, P. (2000b) Genes encoding human killer-cell Ig-like receptors with D1 and D2 extracellular domains all contain untranslated pseudoexons encoding a third Ig-like domain. *Immunogenetics*, 51, 639–646.

Vilches, C., Pando, M.J., Rajalingam, R., Gardiner, C.M., & Parham, P. (2000c) Discovery of two novel variants of KIR2DS5 reveals this gene to be a common component of human KIR "B" haplotypes. *Tissue Antigens*, 56, 453–456.

Vilches, C., & Parham, P. (2002) KIR: diverse, rapidly evolving receptors of innate and adaptive immunity. *Annual Review of Immunology*, 20, 217–251.

Vivier, E., & Biron, C.A. (2002) Immunology. A pathogen receptor on natural killer cells. *Science*, 296, 1248–1249.

Volz, A., Wende, H., Laun, K., & Ziegler, A. (2001) Genesis of the ILT/LIR/MIR clusters within the human leukocyte receptor complex. *Immunological Reviews*, 181, 39–51.

Vyas, Y.M., Maniar, H., & Dupont, B. (2002) Visualization of signaling pathways and cortical cytoskeleton in cytolytic and noncytolytic natural killer cell immune synapses. *Immunological Reviews*, 189, 161–178.

Wagtmann, N., Rajagopalan, S., Winter, C.C., Peruzzi, M., & Long, E.O. (1995) Killer cell inhibitory receptors specific for HLA-C and HLA-B identified by direct binding and by functional transfer. *Immunity*, 3, 801–809.

Watzl, C., & Long, E.O. (2003) Natural killer cell inhibitory receptors block actin cytoskeleton-dependent recruitment of 2B4 (CD244) to lipid rafts. *Journal of Experimental Medicine*, 197, 77–85.

Watzl, C., Peterson, M., & Long, E.O. (2000a) Homogenous expression of killer cell immunoglobulin-like receptors (KIR) on polyclonal natural killer cells detected by a monoclonal antibody to KIR2D. *Tissue Antigens*, 56, 240–247.

Watzl, C., Stebbins, C.C., & Long, E.O. (2000b) NK cell inhibitory receptors prevent tyrosine phosphorylation of the activation receptor 2B4 (CD244). *Journal of Immunology*, **165**, 3545–3548.

Wende, H., Colonna, M., Ziegler, A., & Volz, A. (1999) Organization of the leukocyte receptor cluster (LRC) on human chromosome 19q13.4. *Mammalian Genome*, **10**, 154–160.

Wende, H., Volz, A., & Ziegler, A. (2000) Extensive gene duplications and a large inversion characterize the human leukocyte receptor cluster. *Immunogenetics*, **51**, 703–713.

Whang, D.H., Park, H., Yoon, J.A., & Park, M.H. (2005) Haplotype analysis of killer cell immunoglobulin-like receptor genes in 77 Korean families. *Human Immunology*, **66**, 146–154.

Williams, F., Maxwell, L.D., Halfpenny, I.A., Meenagh, A., Sleator, C., Curran, M.D., & Middleton, D. (2003) Multiple copies of KIR 3DL/S1 and KIR 2DL4 genes identified in a number of individuals. *Human Immunology*, **64**, 729–732.

Wilson, M.J., Torkar, M., Haude, A., Milne, S., Jones, T., Sheer, D., Beck, S. & Trowsdale, J. (2000) Plasticity in the organization and sequences of human KIR/ILT gene families. *Proceedings of the National Academy of Sciences of the United States of America*, **97**, 4778–4783.

Wilson, M.J., Torkar, M., Haude, A., Milne, S., Jones, T., Sheer, D., Beck, S., & Trowsdale, J. (2000) Plasticity in the organization and sequences of human KIR/ILT gene families. *Proceedings of the National Academy of Sciences of the United States of America*, **97**, 4778–4783.

Wilson, M.J., Torkar, M., & Trowsdale, J. (1997) Genomic organization of a human killer cell inhibitory receptor gene. *Tissue Antigens*, **49**, 574–579.

Winter, C.C., Gumperz, J.E., Parham, P., Long, E.O., & Wagtmann, N. (1998) Direct binding and functional transfer of NK cell inhibitory receptors reveal novel patterns of HLA-C allotype recognition. *Journal of Immunology*, **161**, 571–577.

Winter, C.C., & Long, E.O. (1997) A single amino acid in the p58 killer cell inhibitory receptor controls the ability of natural killer cells to discriminate between the two groups of HLA-C allotypes. *Journal of Immunology*, **158**, 4026–4028.

Witt, C.S., Dewing, C., Sayer, D.C., Uhrberg, M., Parham, P., & Christiansen, F.T. (1999) Population frequencies and putative haplotypes of the killer cell immunoglobulin-like receptor sequences and evidence for recombination. *Transplantation*, **68**, 1784–1789.

Witt, C.S., Martin, A., & Christiansen, F.T. (2000) Detection of KIR2DL4 alleles by sequencing and SSCP reveals a common allele with a shortened cytoplasmic tail. *Tissue Antigens*, **56**, 248–257.

Witt, C.S., Whiteway, J.M., Warren, H.S., Barden, A., Rogers, M., Martin, A., Beilin, L., & Christiansen, F.T. (2002) Alleles of the KIR2DL4 receptor and their lack of association with pre-eclampsia. *European Journal of Immunology*, **32**, 18–29.

Yawata, M., Yawata, N., Abi-Rached, L., & Parham, P. (2002a) Variation within the human killer cell immunoglobulin-like receptor (KIR) gene family. *Critical Reviews in Immunology*, **22**, 463–482.

Yawata, M., Yawata, N., McQueen, K.L., Cheng, N.W., Guethlein, L.A., Rajalingam, R., Shilling, H.G., & Parham, P. (2002b) Predominance of group A KIR haplotypes in Japanese associated with diverse NK cell repertoires of KIR expression. *Immunogenetics*, **54**, 543–550.

Yawata, M., Yawata, N., Draghi, M., Little, A. M., Partheniou, F., & Parham, P. (2006) Roles for HLA and KIR polymorphisms in natural killer cell repertoire selection and modulation of effector function. *Journal of Experimental Medicine*, **203**, 633–645.

Young, N.T., Rust, N.A., Dallman, M.J., Cerundolo, V., Morris, P.J., & Welsh, K.I. (1998) Independent contributions of HLA epitopes and killer inhibitory receptor expression to the functional alloreactive specificity of natural killer cells. *Human Immunology*, **59**, 700–712.

Zappacosta, F., Borrego, F., Brooks, A.G., Parker, K.C., & Coligan, J.E. (1997) Peptides isolated from HLA-Cw*0304 confer different degrees of protection from natural killer cell-mediated lysis. *Proceedings of the National Academy of Sciences of the United States of America*, **94**, 6313–6318.

Zinkernagel, R.M., & Doherty, P.C. (1974) Restriction of in vitro T cell-mediated cytotoxicity in lymphocytic choriomeningitis within a syngeneic or semiallogeneic system. *Nature*, **248**, 701–702.

8

Red Blood Cell Genes and Malaria

David Weatherall

Because malaria has long been and continues to be one of the major killers of mankind, and because these parasites spend a critical period of their complex life cycles within red blood cells, it is not surprising that genetic variation in the structure or function of these cells that is deleterious to the parasite has come under intense selection. Indeed, there is now very strong evidence that selective evolutionary pressure of this kind explains why the genetic disorders of the red cell are by far the most common monogenic diseases in man. This chapter briefly describes the common inherited red cell conditions that seem to have come under selection by different forms of malaria, as well as the relevant human loci and their common mutations (table 8.1), and outlines what is known about how these interactions are mediated. Readers who wish to explore particular aspects in more detail, particularly the original sources on which many of its present concepts are based, are referred to a monograph and several more extensive reviews (Weatherall and Clegg, 2001a,

2001b, 2002; Nagel 2001; Luzzatto et al., 2001; Cooke and Hill, 2001; Roberts et al., 2004).

Historical Background

The notion that variation in host response might have a genetic basis is not new (Lederberg, 1999; Cooke and Hill, 2001). But it was not until the late 1940s, and through the remarkable insight of J .B. S. Haldane, that a plausible genetic protective mechanism was first suggested.

During the period just after the Second World War independent studies in Italy and in Mediterranean immigrants in the United States showed that there is a remarkably high frequency of thalassemia in these populations (Valentine and Neel, 1944; Silvestroni and Bianco, 1947). Influenced by the intense interest in human mutation rates following studies of the survivors of the atomic bombs in Hiroshima and Nagasaki,

TABLE 8.1. Some genetic loci affecting the red blood cell implicated in malaria resistance.

Gene ID (NCBI)	Common Name(s)	Entrez Gene ID (Locus Link)	Map Position	Notes on Important SNPs, Indels, Truncations (Region, Reference Sequence [is] Number)	References
HBA1	α-Globin	3039	16p13.3	Single gene deletions	Weatherall and Clegg (2001a)
HBB	β-Globin	3043	11p15.5	Diverse point mutations	Weatherall and Clegg (2001a)
G6PB	Glucose-6-phosphate dehydrogenase	2539	Xq28	Numerous variants with a wide range of enzymatic activity	Luzzatto et al. (2001)
DARC	Duffy blood group/ antigen/chemokine receptor	2532	1q21-q22	Duffy-negative phenotype, at high frequency in Africans, is related to an SNP in a GATA-1– binding site of the promoter	Tournamille et al. (1995)
GYPB	Glycophorin B	2994	4q28-q31	Rare gene deletion underlies the protective blood group S-s-U-	Huang et al. (1987)
GYPC	Glycophorin C	2995	2q14-q21	Exon 3 deletion in Melanesians underlies the protective Gerbich blood group	Chang et al. (1991)
SLC4A1	Erythrocyte band 3; erythroid anion exchange protein	6521	17q21-q22	Nine amino acid deletion underlies southeast Asian and Melanesian ovalocytosis	Mohandas et al. (1992)

workers on both sides of the Atlantic suggested that these high frequencies might reflect a high mutation rate and, because they appeared to be restricted to certain populations, that the mutation rate might differ among different ethnic groups.

At the eighth International Congress of Genetics in Stockhölm in 1948, Neel and Valentine, in order to explain the high frequency of thalassemia in immigrant populations in the United States, calculated a mutation rate for thalassemia of 1:2,500. Haldane felt that this was unlikely and that these remarkable gene frequencies must be the result of heterozygote selection. "The corpuscles [sic] of anemic heterozygotes are smaller than normal, and more resistant to hypertonic solutions. It is at least conceivable that they are also more resistant to attacks by the sporozoa which cause malaria, a disease prevalent in Italy, Sicily and Greece, where the gene is frequent" (Haldane, 1949).

In essence, what became known as the "malaria hypothesis" intimated that diseases like thalassemia can be considered as balanced polymorphisms, that is, conditions in which the gene frequency for the advantageous heterozygous state increases until it is balanced by the loss of homozygotes from the population. Haldane's great contribution to this field was to encourage geneticists and hematologists to analyze the

high frequency of common genetic diseases of the blood as putative polymorphisms of this kind. Although, over the years, the hypothesis has stood the test of time, it has not always been easy to substantiate Haldane's ideas in human populations.

Inherited Disorders of Hemoglobin

Collectively, the inherited disorders of hemoglobin are the commonest monogenic diseases in humans. They are most easily appreciated through an understanding of the structure and genetic control of normal human hemoglobin.

The Genetic Control of Hemoglobin

Different hemoglobins are produced at different stages of human development as an adaptive response to variation in oxygen requirements between embryonic, fetal, and adult life. All the human hemoglobins have the same basic structure. They consist of two different pairs of globin chains; adult and fetal hemoglobins have α-chains associated with β- (Hb A, $\alpha_2\beta_2$), δ- (Hb A_2, $\alpha_2\delta_2$), or γ-chains (Hb F, $\alpha_2\gamma_2$), whereas in the embryo, embryonic α-like chains called ζ-chains combine with γ- (Hb Portland, $\zeta_2\gamma_2$) or ε-chains (Hb Gower 1, $\zeta_2\varepsilon_2$). In addition, in the embryo α- and ε-chains combine to form Hb Gower 2 ($\alpha_2\varepsilon_2$). The α-like genes form a cluster on chromosome 16, while the β-like genes are similarly arranged on chromosome 11. Both clusters contain two genes that are duplicated: There are two α-chain genes, α1 and α2, and two γ-chain genes, $^G\gamma$ and $^A\gamma$. The α1 and α2 genes have identical gene products, while G and A refer to the amino acids glycine and alanine; the products of the two γ genes are identical except at amino acid residue 136, where one contains glycine and the other alanine. Detailed descriptions of the structure and regulation of these gene clusters are given in several recent reviews (Weatherall and Clegg, 2001a; Steinberg et al., 2001).

Hemoglobinopathies

The inherited disorders of hemoglobin, or hemoglobinopathies, consist of the structural hemoglobin variants and the thalassemias, inherited defects in the synthesis of the α- or β-chains of human adult hemoglobin. Although hundreds of structural hemoglobin variants have been identified (Huisman et al., 1998), only three, Hbs S, C, and E, reach polymorphic frequencies.

Although this simple classification of the inherited disorders of hemoglobin is useful in practice it does not tell the whole story. In particular, because Hb E is synthesized at a reduced rate, it has the phenotype of a mild form of β-thalassemia, a fact that has to be borne in mind when discussing its high frequency in relationship to malaria.

Hemoglobin S

Hemoglobin S differs from Hb A by the substitution of valine for glutamic acid at position 6 in the β-globin chain. This causes an increased rate of polymerization of Hb S in its deoxygenated state, which results in deformation of the red blood cells associated with severe anemia and a variety of vascular complications (see Steinberg et al., 2001). Sickle cell anemia, the homozygous state for Hb S, is associated with an extremely high mortality in infancy in Africa and in a reduced life expectancy in immigrants in developed countries.

The Hb S gene can also be co-inherited with Hb C or with different forms of β-thalassemia. Hemoglobin SC disease is milder than sickle cell anemia, while Hb S/β-thalassemia varies in severity depending on the

nature of the β-thalassemia allele; at its most severe, it resembles sickle cell anemia.

Distribution The gene for Hb S is distributed widely throughout sub-Saharan Africa, the Middle East, and parts of the Indian subcontinent, where carrier frequencies range from 5% to 40% or more of the population (Livingstone, 1985; Steinberg et al., 2001) (figure 8.1). Studies of globin gene haplotypes, that is, the patterns of restriction fragment length polymorphisms in the α- or β-globin gene clusters, have provided important information about the evolution of the sickle cell gene. In short, they suggest that the sickle cell mutation may have occurred at least twice, once in Africa and once in either the Middle East or India. It is even possible that the sickle cell gene has arisen more than once in Africa, although a more plausible explanation for much of the haplotype diversity is that it reflects redistribution on different backgrounds by gene conversion and recombination (Flint et al, 1998).

Relationship to Malaria The early studies on the relationship of the high frequency of the Hb S gene to *Plasmodium falciparum* malaria are summarized by Allison (1965). In short, analyses of parasite rates and densities in children with the sickle cell trait and non-affected controls, together with observations of the rarity of sickling in patients with severe malaria and the distribution of the sickle cell gene, combined to provide convincing evidence that the sickle cell trait provides at least some degree of protection against severe malarial infection. More recent studies in West Africa suggest that the greatest impact of Hb S seems to be to protect against either death or severe disease (i.e., profound anemia or cerebral malaria), while having less effect on infection per se (Hill et al., 1991). Indeed, case–control studies suggest that Hb S heterozygotes have a level of protection of approximately 80% against the severe complications of malaria.

Some progress has also been made in determining the mechanisms of protection of those with the sickle cell trait against *P. falciparum* malaria, although certain questions remain unanswered. Luzzatto et al. (1970) demonstrated that the rate of sickling of parasitized red cells in those with the sickle cell trait (AS) is significantly greater than that in normal red cells. The findings were confirmed and extended under more physiological conditions by Roth et al. (1978). These studies suggested that malaria parasites cause a "suicidal infection"; because the parasites increase the rate

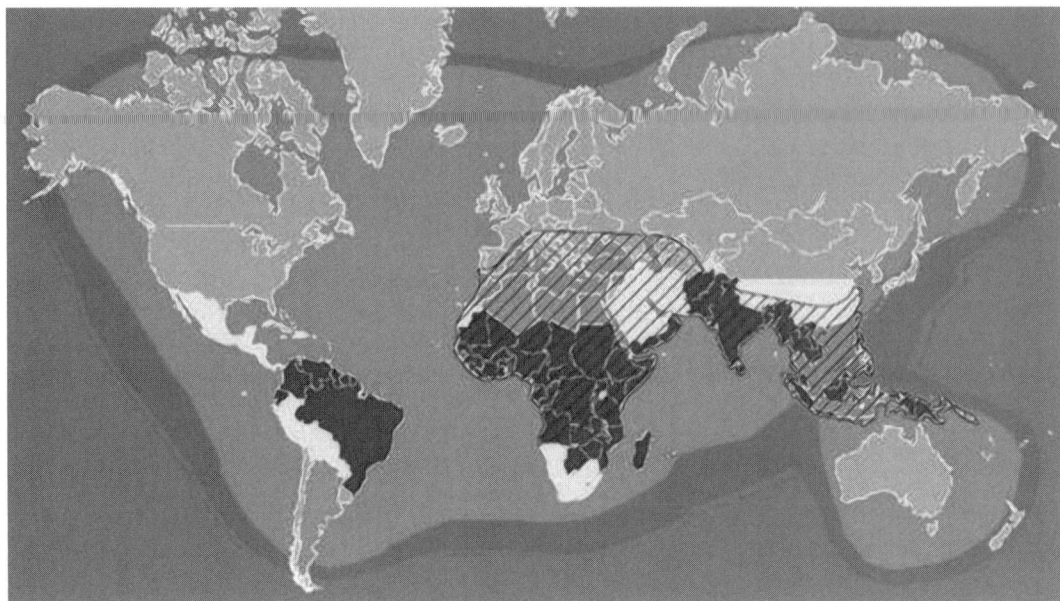

FIGURE 8.1. Global distribution of malaria and red blood cell disorders. Medium gray indicates areas where malaria is present only in a few remote locations (e.g., Argentina and northern Africa, light gray indicates areas with intermediate malaria risk (e.g., Central America, Peru, Bolivia, South Africa, Namibia, Saudi Arabia, Iran, and southern China), and dark gray indicates areas with high malaria risk (e.g., Colombia, Venezuela, Brazil, central Africa, India, and southeast Asia). The hatched area shows the distribution of red blood cell disorders.

of sickling, parasitized AS red cells are more likely to be removed from the circulation. At about the same time, two groups independently demonstrated that parasitized AS cells maintained at low oxygen tension do not support the growth of malarial parasites as effectively as do normal cells at similar tensions (Friedman, 1978; Pasvol et al., 1978). Friedman et al. (1979) suggested that this effect might be due to the increased loss of potassium or water from the sickle-cell–trait cells.

Several possible mechanisms may mediate protection against *P. falciparum* malaria in individuals with the sickle cell trait, and they are not mutually exclusive of each other. Earlier suggestions of an immune protective mechanism (see Allison, 1965) are of great interest; more recent observations of increased protection over the first ten years of life is compatible with an immune process in addition to an intracellular protective mechanism (Williams et al., 2005a).

Hemoglobin C

Hemoglobin C results from the substitution of lysine for glutamic acid at position 6 in the β-globin chain.

Homozygotes have a mild hemolytic anemia, whereas heterozygotes are unaffected except for striking morphological changes of their red cells.

Distribution   Hemoglobin C is found at high frequencies in some parts of West Africa and sporadically in North Africa and other Mediterranean countries.

Relationship to Malaria   Recent studies in West Africa suggest that the relatively high frequencies of Hb C have also been maintained by resistance to *P. falciparum* malaria (Modiano et al., 2001). In this case, both heterozygotes and homozygotes show protection, and unlike the sickle cell mutation, Hb C may be an example of a transient polymorphism that will move to fixation in a population if the selective pressure continues. This supposition is based on the apparent lack of clinical disability or severe hematological changes in Hb C homozygotes. If this were the case, however, it is difficult to understand why the frequency of Hb C is not higher in African populations. Furthermore, whether homozygotes for this variant are completely unaffected is unclear; further work will be required to confirm this interesting suggestion.

Hemoglobin E

Hemoglobin E results from the substitution of lysine for glutamic acid in codon 26 of the β-globin gene. As well as producing a structural hemoglobin variant, this mutation activates a cryptic splice site at the 3′ end of exon 1 of this gene, resulting in an abnormally spliced messenger RNA (Orkin et al., 1982). Thus, less β^E globin is synthesized, and a mild thalassemia phenotype results.

Those homozygous for Hb E have a very mild thalassemia phenotype, very similar to that seen in β-thalassemia trait (see below). Heterozygotes have no clinical or hematological findings.

Distribution   The distribution of Hb E has been reviewed recently (Weatherall and Clegg, 2001b). It occurs at a very high frequency in eastern parts of the Indian subcontinent, in Myanmar, and throughout Southeast Asia. It reaches particularly high frequencies in northern Thailand and Cambodia, the so-called "hemoglobin E triangle." In this region, up to 70% of the population are carriers (figure 8.1).

Relationship to Malaria   Population studies (reviewed in Nagel, 2001; Weatherall and Clegg, 2001a) have been bedeviled by the problems of the very high frequencies of other genetic red cell disorders, particularly α-thalassemia, in many populations where Hb E occurs at a high level. Although some *in vitro* culture data suggest that Hb E–containing red cells may be less able to subserve the growth of *P. falciparum* (Chotivanich et al., 2002), the type of case–control studies that would be required to provide unequivocal evidence of protection have not yet been carried out. Given the distribution of Hb E, its extremely high frequency, and the fact that it behaves like a mild form of thalassemia, it is very likely that, ultimately, it will be found to be protective.

α-Thalassemia

The α-thalassemias are a heterogeneous group of disorders of globin synthesis that result from a defective output of α-globin chains. There are two major varieties, α^o thalassemia, in which both of the linked α-globin genes are deleted, and α^+ thalassemia, in which one of the pair of genes is deleted or inactivated by a point mutation. The homozygous states for the deletional forms of α^o and α^+ thalassemia are represented as $--/--$ and $-\alpha/-\alpha$, respectively. These conditions are extremely heterogeneous at the molecular level, and many different-sized deletions have been found to cause both α^+ and α^o thalassemia.

Distribution α^+ Thalassemia is the commonest monogenic disease in the world population, although, fortunately, in the homozygous state it causes an extremely mild anemia, and heterozygotes show no hematological abnormalities. It occurs in a broad band stretching throughout sub-Saharan Africa and the Mediterranean region, through the Middle East and the Indian subcontinent to Southeast Asia. In these regions, its frequency varies from 5% to 40%, and in parts of northern India and the northern coast of Papua New Guinea, up to 80% of the population are carriers (see Weatherall and Clegg, 2001a, 2001b).

Relationship to Malaria   The frequency of α^+ thalassemia in the Southwest Pacific follows a clinal distribution from north/west to south/east, with the highest frequency in northern New Guinea and the lowest in New Caledonia. These frequencies show a strong correlation with malarial endemicity; similar relations are not observed with other genetic polymorphisms in this region (Flint et al., 1986). The possibility that α-thalassemia has been introduced from the mainland populations of Southeast Asia and that its frequency has been diluted as populations moved south has been excluded by finding that the molecular forms of α-thalassemia in Melanesia and Papua New Guinea are different from those of the mainland and are set in different α-globin haplotypes (Flint et al., 1986). One worrying feature of the distribution of α-thalassemia in this region is that it is also found in Fiji in the west to Tahiti and beyond in the east and in Micronesian atolls, populations in which malaria has never been recorded. However, further studies have shown that in Polynesia and Micronesia, almost 100% of α^+ thalassemia can be accounted for by a single mutation that has been previously defined in Vanuatu, indicating that the occurrence of α-thalassemia in these nonmalarious areas has been the result of population migration (O'Shaughnessy et al., 1990).

These population data have been augmented by a case–control study in northern Papua New Guinea, where it has been found that, compared with normal children, the risk of contracting severe malaria, as defined by WHO guidelines, is 0.4 for α^+ thalassemia homozygotes and 0.66 for α^+ thalassemia heterozygotes

(Allen et al., 1997). Recently, an extensive study of α thalassemia was undertaken in Kilifi, Kenya, where the allele frequency of $α^+$ thalassemia deletions exceeds 0.40. Both heterozygotes and homozygotes were significantly protected from severe malaria and death, with more marked protection for the homozygous and somewhat greater protection against the most severe disease forms, including severe malarial anemia (Williams et al., 2005b). Interestingly, analysis of individuals with both Hb AS and $α^+$ thalassemia (Williams et al., 2005c) produced evidence of negative interaction between the protective effects of these variants (see chapter 24). Taken together, these studies provide strong direct evidence for a very strong protective effect of $α^+$ thalassemia against malaria, in both the heterozygous and homozygous state.

Mechanisms of Protection   Some progress has been made toward an understanding of the mechanisms of protection against malaria afforded by α thalassemia, at both the population and cellular levels.

Studies of a large cohort of children in Vanuatu, an island in which malaria is holoendemic, showed that the incidence with uncomplicated malaria and the prevalence of splenomegaly, an index of malaria infection, was significantly higher in very young children with α-thalassemia than in normal children. Moreover, the effect was most marked in younger children and in those affected by the nonlethal parasite *P. vivax* (Williams et al., 1996). It was suggested that the early susceptibility to *P. vivax*, which may reflect the more rapid turnover of red cells in α-thalassemic infants (Rees et al., 1998), may be acting as a natural vaccine by inducing cross-species protection against *P. falciparum*. These intriguing observations require confirmation in other populations.

How such protection may be mediated at the cellular level is less clear, however. Overall, there is no evidence for a reduced rate of invasion or growth of *P. falciparum* in red cells of the genotype $-α/αα$, $-α/-α$, or $- -/αα$, the mild forms of α-thalassemia that have been shown to be protective in case–control studies. However, it has been found that these cells consistently bind more malaria immune globulin than do normal red cells (Luzzi et al., 1991; Williams et al., 2002). α-Thalassemic red cells infected with parasites appear to be more susceptible to phagocytosis *in vitro* and are less able than normal red cells to form rosettes, an *in vitro* phenomenon whereby uninfected red cells bind to infected cells. Similarly, infected α-thalassemic red cells

are less able to adhere to human umbilical-vein endothelial cells (Yuthavong et al., 1987; Udomsangpetch et al., 1993). Since rosetting and cytoadherence are mechanisms that underlie sequestration of infected red blood cells, these observations suggest that abnormalities of the α-thalassemic red-cell membrane may be involved in malaria protection. In an extensive series of studies to try to define the membrane components involved, it was suggested that altered red-cell membrane band 3 may be a target for enhanced antibody binding to α-thalassemic cells infected with parasites (Williams et al., 2002). A polymorphism of the gene for complement receptor 1 (CR1) reduces rosetting and appears to confer protection against severe malaria, and interestingly, red cells of individuals with $α^+$ thalashalassemia have a reduced expression of CR1 (Cockburn et al, 2004).

Thus, although there are a number of tantalizing clues as to possible mechanisms of protection against malaria by the milder forms of α-thalassemia, a coherent picture of how they fit together remains to be produced. Another important observation also remaining to be explained is that in the case–control studies in Papua New Guinea (Allen et al, 1997), protection was mediated by against not only malaria but also other childhood infections, particularly those involving the upper respiratory tract. Whether this simply reflects better general health in children who are protected against chronic malaria in a holoendemic region or whether it is the result of a more subtle immune mechanism also remains to be determined.

β-Thalassemia

The β-thalassemias are characterized by severe, transfusion-dependent disease in their homozygous or compound heterozygous states, while heterozygotes are usually symptomless. However, a broad spectrum of severity exists between these two extremes (Weatherall and Clegg, 2001a).

Distribution   The distribution of the β-thalassemias is very similar to that described earlier for the α-thalassemias. In high-frequency regions, the carrier states vary between 5% and 20%, although the extremely high levels observed for some forms of α-thalassemia have never been encountered. In parts of the Indian subcontinent and Southeast Asia, because of the very high frequency of Hb E, compound heterozygotes for β-thalassemia and this variant, Hb E β-thalassemia, occur frequently. Indeed, Hb E β-thalassemia is much more common than β-thalassemia major in some countries in this region (e.g., Bangladesh, Myanmar, and Thailand).

Relationship to Malaria   In a series of classical studies conducted in the 1960s, Siniscalco et al. (1961) found that the population frequencies of thalassemia carriers in Sardinia, a considerable number of whom must have been β-thalassemia carriers, correlated with altitude. Although malaria was no longer endemic in Sardinia at this time, historically, its incidence was known to have correlated closely with altitude. Hill et al. (1988) found similar correlations in Melanesia. In addition a relatively small-scale case–control study in northern Liberia suggested that the β-thalassemia trait is protective against severe malaria (Willcox et al., 1983). Thus, although a number of other population studies, mostly analyzing parasite rates or densities, have failed to show any correlations between β-thalassemia and malaria (see Weatherall and Clegg, 2001a), such epidemiological data that are available certainly point to a protective effect of the β-thalassemia trait.

Another major finding in favor of the protective effect of malaria in β-thalassemia is the observation that, in every country in which this disease is common, there is a different set of mutations. Studies of β globin gene haplotypes and their relationship to β-thalassemia mutations have been particularly interesting in this respect. Unlike for α-globin gene haplotypes, there is a "hot-spot" for recombination between the 5′ and 3′ end haplotypes. Over time, there seems to have been admixture between the 5′ and 3′ haplotypes among human populations, but this has not occurred in the case of thalassemia; the thalassemia mutations, which occur in the 3′ haplotype, are almost invariably associated with the same 5′ haplotype, indicating that they are much more recent and that there has not been time for mixing the 5′ and 3′ ends of haplotypes that carry these genes. This suggests a fairly recent selective pressure, possibly about 5,000 years, which is in agreement with current estimations of the time that human populations have been exposed to pathogenic forms of *Plasmodium* (see below).

Mechanisms of Protection   Very little is known about mechanisms of protection against malaria in the case of β-thalassemia. *In vitro* studies have shown that β-thalassemic red cells are invaded at the same rate as normal red cells and that the rate of parasite growth is also indistinguishable from normal. In red cells both in humans and in transgenic mice, those cells that contain human fetal hemoglobin are associated with infective development of *P. falciparum* or *P. yoelii* (Pasvol et al., 1977; Shear et al., 1998). There is strong evidence that the rate of decline of fetal hemoglobin levels after birth is delayed in β-thalassemia heterozygotes (Weatherall and Clegg, 2001a). This could provide a mechanism of protection during the first year of life, but not longer.

Nagel (2001) has suggested a more general hypothesis for why thalassemia heterozygotes might be protected against malaria. In short, because these cells are under increased oxidative stress due to globin-chain imbalance, the further stress imposed by the parasite might render them prone to damage and rapid removal from the circulation. This mechanism is reminiscent of that outlined above for the protective effect of the sickle cell trait; however, no experimental evidence to date either supports or refutes this interesting idea.

The Red Cell Membrane

Considering the complex mechanisms involved in the entry of red cells by malarial parasites, and the equally diverse requirement for their survival in this unfriendly environment, it is not surprising that polymorphisms involving the protein structure of their membranes have come under selection by severe malaria. Indeed, there has been a major interest for many years in the possibility that the distribution of human blood groups has reached its current state through selection by a variety of infective organisms.

Blood Groups

Duffy

Epidemiological studies, first in Africa (Miller et al., 1976) and more recently in Papua New Guinea (Zimmerman et al., 1999), have shown a high frequency of the Duffy-negative phenotype in populations in which malaria is common. The fact that red cells lacking the Duffy determinant are resistant to invasion by *P. knowlesi*, though not to *P. falciparum*, suggested that the Duffy blood group antigen might be the receptor for the related parasite *P. vivax* (Miller et al., 1977). More recent studies showed that the Duffy antigen/chemokine receptor (DARC) is not expressed on red cells when there is a mutation in the promoter of its gene that alters a GATA-1 binding site (Tournamille et al., 1995). In cells carrying this mutation, DARC expression on the surface is abolished, and therefore DARC-mediated entry of *P. vivax* is inhibited.

Malaria due to *P. vivax* is, at least at the present time, much milder than that due to *P. falciparum*. Thus, unless the former was more severe in the past, there may be an additional explanation for the high prevalence of those who do not carry the Duffy antigen in malarious populations.

Gerbich (Ge)

The receptor for the *P. falciparum* red-cell–binding antigen BAEBL (EBA140) is glycophorin C. This interaction may be an important mechanism whereby the parasite invades human erythrocytes (Maier et al., 2003). A deletion of exon 3 of the glycophorin C gene (Chang et al., 1991), which changes the serological phenotype of the Gerbich (Ge) blood group system and results in Ge negativity, reaches a frequency of approximately 45% in coastal areas of Papua New Guinea, where malaria is endemic. These findings strongly suggest that Ge negativity has arisen in Melanesian populations through natural selection by severe malaria. However, although earlier invasion studies indicated that Ge-negative cells are less effectively invaded further population and case–control studies are required to assess the magnitude of protection mediated in this way and the precise mechanisms involved.

S-s-u

Red cells of the S-s-u phenotype are deficient in glycophorin B and relatively resistant to invasion. Early studies suggested that the high frequency of this genotype in certain African populations might have been related to selection by malaria (Mourant, 1968). But although glycophorin B–deficient cells (Huang et al., 1987) are resistant to invasion *in vitro*, a parasite ligand for this protein has not yet been identified.

Other Blood Group Antigens

The suggestion that blood group A is associated with more severe malaria (Fischer and Boone, 1998; Lell et al., 1999) is consistent with the low frequency of this blood group in many areas where malaria is endemic. Such a protective effect could be mediated by the modulation of rosetting, as observed in association with

some strains of *P. falciparum* and different ABO (H) blood groups (Barragan et al., 2000).

Interestingly, removal of sialic acid reduces the invasion of red cells (Miller et al., 1977; Perkins, 1981), and erythrocytes carrying naturally occurring sialic acid–deficient variants are resistant to invasion (Pasvol et al., 1982). However, evidence that red cells carrying these variants reach high frequencies in malarious areas is lacking. Nor have any other variants of glycophorin A reached polymorphic frequencies. This is particularly puzzling because, as discussed above, a ligand for glycophorin A has been identified.

Red-Cell-Membrane Cytoskeletal Proteins

Melanesian Ovalocytosis

This condition, which reaches a frequency of more than 10% in some areas of Papua New Guinea, is an autosomal dominant trait that appears to be lethal in homozygotes. It results from a mutation encoding a nine amino acid deletion in the gene for band 3 of the red cell membrane, the erythrocyte anion transporter (Mohandas et al., 1992). Two case–control studies have shown that this polymorphism is highly protective against severe malaria (Genton et al., 1995; Allen et al., 1999). Remarkably, heterozygotes appear to be prone to attacks of severe malaria yet are almost completely protected against cerebral malaria (Allen et al., 1999). Although it has been suggested that protection may be mediated by a reduced rate of parasite invasion of red cells, this is not consistent with the clinical findings, particularly the observation that parasitemia is not reduced in those who carry the polymorphism (Allen et al., 1999).

Other Red-Cell-Membrane Proteins

Other varieties of elliptocytosis have been reported which involve either the α- or β-chain of spectrin or band 4.1. Two spectrin variants reach polymorphic frequencies in some West African populations (Morle et al., 1989), and it appears that some of them are resistant to invasion by *P. falciparum* (Facer, 1995). Impairment of both invasion by *P. falciparum* and growth has also been reported in elliptocytosis associated with a combined deficiency of protein 4.1, glycophorin C, and P55 (Chishti et al., 1996). Polymorphisms in host receptors for infected erythrocytes are discussed elsewhere (chapter 24).

Red Cell Metabolism

The red cell has two main metabolic pathways: the anaerobic Emden-Meyerhoff pathway, involved in energy metabolism, and the aerobic hexose monophosphate shunt required for reactions of various other pathways, as well as for maintaining the stability of catalase and the preservation and regeneration of the reduced form of glutathione. The latter are essential for the detoxification of hydrogen peroxide.

The only human polymorphism involving these metabolic pathways that is related to resistance to malaria is glucose-6-phosphate-dehydrogenase (G6PD) deficiency. However, recent studies in mice suggest that other enzymes with this property may soon be recognized in humans.

Glucose-6-Phosphate-Dehydrogenase (G6PD) Deficiency

G6PD deficiency is the commonest enzymopathy, affecting an estimated 400 million people worldwide. It is an X-linked disorder, and therefore one of the two G6PD alleles is subject to inactivation in females. Approximately 400 different variants have been reported that differ widely in their effect on G6PD activity in the red cell. The major clinical manifestations of G6PD deficiency are neonatal jaundice, acute hemolytic anemia after ingestion of drugs or certain foodstuffs, and, probably, severe anemia associated with infection.

Distribution   The highest prevalence rates, with gene frequencies in a range of 5–25%, are found in tropical Africa, the Middle East, tropical and subtropical Asia, some parts of the Mediterranean, and Papua New Guinea (Luzzatto et al., 2001). Like the hemoglobinopathies, each of these high-frequency regions has its own particular set of mutations at the G6PD locus.

Relationship to Malaria   The geographical distribution of G6PD deficiency, and its particular high frequency in areas where malaria is holoendemic, suggested that it might be protective against *P. falciparum* malaria. As in the case of the hemoglobinopathies, this hypothesis turned out to be difficult to substantiate by the analysis of parasitemia rates and densities when comparing G6PD-deficient males with normals. These studies are reviewed by Luzzatto et al. (2001); overall, it appears that, at least in Kenya and The Gambia, there is some evidence for protection at the community level. More recent studies suggest that both hemizygous males and heterozygous females are protected in both East and West Africa (Ruwende et al., 1995). Similarly, the existence of multiple G6PD-deficient variants correlates well with malaria endemicity in Vanuatuan archipelago in the southwestern Pacific (Ganczakowski et al., 1995).

Mechanism of Protection   Despite a great deal of work, it is still not absolutely clear how G6PD deficiency protects against malaria. Susceptibility of G6PD-deficient red cells to oxidative stress appears to be a likely mechanism. The observation that deficient red cells undergo phagocytosis by macrophages at an earlier stage than do parasitized normal cells (Cappadoro et al., 1998) raises the possibility that, as for the protective effect mediated by the sickle cell gene, suicidal infection may be at least one protective mechanism (Luzzatto et al., 2001).

Pyruvate Kinase Deficiency

Several genome searches aimed at defining loci that would confer resistance to *P. chabaudi* malaria in mice mapped three potential loci to chromosome 9 (*Char* 1–3). A fourth resistance region was mapped to chromosome 3 (*Char* 4), and sequencing of the latter region localized the effect to the pyruvate kinase gene (Min-Oo et al., 2003). The strain of mice with this loss-of-function mutation at the pyruvate kinase locus almost surely shows the clinical features of mild pyruvate kinase deficiency, that is, a chronic hemolytic anemia with splenomegaly and a high reticulocyte count. Because of the right shift in the oxygen dissociation curve associated with this enzyme deficiency, anemia is well compensated. The analogous condition with low-grade deficiencies could occur in human populations without having been recognized as such.

Conclusion

Haldane's original "malaria hypothesis" has undoubtedly stood the test of time, although the cellular mechanisms for protection of thalassemia heterozygotes against malaria have proved to be much more complex than he proposed. Heterozygote protection not only has resulted in the current high frequency of the hemoglobin disorders and G6PD deficiency, but also has molded the genetic makeup of human populations in many other ways.

Although case–control studies have provided clear evidence about the magnitude of the protection against malaria mediated by the sickle cell gene and α-thalassemia, comparable information is still awaited in the case of β-thalassemia, Hb E, and other common polymorphisms. The cellular mechanisms of heterozygote resistance are still not absolutely clear, but there is increasing evidence that they probably differ between different polymorphisms. While the oxidative damage and suicidal infection mechanisms proposed for the Hb S and G6PD deficiency phenotypes have many attractions, the sparse available evidence indicates that the mechanism operating in α-thalassemia may be quite different.

References

Allen, S.J., O'Donnell, A., Alexander, N.D.E., Alpers, M.P., Peto, T.E.A., Clegg, J.B., & Weatherall, D.J. (1997) α+-Thalassaemia protects children against disease due to malaria and other infections. *Proceedings of the National Academy of Sciences of the United States of America*, **94**, 14736–14741.

Allen, S.J., O'Donnell, A., Alexander, N.D.E., Mgone, C.S., Peto, T.E.A., Clegg, J.B., Alpers, M.P., & Weatherall, D.J. (1999) Prevention of cerebral malaria in children in Papua New Guinea by Southeast Asian ovalocytosis band 3. *American Journal of Tropical Medicine and Hygiene*, **60**, 1056–1060.

Allison, A.C. (1965) Population genetics of abnormal haemoglobins and glucose-6-phosphate dehydrogenase deficiency. In: *Abnormal Haemoglobins in Africa* (ed. J.H.P. Jonxis), p. 365. Oxford: Blackwell Scientific Publications.

Barragan, A., Kremsner, P.G., Wahlgren, M., & Carlson, J. (2000) Blood group A antigen is a coreceptor in *Plasmodium falciparum* rosetting. *Infection and Immunity*, **68**, 2971–2975.

Cappadoro, M., Giribaldi, G., O'Brien, E., Turrini, F., Mannu, F., Ulliers, D., Simula, G., Luzzatto, L., & Arese, P. (1998) Early phagocytosis of glucose-6-phosphate dehydrogenase (G6PD)-deficient erythrocytes parasitized by *Plasmodium falciparum* may explain malaria protection in G6PD deficiency. *Blood*, **92**, 2527–2534.

Chang, S., Reid, M.E., Conboy, J., Kan, Y.W., & Mohandas, N. (1991) Molecular characterization of erythrocyte glycophorin C variants. *Blood*, **77**, 644–648.

Chishti, A.H., Palek, J., Fisher, D., Maalouf, G.J., Liu, S.C. (1996) Reduced invasion and growth of Plasmodium falciparum into elliptocytic red blood cells with a combined deficiency of protein 4.1, glycophorin C, and p55. *Blood*, **87**, 3462–3469.

Chotivanich, K., Udomsangpetch, R., Pattanapanyasat, K., Chierakul, W., Simpson, J., Looareesuwan, S., & White, N. (2002) Hemoglobin E: a balanced polymorphism protective against high parasitemias and thus severe *P. falciparum* malaria. *Blood*, **100**, 1172–1176.

Cockburn, I.A., Mackinnon, M.J., O'Donnell, A., Allen, S.J., Moulds, J.M., Baisor, M., Bockarie, M., Reeder, J.C. & Rowe, J.A. (2004) A human complement receptor 1 polymorphism that reduces *Plasmodium falciparum* rosetting confers protection against severe malaria. *Proceedings of the National Academy of Sciences USA*, **101**, 272–277.

Cooke, G.S., & Hill, A.V.S. (2001) Genetics of susceptibility to human infectious disease. *Nature Reviews Genetics*, **2**, 967–977.

Facer, C.A. (1995) Erythrocytes carrying mutations in spectrin and protein 4.1 show differing sensitivities to invasion by *Plasmodium falciparum*. *Parasitology Research*, **81**, 52–57.

Fischer, P.R., & Boone, P. (1998) Short report: severe malaria associated with blood group. *American Journal of Tropical Medicine and Hygiene*, **58**, 122–123.

Flint, J., Harding, R.M., Boyce, A.J., Clegg, J.B. (1998) The population genetics of the haemoglobinopathies. *Baillieres Clinical Haematology*, **11**, 1–51.

Flint, J., Hill, A.V.S., Bowden, D.K., Oppenheimer, S.J., Sill, P.R., Serjeantson, S.W., Bana Koiri, J., Bhatia, K., Alpers, M.P., Boyce, A.J., Weatherall, D.J., & Clegg, J.B. (1986) High frequencies of α thalassaemia are the result of natural selection by malaria. *Nature*, **321**, 744–749.

Friedman, M.J. (1978) Erythrocytic mechanism of sickle cell resistance to malaria. *Proceedings of the National Academy of Sciences USA*, **75**, 1994.

Friedman, M.J., Roth, E.F., Nagel, R.L., & Trager, W. (1979) *Plasmodium falciparum*: physiological interactions with the human sickle cell. *Experimental Parasitology*, **47**, 73.

Ganczakowski, M., Town, M., Bowden, D.K., Vulliamy, T.J., Kaneko, A., Clegg, J.B., Weatherall, D.J., & Luzzatto, L. (1995) Multiple glucose 6-phosphate dehydrogenase-deficient variants correlate with malaria endemicity in the Vanuatu archipelago (southwestern Pacific). *American Journal of Human Genetics*, **56**, 294–301.

Genton, B., Al-Yaman, F., Mgone, C.S., Alexander, N., Paniu, M.M., & Alpers, M.P. (1995) Ovalocytosis and cerebral malaria. *Nature*, **378**, 564–565.

Haldane, J.B.S. (1949) The rate of mutation of human genes. *Proceedings. VIII International Congress of Genetics. Hereditas*, **35**, 267–273.

Hill, A.V.S., Bowden, D.K., O'Shaughnessy, D.F., Weatherall, D.J., & Clegg, J.B. (1988) β-thalassemia in Melanesia: association with malaria and characterization of a common variant (IVSI nt 5 G-C). *Blood*, **72**, 9.

Hill, A.V.S., Allsopp, C.E.M., Kwiatkowski, D., Anstey, N.M., Twunmasi, P., Rowe, P.A., Bennett, S., Brewster, D., McMichael, A.J., & Greenwood, B.M. (1991) Common West African HLA antigens are associated with protection from severe malaria. *Nature*, **352**, 595–600.

Huang, C.H., Johe, K., Moulds, J.J., Siebert, P.D., Fukuda, M., & Blumenfeld, O.O. (1987) Delta glycophorin (glycophorin B) gene deletion in two individuals homozygous for the S–s–U– blood group phenotype. *Blood*, **70**, 1830–1835.

Huisman, T.H.J., Carver, M.F.H., & Efremov, G.D. (1998) *A Syllabus of Human Hemoglobin Variants*. Augusta, GA: Sickle Cell Foundation.

Lederberg, J. (1999) J.B.S. Haldane (1949) on infectious disease and evolution. *Genetics*, **153**, 1–3.

Lell, B., May, J., Schmidt-Ott, R.J., Lehman, L.G., Luckner, D., Greve, B., Matousek, P., Schmid, D., Herbich, K., Mockenhaupt, F.P., Meyer, C.G., Bienzle, U., & Kremsner, P.G. (1999) The role of red blood cell polymorphisms in resistance and susceptibility to malaria. *Clinical Infectious Diseases*, **28**, 794–799.

Livingstone, F.B. (1985) *Frequencies of hemoglobin variants*. Oxford: Oxford University Press.

Luzzatto, L., Mehta, A., & Vulliamy, T. (2001) Glucose 6-phosphate dehydrogenase. In: *The metabolic and molecular basis of inherited disease* (ed. C.R. Scriver, A.L. Beaudet, W.S. Sly, D. Valle, B. Childs, & B. Vogelstein), pp. 4517–4554. New York: McGraw Hill.

Luzzatto, L., Nwachiku-Jarrett, E.S., & Reddy, S. (1970) Increased sickling of parasitised erythrocytes as mechanism of resistance against malaria in the sickle-cell trait. *Lancet*, **i**, 319.

Luzzi, G.A., Merry, A.H., Newbold, C.I., Marsh, K., Pasvol, G., & Weatherall, D.J. (1991) Surface antigen expression on *Plasmodium falciparum*-infected erythrocytes is modified in α- and β-thalassemia. *Journal of Experimental Medicine*, **173**, 785–791.

Maier, A.G., Duraisingh, M.T., Reeder, J.C., Patel, S.S., Kazura, J.W., Zimmerman, P.A., & Cowman, A.F. (2003) *Plasmodium falciparum* erythrocyte invasion through glycophorin C and selection for Gerbich negativity in human populations. *Nature Medicine*, **9**, 87–92.

Miller, L.H., Mason, S.J., Clyde, D.F., & McGinniss, M.H. (1976) The resistance factor to *Plasmodium vivax* in Blacks. *New England Journal of Medicine*, **295**, 302–304.

Miller, L.H., Haynes, J.D., McAuliffe, F.M., Shiroishi, T., Durocher, J.R., & McGinniss, M.H. (1977) Evidence for differences in erythrocyte surface receptors for the malarial parasites, *Plasmodium falciparum* and *Plasmodium knowlesi*. *Journal of Experimental Medicine*, **146**, 277–281.

Min-Oo, G., Fortin, A., Tam, M.F., Nantel, A., Stevenson, M.M., & Gros, P. (2003) Pyruvate kinase deficiency in mice protects against malaria. *Nature Genetics*, **35**, 357–362.

Modiano, D., Luoni, G., Sirima, B.S., Simporé, J., Verra, F., Konaté, A., Rastrelli, E., Olivieri, A., Calissano, C., Paganotti, G.M., D'Urbano, L., Sanou, I., Sawadogo, A., Modano, G., & Coluzzi, M. (2001) Haemoglobin C protects against clinical *Plasmodium falciparum* malaria. *Nature*, **414**, 305–308.

Mohandas, N., Winardi, R., Knowles, D., Leung, A., Parra, M., George, E., Conboy, J., & Chasis, J. (1992) Molecular basis for membrane rigidity of hereditary ovalocytosis. A novel mechanism involving the cytoplasmic domain of band 3. *Journal of Clinical Investigation*, **89**, 686–692.

Morle, L., Morle, F., Roux, A.F., Godet, J., Forget, B.G., Denoroy, L., Garbarz, M., Dhermy, D., Kastally, R., & Delaunay, J. (1989) Spectrin Tunis (Sp alpha I/78), an elliptocytogenic variant, is due to the CGG–TGG codon change (Arg–Trp) at position 35 of the alpha I domain. *Blood*, **74**, 828–832.

Mourant, A.E. (1968) Genetical polymorphisms and the incidence of disease. *Proceedings of the Royal Society of Medicine*, **61**, 163.

Nagel, R.L. (2001) Malaria and hemoglobinopathies. In: *Disorders of hemoglobin* (ed. M.H. Steinberg, B.G. Forget, D.R. Higgs, & R.L. Nagel), pp. 832–860. Cambridge: Cambridge University Press.

Orkin, S.H., Kazazian, H.H., Antonarakis, S.E., Ostrer, H., Goff, S.C., & Sexton, J.P. (1982) Abnormal RNA processing due to the exon mutation of b^E-globin gene. *Nature*, **300**, 768–769.

O'Shaughnessy, D.F., Hill, A.V.S., Bowden, D.K., Weatherall, D.J., & Clegg, J.B., (1990) Globin genes in Micronesia: origins and affinities of Pacific Island peoples. *American Journal of Human Genetics*, **46**, 144–155.

Pasvol, G., Wainscoat, J.S., & Weatherall, D.J. (1982) Erythrocytes deficiency in glycophorin resist invasion by the malarial parasite *Plasmodium falciparum*. *Nature*, 297, 64–66.

Pasvol, G., Weatherall, D.J., & Wilson, R.J. (1977) Effects of foetal haemoglobin on susceptibility of red cells to *Plasmodium falciparum*. *Nature*, 270, 171–173.

Pasvol, G., Weatherall, D.J., & Wilson, R.J.M. (1978) A mechanism for the protective effect of haemoglobin S against *P. falciparum*. *Nature*, 274, 701–703.

Perkins, M. (1981) Inhibitory effects of erythrocyte membrane proteins on the in vitro invasion of the human malarial parasite (*Plasmodium falciparum*) into its host cell. *Journal of Cell Biology*, 90, 563–567.

Rees, D.C., Williams, T.N., Maitland, K., Clegg, J.B., & Weatherall, D.J. (1998) Alpha thalassemia is associated with increased soluble transferrin receptor levels. *British Journal of Haematology*, 103, 365–370.

Roberts, D.J., Harris, T., & Williams, T.N. (2004) The influence of inherited traits on malaria infection. In: *Susceptibility to infectious diseases: The importance of host genetics* (ed. R. Bellamy), pp. 139–184. Cambridge University Press, Cambridge.

Roth, E.F., Jr., Friedman, M., Ueda, Y., Tellez, L., Trager, W., & Nagel, R.L. (1978) Sickling rates of human AS red cells infected *in vitro* with *Plasmodium falciparum* malaria. *Science*, 202, 650–652.

Ruwende, C., Khoo, S.C., Snow, R.W., Yates, S.N.R., Kwiatkowski, D., Gupta, S., Warn, P., Allsopp, C.E.M., Gilbert, S.C., Peschu, N., Newbold, C.I.N., Greenwood, B.M., Marsh, K. & Hill, A.V.S. (1995) Natural selection of hemi- and heterozygotes for glucose-6-phosphate dehydrogenase deficiency by resistance to severe malaria. *Nature*, 376, 246–249.

Shear, H.L., Grinberg, L., Gilman, J., Fabry, M.E., Stamatoyannopoulos, G., Goldberg, D.E., & Nagel, R.L. (1998) Transgenic mice expressing human fetal globin are protected from malaria by a novel mechanism. *Blood*, 92, 2520–2526.

Silvestroni, E., & Bianco, I. (1947) Sulla frequenza dei porta tori di malatia di morbo di Codey e primi observazioni sulla frequenza dei portatore di microcitemia nel Ferrarese e inakune regioni limitrofe. *Boll Atti Accademia Medica Roma*, 72, 32.

Siniscalco, M., Bernini, L., Latte, B., & Motulsky, A.G. (1961) Favism and thalassaemia in Sardinia and their relationship to malaria. *Nature*, 190, 1179–1180.

Steinberg, M.H., Forget, B.G., Higgs, D.R., & Nagel, R.L. (eds.) (2001) *Disorders of hemoglobin*. New York: Cambridge University Press.

Tournamille, C., Colin, Y., Cartron, J.P., & Le Van Kim C. (1995) Disruption of a GATA motif in the Duffy gene promoter abolishes erythroid gene expression in Duffy-negative individuals. *Nature Genetics*, 10, 224–228.

Udomsangpetch, R., Todd, I., Carlson, J., & Greenwood B.M. (1993) The effects of hemoglobin genotype and ABO blood group on the formation of rosettes by *Plasmodium falciparum*-infected red blood cells. *American Journal of Tropical Medicine and Hygiene*, 48, 149–153.

Valentine, W.N., & Neel, J.V. (1944) Hematologic and genetic study of transmission of thalassemia (Cooley's anemia: Mediterranean anemia). *Archives of Internal Medicine*, 74, 185–196.

Weatherall, D.J., & Clegg, J.B. (2001a) *The thalassaemia syndromes*. 4th ed. Oxford: Blackwell Science.

Weatherall, D.J., & Clegg, J.B. (2001b) Inherited haemoglobin disorders: an increasing global health problem. *Bulletin of the World Health Organisation*, 79, 704–712.

Weatherall, D.J., & Clegg, J.B. (2002) Genetic variability in response to infection. Malaria and after. *Genes and Immunity*, 3, 331–337.

Willcox, M.C., Bjorkman, A., Brohult, J., Persson, P.-O., Rombo, L., & Bengtsson, E. (1983) A case-control study in northern Liberia of *Plasmodium falciparum* malaria in haemoglobin S and b-thalassaemia traits. *Annals of Tropical Medicine and Parasitology*, 77, 239–246.

Williams, T.N., Maitland, K., Bennett, S., Ganczakowski, M., Peto, T.E.A., Newbold, C.I., Bowden, D.K., Weatherall, D.J., & Clegg, J.B. (1996) High incidence of malaria in a-thalassaemic children. *Nature*, 383, 522–525.

Williams, T.N., Mwangi, T.W., Roberts, D.J., Alexander, N.D. Weatherall, D.J., Wambua, S., Kortok, M., Snow, R.W., & Marsh, K. (2005a) An immune basis for malaria protection by the sickle cell trait. *PLoS Medicine*, 2(5), e128.

Williams, T.N., Mwangi, T.W., Wambua, S., Peto, T.E., Weatherall, D.J., Gupta, S., Recker, M., Penman, B.S., Uyoga, S., Macharia, A., Mwacharo, J.K., Snow, R.W., & Marsh, K. (2005c) Negative epistasis between the malaria-protective effects of α^+-thalassaemia and the sickle cell trait. *Nature Genetics* 37, 1253–1257.

Williams, T.N., Wambua, S., Uyoga, S., Macharia, A., Mwacharo, J.K., Newton, C.R., & Maitland, K. (2005b) Both heterozygous and homozygous α^+thalassemia protect against severe and fatal *Plasmodium falciparum* malaria on the coast of Kenya. *Blood*, 106, 368–371.

Williams, T.N., Weatherall, D.J., & Newbold, C.I. (2002) The membrane characteristics of *Plasmodium falciparum*-infected and -uninfected heterozygous α^0-thalassaemic erythrocytes. *British Journal of Haematology*, 118, 663–670.

Yuthavong, Y., Butthep, P., Bunyaratvej, A., & Fucharoen, S. (1987) Inhibitory effect of β^0-thalassaemia/ haemoglobin E erythrocytes on *Plasmodium falciparum* growth *in vitro*. *Transaction of the Royal Society of Tropical Medicine and Hygiene*, 81, 903–906.

Zimmerman, P.A., Woolley, I., Masinde, G.L., Miller, S.M., McNamara, D.T., Hazlett, F., Mgone, C.S., Alpers, M.P., Genton, B., Boatin, B.A., & Kazura, J.W. (1999) Emergence of FY*A(null) in a *Plasmodium vivax*-endemic region of Papua New Guinea. *Proceedings of the National Academy of Sciences of the United States of America*, 96, 13973–13977.

9

Immunoglobulin Fc and Related Receptor Genes

Jennifer A. Croker & Robert P. Kimberly

Fc and Related Receptors

Immunoglobulin Fc receptors (FcRs), members of the immunoglobulin gene superfamily, are membrane-bound glycoproteins that function in the immune system by coupling antibodies to effector functions in a cell. The different FcRs, while each interacting with the constant (Fc) region of an antibody (Ab), may bind to ligand with different affinities. Each FcR utilizes partially overlapping, as well as discrete, signaling mechanisms to elicit cellular immune responses, including phagocytosis, degranulation, endocytosis, immune-complex clearance, Ab-dependent cell cytotoxicity, and transcriptional regulation of cytokine and chemokine expression (Daeron, 1997). Clinically, genetic variants found in several of the FcRs have been implicated in several inflammatory, rheumatic, and autoimmune diseases, such as systemic lupus erythematosus (SLE), rheumatoid arthritis (RA), and vasculitis (Croker and Kimberly, 2005). Recent data also implicate FcR function in susceptibility to infection, particularly in patients

with inflammatory or autoimmune diseases (Kimberly et al., 1988, 1998; Hughes et al., 2004).

Classical FcγR Family

Eight FCGR genes, clustered at the human 1q21-23 chromosomal locus, encode 10 highly homologous, but distinct, classical IgG receptor proteins (FcγR) that can be classified into three groups (FcγRI, FcγRII, and FcγRIII) based on structural homology (Qiu et al., 1990; Oakey et al., 1992; Su et al., 2002). Functionally, activating receptors are characterized by the presence of an immunoreceptor tyrosine-based activation motif (ITAM) in their cytoplasmic tail or by the interaction with other molecules that bear this motif, including the γ-chain of FcεRI. Inhibitory receptors encode a cytoplasmic immunoreceptor tyrosine-based inhibitory motif (ITIM) (Ravetch and Kinet, 1991; Daeron, 1997; Bolland and Ravetch, 1999; Edberg et al., 1999). Cell signaling events result from the balance of cumulative inhibiting and activating effects.

FcγRI Family

Despite three distinct genes and the detection of three corresponding mRNA transcripts, current data suggest that only one protein, FcγRIa, is expressed and has a physiologically relevant role in cellular responses. The 72-kDa transmembrane, activating receptor is expressed in monocytes, macrophages, dendritic cells, and interferon-γ–induced or granulocyte colony stimulating factor–induced polymorphic neutrophils (Ravetch and Bolland, 2001; van Sorge et al., 2003). Three extracellular Ig-like domains contribute to the receptor's high-affinity ($K_a \sim 10^9\,M^{-1}$) binding primarily to monomeric IgG1 and IgG3, and, to a significantly lesser degree, IgG4 (Hulett et al., 1991; Ravetch and Kinet, 1991; van Sorge et al., 2003). Overall, FcγRIa signaling affects phagocytosis, cytokine production (tumor necrosis factor-α [TNFα], interleukin-1 [IL-1], IL-6, and IL-10), Ab-dependent cellular toxicity, generation of a respiratory burst, antigen presentation, and degranulation (Edberg et al., 1999, 2002b; Kimberly et al., 2002). The tyrosine-based signaling cascade activated through FcγRIa's interaction with FcεRI γ-chain can be modulated by the receptor cytoplasmic tail (Edberg et al., 1999).

FcγRII Family

Three genes encode five isoforms of FcγRII family members, differentially expressed in macrophages, neutrophils, platelets, B cells, trophoblasts, and epithelial cells (Cassel et al., 1993). Two extracellular Ig-like domains of the activating FcγRIIa and FcγRIIc receptors bind multimeric human IgG1 and IgG3 with low affinity ($K_a < 10^7\,M^{-1}$), and FcγRIIa can bind human IgG2 in an allele-dependent fashion (Parren et al., 1992). Downstream FcγRII-mediated effects include degranulation, phagocytosis, cytokine production, oxidative burst, and Ab-dependent cellular toxicity (Kimberly et al., 2002).

Interestingly, in addition to IgG, FcγRIIa and, to a lesser extent, FcγRI have been shown to directly interact with C-reactive protein (CRP), an acute-phase serum protein that functions in complement activation, phagocyte chemotaxis, and opsonic activity associated with the innate immune response (Kaplan and Volanakis, 1974; Marnell et al., 1995; Stein et al., 2000b). The characterization of this FcR–opsonin interaction bridges the distinction between innate and acquired immunity.

Two splice variants derived from the single *FCGR2B* gene encode ITIM-containing inhibitory receptors, varying in expression and tissue distribution (Cambier et al., 1994). To properly function, FcγRIIb co-aggregates with ITAM-containing receptors such that the balance of positive and negative signaling determines the cellular response (Salmon and Pricop, 2001). An alternate inhibitory effect, observed in B cells, may involve a pro-apoptotic signal, induced by homotypic aggregation of FcγRIIb, independent of the ITIM (Ravetch and Bolland, 2001).

FcγRIIb has a key role in splenic germinal center–associated follicular dendritic cell (FDC) function (Manser, 2004). FDCs derived from FcγRIIb mutant mice (FcγRIIb$^{-/-}$) or those exposed to an antagonistic anti-FcγRIIb monoclonal Ab failed to efficiently trap immune complexes (ICs) and to elicit effective B-cell recall responses and Ab production (Yoshida et al., 1993; Qin et al., 2000). Additionally, interaction with FDCs enhances IC immunogenicity prior to B-cell presentation (Aydar et al., 2004). Co-ligation of the activating B-cell receptor (BCR) and the inhibitory FcγRIIb on B cells by ICs inhibits B-cell activation and Ab production (Ono et al., 1996, 1997; Tridandapani et al., 1997). Further exploration of FcγRIIb's role in germinal center function and B-cell development is crucial to our understanding of Ab responses to infection and vaccines and in autoimmune conditions.

FcγRIII Family

Two genes encode two members of the FcγRIII family: FcγRIIIa and FcγRIIIb. FcγRIIIa, expressed in macrophages, natural killer (NK) cells, and subsets of T cells and monocytes, preferentially binds multimeric IgG1 and IgG3 complexes with higher affinity ($K_a \sim 10^7\,M^{-1}$), though there is evidence for binding to monomeric IgG1 and IgG3 dependent on cell type and glycosylation state (Huizinga et al., 1989; Kimberly et al., 1989; Vance et al., 1993; Edberg and Kimberly, 1997). Membrane localization and functional signaling of FcγRIIIa require association with and ITAM-tyrosine phosphorylation of FcεRI γ-chain (Wirthmueller et al., 1992; Park et al., 1993; Kimberly et al., 2002).

FcγRIIIb, expressed in neutrophils and eosinophils, has somewhat lower affinity and preferentially binds multimeric IgG1 and IgG3 complexes. It is unique among FcR in that it lacks a transmembrane domain and is expressed on the cell membrane via a glycosylphosphatidylinositol linkage (Kurosaki and Ravetch,

1989). Upon activation, FcγRIIIb initiates tyrosine-phosphorylation–mediated events which lead to degranulation, Ab-dependent cellular cytotoxicity, respiratory bursts, and phagocytosis (Anderson et al., 1990).

Fc-Related Receptors

FcRn

FcRn is an MHC class I–related transmembrane protein that functions in the bidirectional transport of IgG across polarized epithelial mucosal surfaces, including the lung, intestine, and placenta (Lencer and Blumberg, 2005). This process allows for the recycling of IgG from the lysosome and regulation of serum IgG levels, thereby affecting systemic and mucosal immunity (Rodewald and Kraehenbuhl, 1984; Raghavan and Bjorkman, 1996; Ober et al., 2004a, 2004b; Lencer and Blumberg, 2005). Structurally, FcRn is a protein heterodimer of α-chain and β2-microglobulin. The cytosolic domain contains sorting signals that contribute to the trafficking function of the receptor (Simister and Ahouse, 1996).

FcR-Like Gene Family

Homology search strategies have revealed a group of genes with extracellular domains homologous to the classical FcR. Located on human chromosome 1q21-23 centromeric to the classical cluster, these receptors have been termed FcR homologues (FcRH) 1–6, immunoglobulin superfamily–related translocation-associated (IRTA) receptors, immunoglobulin superfamily FcR-GP42 (IFGP), and anti-IgM activating sequence (BXMAS). Currently, FcR-like (FcRL) is the favored nomenclature (Davis et al., 2001, 2002a, 2005; Hatzivassiliou et al., 2001; Nakayama et al., 2001; Guselnikov et al., 2002; Kochi et al., 2005). Collectively, FcRL proteins are primarily expressed on mature B cells, including naive and memory B cells, and to a much lesser extent on germinal center B cells and plasma cells (Davis et al., 2001, 2002b; Hatzivassiliou et al., 2001; Guselnikov et al., 2002; Mechetina et al., 2002; Miller et al., 2002; Leu et al., 2005). FcRL6 (FcRH6/IFGP6) differs in distribution in that it is expressed by T cells and NK cells (Davis et al., 2005).

Given their tissue distribution, it is thought that FcRLs may function in regulating mature B-cell signaling. Preliminary evidence from studies of the ITIM-containing FcRL4 (FcRH4/IRTA1/IFGP2), localized primarily on memory B cells, supports this hypothesis.

Signaling via this receptor can down-regulate B-cell activity, including kinase cascades and calcium mobilization (Ehrhardt et al., 2003). Alternatively, the ITAM containing FcRL1 (FcRH1/IRTA5/IFGP1) can enhance BCR-mediated calcium mobilization, CD69 and CD89 expression, and B-cell proliferation (Leu et al., 2005).

Despite the homology of FcRL with classical FcR extracellular domains, the natural ligands for FcRLs have not yet been determined. Preliminary evidence suggests that FcRLs can weakly bind heat-aggregated IgA(FcRL4/FcRH4/IRTA1/IFGP2)andIgG(FcRL5/FcRH5/IRTA2) (Hatzivassiliou et al., 2001). However these findings remain controversial (Davis et al., 2005; Chistiakov, et al., 2007).

FcR for Other Immunoglobulins

FcαRI

In addition to the FCGR linkage group on chromosome 1, a cluster of Ig superfamily-related receptors, known as the leukocyte receptor complex, exists in the human 19q13.4 chromosomal region (Davis et al., 2002b). As many as 26 genes have been characterized in this region, including FCAR1, which encodes the low-affinity receptor for monomeric IgA (Maliszewski et al., 1990). Multiple transcripts appear to be derived from this gene; however, only two prominent protein isoforms have been detected. FcαRIa2 is expressed exclusively on alveolar macrophages whereas FcαRIa1 has been seen on blood monocytes, macrophages, and neutrophils (Morton et al., 1996, Pleass et al., 1996, Reterink et al., 1996; van Dijk et al., 1996; van Egmond et al., 2001; Monteiro and Van De Winkel, 2003). Although an interaction with FcεRI γ-chain is not required for FcαRI transport to and expression on the cell membrane, FcεRI γ-chain is central to tyrosine-based activation of signal transduction cascades that regulate respiration bursts, phagocytosis, and degranulation (Monteiro and Van De Winkel, 2003).

Polymeric Ig Receptors

Polymeric immunoglobulin receptors (pIgR) are related proteins that function in epithelial transport. Upon binding ligand, mainly IgA (occasionally IgM), the receptor–ligand complex is internalized from the basolateral surface and transcytosed to the apical surface where a proteolytic event releases the ligand-bound portion of the receptor as a secreted IgA (SIgA) molecule. This secreted compound ensures immune exclusion at mucosal surfaces, possibly by preventing bacterial adherence and invasion (Luton and Mostov, 1999; Phalipon and Corthesy, 2003; Traicoff et al., 2003).

Fcα/μ Receptors

Fcα/μR is another receptor capable of binding monomeric IgA and IgM. Expressed in human B cells and macrophages, as well as liver, spleen, kidney, and intestinal cells, the receptor functions in the endocytosis of IgA/M opsonized bacteria (Shibuya et al., 2000). The apparently unique expression of Fcα/μR in human mesangial cells may provide the basis for IgA deposition in IgA nephropathy (McDonald et al., 2002).

FcεRI

FcεRI is a heterotetrameric (α, γ-dimer, and tetraspanin β-chains), transmembrane receptor found on mast cells, Langerhans cells, basophils, eosinophils, and monocytes (Repetto et al., 1996). IgE binds the high-affinity IgE interaction domain in the extracellular region of the FcεR α-chain, and a signal, transmitted via the FcεR γ-chain, activates several cell programs common to the allergic response, including the release of histamine, arachidonic acid metabolites, and cytokines (Hakimi et al., 1990; Ravetch and Kinet, 1991; Beaven and Metzger, 1993).

Role of Ig in Host Defense

Immunoglobulins play a critical role in host defense at the interface between innate and acquired immunity. Seventy-five percent of all immunoglobulins are of the IgG isotype, which includes four subclasses, IgG1, IgG2, IgG3, and IgG4, listed in order of decreasing abundance. IgG subclass deficiencies have been associated with recurrent upper/lower respiratory tract infections (Yount et al., 1970; Stanley et al., 1984). In children, deficiencies of the IgG2 subclass are most common, likely due to delayed onset of IgG2 expression to 5–10 years of age or later, and may relate to recurrent infections of the upper and lower respiratory tracts (Stanley et al., 1984; Soderstrom et al., 1987; Pan and Hammarstrom, 2000). In adults, IgG2 is generally up-regulated, and IgG3 deficiencies are more prevalent, possibly due to reduced isotype switching, though no clear phenotypic associations have been

defined in this case (Pan et al., 1997; Pan and Hammarstrom, 2000). Despite some evidence, the utility of specific IgG subclass deficiencies in predicting infection risk is controversial (Buckley, 2002; Maguire et al., 2002). It may be more likely that disease susceptibility is a function of multiple Ig deficiencies.

IgA is the major immunoglobulin isotype present in mucosal secretions and exists as two subclasses in humans and hominoid primates, IgA1 and IgA2 (Kawamura et al., 1991, 1992). The longer hinge between Fc and Fab regions of IgA1 is more susceptible to proteolytic enzymes expressed by certain pathogens including *Streptococcus pneumoniae*, *Haemophilus influenzae*, or *Neisseria meningitidis*. This susceptibility may facilitate infection by these agents at mucosal surfaces (Senior et al., 1991; Kawamura et al., 1992; Boehm et al., 1999; Furtado et al., 2004). Symptomatic IgA-deficient patients are frequently susceptible to sinopulmonary infections, parasitic infections (giardiasis), and intestinal nodular lymphoid hyperplasia (Gryboski et al., 1968). IgA deficiency is also frequently associated with arthritis, autoimmune endocrinopathies, ulcerative colitis, Crohn's disease, autoimmune hematologic disorders, and lupus-like disorders (Ammann and Hong, 1971; Schaffer et al., 1991; Strober and Sneller, 1991; Heneghan et al., 1997; Cunningham-Rundles, 2001). Chapter 18 reviews immunoglobulin and related deficiencies.

FcR and Infectious Diseases

There are multiple FcR polymorphisms that affect receptor-mediated activation. These polymorphisms can affect the intensity of host response and may be risk factors or determinants for infection (Bredius et al., 1993, 1994; Fijen et al., 1993; Sanders et al., 1994; Yee et al., 1997; Kimberly et al., 2002). Understanding the genetic implications at each locus may offer important insight into individual susceptibility to infection. These polymorphisms may also influence the therapeutic response to Ig-based biologic therapeutics.

FcγR

Polymorphisms in *FCGR2A*, *FCGR3A*, and *FCGR3B*, which impact the extracellular domains of the corresponding proteins, have received the most attention to date. With respect to these "activating" FcγR proteins, lower affinity IgG binding appears to correlate with increased general infection rate (Kimberly et al., 2002). Characteristics of the family of genes encoding FcγRs and associations of polymorphisms in those genes with clinical conditions are summarized in tables 9.1 and 9.2.

FCGR2A

The polymorphism corresponding to residue position 131 in FcγRIIa encodes either histidine (H131) or arginine (R131) in the extracellular domain (EC2). The frequency of the H131 allele is ~0.7 in healthy Asians and ~0.5 in healthy patients of European or African descent (Lehrnbecher et al., 1997; Karassa et al., 2002). Codominantly expressed, the H131 allele has a higher affinity for IgG3 than R131 and is the only FcR variant that binds IgG2 (Warmerdam et al., 1991; Salmon et al., 1992). This property may have a substantial clinical impact. IgG2 is the most important subclass for immune responses against encapsulated bacteria, including N. meningitidis, H. influenzae, and S. pneumoniae, and in the event of an IgG2 response to a pathogen, only neutrophils and monocytes expressing the FcγRIIa-H131 allele would be capable of binding and clearing such ICs. Because the H131 allele may elicit a more effective host response (Salmon and Pricop, 2001), FcγRIIa alleles may represent a risk factor for infection. Indeed, the R131 allele is associated with a higher rate of infection by encapsulated bacteria (e.g., meningococcus) (Bredius et al., 1994; Platonov et al., 1998; Domingo et al., 2002; Kimberly et al., 2002), with bacteremic pneumococcal pneumonia (Yee et al., 2000), and with invasive pneumococcal infection and periodontitis in certain SLE patients (Yee et al., 1997; Kobayashi et al., 2003).

The interaction of FcγRIIa with CRP appears to be allele specific, with greater affinity observed between the opsonin and the R131 receptor variant (Stein et al., 2000a). The functional implications of this interaction suggest the possibility that CRP binding to FcγRIIa-R131 may interfere with IgG IC interactions with the receptor. Another possibility is that the capacity of CRP to interact with capsular polysaccharides of S. pneumoniae and H. influenza might provide some protection to FcγRIIa-R131–homozygous patients in whom IgG2-mediated immune defenses may be significantly compromised (Weiser et al., 1998).

An association of several autoimmune diseases with the FcγRIIa-R131 genotype has been observed in several ethnic populations (Salmon et al., 1996; Zuniga et al., 2001; Gonzalez-Escribano et al., 2002; Kyogoku

et al., 2002b; Lee et al., 2002; Manger et al., 2002). The association of SLE and the R131 allele has been confirmed by linkage, family-based association, and meta-analysis of case–control association studies.

In contrast to the potential benefit of a more vigorous host response to certain acute infections, the H131 allele may also have a role in tissue-specific autoimmune and chronic inflammatory diseases. H131 has been associated with heparin-induced thrombocytopenia, with thrombosis in certain patients with autoimmune antiphospholipid syndrome, and with periodontitis in northern European Caucasians, particularly those who smoke (Burgess et al., 1995; Atsumi et al., 1998; Carlsson et al., 1998; Loos et al., 2003; Yamamoto et al., 2004). The R131 allele has also been associated with a higher rate of acute renal allograft rejection. The molecular basis for this rejection is not fully understood but may serve as an important predictor for rejection risk (Yuan et al., 2004).

FCGR3A

The two codominantly expressed alleles of FCGR3A differ by an amino acid substitution at position 176 of FcγRIIIa encoding either a valine (V176) or phenylalanine (F176). This polymorphism affects the ligand binding site in the membrane proximal EC2 ligand-binding domain (Wu et al., 1997; Koene et al., 1998; Sondermann et al., 2000). The valine allele has higher affinity for monomeric IgG1 and IgG3, and is the only allele able to bind IgG4 (Koene et al., 1997). Hypothetically, this may suggest that the absence of the V176 FcγRIIIa allele may tip the balance of IgG4 signaling toward the inhibitory FcγRIIb. Normally, FcγRIIIa is localized on macrophages and NK cells and can respond to IC involving a variety of pathogens. IgG-induced NK activity is increased in FcγRIIIa-V176 homozygous individuals, likely due to the increased IgG affinity (Vance et al., 1993; Wu et al., 1997; Koene et al., 1998). The lower-affinity F176 allele is enriched in SLE patients and may constitute a risk factor for the disease (Wu et al., 1997; Koene et al., 1998; Edberg et al., 2002a). The FcγRIIIa-F176 allele also has a suggestive association with urinary tract infection (UTI) susceptibility in RA patients (Hughes et al., 2004). It is currently unclear if these results can be extrapolated to normal individuals or to patients with other autoimmune diseases and more diverse ethnicities.

There is some evidence to support a statistically significant overrepresentation of the V176 allele in aggres-

TABLE 9.1. Fcγ receptors, alleles, and infection susceptibility/severity.

Gene Name (NCBI)	Protein Name(s)	Entrez Gene ID	Map Position	UCSC Genome Bioinformatics[a] Position	Alleles (Details)	Allele-associated Infection Susceptibility/Severity	Reference(s)
FCGR2A	FcγRIIa, CD32a	2212	1q21-23	chr1: 158,288,274-158,302,415	H131 / R131 (affects extracellular Ig-binding domain, resulting in markedly reduced IgG2 binding affinity in R131)	H131: Periodontitis R131: N. meningitides, H. influenzae, S. pneumoniae	Loos et al. 2003; Yamamoto et al. 2004 Yee et al. 2000; Domingo et al. 2002; Kimberly et al. 2002
FCGR2B	FcγRIIb, CD32b	2213	1q21-23	chr1: 158,364,610-158,379,618	−386G −120T/−386C −120A (promoter SNPs in two transcription factor binding sites [GATA4 and YY1], resulting in increased transcription factor binding and FcγRIIb expression in −386C −120A) I232/T232 (affects transmembrane domain, resulting in reduced lipid raft association and signaling capacity)	ND	ND
FCGR3A	FcγRIIIa, CD16a	2214	1q21-23	chr1: 158,324,607-158,332,873	V176 / F176 (affects extracellular Ig-binding domain, resulting in reduced IgG1 and IgG3 affinity in F176)	V176: Aggressive / Chronic Periodontitis F176: Urinary tract Infection (UTI) in RA patients	Kobayashi et al. 2001; Meisel et al. 2001; Loos et al. 2003 Hughes et al. 2004
FCGR3B	FcγRIIIb, CD16b	2215	1q21-23	chr1: 158,324,670-158,332,598	NA1/NA2 (affects extracellular Ig-binding domain, resulting in reduced IgG affinity and less activity potential in NA2)	NA2: Upper respiratory tract infection (URI) in rheumatoid arthritis patients	Hughes et al. 2004

ND, not determined.

[a]The UCSC Genome Bioinformatics site (www.genome.ucsc.edu) contains the reference sequence (rs), working draft assemblies, and annotations for several genomes, as well as a variety of tools to analyze the data, including a portal to the National Human Genome Research Institute's ENCODE project (Kent et al. 2002).

TABLE 9.2. FcγR allele-dependent IgG subclass interactions.

Fc Receptor	Allele(s) Affecting Ligand Binding	Distinctive IgG Interaction	Relative IgG Affinity[a]
FcγRIa	None characterized	IgG1, IgG3, IgG4	3 = 1 > 4 >> 2
FcγRIIa	H131	IgG1, IgG2, IgG3	3 = 1, 2 >>> 4
	R131	IgG1, IgG3	3 = 1 >>> 2, 4
FcγRIIb	None characterized	IgG1, IgG3, IgG4	3 = 1 > 4 >> 2
FcγRIIIa	V176	IgG1, IgG3, IgG4	3 = 1 > 4 >> 2
	F176	IgG1, IgG3	3 = 1 >>> 2, 4
FcγRIIIb	NA1	IgG1, IgG3	3 = 1 >>> 2, 4
	NA2	IgG1, IgG3	3 = 1 >>> 2, 4

[a]Relative affinities for IgG subclasses per FcR allele. Generally, FcγRI is considered the "high-affinity" receptor ($K_a \sim 10^8$–10^9 M^{-1}), whereas FcγRII and FcγRIII are considered "low-affinity" receptors ($K_a \sim 10^7$ M^{-1}). Relative IgG affinities correspond to allelic differences. Comparisons between different receptors cannot be drawn from this table. Although FcγRIIIb alleles NA1 and NA2 maintain the same relative IgG affinity order, the NA1 allele binding affinity is overall greater than that of NA2.

sive or chronic periodontitis patients, and the allele may be a risk factor for bone loss in certain ethnicities, though further analysis is needed (Kobayashi et al., 2001; Meisel et al., 2001; Loos et al., 2003).

FCGR3B

In contrast, the polymorphism in FcγRIIIb, originally described as the neutrophil antigen (NA), consists of two alleles that affect signal intensity and IgG affinity (NA1 has higher affinity for IgG1 or IgG3 than NA2) (Huizinga et al., 1990; Salmon et al., 1990; Edberg and Kimberly, 1994). The two alleles differ in the number of functionally relevant N-linked glycosylation sites, which may interfere with protein interactions. The NA1 isoform produces greater phagocytic responses, oxidative bursts, and/or degranulation than the more common NA2 allotype (Kimberly et al., 2002). In RA patients, a significant association between the FcγRIIIb NA2 allele and respiratory tract infections (URI) has been reported, suggesting the allele is the biologically relevant polymorphism having a role in URI susceptibility (Hughes et al., 2004). The role of copy number

variation of FCGR3B in host defense is currently unexplored (Fanciulli, et al., 2007).

Other FcRs: FCGR2B, FCGR1A, and FCGA1

Less is known regarding existing polymorphisms in other related FcRs and their possible role in infection. Single nucleotide polymorphisms (SNPs) have been identified in the regulatory and coding regions of FcγRIIb that may have a functional impact on susceptibility to autoimmune disease and infection (Kyogoku et al., 2002a, 2002b; Li et al., 2003; Siriboonrit et al., 2003; Yasuda et al., 2003; Su et al., 2004). Likewise, an SNP at codon 92 in the exon encoding the extracellular domain of FcγRIa results in a stop codon and a truncated protein; however, no obvious clinical phenotype has been attributed to the change (Chen et al., 2001). Though nonsynonymous SNPs have been identified for FCGR2B and FCGR1A, more work is needed to characterize the functional significance of these polymorphisms with respect to infectious disease.

As for FcαRI (CD89) and its possible role in infection, receptor levels on blood monocytes and neutrophils may be elevated in patients with gram-negative bacteremia; however, the putative role of the receptor in this infection is not well understood (Chiamolera et al., 2001). Likewise, the engagement of myeloid FcαRI by pneumococcal capsular polysaccharide-bound IgA or IgA immune sera from Bordetella pertussis–infected patients, and the efficient activation of effector functions such as phagocytosis, may play a significant role in host defense against S. pneumoniae and B. pertussis, respectively (van der Pol et al., 2000; Hellwig et al., 2001). To date, there are no data on polymorphic differences in FcαRI that may modify the effect of the receptor on susceptibility to or severity of infection.

Interactions Among FCGR and Susceptibility

Susceptibility to infection may be associated with risk alleles at multiple gene loci. These loci may be physically proximate and may be in linkage disequilibrium and constitute a risk haplotype, as may be found in the classical FCGR cluster. Additionally, risk alleles in the FCGR cluster may interact independently without the requirement that they be on the same haplotype. Of course, they may also interact with other gene variants within the genome to enhance susceptibility. For example, the severity of chronic periodontitis is best associated with both FcγRIIIa-V158 and FcγRIIIb-NA2 (Kobayashi et al., 2001). In the case of *N. meningitidis*, as with many gram-negative bacteria, optimal immune clearance necessitates complement activity and phagocytosis. Interestingly, complement-deficient patients homozygous for both low-affinity FcγRIIa (R131) and FcγRIIIb (NA2) alleles are more susceptible to meningococcal infection (Fijen et al., 1993).

FcRL

The frequency of SNPs in human *FcRL* genes is consistent with other coding regions (Bjorkander et al., 1985; Davis et al., 2002b). Some alleles, including a nonconservative substitution in FcRL3 (P660L), have distinct ethnicity-based distributions. The physical location of a nonsynonymous SNP affecting the extracellular domain of FcRL3 (FcRH3/IRTA3/IFGP3) may imply an effect on ligand binding (Davis et al., 2002b). Recently, a significant association was identified between an *FcRL3* promoter SNP, which affects nuclear factor-κB binding, and RA, SLE, and autoimmune thyroid disease (Kochi et al., 2005). Experimental evidence has shown that expression levels and proper function of FcRLs are critical to the balance of B-cell function in immune response (Alizadeh et al., 2000; Hatzivassiliou et al., 2001; Rosenwald et al., 2001, 2003; Wiestner et al., 2003; Attygalle et al., 2004). Though SNP analysis in *FCRL* genes has revealed nonsynonymous alleles, more work is needed to determine their functional significance and a possible relationship with infection susceptibility.

pIgR

Infectious agents, viral and bacterial, frequently colonize on mucosal surfaces of the gastrointestinal, respiratory, and urogenital tracts and initiate systemic infections. The body relies on the adaptive mucosal immune system as a defense against such pathogens. A dominant feature of the mucosal immune system is SIgA, a cleavage product of pIgR–IgA complexes (Mostov et al., 1980).

SIgA binds surface antigens of viral or bacterial pathogens, blocking the interaction of pathogens with epithelial receptors, inhibiting motility, and/or facilitating entrapment in mucus (Childers et al., 1989; Lamm, 1997; Corthesy and Kraehenbuhl, 1999; Phalipon et al., 2002). pIgR may provide the transport of pIgA-bound antigens from the basolateral side of the

epithelium to the lumen, thereby eliminating or neutralizing antigens (Kaetzel et al., 1991; Robinson et al., 2001; Fernandez et al., 2003). Analysis of pIgR$^{-/-}$ mice has shown an essential function of SIgA in protecting gastrointestinal and respiratory surfaces against certain secreted bacterial toxins (Asahi et al., 2002; Sun et al., 2004; Uren et al., 2005). In some cases, there is evidence that mucosal immunity in the upper respiratory tract by natural infection is more effective and more cross-protective against viral infection, particularly with respect to variant viruses, than the systemic immunity induced by parenteral vaccines (Clements et al., 1983; Couch and Kasel, 1983; Johnson et al., 1986; Murphy and Clements, 1989; Asahi et al., 2002). This latter point remains somewhat controversial and is likely pathogen dependent.

Infectious Pathogen Adaptation

As may be expected, microbial pathogens have also developed defense strategies that reduce the ability of FcR to mediate effective host defense. Examples include proteolytic enzymes that can cleave IgA isoforms (Plaut et al. 1977). Similarly, a homolog of CD11b (an α-subunit of the leukocyte integrin) expressed by group A streptococcus interferes with FcγR signaling and promotes pathogen survival (Lei et al., 2001). A glycoprotein secreted by Ebola virus similarly interferes with FcR function (Sanchez et al., 1999). Another strategy, employed by such pathogens as staphylococci, involves the secretion of protein A, which binds both Fab and Fc regions of IgG, affecting the immunoglobulin's ability to bind receptor and initiate the host response (Romagnani et al., 1981). It is likely that allelic differences in receptors and IgG will play a role in this pathogen–host interplay.

Pharmacogenetics

The role of Fc and related receptors in the pathogenesis of autoimmune and infectious disease susceptibility raises the possibility that either receptor expression or function might be modulated for therapeutic intervention. Such strategies may take advantage of differences in immunoglobulin classes and affinity, may target individual FcR with monoclonal antibodies, or may exploit binding interference (van Dijk and van de Winkel, 2001). For example, IgA has been used as immunotherapy to treat malignant diseases (Herberman,

2002; Mota et al., 2003; Otten and van Egmond, 2004; Woof and Kerr, 2004), and receptor-specific bifunctional reagents have been developed to target the high-affinity FcγRIa on macrophages as a potential therapeutic effector receptor in malignancies (Heijnen and Van de Winkel, 1995; Deo et al., 1997; Heijnen et al., 1997; Keler et al., 1997; Pullarkat et al., 1999; Withoff et al., 2001).

Interestingly, FcR alleles may also influence the therapeutic response to some Ig-based biologics. The response of non-Hodgkin's lymphoma and the extent of B-cell depletion in various autoimmune conditions by rituximab, an anti-CD20 monoclonal Ab, varies with host receptor genotype (Cartron et al., 2002). This observation suggests drug treatment, perhaps dose, might be adjusted based on genotype (Anolik et al., 2003; Dall'Ozzo et al., 2004; Kazkaz and Isenberg, 2004; Looney et al., 2004). Other agents, including infliximab and alefacept, are IgG1-based biologics used in a variety of autoimmune disorders (Weinberg, 2003; Kane and FitzGerald, 2004; Haraoui, 2005; Saini et al., 2005). Like rituximab, preliminary evidence suggests that Crohn's disease patients expressing the V158 allele of FcγRIIIa may have a better clinical response to infliximab therapy, a drug that targets TNFα (Louis et al., 2004). Alefacept, a lymphocyte function-associated antigen 3 (LFA-3; CD58)/IgG1 fusion protein, signals in NK cells via FcγRIIIa and CD2 to induce apoptosis (da Silva et al., 2002). An FcγRIIIa allele–dependent response to alefacept has not yet been identified, and well-powered studies are needed to confirm and extend analysis to evaluate the results in additional ethnicities and diseases.

Taken together, it has become very clear that genetic polymorphisms of receptors for antibodies can contribute not only not only to infectious disease susceptibility, but also to other immune-mediated processes and therapeutic responses. Targeting FcRs may be useful in therapeutic modulation of host defense against infectious disease.

Conclusion and Prospects

Genetic diversity plays a significant role in the fundamental bases for biological phenomena regulated by immunoglobulins and their respective receptors in the immune systems. In addition, evidence indicates that these variants also contribute to the efficacy of pharmacogenetic intervention in different patients. Genetic information will assist in the design of therapeutics and the development of better treatment regimens, allowing for the most specific and effective patient care possible.

References

Alizadeh, A.A., Eisen, M.B., Davis, R.E., Ma, C., Lossos, I.S., Rosenwald, A., Boldrick, J.C., Sabet, H., Tran, T., Yu, X., et al. (2000). Distinct types of diffuse large B-cell lymphoma identified by gene expression profiling. Nature 403, 503–511.

Ammann, A.J., and Hong, R. (1971). Selective IgA deficiency and autoimmunity. N Engl J Med 284, 985–986.

Anderson, C.L., Shen, L., Eicher, D.M., Wewers, M.D., and Gill, J.K. (1990). Phagocytosis mediated by three distinct Fc gamma receptor classes on human leukocytes. J Exp Med 171, 1333–1345.

Anolik, J.H., Campbell, D., Felgar, R.E., Young, F., Sanz, I., Rosenblatt, J., and Looney, R.J. (2003). The relationship of FcgammaRIIIa genotype to degree of B cell depletion by rituximab in the treatment of systemic lupus erythematosus. Arthritis Rheum 48, 455–459.

Asahi, Y., Yoshikawa, T., Watanabe, I., Iwasaki, T., Hasegawa, H., Sato, Y., Shimada, S., Nanno, M., Matsuoka, Y., Ohwaki, M., et al. (2002). Protection against influenza virus infection in polymeric Ig receptor knockout mice immunized intranasally with adjuvant-combined vaccines. J Immunol 168, 2930–2938.

Atsumi, T., Caliz, R., Amengual, O., Khamashta, M.A., and Hughes, G.R. (1990). Fcgamma receptor IIA H/R131 polymorphism in patients with antiphospholipid antibodies. Thromb Haemost 79, 924–927.

Attygalle, A.D., Liu, H., Shirali, S., Diss, T.C., Loddenkemper, C., Stein, H., Dogan, A., Du, M.Q., and Isaacson, P.G. (2004). Atypical marginal zone hyperplasia of mucosa-associated lymphoid tissue: A reactive condition of childhood showing immunoglobulin lambda light-chain restriction. Blood 104, 3343–3348.

Aydar, Y., Wu, J., Song, J., Szakal, A.K., and Tew, J.G. (2004). FcgammaRII expression on follicular dendritic cells and immunoreceptor tyrosine-based inhibition motif signaling in B cells. Eur J Immunol 34, 98–107.

Beaven, M.A., and Metzger, H. (1993). Signal transduction by Fc receptors: The Fc epsilon RI case. Immunol Today 14, 222–226.

Bjorkander, J., Bake, B., Oxelius, V.A., and Hanson, L.A. (1985). Impaired lung function in patients with IgA deficiency and low levels of IgG2 or IgG3. N Engl J Med *313*, 720–724.

Boehm, M.K., Woof, J.M., Kerr, M.A., and Perkins, S.J. (1999). The Fab and Fc fragments of IgA1 exhibit a different arrangement from that in IgG: A study by X-ray and neutron solution scattering and homology modelling. J Mol Biol *286*, 1421–1447.

Bolland, S., and Ravetch, J.V. (1999). Inhibitory pathways triggered by ITIM-containing receptors. Adv Immunol *72*, 149–177.

Bredius, R.G., Derkx, B.H., Fijen, C.A., de Wit, T.P., de Haas, M., Weening, R.S., van de Winkel, J.G., and Out, T.A. (1994). Fc gamma receptor IIa (CD32) polymorphism in fulminant meningococcal septic shock in children. J Infect Dis *170*, 848–853.

Bredius, R.G., de Vries, C.E., Troelstra, A., van Alphen, L., Weening, R.S., van de Winkel, J.G., and Out, T.A. (1993). Phagocytosis of *Staphylococcus aureus* and *Haemophilus influenzae* type B opsonized with polyclonal human IgG1 and IgG2 antibodies. Functional hFc gamma RIIa polymorphism to IgG2. J Immunol *151*, 1463–1472.

Buckley, R.H. (2002). Immunoglobulin G subclass deficiency: Fact or fancy? Curr Allergy Asthma Rep *2*, 356–360.

Burgess, J.K., Lindeman, R., Chesterman, C.N., and Chong, B.H. (1995). Single amino acid mutation of Fc gamma receptor is associated with the development of heparin-induced thrombocytopenia. Br J Haematol *91*, 761–766.

Cambier, J., Daeron, M, Fridman, W, Gergely, J, Kinet, J-P, et al. (1994). New nomenclature for the Reth motif (or ARH1/TAM/ARAM/YXXL). Immunol Today *16*, 110.

Carlsson, L.E., Santoso, S., Baurichter, G., Kroll, H., Papenberg, S., Eichler, P., Westerdaal, N.A., Kiefel, V., van de Winkel, J.G., and Greinacher, A. (1998). Heparin-induced thrombocytopenia: New insights into the impact of the FcgammaRIIa-R-H131 polymorphism. Blood *92*, 1526–1531.

Cartron, G., Dacheux, L., Salles, G., Solal-Celigny, P., Bardos, P., Colombat, P., and Watier, H. (2002). Therapeutic activity of humanized anti-CD20 monoclonal antibody and polymorphism in IgG Fc receptor FcgammaRIIIa gene. Blood *99*, 754–758.

Cassel, D.L., Keller, M.A., Surrey, S., Schwartz, E., Schreiber, A.D., Rappaport, E.F., and McKenzie, S.E. (1993). Differential expression of Fc gamma RIIA, Fc gamma RIIB and Fc gamma RIIC in hematopoietic cells: Analysis of transcripts. Mol Immunol *30*, 451–460.

Chen, W., Palanisamy, N., Schmidt, H., Teruya-Feldstein, J., Jhanwar, S.C., Zelenetz, A.D., Houldsworth, J., and Chaganti, R.S. (2001). Deregulation of FCGR2B expression by 1q21 rearrangements in follicular lymphomas. Oncogene *20*, 7686–7693.

Chiamolera, M., Launay, P., Montenegro, V., Rivero, M.C., Velasco, I.T., and Monteiro, R.C. (2001). Enhanced expression of Fc alpha receptor I on blood phagocytes of patients with gram-negative bacteremia is associated with tyrosine phosphorylation of the FcR-gamma subunit. Shock *16*, 344–348.

Chiastiakov, D. A., and Chiastiakov, A. P. (2007). Is FcRL3 a new general autoimmunity gene? Hum Immunol *68*, 375–383.

Childers, N.K., Bruce, M.G., and McGhee, J.R. (1989). Molecular mechanisms of immunoglobulin A defense. Annu Rev Microbiol *43*, 503–536.

Clements, M.L., O'Donnell, S., Levine, M.M., Chanock, R.M., and Murphy, B.R. (1983). Dose response of A/Alaska/6/77 (H3N2) cold-adapted reassortant vaccine virus in adult volunteers: Role of local antibody in resistance to infection with vaccine virus. Infect Immun *40*, 1044–1051.

Corthesy, B., and Kraehenbuhl, J.P. (1999). Antibody-mediated protection of mucosal surfaces. Curr Top Microbiol Immunol *236*, 93–111.

Couch, R.B., and Kasel, J.A. (1983). Immunity to influenza in man. Annu Rev Microbiol *37*, 529–549.

Croker, J.A., and Kimberly, R.P. (2005). Genetics of susceptibility and severity in systemic lupus erythematosus. Curr Opin Rheumatol *17*, 529–537.

Cunningham-Rundles, C. (2001). Physiology of IgA and IgA deficiency. J Clin Immunol *21*, 303–309.

Daeron, M. (1997). Fc receptor biology. Annu Rev Immunol *15*, 203–234.

Dall'Ozzo, S., Tartas, S., Paintaud, G., Cartron, G., Colombat, P., Bardos, P., Watier, H., and Thibault, G. (2004). Rituximab-dependent cytotoxicity by natural killer cells: Influence of FCGR3A polymorphism on the concentration-effect relationship. Cancer Res *64*, 4664–4669.

Davis, R.S., Dennis, G., Jr., Kubagawa, H., and Cooper, M.D. (2002a). Fc receptor homologs (FcRH1-5) extend the Fc receptor family. Curr Top Microbiol Immunol *266*, 85–112.

Davis, R.S., Dennis, G., Jr., Odom, M.R., Gibson, A.W., Kimberly, R.P., Burrows, P.D., and Cooper, M.D. (2002b). Fc receptor homologs: Newest members of a remarkably diverse Fc receptor gene family. Immunol Rev *190*, 123–136.

Davis, R.S., Ehrhardt, G.R., Leu, C.M., Hirano, M., and Cooper, M.D. (2005). An extended family of Fc receptor relatives. Eur J Immunol *35*, 674–680.

Davis, R.S., Wang, Y.H., Kubagawa, H., and Cooper, M.D. (2001). Identification of a family of Fc receptor homologs with preferential B cell expression. Proc Natl Acad Sci USA *98*, 9772–9777.

Deo, Y.M., Graziano, R.F., Repp, R., and van de Winkel, J.G. (1997). Clinical significance of IgG Fc receptors and Fc gamma R-directed immunotherapies. Immunol Today 18, 127–135.

Domingo, P., Muniz-Diaz, E., Baraldes, M.A., Arilla, M., Barquet, N., Pericas, R., Juarez, C., Madoz, P., and Vazquez, G. (2002). Associations between Fc gamma receptor IIA polymorphisms and the risk and prognosis of meningococcal disease. Am J Med 112, 19–25.

Edberg, J.C., and Kimberly, R.P. (1994). Modulation of Fc gamma and complement receptor function by the glycosyl-phosphatidylinositol-anchored form of Fc gamma RIII. J Immunol 152, 5826–5835.

Edberg, J.C., and Kimberly, R.P. (1997). Cell type-specific glycoforms of Fc gamma RIIIa (CD16): Differential ligand binding. J Immunol 159, 3849–3857.

Edberg, J.C., Langefeld, C.D., Wu, J., Moser, K.L., Kaufman, K.M., Kelly, J., Bansal, V., Brown, W.M., Salmon, J.E., Rich, S.S., et al. (2002a). Genetic linkage and association of Fcgamma receptor IIIA (CD16A) on chromosome 1q23 with human systemic lupus erythematosus. Arthritis Rheum 46, 2132–2140.

Edberg, J.C., Qin, H., Gibson, A.W., Yee, A.M., Redecha, P.B., Indik, Z.K., Schreiber, A.D., and Kimberly, R.P. (2002b). The CY domain of the Fcgamma RIa alpha-chain (CD64) alters gamma-chain tyrosine-based signaling and phagocytosis. J Biol Chem 277, 41287–41293.

Edberg, J.C., Yee, A.M., Rakshit, D.S., Chang, D.J., Gokhale, J.A., Indik, Z.K., Schreiber, A.D., and Kimberly, R.P. (1999). The cytoplasmic domain of human FcgammaRIa alters the functional properties of the FcgammaRI,gamma-chain receptor complex. J Biol Chem 274, 30328–30333.

Ehrhardt, G.R., Davis, R.S., Hsu, J.T., Leu, C.M., Ehrhardt, A., and Cooper, M.D. (2003). The inhibitory potential of Fc receptor homolog 4 on memory B cells. Proc Natl Acad Sci USA 100, 13489–13494.

Fanciulli M., Norsworthy P.J., Petretto E., Dong R., Harper L., Kamesh L., Heward J.M., Gough S.C., de Smith A., Blakemore A.I., Froguel P., Owen C.J., Pearce S.H., Teixeira L., Guillevin L., Graham D.S., Pusey C.D., Cook H.T., Vyse T.J., Aitman T.J. (2007) FCGR3B copy number variation is associated with susceptibility to systemic, but not organ-specific, autoimmunity. Nat Genet 39, 721–723.

Fernandez, M.I., Pedron, T., Tournebize, R., Olivo-Marin, J.C., Sansonetti, P.J., and Phalipon, A. (2003). Anti-inflammatory role for intracellular dimeric immunoglobulin A by neutralization of lipopolysaccharide in epithelial cells. Immunity 18, 739–749.

Fijen, C.A., Bredius, R.G., and Kuijper, E.J. (1993). Polymorphism of IgG Fc receptors in meningococcal disease. Ann Intern Med 119, 636.

Furtado, P.B., Whitty, P.W., Robertson A., Eaton J.T., Almogren, A., Kerr, M.A., Woof, J.M., and Perkins, S.J. (2004). Solution structure determination of monomeric human IgA2 by X-ray and neutron scattering, analytical ultracentrifugation and constrained modelling: A comparison with monomeric human IgA1. J Mol Biol 338, 921–941.

Gonzalez-Escribano, M.F., Aguilar, F., Sanchez-Roman, J., and Nunez-Roldan, A. (2002). FcgammaRIIA, FcgammaRIIIA and FcgammaRIIIB polymorphisms in Spanish patients with systemic lupus erythematosus. Eur J Immunogenet 29, 301–306.

Gryboski, J.D., Self, T.W., Clemett, A., and Herskovic, T. (1968). Selective immunoglobulin A deficiency and intestinal nodular lymphoid hyperplasia: Correction of diarrhea with antibiotics and plasma. Pediatrics 42, 833–837.

Guselnikov, S.V., Ershova, S.A., Mechetina, L.V., Najakshin, A.M., Volkova, O.Y., Alabyev, B.Y., and Taranin, A.V. (2002). A family of highly diverse human and mouse genes structurally links leukocyte FcR, gp42 and PECAM-1. Immunogenetics 54, 87–95.

Hakimi, J., Seals, C., Kondas, J.A., Pettine, L., Danho, W., and Kochan, J. (1990). The alpha subunit of the human IgE receptor (FcERI) is sufficient for high affinity IgE binding. J Biol Chem 265, 22079–22081.

Haraoui, B. (2005). The anti-tumor necrosis factor agents are a major advance in the treatment of rheumatoid arthritis. J Rheumatol 72(suppl), 46–47.

Hatzivassiliou, G., Miller, I., Takizawa, J., Palanisamy, N., Rao, P.H., Iida, S., Tagawa, S., Taniwaki, M., Russo, J., Neri, A., et al. (2001). IRTA1 and IRTA2, novel immunoglobulin superfamily receptors expressed in B cells and involved in chromosome 1q21 abnormalities in B cell malignancy. Immunity 14, 277–289.

Heijnen, I.A., Rijks, L.J., Schiel, A., Stockmeyer, B., van Ojik, H.H., Dechant, M., Valerius, T., Keler, T., Tutt, A.L., Glennie, M.J., et al. (1997). Generation of HER-2/neu-specific cytotoxic neutrophils in vivo: Efficient arming of neutrophils by combined administration of granulocyte colony-stimulating factor and Fcgamma receptor I bispecific antibodies. J Immunol 159, 5629–5639.

Heijnen, I.A., and Van de Winkel, J.G. (1995). A human Fc gamma RI/CD64 transgenic model for in vivo analysis of (bispecific) antibody therapeutics. J Hematother 4, 351–356.

Hellwig, S.M., van Spriel, A.B., Schellekens, J.F., Mooi, F.R., and van de Winkel, J.G. (2001). Immunoglobulin A-mediated protection against *Bordetella pertussis* infection. Infect Immun 69, 4846–4850.

Heneghan, M.A., Stevens, F.M., Cryan, E.M., Warner, R.H., and McCarthy, C.F. (1997). Celiac sprue and immunodeficiency states: A 25-year review. J Clin Gastroenterol 25, 421–425.

Herberman, R.B. (2002). Cancer immunotherapy with natural killer cells. Semin Oncol 29, 27–30.

Hughes, L.B., Criswell, L.A., Beasley, T.M., Edberg, J.C., Kimberly, R.P., Moreland, L.W., Seldin, M.F., and Bridges, S.L. (2004). Genetic risk factors for infection in patients with early rheumatoid arthritis. Genes Immun 5, 641–647.

Huizinga, T.W., Kerst, M., Nuyens, J.H., Vlug, A., von dem Borne, A.E., Roos, D., and Tetteroo, P.A. (1989). Binding characteristics of dimeric IgG subclass complexes to human neutrophils. J Immunol 142, 2359–2364.

Huizinga, T.W., Kleijer, M., Tetteroo, P.A., Roos, D., and von dem Borne, A.E. (1990). Biallelic neutrophil Na-antigen system is associated with a polymorphism on the phospho-inositol-linked Fc gamma receptor III (CD16). Blood 75, 213–217.

Hulett, M.D., Osman, N., McKenzie, I.F., and Hogarth, P.M. (1991). Chimeric Fc receptors identify functional domains of the murine high affinity receptor for IgG. J Immunol 147, 1863–1868.

Johnson, P.R., Feldman, S., Thompson, J.M., Mahoney, J.D., and Wright, P.F. (1986). Immunity to influenza A virus infection in young children: A comparison of natural infection, live cold-adapted vaccine, and inactivated vaccine. J Infect Dis 154, 121–127.

Kaetzel, C.S., Robinson, J.K., Chintalacharuvu, K.R., Vaerman, J.P., and Lamm, M.E. (1991). The polymeric immunoglobulin receptor (secretory component) mediates transport of immune complexes across epithelial cells: A local defense function for IgA. Proc Natl Acad Sci USA 88, 8796–8800.

Kane, D., and FitzGerald, O. (2004). Tumor necrosis factor-alpha in psoriasis and psoriatic arthritis: A clinical, genetic, and histopathologic perspective. Curr Rheumatol Rep 6, 292–298.

Kaplan, M.H., and Volanakis, J.E. (1974). Interaction of C-reactive protein complexes with the complement system. I. Consumption of human complement associated with the reaction of C-reactive protein with pneumococcal C-polysaccharide and with the choline phosphatides, lecithin and sphingomyelin. J Immunol 112, 2135–2147.

Karassa, F.B., Trikalinos, T.A., and Ioannidis, J.P. (2002). Role of the Fcgamma receptor IIa polymorphism in susceptibility to systemic lupus erythematosus and lupus nephritis: A meta-analysis. Arthritis Rheum 46, 1563–1571.

Kawamura, S., Saitou, N., and Ueda, S. (1992). Concerted evolution of the primate immunoglobulin alpha-gene through gene conversion. J Biol Chem 267, 7359–7367.

Kawamura, S., Tanabe, H., Watanabe, Y., Kurosaki, K., Saitou, N., and Ueda, S. (1991). Evolutionary rate of immunoglobulin alpha noncoding region is greater in hominoids than in Old World monkeys. Mol Biol Evol 8, 743–752.

Kazkaz, H., and Isenberg, D. (2004). Anti B cell therapy (rituximab) in the treatment of autoimmune diseases. Curr Opin Pharmacol 4, 398–402.

Keler, T., Graziano, R.F., Mandal, A., Wallace, P.K., Fisher, J., Guyre, P.M., Fanger, M.W., and Deo, Y.M. (1997). Bispecific antibody-dependent cellular cytotoxicity of HER2/neu-overexpressing tumor cells by Fc gamma receptor type I-expressing effector cells. Cancer Res 57, 4008–4014.

Kent, W.J., Sugnet, C.W., Furey, T.S., Roskin, K.M., Pringle, T.H., Zahler, A.M., and Haussler, D. (2002). The human genome browser at UCSC. Genome Res 12, 996–1006.

Kimberly, R., Moreland, L.W., Gibson, A.W., Weinblatt, M.E., and Blosch, C. (1998). Susceptibility to infection may vary with TNF promoter genotype. Arthritis Rheum 41, S273.

Kimberly, R., Moreland, L.W., Wu, J., Edberg, J.C., Weinblatt, M.E., and Blosch, C. (1988). Occurrence of infection varies with Fc receptor genotype. Arthritis Rheum 41, S273.

Kimberly, R.P., Tappe, N.J., Merriam, L.T., Redecha, P.B., Edberg, J.C., Schwartzman, S., and Valinsky, J.E. (1989). Carbohydrates on human Fc gamma receptors. Interdependence of the classical IgG and nonclassical lectin-binding sites on human Fc gamma RIII expressed on neutrophils. J Immunol 142, 3923–3930.

Kimberly, R.P., Wu, J., Gibson, A.W., Su, K., Qin, H., Li, X., and Edberg, J.C. (2002). Diversity and duplicity: Human FCgamma receptors in host defense and autoimmunity. Immunol Res 26, 177–189.

Kobayashi, T., Ito, S., Yamamoto, K., Hasegawa, H., Sugita, N., Kuroda, T., Kaneko, S., Narita, I., Yasuda, K., Nakano, M., et al. (2003). Risk of periodontitis in systemic lupus erythematosus is associated with Fcgamma receptor polymorphisms. J Periodontol 74, 378–384.

Kobayashi, T., Yamamoto, K., Sugita, N., van der Pol, W.L., Yasuda, K., Kaneko, S., van de Winkel, J.G., and Yoshie, H. (2001). The Fc gamma receptor genotype as a severity factor for chronic periodontitis in Japanese patients. J Periodontol 72, 1324–1331.

Kochi, Y., Yamada, R., Suzuki, A., Harley, J.B., Shirasawa, S., Sawada, T., Bae, S.C., Tokuhiro, S.,

Chang, X., Sekine, A., et al. (2005). A functional variant in FCRL3, encoding Fc receptor-like 3, is associated with rheumatoid arthritis and several autoimmunities. Nat Genet 37, 478–485.

Koene, H.R., Kleijer, M., Algra, J., Roos, D., von dem Borne, A.E., and de Haas, M. (1997). Fc gamma-RIIIa-158V/F polymorphism influences the binding of IgG by natural killer cell Fc gammaRIIIa, independently of the Fc gammaRIIIa-48L/R/H phenotype. Blood 90, 1109–1114.

Koene, H.R., Kleijer, M., Swaak, A.J., Sullivan, K.E., Bijl, M., Petri, M.A., Kallenberg, C.G., Roos, D., von dem Borne, A.E., and de Haas, M. (1998). The Fc gammaRIIIA-158F allele is a risk factor for systemic lupus erythematosus. Arthritis Rheum 41, 1813–1818.

Kurosaki, T., and Ravetch, J.V. (1989). A single amino acid in the glycosyl phosphatidylinositol attachment domain determines the membrane topology of Fc gamma RIII. Nature 342, 805–807.

Kyogoku, C., Dijstelbloem, H.M., Tsuchiya, N., Hatta, Y., Kato, H., Yamaguchi, A., Fukazawa, T., Jansen, M.D., Hashimoto, H., van de Winkel, J.G., et al. (2002a). Fcgamma receptor gene polymorphisms in Japanese patients with systemic lupus erythematosus: Contribution of FCGR2B to genetic susceptibility. Arthritis Rheum 46, 1242–1254.

Kyogoku, C., Tsuchiya, N., Matsuta, K., and Tokunaga, K. (2002b). Studies on the association of Fc gamma receptor IIA, IIB, IIIA and IIIB polymorphisms with rheumatoid arthritis in the Japanese: Evidence for a genetic interaction between HLA-DRB1 and FCGR3A. Genes Immun 3, 488–493.

Lamm, M.E. (1997). Interaction of antigens and antibodies at mucosal surfaces. Annu Rev Microbiol 51, 311–340.

Lee, E.B., Lee, Y.J., Baek, H.J., Kang, S.W., Chung, E.S., Shin, C.H., Hong, K.M., Tsao, B.P., Hahn, B.H., and Song, Y.W. (2002). Fcgamma receptor IIIA polymorphism in Korean patients with systemic lupus erythematosus. Rheumatol Int 21, 222–226.

Lehrnbecher, T., Foster, C., Vazquez, N., Mackall, C.L., and Chanock, S.J. (1997). Therapy-induced alterations in host defense in children receiving therapy for cancer. J Pediatr Hematol Oncol 19, 399–417.

Lei, B., DeLeo, F.R., Hoe, N.P., Graham, M.R., Mackie, S.M., Cole, R.L., Liu, M., Hill, H.R., Low, D.E., Federle, M.J., et al. (2001). Evasion of human innate and acquired immunity by a bacterial homolog of CD11b that inhibits opsonophagocytosis. Nat Med 7, 1298–1305.

Lencer, W.I., and Blumberg, R.S. (2005). A passionate kiss, then run: Exocytosis and recycling of IgG by FcRn. Trends Cell Biol 15, 5–9.

Leu, C.M., Davis, R.S., Gartland, L.A., Fine, W.D., and Cooper, M.D. (2005). FcRH1: An activation coreceptor on human B cells. Blood 105, 1121–1126.

Li, X., Wu, J., Carter, R.H., Edberg, J.C., Su, K., Cooper, G.S., and Kimberly, R.P. (2003). A novel polymorphism in the Fcgamma receptor IIB (CD32B) transmembrane region alters receptor signaling. Arthritis Rheum 48, 3242–3252.

Looney, R.J., Anolik, J.H., Campbell, D., Felgar, R.E., Young, F., Arend, L.J., Sloand, J.A., Rosenblatt, J., and Sanz, I. (2004). B cell depletion as a novel treatment for systemic lupus erythematosus: A phase I/II dose-escalation trial of rituximab. Arthritis Rheum 50, 2580–2589.

Loos, B.G., Leppers-Van de Straat, F.G., Van de Winkel, J.G., and Van der Velden, U. (2003). Fcgamma receptor polymorphisms in relation to periodontitis. J Clin Periodontol 30, 595–602.

Louis, E., El Ghoul, Z., Vermeire, S., Dall'Ozzo, S., Rutgeerts, P., Paintaud, G., Belaiche, J., De Vos, M., Van Gossum, A., Colombel, J.F., and Watier, H. (2004). Association between polymorphism in IgG Fc receptor IIIa coding gene and biological response to infliximab in Crohn's disease. Aliment Pharmacol Ther 19, 511–519.

Luton, F., and Mostov, K.E. (1999). Transduction of basolateral-to-apical signals across epithelial cells: Ligand-stimulated transcytosis of the polymeric immunoglobulin receptor requires two signals. Mol Biol Cell 10, 1409–1427.

Maguire, G.A., Kumararatne, D.S., and Joyce, H.J. (2002). Are there any clinical indications for measuring IgG subclasses? Ann Clin Biochem 39, 374–377.

Maliszewski, C.R., March, C.J., Schoenborn, M.A., Gimpel, S., and Shen, L. (1990). Expression cloning of a human Fc receptor for IgA. J Exp Med 172, 1665–1672.

Manger, K., Repp, R., Jansen, M., Geisselbrecht, M., Wassmuth, R., Westerdaal, N.A., Pfahlberg, A., Manger, B., Kalden, J.R., and van de Winkel, J.G. (2002). Fcgamma receptor IIa, IIIa, and IIIb polymorphisms in German patients with systemic lupus erythematosus: Association with clinical symptoms. Ann Rheum Dis 61, 786–792.

Manser, T. (2004). Textbook germinal centers? J Immunol 172, 3369–3375.

Marnell, L.L., Mold, C., Volzer, M.A., Burlingame, R.W., and Du Clos, T.W. (1995). C-reactive protein binds to Fc gamma RI in transfected COS cells. J Immunol 155, 2185–2193.

McDonald, K.J., Cameron, A.J., Allen, J.M., and Jardine, A.G. (2002). Expression of Fc alpha/mu receptor by human mesangial cells: A candidate receptor for immune complex deposition in IgA nephropathy. Biochem Biophys Res Commun 290, 438–442.

Mechetina, L.V., Najakshin, A.M., Volkova, O.Y., Guselnikov, S.V., Faizulin, R.Z., Alabyev, B.Y., Chikaev, N.A., Vinogradova, M.S., and Taranin, A.V. (2002). FCRL, a novel member of the leukocyte Fc receptor family possesses unique structural features. Eur J Immunol 32, 87–96.

Meisel, P., Carlsson, L.E., Sawaf, H., Fanghaenel, J., Greinacher, A., and Kocher, T. (2001). Polymorphisms of Fc gamma-receptors RIIa, RIIIa, and RIIIb in patients with adult periodontal diseases. Genes Immun 2, 258–262.

Miller, I., Hatzivassiliou, G., Cattoretti, G., Mendelsohn, C., and Dalla-Favera, R. (2002). IRTAs: A new family of immunoglobulinlike receptors differentially expressed in B cells. Blood 99, 2662–2669.

Monteiro, R.C., and Van De Winkel, J.G. (2003). IgA Fc receptors. Annu Rev Immunol 21, 177–204.

Morton, H.C., Schiel, A.E., Janssen, S.W., and van de Winkel, J.G. (1996). Alternatively spliced forms of the human myeloid Fc alpha receptor (CD89) in neutrophils. Immunogenetics 43, 246–247.

Mostov, K.E., Kraehenbuhl, J.P., and Blobel, G. (1980). Receptor-mediated transcellular transport of immunoglobulin: Synthesis of secretory component as multiple and larger transmembrane forms. Proc Natl Acad Sci USA 77, 7257–7261.

Mota, G., Manciulea, M., Cosma, E., Popescu, I., Hirt, M., Jensen-Jarolim, E., Calugaru, A., Galatiuc, C., Regalia, T., Tamandl, D., et al. (2003). Human NK cells express Fc receptors for IgA which mediate signal transduction and target cell killing. Eur J Immunol 33, 2197–2205.

Murphy, B.R., and Clements, M.L. (1989). The systemic and mucosal immune response of humans to influenza A virus. Curr Top Microbiol Immunol 146, 107–116.

Nakayama, Y., Weissman, S.M., and Bothwell, A.L. (2001). BXMAS1 identifies a cluster of homologous genes differentially expressed in B cells. Biochem Biophys Res Commun 285, 830–837.

Oakey, R.J., Howard, T.A., Hogarth, P.M., Tani, K., and Seldin, M.F. (1992). Chromosomal mapping of the high affinity Fc gamma receptor gene. Immunogenetics 35, 279–282.

Ober, R.J., Martinez, C., Lai, X., Zhou, J., and Ward, E.S. (2004a). Exocytosis of IgG as mediated by the receptor, FcRn: An analysis at the single-molecule level. Proc Natl Acad Sci USA 101, 11076–11081.

Ober, R.J., Martinez, C., Vaccaro, C., Zhou, J., and Ward, E.S. (2004b). Visualizing the site and dynamics of IgG salvage by the MHC class I-related receptor, FcRn. J Immunol 172, 2021–2029.

Ono, M., Bolland, S., Tempst, P., and Ravetch, J.V. (1996). Role of the inositol phosphatase SHIP in negative regulation of the immune system by the receptor Fc(gamma)RIIB. Nature 383, 263–266.

Ono, M., Okada, H., Bolland, S., Yanagi, S., Kurosaki, T., and Ravetch, J.V. (1997). Deletion of SHIP or SHP-1 reveals two distinct pathways for inhibitory signaling. Cell 90, 293–301.

Otten, M.A., and van Egmond, M. (2004). The Fc receptor for IgA (FcalphaRI, CD89). Immunol Lett 92, 23–31.

Pan, Q., and Hammarstrom, L. (2000). Molecular basis of IgG subclass deficiency. Immunol Rev 178, 99–110.

Pan, Q., Lindersson, Y., Sideras, P., and Hammarstrom, L. (1997). Structural analysis of human gamma 3 intervening regions and switch regions: implication for the low frequency of switching in IgG3-deficient patients. Eur J Immunol 27, 2920–2926.

Park, J.G., Murray, R.K., Chien, P., Darby, C., and Schreiber, A.D. (1993). Conserved cytoplasmic tyrosine residues of the gamma subunit are required for a phagocytic signal mediated by Fc gamma RIIIA. J Clin Invest 92, 2073–2079.

Parren, P.W., Warmerdam, P.A., Boeije, L.C., Arts, J., Westerdaal, N.A., Vlug, A., Capel, P.J., Aarden, L.A., and van de Winkel, J.G. (1992). On the interaction of IgG subclasses with the low affinity Fc gamma RIIa (CD32) on human monocytes, neutrophils, and platelets. Analysis of a functional polymorphism to human IgG2. J Clin Invest 90, 1537–1546.

Phalipon, A., Cardona, A., Kraehenbuhl, J.P., Edelman, L., Sansonetti, P.J., and Corthesy, B. (2002). Secretory component: A new role in secretory IgA-mediated immune exclusion in vivo. Immunity 17, 107–115.

Phalipon, A., and Corthesy, B. (2003). Novel functions of the polymeric Ig receptor: well beyond transport of immunoglobulins. Trends Immunol 24, 55–58.

Platonov, A.E., Shipulin, G.A., Vershinina, I.V., Dankert, J., van de Winkel, J.G., and Kuijper, E.J. (1998). Association of human Fc gamma RIIa (CD32) polymorphism with susceptibility to and severity of meningococcal disease. Clin Infect Dis 27, 746–750.

Plaut, A.G., Gilbert, J.V., and Wistar, R., Jr. (1977). Loss of antibody activity in human immunoglobulin A exposed extracellular immunoglobulin A proteases of Neisseria gonorrhoeae and Streptococcus sanguis. Infect Immun 17, 130–135.

Pleass, R.J., Andrews, P.D., Kerr, M.A., and Woof, J.M. (1996). Alternative splicing of the human IgA Fc receptor CD89 in neutrophils and eosinophils. Biochem J 318(pt 3), 771–777.

Pullarkat, V., Deo, Y., Link, J., Spears, L., Marty, V., Curnow, R., Groshen, S., Gee, C., and Weber, J.S. (1999). A phase I study of a HER2/neu bispecific antibody with granulocyte-colony-stimulating factor in patients with metastatic breast cancer that over-expresses HER2/neu. Cancer Immunol Immunother 48, 9–21.

Qin, D., Wu, J., Vora, K.A., Ravetch, J.V., Szakal, A.K., Manser, T., and Tew, J.G. (2000). Fc gamma receptor IIB on follicular dendritic cells regulates the B cell recall response. J Immunol 164, 6268–6275.

Qiu, W.Q., de Bruin, D., Brownstein, B.H., Pearse, R., and Ravetch, J.V. (1990). Organization of the human and mouse low-affinity Fc gamma R genes: Duplication and recombination. Science 248, 732–735.

Raghavan, M., and Bjorkman, P.J. (1996). Fc receptors and their interactions with immunoglobulins. Annu Rev Cell Dev Biol 12, 181–220.

Ravetch, J.V., and Bolland, S. (2001). IgG Fc receptors. Annu Rev Immunol 19, 275–290.

Ravetch, J.V., and Kinet, J.P. (1991). Fc receptors. Annu Rev Immunol 9, 457–492.

Repetto, B., Bandara, G., Kado-Fong, H., Larigan, J.D., Wiggan, G.A., Pocius, D., Basu, M., Gilfillan, A.M., and Kochan, J.P. (1996). Functional contributions of the FcepsilonRIalpha and FepsilonRIgamma sub-unit domains in FcepsilonRI-mediated signaling in mast cells. J Immunol 156, 4876–4883.

Reterink, T.J., Verweij, C.L., van Es, L.A., and Daha, M.R. (1996). Alternative splicing of IgA Fc receptor (CD89) transcripts. Gene 175, 279–280.

Robinson, J.K., Blanchard, T.G., Levine, A.D., Emancipator, S.N., and Lamm, M.E. (2001). A mucosal IgA-mediated excretory immune system in vivo. J Immunol 166, 3688–3692.

Rodewald, R., and Kraehenbuhl, J.P. (1984). Receptor-mediated transport of IgG. J Cell Biol 99, 159s–164s.

Romagnani, S., Giudizi, M.G., Biagiotti, R., Almerigogna, F., Maggi, E., Del Prete, G., and Ricci, M. (1981). Surface immunoglobulins are involved in the interaction of protein A with human B cells and in the triggering of B cell proliferation induced by protein A-containing Staphylococcus aureus. J Immunol 127, 1307–1313.

Rosenwald, A., Alizadeh, A.A., Widhopf, G., Simon, R., Davis, R.E., Yu, X., Yang, L., Pickeral, O.K., Rassenti, L.Z., Powell, J., et al. (2001). Relation of gene expression phenotype to immunoglobulin mutation genotype in B cell chronic lymphocytic leukemia. J Exp Med 194, 1639–1647.

Rosenwald, A., Wright, G., Wiestner, A., Chan, W.C., Connors, J.M., Campo, E., Gascoyne, R.D., Grogan, T.M., Muller-Hermelink, H.K., Smeland, E.B., et al. (2003). The proliferation gene expression sig-

nature is a quantitative integrator of oncogenic events that predicts survival in mantle cell lymphoma. Cancer Cell 3, 185–197.

Saini, R., Tutrone, W.D., and Weinberg, J.M. (2005). Advances in therapy for psoriasis: An overview of infliximab, etanercept, efalizumab, alefacept, adalimumab, tazarotene, and pimecrolimus. Curr Pharm Des 11, 273–280.

Salmon, J.E., Edberg, J.C., Brogle, N.L., and Kimberly, R.P. (1992). Allelic polymorphisms of human Fc gamma receptor IIA and Fc gamma receptor IIIB. Independent mechanisms for differences in human phagocyte function. J Clin Invest 89, 1274–1281.

Salmon, J.E., Edberg, J.C., and Kimberly, R.P. (1990). Fc gamma receptor III on human neutrophils. Allelic variants have functionally distinct capacities. J Clin Invest 85, 1287–1295.

Salmon, J.E., Millard, S., Schachter, L.A., Arnett, F.C., Ginzler, E.M., Gourley, M.F., Ramsey-Goldman, R., Peterson, M.G., and Kimberly, R.P. (1996). Fc gamma RIIA alleles are heritable risk factors for lupus nephritis in African Americans. J Clin Invest 97, 1348–1354.

Salmon, J.E., and Pricop, L. (2001). Human receptors for immunoglobulin G: key elements in the pathogenesis of rheumatic disease. Arthritis Rheum 44, 739–750.

Sanchez, A., Ksiazek, T.G., Rollin, P.E., Miranda, M.E., Trappier, S.G., Khan, A.S., Peters, C.J., and Nichol, S.T. (1999). Detection and molecular characterization of Ebola viruses causing disease in human and nonhuman primates. J Infect Dis 179(suppl 1), S164–169.

Sanders, L.A., van de Winkel, J.G., Rijkers, G.T., Voorhorst-Ogink, M.M., de Haas, M., Capel, P.J., and Zegers, B.J. (1994). Fc gamma receptor IIa (CD32) heterogeneity in patients with recurrent bacterial respiratory tract infections. J Infect Dis 170, 854–861.

Schaffer, F.M., Monteiro, R.C., Volanakis, J.E., and Cooper, M.D. (1991). IgA deficiency. Immunodefic Rev 3, 15–44.

Senior, B., Loomes, L.M., and Kerr, M.A. (1991). Microbial IgA proteases and virulence. Rev Med Microbiol 2, 200–207.

Shibuya, A., Sakamoto, N., Shimizu, Y., Shibuya, K., Osawa, M., Hiroyama, T., Eyre, H.J., Sutherland, G.R., Endo, Y., Fujita, T., et al. (2000). Fc alpha/mu receptor mediates endocytosis of IgM-coated microbes. Nat Immunol 1, 441–446.

Simister, N.E., and Ahouse, J.C. (1996). The structure and evolution of FcRn. Res Immunol 147, 333–337; discussion 353.

Siriboonrit, U., Tsuchiya, N., Sirikong, M., Kyogoku, C., Bejrachandra, S., Suthipinittharm, P., Luangtrakool,

K., Srinak, D., Thongpradit, R., Fujiwara, K., et al. (2003). Association of Fcgamma receptor IIb and IIIb polymorphisms with susceptibility to systemic lupus erythematosus in Thais. Tissue Antigens 61, 374–383.

Soderstrom, T., Soderstrom, R., Avanzini, A., Brandtzaeg, P., Karlsson, G., and Hanson, L.A. (1987). Immunoglobulin G subclass deficiencies. Int Arch Allergy Appl Immunol 82, 476–480.

Sondermann, P., Huber, R., Oosthuizen, V., and Jacob, U. (2000). The 3.2-A crystal structure of the human IgG1 Fc fragment-Fc gammaRIII complex. Nature 406, 267–273.

Stanley, P.J., Corbo, G., and Cole, P.J. (1984). Serum IgG subclasses in chronic and recurrent respiratory infections. Clin Exp Immunol 58, 703–708.

Stein, M.P., Edberg, J.C., Kimberly, R.P., Mangan, E.K., Bharadwaj, D., Mold, C., and Du Clos, T.W. (2000a). C-reactive protein binding to FcgammaRIIa on human monocytes and neutrophils is allele-specific. J Clin Invest 105, 369–376.

Stein, M.P., Mold, C., and Du Clos, T.W. (2000b). C-reactive protein binding to murine leukocytes requires Fc gamma receptors. J Immunol 164, 1514–1520.

Strober, W., and Sneller, M.C. (1991). IgA deficiency. Ann Allergy 66, 363–375.

Su, K., Li, X., Edberg, J.C., Wu, J., Ferguson, P., and Kimberly, R.P. (2004). A promoter haplotype of the immunoreceptor tyrosine-based inhibitory motif-bearing FcgammaRIIb alters receptor expression and associates with autoimmunity. II. Differential binding of GATA4 and Yin-Yang1 transcription factors and correlated receptor expression and function. J Immunol 172, 7192–7199.

Su, K., Wu, J., Edberg, J.C., McKenzie, S.E., and Kimberly, R.P. (2002). Genomic organization of classical human low-affinity Fcgamma receptor genes. Genes Immun 3(suppl 1), S51–56.

Sun, K., Johansen, F.E., Eckmann, L., and Metzger, D.W. (2004). An important role for polymeric Ig receptor-mediated transport of IgA in protection against Streptococcus pneumoniae nasopharyngeal carriage. J Immunol 173, 4576–4581.

Traicoff, J.L., De Marchis, L., Ginsburg, B.L., Zamora, R.E., Khattar, N.H., Blanch, V.J., Plummer, S., Bargo, S.A., Templeton, D.J., Casey, G., and Kaetzel, C.S. (2003). Characterization of the human polymeric immunoglobulin receptor (PIGR) 3'UTR and differential expression of PIGR mRNA during colon tumorigenesis. J Biomed Sci 10, 792–804.

Tridandapani, S., Kelley, T., Pradhan, M., Cooney, D., Justement, L.B., and Coggeshall, K.M. (1997). Recruitment and phosphorylation of SH2-containing inositol phosphatase and Shc to the B-cell Fc gamma immunoreceptor tyrosine-based inhibition motif peptide motif. Mol Cell Biol 17, 4305–4311.

Uren, T.K., Wijburg, O.L., Simmons, C., Johansen, F.E., Brandtzaeg, P., and Strugnell, R.A. (2005). Vaccine-induced protection against gastrointestinal bacterial infections in the absence of secretory antibodies. Eur J Immunol 35, 180–188.

Vance, B.A., Huizinga, T.W., Wardwell, K., and Guyre, P.M. (1993). Binding of monomeric human IgG defines an expression polymorphism of Fc gamma RIII on large granular lymphocyte/natural killer cells. J Immunol 151, 6429–6439.

van der Pol, W., Vidarsson, G., Vile, H.A., van de Winkel, J.G., and Rodriguez, M.E. (2000). Pneumococcal capsular polysaccharide-specific IgA triggers efficient neutrophil effector functions via FcalphaRI (CD89). J Infect Dis 182, 1139–1145.

van Dijk, M.A., and van de Winkel, J.G. (2001). Human antibodies as next generation therapeutics. Curr Opin Chem Biol 5, 368–374.

van Dijk, T.B., Bracke, M., Caldenhoven, E., Raaijmakers, J.A., Lammers, J.W., Koenderman, L., and de Groot, R.P. (1996). Cloning and characterization of Fc alpha Rb, a novel Fc alpha receptor (CD89) isoform expressed in eosinophils and neutrophils. Blood 88, 4229–4238.

van Egmond, M., Damen, C.A., van Spriel, A.B., Vidarsson, G., van Garderen, E., and van de Winkel, J.G. (2001). IgA and the IgA Fc receptor. Trends Immunol 22, 205–211.

van Sorge, N.M., van der Pol, W.L., and van de Winkel, J.G. (2003). FcgammaR polymorphisms: Implications for function, disease susceptibility and immunotherapy. Tissue Antigens 61, 189–202.

Warmerdam, P.A., van de Winkel, J.G., Vlug, A., Westerdaal, N.A., and Capel, P.J. (1991). A single amino acid in the second Ig-like domain of the human Fc gamma receptor II is critical for human IgG2 binding. J Immunol 147, 1338–1343.

Weinberg, J.M. (2003). An overview of infliximab, etanercept, efalizumab, and alefacept as biologic therapy for psoriasis. Clin Ther 25, 2487–2505.

Weiser, J.N., Pan, N., McGowan, K.L., Musher, D., Martin, A., and Richards, J. (1998). Phosphorylcholine on the lipopolysaccharide of Haemophilus influenzae contributes to persistence in the respiratory tract and sensitivity to serum killing mediated by C-reactive protein. J Exp Med 187, 631–640.

Wiestner, A., Rosenwald, A., Barry, T.S., Wright, G., Davis, R.E., Henrickson, S.E., Zhao, H., Ibbotson, R.E., Orchard, J.A., Davis, Z., et al. (2003). ZAP-70 expression identifies a chronic lymphocytic leukemia subtype with unmutated immunoglobulin genes, inferior clinical outcome, and distinct gene expression profile. Blood *101*, 4944–4951.

Wirthmueller, U., Kurosaki, T., Murakami, M.S., and Ravetch, J.V. (1992). Signal transduction by Fc gamma RIII (CD16) is mediated through the gamma chain. J Exp Med *175*, 1381–1390.

Withoff, S., Helfrich, W., de Leij, L.F., and Molema, G. (2001). Bi-specific antibody therapy for the treatment of cancer. Curr Opin Mol Ther *3*, 53–62.

Woof, J.M., and Kerr, M.A. (2004). IgA function—variations on a theme. Immunology *113*, 175–177.

Wu, J., Edberg, J.C., Redecha, P.B., Bansal, V., Guyre, P.M., Coleman, K., Salmon, J.E., and Kimberly, R.P. (1997). A novel polymorphism of FcgammaRIIIa (CD16) alters receptor function and predisposes to autoimmune disease. J Clin Invest *100*, 1059–1070.

Yamamoto, K., Kobayashi, T., Grossi, S., Ho, A.W., Genco, R.J., Yoshie, H., and De Nardin, E. (2004). Association of Fcgamma receptor IIa genotype with chronic periodontitis in Caucasians. J Periodontol *75*, 517–522.

Yasuda, K., Sugita, N., Kobayashi, T., Yamamoto, K., and Yoshie, H. (2003). FcgammaRIIB gene polymorphisms in Japanese periodontitis patients. Genes Immun *4*, 541–546.

Yee, A.M., Ng, S.C., Sobel, R.E., and Salmon, J.E. (1997). Fc gammaRIIA polymorphism as a risk factor for invasive pneumococcal infections in systemic lupus erythematosus. Arthritis Rheum *40*, 1180–1182.

Yee, A.M., Phan, H.M., Zuniga, R., Salmon, J.E., and Musher, D.M. (2000). Association between FcgammaRIIa-R131 allotype and bacteremic pneumococcal pneumonia. Clin Infect Dis *30*, 25–28.

Yoshida, K., van den Berg, T.K., and Dijkstra, C.D. (1993). Two functionally different follicular dendritic cells in secondary lymphoid follicles of mouse spleen, as revealed by CR1/2 and FcR gamma II-mediated immune-complex trapping. Immunology *80*, 34–39.

Yount, W.J., Seligmann, M., Hong, R., Good, R., and Kunkel, H.G. (1970). Imbalances of gamma globulin subgroups and gene defects in patients with primary hypogammaglobulinemia. J Clin Invest *49*, 1957–1966.

Yuan, F.F., Watson, N., Sullivan, J.S., Biffin, S., Moses, J., Geczy, A.F., and Chapman, J.R. (2004). Association of Fc gamma receptor IIA polymorphisms with acute renal-allograft rejection. Transplantation *78*, 766–769.

Zuniga, R., Ng, S., Peterson, M.G., Reveille, J.D., Baethge, B.A., Alarcon, G.S., and Salmon, J.E. (2001). Low-binding alleles of Fcgamma receptor types IIA and IIIA are inherited independently and are associated with systemic lupus erythematosus in Hispanic patients. Arthritis Rheum *44*, 361–367.

10

Mannose-Binding Lectin Genes

Richard Bellamy

Product in Infection: Structure and Function of the MBL Protein

Mannose-binding lectin (MBL) is an important component of the innate immune system. MBL belongs to the family of proteins called collectins, which contain both collagen-like domains and C-type lectin domains. The human collectin family includes MBL and lung surfactant proteins A and D (Holmskov et al., 1994; Lu, 1997; Lu et al., 2002).

The MBL gene (table 10.1) product contains 248 amino acids, organized in four domains. The first domain is a cysteine-rich, N-terminal region. Adjacent to this is a long collagen-like domain, which is followed by a short α-helical neck region. The fourth domain is a C-terminal C-type lectin (Sastry et al., 1989; Taylor et al., 1989). Each peptide chain is around 32 kDa. The MBL protein contains three of these identical peptide chains, where the collagen-like domains are coiled to form a triple helix (Weis and Drickamer, 1994). The three lectin domains of each homotrimeric molecule give MBL a large globular head, which serves as the carbohydrate recognition domain. The three lectin domains form a flat platform with a constant distance between the carbohydrate-binding sites of 45 Å in humans (Sheriff et al., 1994). This platform facilitates binding to the 3- and 4-hydroxyl groups of *N*-acetyl glucosamine, mannose, *N*-acetyl mannosamine, fucose and glucose. D-Galactose does not bind effectively (Weis et al., 1992; Drickamer, 1992).

The homotrimeric subunits of MBL form larger oligomers via disulfide bonds between the N-terminal domains. This gives MBL a bouquet-like structure similar to C1q (Kawasaki, 1999). In plasma, MBL occurs as a mixture of dimers (i.e., consisting of two molecules of the homotrimeric subunit), trimers, tetramers, and other higher oligomers (Lu et al., 1990; Lipscombe et al., 1995; Garred et al., 2003a). The repetitive carbohydrate structures found on microorganisms can bind to high-molecular-weight MBL with high avidity because of the large number of lectin–carbohydrate interactions. Simultaneous binding to

TABLE 10.1 *MBL2* gene summary.

Gene ID (NCBI)	Common Name(s)	Entrez Gene ID (Locus Link)	Map Position	Notes on Important SNPs, Indels, Truncations (Region, Reference Sequence [rs] Number)	References
MBL2	Mannose-binding lectin Mannose-binding protein Mannan-binding protein	(4153)	10q11.2	Coding changes at amino acids 52, 54, 57 Functional promoter polymorphisms	Sumiya et al. (1991) Lipscombe et al. (1992) Madsen et al. (1994, 1995, 1998a)

multiple sites is required because each individual MBL–sugar interaction is relatively weak (Iobst et al., 1994).

MBL has four distinct functions (Turner, 2003): (1) activation of complement via a third pathway independent of the classical and alternative pathways (figure 10.1); (2) direct promotion of opsonophagocytosis, independent of complement activation; (3) modulation of the inflammatory response; and (4) promotion of apoptosis.

In human plasma, MBL is found in association with four structurally related proteins: MASP-1, MASP-2, MASP-3 (the MBL-associated proteases), and MAp19 (a truncated version of MASP-2) (Matsushita and Fujita, 1992; Thiel et al., 1997; Stover et al., 1999;

Takahashi et al., 1999; Dahl et al., 2000). MASP-2 is believed to be the most important for complement activation (Thiel et al., 1997). The MBL-MASP-2 complex becomes activated when bound to the sugar-coated surface of microorganisms (Thiel et al., 2000). Activated MBL-MASP-2 cleaves C4 and C2, and the resultant C4b2a complex cleaves C3 and activates the complement cascade (Ikeda et al., 1987). Only the high-molecular-weight forms of MBL (made up of higher order oligomers) are able to bind mannan effectively and active complement (Yokota et al., 1995; Garred et al., 2003a).

The possibility that MBL could bind to cell-surface receptors and promote opsonophagocytosis was first suggested by Kuhlmann et al. (1989). A number of re-

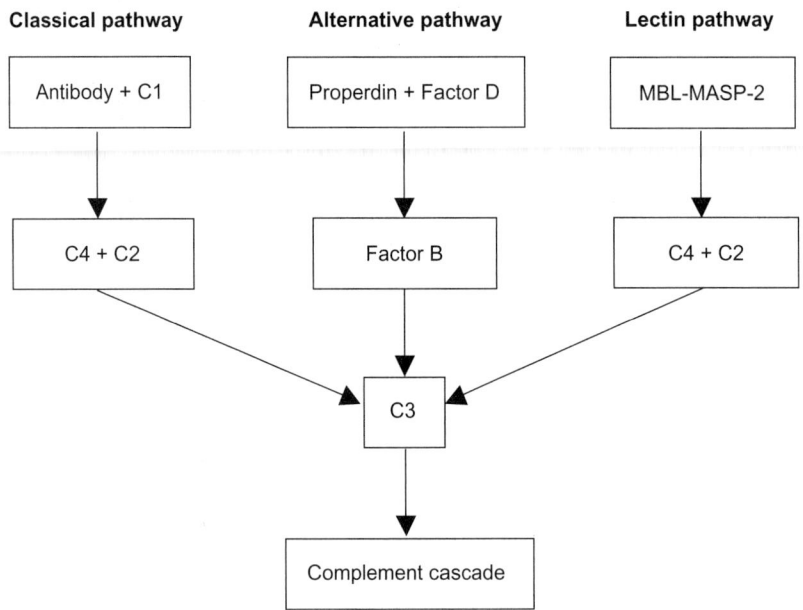

FIGURE 10.1. Complement activation via the classical, alternative, and lectin pathways. MBL-MASP-2 can activate the complement cascade independently of C1q.

ceptors have been suggested as mediators of opsono-phagocytosis, including cC1qR (calreticulin) (Malhotra et al., 1990), C1qR$_p$ (Tenner et al., 1995), and CR1 (Ghiran et al., 2000). However, it remains controversial whether MBL is directly acting as an opsonin or whether it is promoting complement or antibody-mediated phagocytosis (Jack et al., 2001a).

MBL may also play a role in the regulation of the inflammatory response (Turner, 2003). Jack et al. (2001b) found that high MBL concentrations inhibit the release of tumor necrosis factor-α, interleukin 1β, and interleukin-6 from monocytes cultured with Neisseria meningitidis. This finding may explain some of the associations observed between MBL genotypes and the severity of autoimmune diseases.

It has also been suggested that MBL can bind to apoptotic T cells and stimulate macropinocytosis by mononuclear phagocytes (Ogden et al., 2001). This process is said to require the collagenous region of MBL to interact with CD91 (the α$_2$-macroglobulin receptor) and cC1qR on the surface of the mononuclear cell (Ogden et al., 2001).

The serum MBL concentration is normally greater than 1 μg/ml, but there is a substantial minority of the population with a much lower level (Garred et al., 2003a). MBL is an acute phase reactant, but plasma protein levels only rise 2- to 3-fold during the acute phase response (Thiel et al., 1992). Therefore for the majority of the population variation in circulating MBL reflects inherited rather than acquired differences.

Pathogenesis of MBL Deficiency

Low serum MBL has been described as the world's commonest immune deficiency (Thompson 1995). The first clearly documented case of MBL deficiency was described in 1968 (Miller et al., 1968). During the first two years of her life, a young girl had experienced severe dermatitis, persistent diarrhea, and recurrent upper respiratory tract infections. Antibiotic and steroid therapy had been of little benefit. The patient did not have an identifiable immunoglobulin defect. However, when polymorphonuclear leukocytes from human donors were incubated with the patient's serum, they were unable to phagocytose heat-killed yeast particles from Saccharomyces cerevisiae (baker's yeast) efficiently. In contrast, when the patient's polymorphonuclear leukocytes were incubated with autologous

serum, they were able to phagocytose efficiently. This indicated that the girl had an opsonic defect due to deficiency of some component of her serum. A similar phagocytic defect was identified in the patient's mother and several other adult relatives, who were apparently healthy. The familial nature of the defect suggested that it was inherited. The girl was treated with plasma infusions, and her condition improved (Miller et al., 1968).

During the next 20 years, this opsonic defect was described in association with recurrent respiratory tract infections, persistent diarrhea, atopy, and failure to thrive (Candy et al., 1980; Richardson et al., 1983; Soothill and Harvey, 1976; Turner et al., 1978). However, it was also found that the defect was present in 5–8% of healthy adults (Soothill and Harvey, 1976). When serum from those with the opsonic defect was incubated with yeast cells, it was found that reduced C3b/iC3b was deposited on the yeast's surface compared to when serum from normal individuals was used (Turner et al., 1981, 1986). No complement defect could be found, indicating that the defect must lie in some important mediator of the complement cascade (Turner et al., 1985). After it was shown that MBL could activate complement, it was proven that reconstituting defective serum with purified MBL could correct the opsonic defect (Super et al., 1989). This indicated that the opsonic defect was caused by MBL deficiency.

Pediatricians at a major referral center for children with immune deficiencies have reported that MBL deficiency typically presents as recurrent infections, frequently of the upper and lower respiratory tract (Jack et al., 2004). The infections begin between 3 and 6 months of age. Despite the infections the children continue to thrive, although they generally require frequent courses of antibiotics. After the child has reached 2–3 years of age, the frequency of the infections declines (Jack et al., 2004). These observations are consistent with the theory that MBL is most important during the "window of vulnerability," between the ages of 6 months (following the decline in maternal antibody levels) and 2 years (when the child has acquired a more effective acquired immune response) (Turner, 1996). It has been suggested that MBL may also be important in adults in the initial stages of an infection before the specific immune response is activated (Ezekowitz, 1991). The term "ante-antibody" has been suggested to describe this function (Ezekowitz,

1991). An alternative theory is that MBL deficiency is only relevant in the presence of an additional immune defect. Examples of such defects include IgG subclass deficiency (Aittoniemi et al., 1998), a chemotaxis defect (Ten et al., 1999), chemotherapy-induced neutropenia (Neth et al., 2001; Peterslund et al., 2001; Horiuchi et al. 2005), systemic lupus erythematosus (Garred et al., 1999a), AIDS (Hundt et al., 2000; Kelly et al., 2000), and cystic fibrosis (Garred et al., 1999b).

MBL deficiency does not have a close relationship with susceptibility to specific pathogens (Jack et al., 2004). This may be because MBL can bind to a wide range of microorganisms, including bacteria, viruses, fungi, protozoa, and helminths (table 10.2).

TABLE 10.2. Microorganisms that bind to MBL.

Type of Microorganism	Positive for Binding to MBL	Negative or Low Binding to MBL
Bacteria	Actinomyces israelii	Clostridium spp.
	Bacteroides spp.	Enterococcus spp.
	Bifidobacterium bifidum	Pseudomonas aeruginosa
	Burkholderia cepacia	Neisseria mucosa
	Chlamydia pneumoniae	Neisseria gonorrhoeae (LOS sialylated)
	Escherichia coli	Neisseria meningitidis groups B and C
	Eubacterium spp.	(LOS sialylated)
	Fusobacterium spp.	Salmonella typhimurium (smooth chemotype)
	Haemophilus influenzae	Staphylococcus epidermidis
	Klebsiella spp.	Group B β-hemolytic Streptococcus
	Leptotrichia buccalis	Streptococcus agalactiae[1]
	Listeria monocytogenes	Streptococcus sanguis
	Mycobacterium avium	
	Neisseria cinerea	
	Neisseria gonorrhoeae (LOS nonsialylated)	
	Neisseria meningitidis groups B and C (LOS nonsialylated)	
	Neisseria meningitidis group A	
	Neisseria subflava	
	Propionibacterium acnes	
	Salmonella montevideo	
	Salmonella typhimurium (rough chemotype)	
	Staphylococcus aureus	
	Group A.. β-hemolytic Streptococcus	
	Streptococcus pneumoniae	
	Streptococcus suis	
	Veillonella dispar	
Fungi	Aspergillus fumigatus	Cryptococcus neoformans (encapsulated)
	Candida albicans	
	Cryptococcus neoformans (nonencapsulated)	
Viruses	Influenza A	
	HIV-1	
	Herpes simplex 2	
Protozoa	Cryptosporidium parvum	
	Plasmodium falciparum	
	Trypanosoma cruzi	
Helminths	Schistosoma mansoni	

LOS, lipo-oligosaccharide.
Based on Jack et al. (2001a, 2004) and Kilpatrick (2002).

Within a single species of some bacteria, a proportion of the organisms exhibit MBL binding and a proportion do not bind to MBL (Neth et al., 2000). In the case of *Neisseria meningitidis* and *Neisseria gonorrhoeae*, it has been found that bacteria with sialylation of lipo-oligosaccharide structures are resistant to MBL and nonsialylated organisms bind MBL (Jack et al., 1998, 2001c, 2004; Devyatyarova-Johnson et al., 2000). For *Salmonella typhimurium*, the rough chemotype binds to MBL, whereas the smooth chemotype does not facilitate MBL binding (Devyatyarova-Johnson et al., 2000). It appears that the three-dimensional structure of the lipopolysaccharides on the bacterial surface is the major determinant of whether MBL binding can occur (Turner, 2003). As MBL binding correlates with complement activation, it appears that bacterial expression of particular lipopolysaccharide structures may be a virulence mechanism to escape MBL binding and thus evade the host's innate immune response (Turner, 2003).

The term "MBL deficiency" is not clearly defined (Kilpatrick, 2002). The failure to opsonize baker's yeast is found in serum from more than 5% of the population, and this corresponds to a detectable level of <0.1 μg/ml of serum MBL. However, in many studies, MBL deficiency has been defined by variant genotypes associated with MBL deficiency (see below) or by the measured serum MBL concentration. Not all individuals defined by these criteria will have the functional opsonic defect. Moreover, it has recently been found that some of those with "MBL deficiency" actually do have acceptable levels of serum MBL, but the variant MBL they possess is present in a lower molecular weight form (Garred et al., 2003a). This variant MBL is less stable (Super et al., 1992), does not form higher oligomers (Wallis and Cheng, 1999), and is unable to bind mannan efficiently and activate complement (Super et al., 1992; Garred et al., 2003a). Thus, "MBL deficiency" may be more appropriately considered as "dysfunctional MBL." However, in keeping with the accepted terminology, the term "MBL deficiency" is used throughout this review. A description of the genetic basis of MBL deficiency follows a brief characterization of the gene encoding MBL protein. The term "variant allele" refers specifically to any of several polymorphisms encoding the alternative molecular forms leading to MBL deficiency.

Gene Organization and Sequence

In 1986, the rat MBL gene was cloned by probing a rat liver cDNA library using a cDNA probe, whose sequence was deduced from the known polypeptide sequence of the rat MBL carbohydrate recognition domain (Drickamer et al., 1986). This same cDNA probe was subsequently used to probe a human liver cDNA library. This enabled identification of the cDNA encoding the human MBL protein (Ezekowitz et al., 1988). The human cDNA was then used to screen a λ-phage library (Sastry et al., 1989) and a cosmid library (Taylor et al., 1989). The human MBL gene (called *MBL2*) was then cloned and sequenced independently by the two groups (Sastry et al., 1989; Taylor et al., 1989). The *MBL2* gene was localized to the same region that contains the genes for the other human collectins (lung surfactant protein A and lung surfactant protein D), 10q11.2-q21 (Sastry et al., 1989).

The MBL gene contains four exons, separated by introns of 600, 1,350, and 800 bp (Taylor et al., 1989). Exon 1 encodes the signal peptide, the N-terminal cysteine-rich region and the first seven glycine-X-Y repeats of the collagenous domain. Exon 2 encodes an additional 12 glycine-X-Y repeats. Exon 3 encodes the α-coiled neck region, and exon 4 encodes the lectin domain. The TATAA box is located at −38 bp, and the CAAT box is at −79 bp. There is a heat-shock element at −592 bp and glucocorticoid-responsive elements at −245, −656, and −736 bp.

Polymorphisms and Populations

Three identified mutations produce structural changes in the MBL protein (see figure 10.2, table 10.3). The first mutation was identified by sequencing the MBL gene in three unrelated children with recurrent infections, low serum MBL, and the opsonic defect (Sumiya et al., 1991). All three children possessed the same single amino acid substitution of glycine with aspartic acid (due to a GGC → GAC mutation) at codon 54 of exon 1 (Sumiya et al., 1991). The second mutation causing a structural variant of MBL was described in 1992. This was a single amino acid substitution of glycine with glutamic acid (due to a GGA → GAA mutation) at codon 57 of exon 1 (Lipscombe et al., 1992). The third mutation causing a structural variant of MBL was described two years later. This was

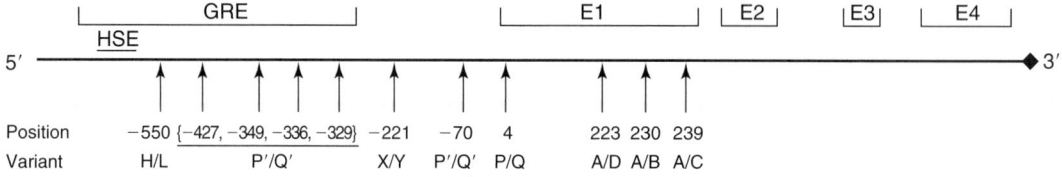

FIGURE 10.2. Polymorphic sites in the *MBL2* gene. P′/Q′ represents a series of promoter polymorphisms in strong linkage disequilibrium with the P/Q dimorphism. HSE, heat shock element; GRE, glucorticocoid-responsive elements; E, exon. Diagram not drawn to scale.

a single amino acid substitution of arginine with cysteine (due to a CGT → TGT mutation) at codon 52 of exon 1 (Madsen et al., 1994). The wild-type allele is now commonly known as "A," the codon 54 mutation as "B," the codon 57 mutation as "C," and the codon 52 mutation as "D."

Individuals who possess two variant alleles (whether homozygotes or compound heterozygotes) were initially found to have virtually undetectable MBL in their serum. Heterozygous individuals were found to have approximately 1/10th the normal MBL concentration. It was suggested that this was because if half of the MBL polypeptides produced are of the variant type, only one in eight ($\frac{1}{2} \times \frac{1}{2} \times \frac{1}{2}$) of the homotrimeric units would not contain a variant chain (Sumiya et al., 1991). As discussed above, it is now known that those who are homozygous for the variant alleles do have MBL in serum, but it is of the low-molecular-weight type and is not detectable by the commonly used assays (Garred et al., 2003a). This low-molecular-weight MBL is dysfunctional because it does not bind mannan effectively and does not activate complement (Garred et al., 2003a).

Several polymorphisms have been identified in the promoter region of the *MBL2* gene (table 10.3, figure 10.2) and found to be associated with the level of circulating MBL (Madsen et al., 1995, 1998a). The H/L polymorphism is located at −550 bp (respectively, G or C), the X/Y polymorphism is at −221 bp (C or G), and the P/Q polymorphism is at +4 bp in an untranslated region of exon 1 (C or T). The P/Q polymorphism is in strong linkage disequilibrium with a number of other polymorphisms located at −427 bp (A or C), −349 bp (A or G), −329 to −324 bp (absence or presence of a 6-bp deletion), and −70 bp (C or T). The HYP haplotype is associated with the highest serum levels of MBL, and the LXP haplotype is associated with the lowest. A person who is homozygous for HYPA has a protein level that is on average six times higher than a person who is homozygous for LXPA (Madsen et al., 1998a).

The *MBL2* haplotypes are in strong linkage disequilibrium with each other. The seven haplotypes that have been commonly described are HYPA, LYQA, LYPA, LXPA, LYPB, LYQC, and HYPD. Garred et al. (2003a) have suggested that for ease of interpretation, it

TABLE 10.3. Genetic variants of human *MBL2*.

Gene Variant	Position	Gene Location	Amino Acid Substitution	Effect on MBL
A	—	—	—	Wild-type allele
B	230	Codon 54 of exon 1	Glycine to aspartic acid	Structurally abnormal MBL
C	239	Codon 57 of exon 1	Glycine to glutamic acid	Structurally abnormal MBL
D	223	Codon 52 of exon 1	Arginine to cysteine	Structurally abnormal MBL
H/L	−550	Promoter region	—	L variant associated with lower MBL levels
X/Y	−221	Promoter region	—	X variant associated with lower MBL levels
P/Q	4	Untranslated exon 1	—	P variant associated with lower MBL levels

Linkage disequilibrium between variants results in seven haplotypes: HYPA, LYQA, LYPA, LXPA, LYPB, LYQC, and HYPD. Among the promoter variants, HYP is associated with the highest MBL levels and LXP is associated with the lowest. Data derived from Madsen et al. (1995, 1998a).

is simpler to pool the structural alleles B, C, and D as a single null allele named "O" and to describe only the most important promoter allele (X/Y) when it occurs on the A type background. There are then just three functional allele designations, O, XA, and YA, respectively, representing zero functional MBL, low MBL, and high MBL (Garred et al., 2003a). This classification system simplifies analysis of potential MBL disease associations.

The frequencies of the *MBL2* variant alleles vary widely among populations (Turner, 1996). The B variant occurs in 22–28% of the Eurasian population but is rare in Africans. The C variant is found in more than 50% of the population in sub-Saharan Africa but is rare in Europeans. The D variant is found in many populations; it is found in up to 14% of some European populations, but in other racial groups it is less common. The substantial racial variation in the frequency of *MBL2* variant alleles means that it is essential to match carefully for ethnic group in any case–control study testing for associations between MBL deficiency and disease.

Two large, adequately powered studies have found that children who carry two MBL variant alleles (i.e., genotype OO) have increased risk of infections during the early years of life (Summerfield et al., 1997; Koch et al., 2001). These results are consistent with the theory that MBL is an important component of the innate immune response and that its main role is to protect against infections during the "window of vulnerability" before the acquired immune response is fully developed. Adults who carry two MBL variant alleles have also been found to have a generalized increased risk of infections (Garred et al., 1995; Summerfield et al., 1995). This finding is more surprising but could perhaps be explained by the ante-antibody function of MBL, fighting infections before the acquired immune response is activated. MBL deficiency has also been reported to be a risk factor in disease progression for infectious diseases such as HIV (Garred et al., 1997a; Maas et al., 1998) and noninfectious diseases such as rheumatoid arthritis (Graudal et al., 1998, 2000; Garred et al., 2000; Ip et al., 2000; Jacobsen et al., 2001; Saevarsdottir et al., 2001) and systemic lupus erythematosus (Garred et al., 2001). These findings and the report that MBL deficiency is a risk factor for the systemic inflammatory response syndrome (Garred et al., 2003b) are consistent with the hypothesis that MBL is a regulator of the inflammatory response (Turner, 2003).

A large number of specific infectious and noninfectious diseases have been reported to be associated with MBL deficiency (or *MBL2* variant alleles) (table 10.4). Many of these associations have been reported in only a single study, or when replication has been attempted, the results have been contradictory. For example, there have been contradictory findings for MBL deficiency and meningococcal disease (Garred et al., 1993; Hibberd et al., 1999). The striking racial variation in the frequency of *MBL2* variant alleles

TABLE 10.4. A selection of diseases for which an association between MBL deficiency (or *MBL2* gene variants) and disease risk (or severity) has been described.

Disease	Selected References
Aspergillosis (pulmonary)	Crosdale et al. (2001)
Atopic dermatitis	Brandrup et al. (1999)
Atherosclerosis	Madsen et al. (1998b)
Celiac disease	Boniotto et al. (2002)
Chronic diarrhea in children	Candy et al. (1980)
Chronic hepatitis B carriage and disease progression	Thomas et al. (1996) Chong et al. (2005)
Chronic hepatitis C carriage	Matsushita et al. (1998)
Cryptosporidiosis in patients with AIDS	Kelly et al. (2000)
Cystic fibrosis (survival)	Garred et al. (1999b)
Dermatomyositis	Werth et al. (2002)
Giant cell arteritis	Jacobsen et al. (2002)
HIV disease	Nielsen et al. (1995) Garred et al. (1997a)
Ischemia-reperfusion injury	Collard et al. (2001)
Kawasaki disease	Biezeveld et al. (2003)
Leishmaniasis (visceral)	Santos et al. (2001)
Malaria	Luty et al. (1998)
Meningococcal disease	Hibberd et al. (1999)
Otitis media	Richardson et al. (1983)
Pneumococcal disease (invasive)	Roy et al. (2002)
Recurrent infections in adults	Garred et al. (1995) Summerfield et al. (1995)
Recurrent infections in children	Summerfield et al. (1997) Koch et al. (2001)
Rheumatoid arthritis	Graudal et al. (1998)
Systemic inflammatory response syndrome	Garred et al. (2003b)
Spontaneous abortion (recurrent)	Kilpatrick et al. (1995)
Systemic lupus erythematosus	Garred et al. (2001)
Tuberculosis	Selvaraj et al. (1999) El Sahly et al. (2004)
Vulvovaginal candidiasis	Babula et al. (2003)

means that inadequate ethnic group matching is more likely to produce spurious associations than for most other candidate gene studies. Conversely, inadequate matching by ethnic group can also result in negative confounding, preventing a true association being detected. Therefore, many of the potential associations listed in table 10.4 should be regarded with some caution until further evidence is produced to support them. Initially, pneumococcal disease also appeared to show inconsistent findings, with a large Oxford study showing clear susceptibility for those of genotype OO (Roy et al., 2002) but no association in Denmark (Kronborg et al., 2002). However, reanalysis of the Danish study revealed evidence of susceptibility for those with OO genotypes (Kronborg and Garred 2002).

If MBL deficiency predisposes to a large number of potentially fatal diseases, there must be some selective advantage in carriage of the variant alleles to explain their high population frequency. The most plausible explanation is that low MBL (as occurs in AO heterozygotes) provides some protection against mycobacterial infections (Garred et al., 1994). This theory has been given support from studies of tuberculosis (Garred et al., 1997b; Bellamy et al., 1998; Hoal-van Helden et al., 1999; Soborg et al., 2003), leprosy (Garred et al., 1994), *Mycobacterium avium* (Polotsky et al., 1997), and visceral leishmaniasis (Santos et al., 2001). However, there is also some limited contradictory evidence that MBL deficiency is a risk factor for tuberculosis (Selvaraj et al., 1999; El Sahly et al., 2004). An alternative explanation for the high frequency of *MBL2* variant alleles is that reduced MBL levels limit host damage from the inflammatory response (Lipscombe et al., 1992). However, this theory is not supported by the recent finding that carriage of *MBL2* variant alleles increases the risk of a fatal outcome in patients with the systemic inflammatory response syndrome (Garred et al., 2003b). Until it is known whether low-molecular-weight MBL serves any useful function, it will be difficult to draw firm conclusions regarding the reasons for the high frequency of *MBL2* variant alleles.

Pharmacogenetics: MBL Replacement Therapy

MBL replacement therapy was first used in 1968 when fresh-frozen plasma was given to correct the opsonic defect found in a young girl with recurrent infections (Miller et al., 1968). It was reported that the treatment produced clinical improvement. Soothill and Harvey (1976) used plasma infusions to treat two further patients with the opsonic defect. One patient died a short time later, and the second patient had only a short lived benefit. Four children with chronic diarrhea, failure to thrive, and the opsonic defect were treated by plasma infusions (Candy et al., 1980). Clinical benefit was reported for three patients. Although promising, these early studies did not prove that the plasma infusions were an effective treatment for MBL deficiency, nor did they prove that it was the MBL (rather than some other component of plasma) that produced the clinical benefits claimed.

Valdimarsson et al. (1998) administered MBL, purified from pooled donor plasma, to two MBL-deficient persons. One of the recipients was an adult volunteer who did not have a history of recurrent infections. The other recipient was a 2-year-old girl who suffered from recurrent infections. The MBL did not elicit any side effects and achieved normalization of complement-mediated opsonization. After several MBL infusions, there was no evidence that anti-MBL antibodies were being produced. Following MBL therapy, the young girl ceased experiencing recurrent infections, although the authors rightly concluded that this may simply have been coincidental (Valdimarsson et al., 1998). There is also a report of a patient with cystic fibrosis being treated with plasma-derived MBL, resulting in stabilization of his rapidly deteriorating condition (Garred et al., 2002).

A phase I safety and pharmacokinetic study of plasma-derived MBL has now been carried out in 20 MBL-deficient, healthy, adult volunteers (Valdimarsson et al., 2004). No adverse events occurred, there was no evidence of infusion-associated complement activation, and no patient produced anti-MBL antibodies. The half-life was 18 to 115 hours, suggesting that adults would need to be given 6 mg of purified MBL two to three times per week to maintain MBL levels above 1 μg/ml (Valdimarsson et al., 2004).

Recombinant human MBL has now been produced by two independent groups (Ohtani et al., 1999; Vorup-Jensen et al., 2001a, 2001b). The recombinant MBL product is reported to be biologically equivalent to plasma-derived MBL (Vorup-Jensen et al., 2001b). The potential advantages of recombinant MBL are that there should be no risk of prion or viral contamination, the production could be performed on a large scale, and the product could theoretically be modified to achieve additional desirable properties (e.g., prolonged biological half-life). The potential disadvantage of recombinant MBL is that there may be a different distribution of oligomers, and this may result in different biological properties from plasma-derived MBL (Kilpatrick, 2002).

A consensus statement on the future of MBL replacement therapy was recently produced following a conference of the U.K. Biochemical Society (Kilpatrick, 2003). The conference delegates concluded that the future of MBL therapy will depend on proof of its efficacy in randomized controlled trials (RCT). They suggested that before an RCT is performed for a specific clinical indication, there should be at least two independent studies showing a relationship between MBL deficiency and the disease in question. They also suggested that a clear and objective end point of the therapy should be defined and achievable within a relatively short time. They recommended that at least 20 patients would be required for a phase II trial and 100–200 for a phase III trial (depending on power calculations) (Kilpatrick, 2003). The conference delegates recommended RCTs of MBL therapy in MBL-deficient patients with several target disorders including immunodeficiency secondary to chemotherapy or HIV disease, rheumatoid arthritis, cystic fibrosis, recurrent spontaneous abortion, and young children with recurrent debilitating infections. The delegates believed that to establish efficacy, RCTs should generally be performed using plasma-derived MBL prior to studies with recombinant MBL, but they did not think this was an absolute requirement (Kilpatrick, 2003).

It is conceivable that once studies have commenced, previously unforeseen applications of MBL therapy may be developed, as has occurred with intravenous immunoglobulin G (Kilpatrick, 2002).

Summary and Conclusions

MBL deficiency is the world's commonest inherited immune defect. Some persons with the condition remain completely healthy, while others suffer from severe, recurrent infections. Why there should be such a wide range of expression of the clinical phenotype remains unexplained. The possibility that MBL deficiency manifests clinically only when it occurs with other causes of immune deficiency has been insufficiently investigated and warrants further study (Turner, 2003).

It has been proposed that MBL deficiency is a contributing factor to the etiology of a wide range of infectious and noninfectious diseases. Some of these associations may eventually prove to be unfounded, although the current evidence suggests that MBL deficiency is a genuine risk factor for a wide range of infectious diseases. Future case–control studies of MBL deficiency and specific diseases should ensure that adequate ethnic matching occurs to reduce the risk of confounding producing false-negative or false-positive results. It is simply not adequate to classify racial groups as "European," "African," or "Asian," as such groupings can hide considerable ethnic differences.

There is still much uncertainty about the reasons for the high frequency of *MBL2* variant alleles. Further studies of mycobacterial infections are indicated to resolve the conflicting results found in this area. Determining in what situations low MBL levels are beneficial may provide valuable insights into the treatment or prevention of important diseases.

MBL replacement therapy offers much promise for the future. It is now appropriate to commence trials of MBL replacement therapy in a small number of specific situations. Further research is required to identify additional conditions which fulfill the criteria for an RCT of MBL replacement therapy (Kilpatrick, 2003). Trials of MBL replacement therapy will prove to be the ultimate test of whether MBL is an important component of host immune defenses.

References

Aittoniemi J, Baer M, Soppi E, Vesikari T, & Miettinen A. (1998) Mannan binding lectin deficiency and concomitant immunodefects. *Archives of Disease in Childhood* 78, 245–248.

Babula O, Lazdane G, Kroica J, Ledger WJ, & Witkin SS. (2003) Relation between recurrent vulvovaginal candidiasis, vaginal concentrations of mannose-binding lectin, and a mannose-binding lectin gene polymorphism in Latvian women. *Clinical Infectious Diseases* 37, 733–737.

Bellamy R, Ruwende C, McAdam KPWJ, et al. (1998) Mannose binding protein deficiency is not associated with increased susceptibility to malaria, hepatitis B carriage nor tuberculosis in Africans. *Quarterly Journal of Medicine* 91, 13–18.

Biezeveld MH, Kuipers IM, Geissler J, et al. (2003) Association of mannose-binding lectin genotype with cardiovascular abnormalities in Kawasaki disease. *Lancet* 361, 1268–1270.

Boniotto M, Braida L, Spano A, et al. (2002) Variant mannose-binding lectin alleles are associated with celiac disease. *Immunogenetics* 54, 596–598.

Brandrup F, Homburg KM, Wang P, Garred P, & Svejgaard A. (1999) Mannan-binding lectin deficiency associated with recurrent cutaneous abscesses, prurigo and possibly atopic dermatitis. A family study. *British Journal of Dermatology* **140**, 168–192.

Candy DCA, Larcher VF, Tripp JH, Harries JT, Harvey BAM, & Soothill JF. (1980) Yeast opsonisation in children with chronic diarrhoeal states. *Archives of Disease in Childhood* **55**, 189–193.

Chong WP, To YF, Ip WK, et al. (2005) Mannose-binding lectin in chronic hepatitis B virus infection. *Hepatology* **42**, 1037–1045.

Collard CD, Montalto MC, Reenstra WR, Buras JA, & Stahl GL. (2001) Endothelial oxidative stress activates the lectin complement pathway—role of cytokeratin 1. *American Journal of Pathology* **159**, 1045–1054.

Crosdale DJ, Poulton KV, Ollier WER, Thomson W, & Denning DW. (2001) Mannose-binding lectin gene polymorphisms as a susceptibility factor for chronic necrotizing pulmonary aspergillosis. *Journal of Infectious Diseases* **184**, 653–656.

Dahl MR, Thiel S, Willis AC, et al. (2000) Mannan-binding lectin associated serine protease 3 (MASP-3)—a new component of the lectin pathway of complement activation. *Immunopharmacology* **49**, 79.

Devyatyarova-Johnson M, Rees IH, Robertson BD, et al. (2000) The lipopolysaccharide structures of *Salmonella enterica* serovar *typhimurium* and *Neisseria gonorrhoeae* determine the attachment of human mannose-binding lectin to intact organisms. *Infection and Immunity* **68**, 3894–3899.

Drickamer K. (1992) Engineering galactose-binding activity into a C-type mannose-binding protein. *Nature* **360**, 183–186.

Drickamer K, Dordal MS, & Reynolds L. (1986) Mannose-binding proteins from rat liver contain carbohydrate recognition domains linked to collagenous tails. *Journal of Biological Chemistry* **261**, 6878–6887.

El Sahly HM, Reich RA, Dou SJ, Musser JM, & Graviss EA. (2004) The effect of mannose binding lectin gene polymorphisms on susceptibility to tuberculosis in different ethnic groups. *Scandinavian Journal of Infectious Diseases* **36**, 106–108.

Ezekowitz RAB. (1991) Ante-antibody immunity. *Current Opinion in Immunology* **1**, 60–62.

Ezekowitz RAB, Day L, & Herman G. (1988) A human mannose-binding protein is an acute phase reactant that shares sequence homology with other vertebrate lectins. *Journal of Experimental Medicine* **167**, 1034–1046.

Garred P, Harboe M, Oettinger T, et al. (1994) Dual role of mannan-binding protein in infections: another case of heterosis? *European Journal of Human Genetics* **21**, 125–131.

Garred P, Larsen F, Madsen HO, & Koch C. (2003a) Mannose-binding lectin deficiency—revisited. *Molecular Immunology* **40**, 73–84.

Garred P, Madsen HO, Balslev U, et al. (1997a) Susceptibility to HIV infection and progression to AIDS in relation to variant alleles of mannose-binding lectin. *Lancet* **349**, 236–240.

Garred P, Madsen HO, Halber P, et al. (1999a) Mannose-binding lectin polymorphisms and susceptibility to infection in systemic lupus erythematosus. *Arthritis and Rheumatism* **42**, 2145–2152.

Garred P, Madsen HO, Hoffmann B, et al. (1995) Increased frequency of homozygosity of abnormal mannan-binding protein alleles in patients with suspected immunodeficiency. *Lancet* **346**, 941–943.

Garred P, Madsen HO, Marquet H, et al. (2000) Two edged role of mannose binding lectin in rheumatoid arthritis: a cross sectional study. *Journal of Rheumatology* **27**, 26–34.

Garred P, Michaelsen TE, Bjune G, et al. (1993) A low serum concentration of mannan-binding protein is not associated with serogroup B or C meningococcal disease. *Scandinavian Journal of Immunology* **37**, 468–470.

Garred P, Pressler T, Lanng S, et al. (2002) Mannose-binding lectin (MBL) substitution in an MBL deficient patient with severe cystic fibrosis. *Pediatric Pulmonology* **33**, 201–207.

Garred P, Pressler T, Madsen HO, et al. (1999b) Association of mannose-binding lectin gene heterogeneity with severity of lung disease and survival in cystic fibrosis. *Journal of Clinical Investigation* **104**, 431–437.

Garred P, Richter C, Andersen AB, et al. (1997b) Mannan-binding lectin in the sub-Saharan HIV and tuberculosis epidemics. *Scandinavian Journal of Immunology* **46**, 204–208.

Garred P, Strom J, Quist L, Taaning E, & Madsen HO. (2003b) Association of mannose-binding lectin polymorphisms with sepsis and fatal outcome in patients with systemic inflammatory response syndrome. *Journal of Infectious Diseases* **188**, 1394–1403.

Garred P, Voss A, Madsen HO, & Junker P. (2001) Association of mannose-binding lectin gene variation with disease severity and infections in a population-based cohort of systemic lupus erythematosus patients. *Genes and Immunity* **2**, 442–450.

Ghiran I, Barbashow SF, Klickstein LB, Tas SW, Jenenius JC, & Nicholson-Weller A. (2000) Complement receptor 1/CD35 is a receptor for mannan-binding lectin. *Journal of Experimental Medicine* **192**, 1797–1807.

Graudal NA, Homann C, Madsen HO, et al. (1998) Mannan binding lectin in rheumatoid arthritis, a longitudinal study. *Journal of Rheumatology* **25**, 629–635.

Graudal N, Madsen HO, Tarp U, et al. (2000) The association of variant mannose binding lectin genotypes with radiographic outcome in rheumatoid arthritis. *Arthritis and Rheumatism* **43**, 515–521.

Hibberd ML, Sumiya M, Summerfield JA, Booy R, Levin M, & the Meningococcal Research Group. (1999) Association of variants of the gene for mannose-binding lectin with susceptibility to meningococcal disease. *Lancet* **353**, 1049–1053.

Hoal-van Helden, Epstein J, Victor TC, et al. (1999) Mannose-binding protein B allele confers protection against tuberculosis meningitis. *Pediatric Research* **45**, 459–464.

Holmskov U, Malhotra R, Sim RB, & Jensenius JC. (1994) Collectins: collagenous C-type lectins of the innate immune system. *Immunology Today* **15**, 67–74.

Horiuchi T, Gondo H, Miyagawa H, et al. (2005) Association of MBL gene polymorphisms with major bacterial infection in patients treated with high-dose chemotherapy and autologous PBSCT. *Genes and Immunity* **6**, 162–166.

Hundt M, Heiken D, & Schmidt RE. (2000) Association of low mannose-binding lectin serum concentrations and bacterial pneumonia in HIV infection. *AIDS* **14**, 1853–1854.

Ikeda K, Sannoh H, Kawasaki N, Kawasaki T, & Yamashina I. (1987) Serum lectin with known structure activates complement through the classical pathway. *Journal of Biological Chemistry* **262**, 7451–7454.

Iobst ST, Wormald MR, Weis WI, Dwek RA, & Drickamer K. (1994) Binding of sugar ligands to Ca^{2+}-dependent animal lectins. I. Analysis of mannose binding by site-directed mutagenesis and NMR. *Journal of Biological Chemistry* **269**, 15505–15511.

Ip WK, Lau YL, Chan SY, et al. (2000) Mannose binding lectin and rheumatoid arthritis in southern Chinese. *Arthritis and Rheumatism* **43**, 1679–1687.

Jack DL, Dodds AW, Anwar N, et al. (1998) Activation of complement by mannose-binding lectin on isogenic mutants of *Neisseria meningitidis* serogroup B. *Journal of Immunology* **160**, 1346–1353.

Jack DL, Jarvis GA, Booth CL, et al. (2001c) Mannose-binding lectin accelerates complement activation and increases serum killing of *Neisseria meningitidis* serogroup C. *Journal of Infectious Diseases* **184**, 836–845.

Jack D, Klein NJ, & Turner MW. (2001a) Mannose-binding lectin: targeting the microbial world for complement attack and opsonophagocytosis. *Immunological Reviews* **180**, 86–99.

Jack DL, Klein NJ, & Turner MW. (2004) Mannose-binding lectin deficiency and susceptibility to infectious disease. In: *Susceptibility to Infectious Diseases: The Importance of Host Genetics*. Advances in cellular and molecular microbiology series. Bellamy R., ed. Cambridge: Cambridge University Press, pp. 279–307.

Jack DL, Read RC, Tenner AJ, Frosch M, Turner MW, & Klein NJ. (2001b) Mannose-binding lectin regulates the inflammatory response of human professional phagocytes to *Neisseria meningitidis* serogroup B. *Journal of Infectious Diseases* **184**, 1152–1162.

Jacobsen S, Baslund B, Madsen HO, Tvede N, Svejgaard A, & Garred P. (2002) Mannose-binding lectin variant alleles and HLA-DR4 alleles are associated with giant cell arteritis. *Journal of Rheumatology* **29**, 2148–2153.

Jacobsen S, Madsen HO, Klarlund M, et al. (2001) The influence of mannose binding lectin polymorphisms on disease outcome in early polyarthritis. TIRA Group. *Journal of Rheumatology* **28**, 935–942.

Johnson CA, Densen P, Hurford RK, Colten HR, & Wetsel RA. (1992) Type 1 human complement C2 deficiency. A 28-base pair gene deletion causes skipping of exon 6 during RNA splicing. *J Biol Chem* **267**, 9347–9353.

Kawasaki T. (1999) Structure and biology of mannan-binding protein, MBP, an important component of innate immunity. *Biochimica et Biophysica Acta* **1473**, 186–195.

Kelly P, Jack DL, Naeem A, et al. (2000) Mannose-binding lectin is a component of innate mucosal defence against *Cryptosporidium parvum* in AIDS. *Gastroenterology* **119**, 1236–1242.

Kilpatrick DC. (2002) Mannan-binding lectin and its role in innate immunity. *Transfusion Medicine* **12**, 335–351.

Kilpatrick DC. (2003) Consensus statement on the future of mannan-binding lectin (MBL)-replacement therapy. *Biochemical Society Transactions* **31**, 776.

Kilpatrick DC, Bevan BH, & Liston WA. (1995) Association between mannan-binding protein deficiency and recurrent miscarriage. *Human Reproduction* **10**, 2501–2505.

Koch A, Melbye M, Sorensen P, et al. (2001) Acute respiratory tract infections and mannose binding lectin insufficiency during early childhood. *Journal of the American Medical Association* **285**, 1316–1321.

Kronborg C, Garred P. (2002) Mannose-binding lectin genotype as a risk factor for invasive pneumococcal infection. *Lancet* **360**, 1176.

Kronborg C, Weis N, Madsen HO, et al. (2002) Variant mannose binding lectin alleles are not associated with susceptibility to or outcome of invasive pneumococcal infection in randomly included patients. *Journal of Infectious Diseases* **185**, 1517–1520.

Kuhlmann M, Joiner K, & Ezekowitz RAB. (1989) The human mannose-binding protein functions as an opsonin. *Journal of Experimental Medicine* **169**, 6848–6859.

Lipscombe RJ, Sumiya M, Hill AV, et al. (1992) High frequencies in African and non-African populations of independent mutations in the mannose binding protein gene. *Human Molecular Genetics* **1**, 709–715.

Lipscombe RJ, Sumiya M, Summerfield JA, & Turner MW. (1995) Distinct physicochemical characteristics of human mannose binding protein expressed by individuals of differing genotype. *Immunology* **85**, 660–667.

Lu J. (1997) Collectins: collectors of microorganisms for the innate immune system. *Bioessays* **19**, 509–518.

Lu J, Teh C, Kishore U, & Reid KBM. (2002) Collectins and ficolins: sugar pattern recognition molecules of the mammalian innate immune system. *Biochimica et Biophysica Acta* **1572**, 387–400.

Lu J, Thiel S, Wiederman H, Timpl R, & Reid KBM. (1990) Binding of the pentamer/hexamer forms of mannan-binding protein to zymosan activates the proenzyme $C1r_2 C1s_2$ complex, of the classical pathway of complement, without involvement of C1q. *Journal of Immunology* **144**, 2287–2294.

Luty AJF, Kun JFJ, & Kremsner PG. (1998) Mannose-binding lectin plasma levels and gene polymorphisms in *Plasmodium falciparum* malaria. *Journal of Infectious Diseases* **178**, 1221–1224.

Maas J, de Roda H, Brouwer M, et al. (1998) Presence of the variant mannose binding lectin alleles associated with slower progression to AIDS. Amsterdam Cohort Study. *AIDS* **12**, 2275–2280.

Madsen HO, Garred P, Kurtzhals JAL, et al. (1994) A new frequent allele is the missing link in the structural polymorphism of the human mannan-binding protein. *Immunogenetics* **40**, 37–44.

Madsen HO, Garred P, Thiel S, et al. (1995) Interplay between promoter and structural gene variants control basal serum level of mannan-binding protein. *Journal of Immunology* **155**, 3013–3020.

Madsen HO, Satz ML, Hogh B, Svejgaard A, & Garred P. (1998a) Different molecular events result in low protein levels of mannan binding lectin in populations from southeast Africa and South America. *Journal of Immunology* **161**, 3169–3175.

Madsen HO, Videm V, Svejgaard A, Svennevig JL, & Garred P. (1998b) Association of mannose-binding lectin deficiency with severe atherosclerosis. *Lancet* **352**, 959–960.

Malhotra R, Thiel S, Reid KBM, & Sim RB. (1990) Human leukocyte C1q receptor binds other soluble proteins with collagen domains. *Journal of Experimental Medicine* **172**, 955–959.

Matsushita M, & Fujita T. (1992) Activation of the classical complement pathway by mannose-binding protein in association with a novel C1s-like serine protease. *Journal of Experimental Medicine* **176**, 1497–1502.

Matsushita M, Hijikata M, Ohta Y, & Mishiro S. (1998) Association of mannose-binding lectin gene haplotype LXPA and LYPB with interferon-resistant hepatitis C virus infection. *Journal of Hepatology* **29**, 695–700.

Miller ME, Seals J, Kaye R, & Levitsky LC. (1968) A familial, plasma associated defect of phagocytosis: new cause of recurrent bacterial infection. *Lancet* **ii**, 60–63.

Neth O, Jack DL, Dodds AW, Holzel H, Klein NJ, & Turner MW. (2000) Mannose-binding lectin binds a range of clinically relevant microorganisms and promotes complement deposition. *Infection and Immunity* **68**, 688–693.

Neth O, Hann I, Turner MW, & Klein NJ. (2001) Deficiency of mannose-binding lectin and burden of infection in children with malignancy: a prospective study. *Lancet* **358**, 614–618.

Nielsen SL, Andersen PL, Koch C, Jensenius JC, & Thiel S. (1995) The level of the serum opsonin, mannan-binding protein in HIV-1 antibody-positive patients. *Clinical and Experimental Immunology* **100**, 219–222.

Nishizaka H, Horiuchi T, Zhu ZB, et al. (1996a) Molecular bases for inherited complement component C6 deficiency in two unrelated individuals. *Journal of Immunology* **156**, 2309–2315.

Nishizaka H, Horiuchi T, Zhu ZB, et al. (1996b) Genetic bases of human complement C7 deficiency. *Journal of Immunology* **157**, 4239–4243.

Ogden CA, deCathelineau A, Hoffmann PR, et al. (2001) C1q and mannose-binding lectin engagement of cell surface calreticulin and CD91 initiates macropinocytosis and uptake of apoptotic cells. *Journal of Experimental Medicine* **194**, 781–795.

Ohtani K, Suzuki Y, Eda S, et al. (1999) High-level and effective production of human mannan-binding lectin (MBL) in Chinese hamster ovary (CHO) cells. *Journal of Immunological Methods* **222**, 135–144.

Peterslund NA, Koch C, Jensenius JC, & Thiel S. (2001) Association between deficiency of mannose-binding lectin and severe infections after chemotherapy. *Lancet* **358**, 637–638.

Polotsky VY, Belisle BT, Mukosova K, Ezekowitz RAB, & Joiner KA. (1997) Interaction of human mannose-binding lectin with *Mycobacterium avium*. *Journal of Infectious Diseases* **175**, 1159–1168.

Richardson VF, Larcher VF, & Price JF. (1983) A common congenital immunodeficiency predisposing to infection and atopy in infancy. *Archives of Disease in Childhood* 58, 799–802.

Roy S, Knox K, Segal S, et al. (2002) MBL genotype and risk of invasive pneumococcal disease: a case-control study. *Lancet* 359, 1569–1573.

Saevarsdottir S, Vikingsdottir T, Vikingsson A, Manfredsdottir V, Geirsson AJ, & Valdimarsson H. (2001) Low mannose binding lectin predicts poor prognosis in patients with early rheumatoid arthritis. *Journal of Rheumatology* 28, 728–734.

Santos IK, Costa CH, Krieger H, et al. (2001) Mannan-binding lectin enhances susceptibility to visceral leishmaniasis. *Infection and Immunity* 69, 5212–5215.

Sastry K, Herman GA, Day L, et al. (1989) The human mannose-binding protein gene: exon structure reveals its evolutionary relationship to a human pulmonary surfactant gene and localization to chromosome 10. *Journal of Experimental Medicine* 170, 1175–1189.

Selvaraj P, Narayanan PR, & Reetha AM. (1999) Association of functional mutant homozygotes of the mannose binding protein gene with susceptibility to pulmonary tuberculosis in India. *Tubercle and Lung Disease* 79, 221–227.

Sheriff S, Chang CY, & Ezekowitz RAB. (1994) Human mannose-binding protein carbohydrate recognition domain trimerizes through a triple α-helical coiled-coil. *Nature Structural Biology* 1, 789–794.

Sjoholm AG, Braconier JH, & Soderstrom C. (1982) Properdin deficiency in a family with fulminant meningococcal infections. *Clinical Experimental Immunology* 50, 291–297.

Sjoholm AG, Soderstrom C, & Nilsson LA. (1988) A second variant of properdin deficiency: the detection of properdin in low concentrations in affecetd males. *Complement* 5, 130–140.

Soborg C, Madsen HO, Andersen AB, Lillebaek T, Kok-Jensen A, & Garred P. (2003) Mannose-binding lectin polymorphisms in clinical tuberculosis. *Journal of Infectious Diseases* 188(5):777–782.

Soothill JF, & Harvey BAM. (1976) Defective opsonization. A common immune deficiency. *Archives of Disease in Childhood* 51, 91–99.

Stover CM, Thiel S, Thelen M, et al. (1999) Two constituents of the initiation complex of the mannan-binding lectin activation pathway of complement are encoded by a single structural gene. *Journal of Immunology* 162, 3481–3490.

Sumiya M, Super M, Tabona P, et al. (1991) Molecular basis of opsonic defect in immunodeficient children. *Lancet* 337, 1569–1570.

Summerfield JA, Ryder S, Sumiya M, et al. (1995) Mannose-binding protein gene-mutations associated with unusual and severe infections in adults. *Lancet* 345, 886–889.

Summerfield JA, Sumiya M, Levin M, et al. (1997) Mannose-binding protein gene mutations are associated with childhood infections in a consecutive hospital series. *BMJ* 314, 1229–1232.

Super M, Gillies SD, Foley S, et al. (1992) Distinct and overlapping functions of allelic forms of human mannose binding protein. *Nature Genetics* 2, 50–55.

Super M, Thiel S, Lu J, Levinsky RJ, & Turner MW. (1989) Association of low levels of mannan-binding protein with a common defect in opsonisation. *Lancet* ii, 1236–1239.

Takahashi M, Endo Y, Fujita T, & Matsushita M. (1999) A truncated form of mannose-binding lectin-associated protease (MASP)-2 expressed by alternative polyadenylation is a component of the lectin complement pathway. *International Immunology* 11, 859–863.

Taylor ME, Brickell PM, Craig RK, & Summerfield JA. (1989) Structure and evolutionary origin of the gene encoding a human serum mannose-binding protein. *Biochemical Journal* 262, 763–771.

Ten RM, Carmona EM, Babovic-Vuksanovic D, & Katzmann JA. (1999) Mannose-binding lectin deficiency associated with neutrophil chemotactic unresponsiveness to C5a. *Journal of Allergy and Clinical Immunology* 104, 419–424.

Tenner AJ, Robinson SL, & Ezekowitz RAB. (1995) Mannose-binding protein (MBP) enhances mononuclear phagocyte function via a receptor that contains the 126,000 M_r component of the C1q receptor. *Immunity* 3, 485–493.

Thiel S, Holmskov U, Hviid L, Laursen SB, & Jensenius JC. (1992) The concentration of the C-type lectin, mannan-binding protein, in human plasma increases during an acute phase response. *Clinical and Experimental Immunology* 90, 31–35.

Thiel S, Petersen SV, Vorup-Jensen T, et al. (2000) Interaction of C1q and mannan-binding lectin (MBL) with C1r, C1s, MBL-associated serine proteases 1 and 2, and the MBL-associated protein MAp19. *Journal of Immunology* 165, 878–887.

Thiel S, Vorup-Jensen T, Stover CM, et al. (1997) A second serine protease associated with mannan-binding lectin that activates complement. *Nature* 386, 506–510.

Thomas HC, Foster GR, Sumiya M, et al. (1996) Mutation of gene for mannose-binding protein associated with chronic hepatitis B viral infection. *Lancet* 348, 1417–1419.

Thompson C. (1995) Protein proves to be a key link in innate immunity. *Science* 269, 301–302.

Turner MW. (1996) Mannose-binding lectin: the pluripotent molecule of the innate immune system. *Immunology Today* **17**, 532–540.

Turner MW. (2003) The role of mannose-binding lectin in health and disease. *Molecular Immunology* **40**, 423–429.

Turner MW, Grant C, Seymour ND, et al. (1986) Evaluation of C3b/C3bi opsonization and chemiluminescence with selected yeasts and bacteria using sera of different opsonic potential. *Immunology* **58**, 111–115.

Turner MW, Mowbray JF, Harvey BAM, Brostoff J, Wells RS, & Soothill JF. (1978) Defective yeast opsonization and C2 deficiency in atopic patients. *Clinical and Experimental Immunology* **34**, 253–259.

Turner MW, Mowbray JF, & Robertson DR. (1981) A study of C3b deposition on yeast surfaces by sera of known opsonic potential. *Clinical and Experimental Immunology* **34**, 253–259.

Turner MW, Seymour ND, Kazatchkine MD, et al. (1985) Suboptimal C3b/C3bi deposition and defective yeast opsonization. II Partial purification and preliminary characterisation of an opsonic co-factor able to correct sera with the defect. *Clinical and Experimental Immunology* **62**, 435–441.

Valdimarsson H, Stefansson M, Vikingsdottir T, et al. (1998) Reconstitution of opsonizing activity by infusion of mannan-binding lectin (MBL) to MBL-deficient humans. *Scandinavian Journal of Immunology* **48**, 116–123.

Valdimarsson H, Vikingsdottir T, Bang P, et al. (2004) Human plasma-derived mannose-binding lectin: a phase I safety and pharmacokinetic study. *Scandinavian Journal of Immunology* **59**, 97–102.

Vorup-Jensen T, Jensen UB, Lui A, et al. (2001a) Tail-vein injection of human mannan-binding lectin DNA leads to high expression levels of multimeric protein in liver. *Molecular Therapy* **3**, 867–874.

Vorup-Jensen T, Sorensen E-S, Jensen UB, et al. (2001b) Recombinant expression of human mannan-binding lectin. *International Immunopharmacology* **1**, 677–687.

Wallis R, & Cheng JT. (1999) Molecular defects in variant forms of mannose-binding protein associated with immunodeficiency. *Journal of Immunology* **163**, 4953–4959.

Weis WI, & Drickamer K. (1994) Trimeric structure of a C-type mannose-binding protein. *Structure* **2**, 1227–1240.

Weis WI, Drickamer K, & Hendrickson WA. (1992) Structure of a C-type mannose-binding protein complexed with an oligosaccharide. *Nature* **360**, 127–134.

Werth VP, Berlin JA, Callen JP, Mick R, & Sullivan KE. (2002) Mannose binding lectin (MBL) polymorphisms associated with low MBL production in patients with dermatomyositis. *Journal of Investigative Dermatology* **119**, 1394–1399.

Yokota Y, Arai T, & Kawasaki T. (1995) Oligomeric structures required for complement activation of serum mannan-binding proteins. *Journal of Biochemistry* **117**, 414–419.

11

Complement Genes

Keith D. Crawford & Chester A. Alper

This chapter provides a broad overview of the human complement system, its component proteins and interactions, and the functions generated by its activation. We broadly outline the genetics of complement proteins with special emphasis on inherited deficiencies. We seek thereby to explain some of the clinical consequences of genetic defects in the system. For more details on the complement system and its components, see the comprehensive reviews in Müller-Eberhard (1988) and Volanakis and Arlaud (1998).

Components and Interactions of the Human Complement System

The human complement system consists of more than 40 serum and cell-surface proteins, including nine numbered components and a variety of serum and cell-surface regulators (table 11.1). It provides effector functions in both innate and adaptive immunity. There are three arms, any of which can cleave and activate

C3 to generate C3b and C3a. C3b, in turn, in complexes with C4bC2a or C3bBb activates a final common pathway, resulting in the generation of the membrane attack complex (MAC), consisting of C5b-C6-C7-C8-$(C9)_n$. The MAC has the ability to insert into cell membranes (bacterial or mammalian), generating perforin-like pores that result in cell lysis and necrosis. The MAC is inhibited by the membrane inhibitor of reactive lysis (CD59).

The first of the activating pathways to be elucidated was the classical pathway: C1, C4, C2, and the C1 inhibitor. It is an effector system for adaptive immunity, being activated by aggregated antibodies, chiefly of the IgM and IgG classes.

C1 consists of a Ca^{2+}-mediated complex of three subcomponents, C1q, C1r, and C1s. C1q has six sets of three kinds of polypeptide chains (A, B, and C) synthesized from three adjacent genes on chromosome 1. The N-terminal collagen-like stalk of a C1q molecule ends in six tuliplike C-terminal globular regions. Each C1q molecule associates with two

151

TABLE 11.1. Complement components.

Gene ID	Protein Product Accession No. Map Position	Mutations	Pathogenesis
Alternative pathway			
C3	Third complement component NM_000064 19p13.3-p13.2	C3s/C3F polymorphism: Arg102 → Gly (Botto, 1990) C3 polymorphism: Hav 4-1 plus/minus type C3: Leu314 → Pro (Botto, 1990) C3 deficiency: 61-bp del, exon 18, 800-bp del, exons 22, 23 (Botto, 1992)	Partial lipodystrophy (McLean and Hoefnagel, 1980) MPG (Alper et al., 1972; Berger et al., 1983; Borzy et al., 1988; Pussell et al., 1980) SLE-like syndrome, meningococcal meningitis (Botto, 1990, 1992; Nilsson, 1992)
CFB	Complement factor B NM_001710 6p21.3	Factor B fast-slow polymorphism BF*Fa/S BF, Arg8 → Gln (Mejia et al., 1994) Polymorphism BF*Fb/S BF, Arg8 → Trp (Campbell, 1987)	
CFD	Complement factor D (adipsin) NM_001928 19p13.3		Obesity (Rosen et al., 1989)
PFC	Properdin NM_002621 Xp11.4-p11.2	Properdin deficiency: Gly271 → Val (Van den Bogaard et al., 2000) Arg73 → Trp (Sjoholm, 1988; Westberg et al., 1995) Ser179 → Ter; Tyr387 → Tsp (Van den Bogaard et al., 2000) Arg134 → Ter (Sjoholm, 1982; Westberg et al., 1995)	Low serum properdin levels (Sjoholm, 1982; 1988) Meningococcal infection (Ross and Densen, 1984)
Classical pathway			
C1QA	C1q subcomponent, α-chain NM_015991 1p36.3-p34.1	Gln186 → Ter (Topaloglu et al., 1996; Petry et al., 1997)	SLE, glomerulonephritis (Topaloglu et al., 1996)
C1QB	C1q subcomponent, β-chain NM_000491 1p36.3-p34.1	G150 → A (McAdam et al., 1988)	
C1QC	C1q subcomponent γ-chain NM_172369 1p36.11	C41 → T (Slingsby et al., 1996) G6 → A (Slingsby et al., 1996; Kirschfink et al., 1993)	SLE (Kirschfink et al., 1993)
C1R	C1r subcomponent NM_001733 12p13		SLE-like disease (Lee et al., 1978; Day et al., 1972)
C1S	C1s subcomponent NM_001734 12p13	4-bp del, NT1087 (Inoue et al., 1998) Arg534 → Ter (Dragon-Durey et al., 2001)	SLE-like disease (Inoue et al., 1998 ; Dragon-Durey et al., 2001)

TABLE 11.1. (continued)

Gene ID	Protein Product Accession No. Map Position	Mutations	Pathogenesis
C4A	C4A (Rodgers blood group) NM_007293 6p21.3		SLE, type I diabetes mellitus (Huang et al., 1995; Lhotta et al., 1990)
C4B	C4B (Chido blood group) NM_000592 p21.3		Glomerular nephritis (Wank et al., 1984) SLE (Wilson and Perez, 1988)
C2	C2 NM_000063 6p21.3	Type I C2, 28-bp del (Johnson, 1992) Type II C2, Ser189 → Phe; Gly444 → Arg (Wetsel et al., 1996)	SLE, MPG (Kim et al., 1977; Friend et al., 1975; Gewurz et al., 1978)

Lectin pathway

Gene ID	Protein Product Accession No. Map Position	Mutations	Pathogenesis
MBL2	Mannose-binding lectin GDB:120167 10q11.2-q21		
MASP1	Mannan-binding lectin serine peptidase 1 D28593 3q27-q28		
MASP2	Mannan-binding lectin serine protease 2 NM_006610 1p36.3-p36.2	Asp105 → Gly (Stengaard-Pedersen et al., 2003)	Chronic infection

Terminal pathway

Gene ID	Protein Product Accession No. Map Position	Mutations	Pathogenesis
C5	C5 NM_001735 9q33-q34		Recurrent systemic infections, usually of gram-negative bacteria
C6	C6 NM_000065 5p13	C6 A/B polymorphism Glu98 → Ala (Fernie et al., 1993) C6 deficiency, total C6: IVS15DS, T-C, +2 (Wurzner et al., 1995) 1-bp del, 879G (Hobart et al., 1998) 1-bp del, 1195C (Zhu et al., 1998) 1-bp del, 1936G (Nishizaka et al., 1996a)	Sporadic meningococcal disease (Ellison et al., 1983)
C7	C7 NM_000587 5p13	C7 deficiency: Cys728 → Ter (Nishizaka, 1996b) 2-bp del, 2137TG (Nishizaka, 1996b)	Raynaud phenomenon, sclerodactyly, and telangiectasia (incomplete CRST syndrome) (Boyer et al., 1975)

(continued)

TABLE 11.1. (continued)

Gene ID	Protein Product Accession No. Map Position	Mutations	Pathogenesis
		Arg499 → Ser (Fernie et al., 1996) C7 deficiency, total: Ivs1, G-A, −1 (Fernie et al., 1997) Exon 7–8 del (Fernie et al., 1997) Gly357 → Arg (Fernie et al., 1997)	
C8A	C8, α-chain NM_000562 1p36.2-p22.1	A/B polymorphism C8A, Gln → Lys (Zhang et al., 1995)	Gonococcal infection (Schlesinger et al., 1990)
C8B	C8, β-chain hCG23458 1p36.2-p22.1	Complement C8b deficiency C8b, Arg374 → Ter (Kaufmann et al., 1993)	Neisserial infection (Schlesinger et al., 1990)
C8G	C8, γ-chain NM_0006065 9q22.3-q32		
C9	C9 NM_001737 5p14-p12	Arg95 → Ter; Cys33 → Ter (Horiuchi et al., 1998) Cys98 → Gly; Ser406 → Ter (Witzel-Schlomp et al., 1997) Ser 406 → Ter Ter (Witzel-Schlomp et al., 1997)	Meningococcal meningitis (Nagata et al., 1989)

MPG, membranoproliferative glomerulonephritis; SLE, systemic lupus erythematosus; Ter, terminal amino acid

C1r and two C1s zymogen molecules. Aggregated Ig as in antigen–antibody immune complexes is bound by the C1q subcomponent of C1, which in turn results in activation of the serine protease C1r and C1s subcomponents. C1 inhibitor is the naturally occurring inhibitor of these proteases, as well as proteins in the contact and coagulation pathways. Activated C1s cleaves C4 and C2 to yield fragments C4b and C2a that form a complex in which C2a is a serine protease for which C3 is a specific substrate. When C3 is cleaved, C3a, a low-molecular-weight smooth-muscle–contracting anaphylatoxin, and C3b are generated. The latter fragment is highly chemically reactive, by virtue of an internal thiolester, and forms covalent bonds with cell-surface proteins, antigens, or, by default, water. C5b, generated by the activated C4b2a3b complex, associates with the latter, but it is only after the addition of C6 and C7 that the C4b2a3b5b67 complex is stable. Thus, cell-surface–attached C3b is the nidus for MAC formation. The addition of C8 results in low-level pore formation and cell lysis that is very much potentiated by the addition of poly-C9.

C3b also serves as the initiator of the alternative complement pathway, an amplifier of complement activation and C3b generation by any pathway, including the alternative pathway. Natural activators of the alternative pathway include zymosan and inulin and analogous structures on microorganisms. C3b, in the presence of factors B, D (a protease that circulates in active form), and magnesium, cleaves factor B (BF) to form C3bBb complexes, which in turn cleave C3 to generate more C3b and thus is part of a self-contained amplification loop. In the bimolecular C3bBb complex, Bb is a serine protease with C3 as its substrate (analogous to C2a of the C4bC2a of the classical pathway). Also, as in the classical pathway, the C3bBbC3b complex can cleave C5 and lead to MAC generation. Properdin (P) stabilizes the complex. Factor I (IF), with factor H (HF) as a co-factor (in the fluid phase, as well as on cell surfaces), cleaves and inactivates C3b in the fluid phase, and HF, decay-accelerating factor

(DAF), and membrane co-factor protein (MCP) down-regulate the pathway on cell surfaces.

The most recently recognized pathway of complement activation involves recognition of carbohydrate structures on microbes by mannose-binding lectin (MBL), L-ficolin and H-ficolin, and activation of the potential serine proteases MASP-1 and MASP-2 (Holmskov et al., 2003). This results in cleavage of C4 and C2 to generate C4bC2a, a C3 convertase. (For more on MBL, see chapter 10.)

Complement-Mediated Functions

The human complement system mediates a large number of functions and has a role in many physiologic and pathologic situations, some only recognized in the past few years (Barrington et al., 2001). In the innate immune system, complement is part of the first line of defense against pathogenic organisms, including bacteria, viruses (many of which use complement receptors to adhere to and enter host cells), yeasts, fungi, and protozoa. The lectin and alternative complement pathways are activated by carbohydrate structures on the surface of pathogens.

Complement plays an important part in normal B-cell development and the normal antibody response to T-cell–dependent antigens as well as in the maintenance of B-cell tolerance (Prodeus et al., 1998; Carroll, 2000); the failure of B-cell tolerance is implicated in autoimmune disease. The classical pathway and the complement receptor CR2 (CD21, C3d receptor) (Nussenzweig et al., 1971; Melchers et al., 1985) are of particular importance in this function. Co-ligation of the B-cell receptor and CR2 results in a striking lowering of the threshold for B-cell activation and enhances B-cell survival. CR2 and CR1 (C3b, C4b receptor; CD35) probably initiate classical pathway activation in the naive host because of the presence of IgM-class natural antibodies. Another important function of CR1, CR2, CR3, and CR4 (gp150,95) is in the clearance of immune complexes. CR3 (Mac-1, Mo-1, αMβ2 integrin, CD11bCD18) is expressed predominantly on neutrophils and mononuclear phagocytes. It is a pattern-recognition receptor for lipopolysaccharide and other bacterial carbohydrates and proteins that activates leukocytes, promotes their transmigration, and, via ligation with iC3b, mediates phagocytosis.

A number of complement regulatory proteins are encoded by closely situated genes in the regulators of complement activation (RCA) region of chromosome 1q32: CR1, CR2, C4 binding protein (C4bp), MCP, HF, and DAF (Rodriguez de Cordoba et al., 1985). These proteins are all cell-surface receptors of C3 or C4 fragments produced by complement activation that serve to modulate the effects of such activation and protect the host's tissues.

Ischemia/reperfusion injury depends on intact classical and alternative complement pathways, as does acute allograft rejection (Kirschfink, 1997). It seems likely that ischemia/reperfusion is initiated by natural antibody to self molecules altered by ischemic injury, with engagement of C1q and MBL.

Small biologically active fragments are generated by complement activation. C4a, C3a, and C5a are smooth-muscle–contracting anaphylatoxins that degranulate mast cells. Recent experiments suggest that C3a has a role in bone marrow localization of B cells. C5a is a potent chemoattractant for neutrophils and can mediate adult acute respiratory distress syndrome. The naturally occurring carboxypeptidase B spontaneously cleaves the terminal arginine from C5a, resulting in a loss of anaphylatoxic but retention of chemotactic activity. C3b is a powerful inducer of phagocytosis. There are cell-surface receptors (CR1–CR4) for the C4b and C3b fragments (and the inactive form of C3b, iC3b, and the fragment C3dg), as well as specific receptors for the C3a, C4a, and C5a fragments.

Patients with deficiencies of C1, C4, and, to a lesser extent, C2 have an increased frequency of lupus-like disease. An intriguing possible reason for this is that C1q and perhaps other early components are involved in the clearance of immune complexes or apoptotic cells or cell products (Walport et al., 1998). The creation of a C1q knockout mouse has been helpful in exploring these possibilities. Half of such mice on a mixed genetic background have anti-C1q antibodies, and a quarter have glomerulonephritis.

Patients with deficiencies of the proteins that form the MAC have increased susceptibility to infection by *Neisseria* species, because of deficient bacteriolysis (Densen, 1991; Würzner, 2003). C5 deficiency has the added disadvantage of the lack of C5a generation and consequent deficient neutrophil chemotaxis. On the other hand, subtotal deficiency of C6/C7 may protect against autoimmune disease severity, and patients may have less severe neisserial infections. Another intriguing recent observation is that C1 inhibitor functions to regulate leukocyte adhesion, not through the protease inhibitory site, but rather through the molecule's abundant carbohydrate (Cai et al., 2005).

Genetics of the Complement System

In the late nineteenth and early twentieth century, such brilliant scientists as Jules Bordet (Bordet and Gengou, 1901) and Paul Ehrlich (Ehrlich and Morgenroth, 1899), with very few technical tools, recognized not only that the system had at least two components but also that the two reacted sequentially in the lysis of antibody-coated red cells and, more to the point, bacteria. The first report of deficiency of a complement component (or of any serum protein in a mammal) came from a Vermont guinea pig colony (Moore, 1919). These animals appeared to be healthy and survived a streptococcal epidemic of the colony in the same proportions as complement-normal animals (Hyde, 1932). Which component was lacking is unknown since the strain was lost in the 1940s.

Two groups of investigators who identified the third component (Sachs, 1911; Browning and Mackie, 1913) came eerily close to discovering the alternative pathway more than 40 years before that task was finally accomplished (Pillemer, 1954). In 1971, the "properdin pathway" to C3 activation was rediscovered as the alternative complement pathway. In the first patient recognized to have factor I (IF) deficiency, all of his abnormalities resulted from his inherited lack of the major inhibitor of the alternative pathway, IF (Alper et al., 1970). But this patient also had strikingly increased susceptibility to infection. A homozygous C3-deficient patient discovered soon thereafter (Alper et al., 1972) also had frequent infections by pyogens such as *Streptococcus* species and *Staphylococcus aureus*, as well as *Neisseria meningitidis*. This led to many reports of increased frequency of infections among complement-deficient patients and to the legitimization of complementology as a bona fide part of immunology. Still more recently, the third pathway to C3 activation was discovered among patients with increased susceptibility to infection due to remarkably common defects in the MBL.

Naturally occurring deficiency states for many of the proteins of the human complement system are now known (Frank, 2000). These (many discovered before the availability of knockout mice) are associated with clinical abnormalities and have taught us much about the natural functions of the system as well as how its proteins interact. The clinical consequences of complement deficiency are dependent on the deficient component or inhibitor but include (1) hereditary angioedema (C1 inhibitor defects) with painless, non-pruritic swelling of the skin, swelling of the larynx (with potentially life-threatening obstruction), and swelling of the gastrointestinal tract, with diarrhea and abdominal pain; (2) systemic lupus erythematosus (SLE)-like disease with deficiency of C1 subcomponents, C4, and, to a lesser extent, C2; (3) increased susceptibility to infections with deficiencies of all of the components of the complement system, including the common pathway; (4) glomerulonephritis in C3 deficiency and some early component deficiencies; and (5) atypical hemolytic-uremic syndrome with HF deficiency. Except for properdin deficiency (X-linked recessive) and C1 inhibitor deficiency (autosomal dominant), complement deficiencies are uncommon autosomal recessive traits that tend to vary in frequency in different ethnic groups.

The influence of complement on B-cell development and function was recognized with the discovery of a C3 receptor on the surface of B cells (Nussenzweig et al., 1971). Subsequently, observations that mice treated with cobra venom factor to render them hypocomplementemic had a poor antibody response (Pepys, 1976), and that patients with C3 or C4 deficiency had weak antibody responses to certain antigens clarified the role for classical complement components in B-cell maturation and activation. This role has been convincingly demonstrated in C2 and C4 gene knockout mice.

Another group of patients, with deficiencies of classical complement components or C3 but not of other components, had markedly decreased serum IgG4 concentrations (Bird and Lachmann, 1988). This phenomenon was confirmed in a large number of C2-deficient homozygotes (Alper et al., 2003), along with deficiencies of IgG2 and IgD. In the C2-deficient patients with increased susceptibility to infections, serum concentrations of IgG4 and IgA were significantly lower. C2-deficient heterozygotes had normal levels of immunoglobulins and factor B (BF) but lower than normal levels of IgD, probably not related to half-normal C2 levels but more likely to a dominantly expressed gene on the conserved extended haplotype (CEH) that carries the C2 deficiency gene (see below).

Genetic polymorphisms in coding regions of many complement proteins, almost all without clinical consequences, have been known for decades (Marcus-

Bagley and Alper, 1992; Crawford and Alper, 2000). Recently, genomewide scans have revealed the presence of single nucleotide polymorphisms (SNPs) in essentially all genes, including the complement genes. Genes for complement proteins of related function or structure may be closely linked and form clusters. Examples include the four complement genes of the MHC (Carroll et al., 1987) on chromosome 6 (complotypes), genes for the RCA complex on chromosome 1, the three genes for subunits of C1q on chromosome 1, and the *C1R* and *C1S* genes on chromosome 12.

C1q, C1r, and C1s

C1q deficiency may be the result of no secreted C1q owing to mutation, deletion, or similar mechanism or to a dysfunctional molecule as a result of mutation. Patients with C1q deficiency are markedly prone to SLE-like disease, currently attributed to the natural role for C1q in the clearance of apoptotic cell debris (Thompson et al., 1980). As expected for any rare recessive inherited disease, incidence is particularly high among certain ethnic groups (Turks, in this case), and consanguinity is common.

The genes for C1r and C1s are immediately next to one another on chromosome 12p13 and show considerable sequence identity, suggesting that they arose by gene duplication. Deficiencies for the two proteins often co-occur. C1r and C1s deficiency is often associated with SLE-like disease.

C4

C4 is synthesized as a single 200-kDa polypeptide chain that is processed by limited proteolysis to form the final three chain (α, β, γ) disulfide-linked structure. There are two kinds of C4, C4A, and C4B, synthesized by two distinct adjacent genes (*C4A* and *C4B*) that are closely similar in nucleotide sequence, having presumably arisen from gene duplication in a nonhuman primate ancestor. Interestingly, the mouse C4 gene is also duplicated, but by a separate event. C4, like C3, is highly chemically reactive owing to the presence of an internal thiolester group. The chemical and biologic reactivities of C4A and C4B differ. C4B reacts with hydroxyl groups and is hemolytically active, whereas C4A reacts with amide groups and is not. As detected in the protein, there are four common variants, C4B 1, 2, 3, and 5. Three forms of *C4*A3* (*C4A*3a*, *C4A*3b*, and *C4A*3c*) and three of *C4B1* (*C4B1*1a*, *C4B1*1b*, and *C4B1*1c*) have been found at the DNA level

(Blanchong et al., 2001). Null *C4A* and *C4B* genes, *C4A*Q0* and *C4B*Q0*, are remarkably common, with normal Boston Caucasian frequencies of 0.17 and 0.14. Similarly, there are four common protein variants, C4A 2, 3, 4, and 6. Both *C4A*Q0* and *C4B*Q0* have two forms, deleted and nondeleted. Rare variants of C4A and C4B total more than 35 each.

In addition to electrophoretic analysis to recognize C4 variants, analysis for the Rodgers (Rg) and Chido (Ch) blood group antigens with specific human and mouse monoclonal antisera has also been useful. There are two Rg specificities, Rg1 and Rg2, and six Ch specificities, Ch1–Ch6. Rg epitopes are largely carried by C4A variants and Ch epitopes by C4B variants. The amino acid sequences 1101–1106 of the C4d fragment of C4A and C4B differ by only four residues: <u>PCPVLD</u> (C4A) versus <u>LSPVIH</u> (C4B). In both *C4A* and *C4B* genes there is also polymorphism reflecting the presence or absence of HERV-K (C4), a retroviral DNA insertion of approximately 6.5 kb. For the most part, this affects *C4B* genes and results in long (L) and short (S) variants.

Because there are two C4 genes in the majority of MHC haplotypes in the population, C4 deficiency may involve different genetic mechanisms in the same individual and in the same haplotype. The majority of cases of complete C4 deficiency have had SLE-like disease.

C2

C2 is the least polymorphic of the chromosome 6 complement loci at the protein level with the common allele, C2*C ("C" for common), having a frequency of around 0.90 or more in most populations. There is a less common structural allele, C2*B ("B" for basic), with a frequency of 0.06–0.12 in Caucasian and Asian populations. A number of rare acidic and basic variant alleles are found in many populations. In genomic DNA, the C2 exhibits considerable polymorphism in an SstI restriction fragment length polymorphism (RFLP) with size variation from 2.40 to 2.75 kb. Frequencies of the five alleles found in Caucasians vary from 0.02 to 0.53. The polymorphism reflects differences in the size of a presumably ancient retroposon.

C2 deficiency is the most common complement deficiency among Caucasians, with an estimated incidence of 1 in 10,000. Many C2-deficient persons are healthy (Silverstein, 1960; Klemperer et al., 1966). Some develop SLE-like disease (Agnello et al., 1972), although this appears to be less frequent than in C1- and C4-deficient subjects. However, around 25% of C2-deficient persons have increased susceptibility to severe infection with repeated attacks of meningitis or pneumonia involving bacteria such as *S. pneumoniae*, *N. meningitidis*, and *H. influenzae*.

The most common (type I) null gene for C2 (C2*Q0 for quantity zero) (Johnson et al., 1992) has a frequency of nearly 0.01 among European Caucasians. Homozygotes represent 1 in 10,000 Caucasians and have complete C2 deficiency. Type I C2*Q0 has a 28-bp deletion in the sixth exon of the C2 gene that results in premature chain termination and the failure to synthesize any C2 protein. Type I C2 deficiency occurs in the conserved extended haplotype (see below) (HLA-A25, B18, S042, DR2) or its fragments. Type II C2*Q0 genes are rare and heterogeneous.

Factor B

In Caucasians there are three common (BF*S, BFA, and BF*FB) and two less common (frequencies near 0.01; BF*F1 and BF*S1) alleles of factor B (BF) of the alternative pathway (Crawford and Alper, 2000). The clinical consequences of this allelic variation are not yet known. In addition, more than two dozen rare variants have been observed, including some with lower than normal hemolytic activity. Studies of the nucleotide sequences of BF*S, BF*FA, and BF*FB have shown that they differ within a single codon (codon 7 of the Ba fragment): CGG, CAG, and TGG, respectively. Although heterozygotes for BF*Q0 have been identified, no homozygous BF deficients are known. BF-deficient mice have been created and used to explore the role of the alternative pathway in a number of situations.

Complotypes

Complotypes (Alper et al., 1983) constitute the first small haplotype block to be identified in the human genome. They contain the four complement genes, C2, *BF*, *C4A*, and *C4B* and occupy 80–120 kb of DNA in the MHC region (Carroll et al., 1987). The variability in size reflects duplications and deletions of the C4 and immediately adjacent cytochrome P450 21-hydroxylase genes such that any given individual may have one to six C4-containing cassettes (called RCCX for the limiting *RP1* and *TNXB* genes) (Blanchong et al., 2001). Complotypes are designated in abbrevi-ated form by their *BF*, *C2*, *C4A*, and *C4B* variant genes. Thus, SC01 represents the complotype BF*S, C2*C, C4A*Q0 (for quantity zero), and C4B*1, and FC(3,2)0 represents a complotype in which, owing to a presumed gene conversion of *C4B* to *C4A*, there are two *C4A* genes. Type I C2 deficiency occurs in the complotype S042 in all known cases. Type II C2 deficiency occurs in a variety of complotypes, including F030 and S031.

Through the use of restriction enzyme digestion and agarose gel electrophoresis to detect SNPs and intrinsic size differences (insertions, deletions, duplications), complotypes can be further subdivided according to complement RFLP constellations (CRCs) (Crawford and Alper, 2000). In this way, 14 CRCs in Caucasians with a frequency ≥ 0.01 are identified. Most important, the very common complotype SC31 (which accounts for around 40% of complotypes) can be divided into three subsets.

Conserved Extended Haplotypes

It is necessary to understand the population structure of the MHC in order to interpret associations of individual alleles, including null alleles, with diseases or other clinical features. Among 2,000 normal MHC haplotypes determined from family studies in Boston, approximately half have fixed *HLA-B*, complotype, DR/DQ alleles. They have been called conserved extended haplotypes (CEHs) (Awdeh et al., 1983) or ancestral haplotypes. Although recognized by these alleles that define a stretch of about 1 Mb, intervening sequences are also fixed and, to a haplotype-specific extent, so are predominant alleles at neighboring loci. For example, the *HLA-A* allele of the CEH [HLA-B18, F1C30, DR3] is HLA-A30 on about 40% and *DPB1* *0202 on about 80% of instances (among Basques, where it is particularly common) for a stretch of fixity of more than 3 Mb. As indicated by this statement, CEHs are ethnic group characteristic, and often sub-ethnic group characteristic. Many MHC allele associations with disease or immune phenomena involve markers on CEHs, making identification of specific susceptibility alleles highly problematic.

Illustrative of this problem is the finding that there are two common CEHs that are increased in frequency among nonresponders to the HBsAg vaccine: [HLA-B8, SC01, DR3] and [HLA-B44, FC31, DR7]. One might focus on the C4A*Q0 of the first CEH rather than the whole CEH and conclude that it is responsible for nonresponse. If that were so, it would be difficult to explain the second haplotype, which usually, but not always, has a C4A*3 gene. However, although the [HLA-B44, FC31, DR7] CEH actually shows microvariation at HLA-Cw and in the complotype, it does not generally include C4A*Q0, which is therefore less likely to account for HBsAg nonresponse.

C3

C3 occupies a central position in the complement system. Its activation through any of the three pathways can result in C5 cleavage and assembly of the MAC in the common pathway. Like C4, the C3 molecule is synthesized as a single polypeptide chain (pro-C3) that is processed by limited proteolysis to give the final structure with two disulfide-linked (α and β) chains. Also like C4, the C3 molecule has a reactive internal thiolester that is activated when C3 is cleaved and C3b is generated.

Genetic polymorphism in C3 was the first to be discovered in the complement system (Alper and Propp, 1969). Two major alleles, C3*S and C3*F, occur in Caucasians, with C3*S at a frequency of 0.80. In other populations, C3*S is nearly universal. The C3*S to C3*F difference is in nucleotide position 394 (C $\rightarrow$ G), resulting in amino acid R $\rightarrow$ G. A second polymorphism in the coding region of C3 involves a substitution in the amino acid sequence (P314L).

C3 deficiency has been described throughout the world but was first detected in a family with heterozygotes only because of half-normal serum levels and anomalous inheritance of structural variants. An unrelated homozygote (Alper et al., 1972) had markedly increased susceptibility to gram-positive bacterial infection but, remarkably, no neutrophilia. This may be somehow related to the recent demonstration that C3a is involved in lymphocyte homing to the bone marrow. Most C3-deficient patients have immune-complex–mediated phenomena involving the skin and the kidney, most likely representing failure to clear immune complexes.

The originally described C3 deficiency was the result of a mutation involving the 5' donor splice site in intron 18 of the C3 gene. This produces a cryptic 5' splice site in exon 18, a 61-bp deletion in the processed mRNA, and a frame shift producing a premature stop codon, but other mutations have been described in other patients.

Late-Acting Complement Components (C5–C9)

Deficiencies of late-acting components of the common pathway may produce increased susceptibility to systemic infection with *Neisseria* species; however, some late-acting complement-component–deficient patients seem surprisingly healthy.

C5

C5 is largely monomorphic at both the protein and DNA levels throughout the world. Although rare, C5 deficiency has been reported, largely in African-American patients. Bactericidal activity for gram-negative bacteria is severely reduced in C5-deficient serum and is restored by the addition of purified C5. Patients have repeated bouts of meningococcal and sometimes gonococcal bacteremia.

C6, C7

The genes for C6, C7, and C9 are closely linked on chromosome 5p13, show closely related structural features, and probably arose by gene duplication and modification of a common precursor gene (Würzner, 2003). C6 shows a common structural polymorphism detectable by isoelectric focusing in acrylamide gels. Inherited deficiency is rare but in many cases involves both proteins as subtotal deficiency. Although isolated C6 deficiency occurs largely in blacks, C7 deficiency is primarily in whites, with Moroccan Jews having a particularly high frequency. Again, patients have neisserial infection.

C8

The C8 molecule consists of three chains, α, γ, and β encoded by three genes, C8A, C8B, and C8G such that the C8 α-γ chains are noncovalently bound to the C8 β-chains. The C8 β-chain has the binding site for poly C9. There are common genetic polymorphisms in the exons of both C8A and C8B. Homozygous deficiency of either C8A or C8B (C8A*Q0 or C8B*Q0) results in deficiency of the active complete molecule. There is a sharp difference in the ethnic distribution of the two forms of C8 deficiency, with C8A*Q0 in Caucasians but C8B*Q0 in African Americans. As with other late-acting component deficiencies, all forms of C8 deficiency are associated with increased susceptibility to neisserial infection.

C9

Homozygous C9 deficiency has a remarkably high prevalence in Japan (1 per 1,000 persons). Perhaps because of the slow spontaneous lysis by C5b-8 cells, C9-deficient persons are commonly healthy, although a few have been reported to have neisserial infections.

Complement Receptor Deficiency

CR1 has a structure consisting of 30 short consensus repeats (SCRs) with four conserved cysteines. SCRs are also found in a number of proteins that bind activation fragments of C3 or C4: CR2, C1r, C1s, C2, BF, C4BP, MCP and DAF. Genetic variants of CR1 differ in molecular mass by virtue of having varying numbers of SCRs. The variants, in turn, vary in density on the blood cells (in humans, these include red cells and platelets). Deficiencies in CR1 occur commonly in SLE patients. However, since the extent of deficiency may vary with disease activity, the pathogenetic relationships are uncertain.

Deficiency of CR3 is the result of homozygosity for a null gene for CD18. Since this subunit is common to several other biologically important molecules, such as the β-integrin LFA-1 (CD11a, CD18), as well as CR4 (CD11c, CD18), patients with CD18 deficiency have severe impairments of host defense: neutrophil and macrophage dysfunction including phagocytosis, impaired adhesion and migration, and poor pus formation. Mouse experiments with selected CD11a and -b knockouts have helped to define the contributions of LFA-1 and CR3, although interpretations have been controversial.

C1 Inhibitor

There are two varieties of C1 inhibitor deficiency (hereditary angioedema) (Landerman et al., 1962; Donaldson and Evans, 1963), a deficiency of the protein or a mutated dysfunctional C1 inhibitor. Most cases represent new mutations (forebears do not have disease, although 50% of offspring are affected). It is estimated that new cases occur with a frequency of 1 per 300,000. Fortunately, there is treatment and prophylaxis of hereditary angioedema in the form of intravenous purified C1 inhibitor and oral impeded androgens such as stanozolol.

The Lectin Pathway

The recognition protein of the lectin pathway is the collectin MBL (Holmskov et al., 2003), which is described in detail in chapter 10. It shares structural features with C1q (which is not a lectin). Like C1q, MBL has a collagen-like stalk, but in contrast to C1q, this consists of an α-helical coil–coiled trimer of a single polypeptide chain ending in three (rather than six) globular heads. MBL associates with four proteins: MASP-1, MASP-3, MASP-2, and Map19. Remarkably, one gene, on chromosome 3, encodes the first two serine proteases by alternative mRNA splicing, and another gene, on chromosome 1, encodes the protease MASP-2 and Map19 (which lacks a serine protease domain) also by alternative splicing. All four proteins form aggregates with MBL. Although the MASPs and C1r/C1s have identical domain structures, there is no cross-binding of the MASPs with C1q. The MASPs and Map19 also form complexes with L-, M-, and H-ficolins, which can function like MBL in activating complement.

Factor I

The infectious organisms to which IF-deficient patients are particularly susceptible are more varied than those affecting patients with late-acting component deficiencies and include streptococci, *H. influenzae*, and other bacteria, such as *Neisseria*. Clinical manifestations include pneumonia, meningitis, and otitis media. This probably reflects the absence of a functioning alternative pathway, as well as low (but not absent) serum levels of native C3 and the lack of generation of C3 degradation products beyond C3b.

IF is polymorphic in the Japanese, with a frequency of the minor allele (IF*A) of 0.10, but there is no common variation among Caucasians. Although IF deficiency is rare, a number of IF-deficient patients have been identified in many parts of the world.

Factor H

HF is one of several factor H-like genes; it is functional, and the others may be, as well. Deficiency of HF gives a clinical picture similar to that of IF deficiency, with increased susceptibility to a variety of pyogenic organisms. In addition, patients and even heterozygous carriers (who do not have an increased frequency of infections) may have atypical hemolytic-uremic syndrome, for reasons that are unclear.

Factor D and Properdin

Factor D (adipsin) circulates as an active enzyme. Factor D deficiency has been described in several families and is associated with increased susceptibility to pyogenic infection. Properdin deficiency is unique among the complement protein deficiencies in its inheritance as an X-linked recessive trait. Affected males have increased susceptibility to infections with *Neisseria*.

Summary

The complement system includes more than three dozen proteins and three pathways to activation of C3 and generation of the MAC. The system has myriad functions. Certain known human complement deficiency states relate to genetic polymorphism and clinical abnormalities, and knockout mouse models have assisted in their elucidation.

Patients with inherited selective deficiencies of almost all complement proteins have uniformly increased susceptibility to infection by *Neisseria*. Those with deficiencies of classical complement components, particularly those with deficiency of or affecting C3 and the alternative pathway, are also susceptible to infection by pyogenic bacteria. The increased susceptibility to infection is clearly related to impairment of such complement-mediated functions as phagocytosis, lysis of organisms (whether antibody coated or not), chemotaxis for leukocytes, and clearance of antibody-sensitized pathogens. In addition, with deficiencies of C1, C4, C2, and C3, susceptibility involves the participation of these components in B-cell maturation, normal antibody response, and maintenance of normal immunoglobulin levels.

Acknowledgments

This work was supported by grants from the National Heart, Lung, and Blood Institute, National Institute of Allergy and Infectious Diseases, and National Cancer Institute of the National Institutes of Health (HL29583, AI14157, and CA09141) and by a grant from the Department of Defense (DAMD17–03–2–0054).

References

Agnello, V., de Bracco, M.M.E., Kunkel, H.G. 1972. Hereditary C2 deficiency with some manifestations of systemic lupus erythematosis. J. Immunol. 108: 837–840.

Alper, C.A., Abramson, N., Johnston, R.B., Jr, Jandl, J.H., Rosen, F.S. 1970. Increased susceptibility to infection associated with abnormalities of complement-mediated functions and of the third component of complement (C3). N. Engl. J. Med. 282:349–354.

Alper, C.A., Colten, H.R., Rosen, F.S., Rabson, A.R., Macnab, G.M., Gear, J.S.S. 1972. Homozygous deficiency of C3 in a patient with repeated infections. Lancet ii:1179–1181.

Alper, C.A., Propp, R.P. 1968. Genetic polymorphism of the third component of human complement (C'3). J. Clin. Invest. 47:2181–2191.

Alper, C.A., Raum, D., Karp, S., Awdeh, Z.L., and Yunis, E.J. 1983. Serum complement "supergenes" of the major histocompatibility complex in man (complotypes). Vox Sang. 45:62–67.

Alper, C.A., Xu, J., Cosmopoulos, K., Dolinski, B., Stein, R., Uko, G., Larsen, C.E., Dubey, D.P., Densen, P., Truedsson, L., Sturfelt, G., Sjöholm, A.G. 2003. Immunoglobulin deficiencies and susceptibility to infections among homozygotes and heterozygotes for C2 deficiency. J. Clin. Immunol. 23:297–305.

Awdeh, Z.L., Raum, D., Yunis, E.J., Alper, C.A. 1983. Extended HLA/complement allele haplotypes: Evidence for T/t-like complex in man. Proc. Natl. Acad. Sci. U. S. A. 80:259–263.

Barrington, R., Zhang, M., Fischer, M., Carroll, M.C. 2001. The role of complement in inflammation and adaptive immunity. Immunol. Rev. 180:5–15.

Berger, M., Balow, J.E., Wilson, C.B., Frank, M.M. 1983. Circulating immune complexes and glomerulonephritis in a patient with congenital absence of the third component of complement. N. Engl. J. Med. 308:1009–1012.

Bird, P., Lachmann, P.J. 1988. The regulation of IgG subclass production in man: Low serum IgG4 in inherited deficiencies of the classical pathway of C3 activation. Eur. J. Immunol. 18:1217–1222.

Blanchong, C.A., Chung, E.K., Rupert, K.L., Yang, Y., Yang, Z., Zhou, B., Moulds, J.M., Yu, C.Y. 2001. Genetic, structural and functional diversities of human complement components C4A and C4B and their mouse homologues, Slp and C4. Int. Immunopharmacol. 1:365–392.

Bordet, J., Gengou, O. 1901. Sur l'existence de substances sensabilisatrices dans la plupart des sérums antimicrobiens. Ann. Inst. Pasteur 15:289–302.

Borzy, M.S., Gewurz, A., Wolff, L., Houghton, D., Lovrien, E. 1988. Inherited C3 deficiency with recurrent infections and glomerulonephritis. Am. J. Dis. Child. 142:79–83.

Botto, M., Fong, K.Y., So, A.K., Koch, C., Walport, M.J. 1990. Molecular basis of polymorphisms of human complement component C3. J. Exp. Med. 172: 1011–1017.

Botto, M., Fong, K.Y., So, A.K., et al. 1992. Homozygous hereditary C3 deficiency due to a partial gene deletion. Proc. Natl. Acad. Sci. U.S.A. 89:4957–4961.

Boyer, J.T., Gall, E.P., Norman, M.E., Nilsson, U.R., Zimmerman, T.S. 1975. Hereditary deficiency of the seventh component of complement. J. Clin. Invest. 56:905–913.

Browning, C.H., Mackie, T.J. 1913. The relationship of the complementing action of fresh serum along with immune body to its haemolytic effect with cobra venom—a contribution on the structure of complement. Z. Immun. Forsch. 17:1–20.

Cai, S., Dole, V.S., Bergmeier, W., Scafidi, J., Feng, H., Wagner, D., Davis, A.E., III. 2005. A direct role for C1 inhibitor in regulation of leukocyte adhesion. J. Immunol. 174:6462–6466.

Campbell, R.D. 1987. The molecular genetics and polymorphism of C2 and factor B. Br. Med. Bull. 43:37–49.

Carroll, M.C. 2000. The role of complement in B cell activation and tolerance. Adv. Immunol. 74:61–88.

Carroll, M.C., Katzman, P., Alicot, E.M., Koller, B.H., Geraghty, D.E., Orr, H.T., Strominger, J.L., Spies, T. 1987. Linkage map of the human major histocompatibility complex including the tumor necrosis factor genes. Proc. Natl. Acad. Sci. U.S.A. 84: 8535–8539.

Crawford, K.D., Alper, C.A. 2000. Genetics of the complement system. Rev. Immunogenet. 2:323–338.

Day, N.K., Geiger, H., Stroud, R., et al. 1972. C1r deficiency: An inborn error associated with cutaneous and renal disease. J. Clin. Invest. 51:1102–1108.

Densen, P. 1991. Complement deficiencies and meningococcal disease. Clin. Exp. Immunol. 86(suppl. 1): 57–62.

Donaldson, V.H., Evans, R.R. 1963. A biochemical abnormality in hereditary angioneurotic edema: Absence of serum inhibitor of C'1 esterase. Am. J. Med. 35:37–44.

Dragon-Durey, M.A., Quartier, P., Fremeaux-Bacchi, V., et al. 2001. Molecular basis of a selective C1s deficiency associated with early onset multiple autoimmune diseases. J. Immunol. 166:7612–7616.

Ehrlich, P., Morgenroth, J. 1899. Zur Theorie der Lysin-Wirkung. Berl. Klin. Wschr. 36:6–9.

Ellison, R.T., III, Kohler, P.F., Curd, J.G., Judson, F.N., Reller, L.B. 1983. Prevalence of congenital or acquired complement deficiency in patients with sporadic meningococcal disease. N. Engl. J. Med. 308:913–916.

Fernie, B.A., Delbridge, G., Hobart, M.J. 1993. Correlation of a Glu/Ala substitution at position 98 with the complement C6 A/B phenotypes. Hum. Mol. Genet. 2:591–592.

Fernie, B.A., Wurzner, R., Orren, A., et al. 1996. Molecular bases of combined subtotal deficiencies of C6 and C7: Their effects in combination with other C6 and C7 deficiencies. J Immunol. 157:3648–3657.

Fernie, B.A., Orren, A., Sheehan, G., Schlesinger, M., Hobart, M.J. 1997. Molecular bases of C7 deficiency: Three different defects. J. Immunol. 159:1019–1026.

Frank, M.M. 2000. Complement deficiencies. Pediatr. Clin. N. Am. 47:1339–1354.

Friend, P., Repine, J.E., Clawson, C.C., Michael, A.F. 1975. Deficiency of the second component of complement (C2) with chronic vasculitis. Ann. Intern. Med. 83:813–816.

Gewurz, A., Lint, T.F., Roberts, J.L., Zeitz, H., Gewurz H. 1978. Homozygous C2 deficiency with fulminant lupus erythematosus: Severe nephritis via the alternative complement pathway. Arthritis Rheum. 21: 28–36.

Hobart, M.J., Fernie, B.A., Fijen, K.A., Orren A. 1998. The molecular basis of C6 deficiency in the western Cape, South Africa. Hum. Genet. 103:506–512.

Holmskov, U., Thiel, S., Jensenius, J. 2003. Collectins and ficolins: Humoral lectins of the innate immune defense. Annu. Rev. Immunol, 21:547–578.

Horiuchi, T., Nishizaka, H., Kojima, T., et al. 1998. A non-sense mutation at Arg95 is predominant in complement 9 deficiency in Japanese. J. Immunol. 160: 1509–1513.

Huang, D.F., Siminovitch, K.A., Liu, X.Y., et al. 1995. Population and family studies of three disease-related polymorphic genes in systemic lupus erythematosus. J. Clin. Invest. 95:1766–1772.

Hyde, R.R. 1932. The complement deficient guinea pig: A study of an inheritable factor in immunity. Am. J. Hyg. 15:824–836.

Inoue, N., Saito, T., Masuda, R., et al. 1998. Selective complement C1s deficiency caused by homozygous four-base deletion in the C1s gene. Hum. Genet. 103:415–418.

Johnson, C.A., Densen, P., Hurford, R.K., Jr., Colten, H.R., and Wetsel, R.A. 1992. Type I human complement C2 deficiency. A 28-basepair gene deletion causes skipping of exon 6 during RNA splicing. J. Biol. Chem. 267:9347–9353.

Kaufmann T, Hansch G, Rittner C., et al. 1993. Genetic basis of human complement C8 beta deficiency. J. Immunol. 150:4943–4947.

Kim, Y., Friend, P.S., Dresner, I.G., Yunis, E.J., Michael, A.F. 1977. Inherited deficiency of the second component of complement (C2) with membranoproliferative glomerulonephritis. Am. J. Med. 62:765–771.

Kirschfink, M. 1997. Controlling the complement system in inflammation. Immunopharmacol. 38:51–62.

Kirschfink, M., Petry, F., Khirwadkar, K., et al. 1993. Complete functional C1q deficiency associated with systemic lupus erythematosus (SLE). Clin. Exp. Immunol. 94:267–272.

Klemperer, M.R., Woodworth, H.C., Rosen, F.S., Austen, K.F. 1966. Hereditary deficiency of the second component of complement in man. J. Clin. Invest. 45:880–890.

Landerman, N.S., Webster, M.E., Becker, E.L., Ratcliffe, H.E. 1962. Hereditary angioneurotic edema. II. Deficiency of inhibitor for serum globulin permeability factor and/or plasma kallikrein. J. Allergy. 33: 330–341.

Lee, S.L., Wallace, S.L., Barone, R., Blum, L., Chase, P.H. 1978. Familial deficiency of two subunits of the first component of complement. C1r and C1s associated with a lupus erythematosus-like disease. Arthritis Rheum. 21:958–967.

Lhotta, K., Konig, P., Hintner, H., Spielberger, M., Dittrich, P. 1990. Renal disease in a patient with hereditary complete deficiency of the fourth component of complement. Nephron. 56:206–211.

Marcus-Bagley, D., Alper, C.A. 1992. Methods for allotyping complement proteins. In *Manual of Clinical Laboratory Immunology*, 4th ed. Rose, N.R., Conway de Macario, E., Fahey, J.L., Friedman, H., and Penn, G.M., eds. American Society for Microbiology, Washington, D.C., pp. 124–141.

McAdam, R.A., Goundis, D., Reid, K.B. 1988. A homozygous point mutation results in a stop codon in the C1q B-chain of a C1q-deficient individual. Immunogenetics. 27:259–264.

McLean, R.H., Hoefnagel, D. 1980. Partial lipodystrophy and familial C3 deficiency. Hum. Hered. 30:149–154.

Mejia, J.E., Jahn I., de la Salle, H., Hauptmann, G. 1994. Human factor B. Complete cDNA sequence of the BF*S allele. Hum. Immunol. 39:49–53.

Melchers, F., Erdai A., Schulz, T., Dierich, M.P. 1985. Growth control of activated, synchronized murine B cells by the C3d fragment of human complement. Nature 317:264–267.

Moore, H.D. 1919. Complementary and opsonic functions in their relation to immunity. A study of the serum of guinea pigs naturally deficient in complement. J. Immunol. 4:425–441.

Müller-Eberhard, H.J. 1988. Molecular organization and function of the complement system. Annu. Rev. Biochem. 57:321–347.

Nagata, M., Hara, T., Aoki, T., et al. 1989. Inherited deficiency of ninth component of complement: An increased risk of meningococcal meningitis. J. Pediatr. 114:260–264.

Nilsson, U.R., Nilsson, B., Storm, K.E., Sjolin-Forsberg, G., Hallgren, R. 1992. Hereditary dysfunction of the third component of complement associated with a systemic lupus erythematosus-like syndrome and meningococcal meningitis. Arthritis Rheum. 35: 580–586.

Nishizaka, H., Horiuchi, T., Zhu, Z.B., et al. 1996a. Molecular bases for inherited human complement component C6 deficiency in two unrelated individuals. J. Immunol. 156:2309–2315.

Nishizaka, H., Horiuchi, T., Zhu, Z.B., Fukumori, Y., Volanakis, J.E. 1996b. Genetic bases of human complement C7 deficiency. J. Immunol. 157:4239–4243.

Nussenzweig, V., Bianco, C., Dukor, P., Eden, A. 1971. Receptors for C3 on B lymphocytes: Possible role in the immune response. Academic Press, New York.

Pepys, M.B. 1976. Role of complement in the induction of immunological responses. Transpl. Rev. 32:93–120.

Petry, F., Hauptmann, G., Goetz, J., Grosshans, E., Loos, M. 1997. Molecular basis of a new type of C1q-deficiency associated with a non-functional low molecular weight (LMW) C1q: Parallels and differences to other known genetic C1q-defects. Immunopharmacology 38:189–201.

Pillemer, L., Blum, L., Lepow, I.H., Ross, O.A., Todd, E.W., Wardlaw, A.C. 1954. The properdin system and immunity. I. Demonstration and isolation of a new serum protein, properdin, and its role in immune phenomena. Science 120, 279–285.

Prodeus, A.P., Shen, L.M., Pozdnyakova, O.O., Chu, L., Alicot, E.M. 1998. A critical role for complement in maintenance of self-tolerance. Immunity 9:721–731.

Pussell, B.A., Bourke, E., Nayef, M., Morris, S., Peters, D.K. 1980. Complement deficiency and nephritis. A report of a family. Lancet i:675–677.

Rodriguez de Cordoba, S., Lublin, D.M., Rubinstein, P., Atkinson, J.P. 1985. Human genes for three complement components that regulate the activation of C3 are tightly linked. J. Exp. Med. 161:1189–1195.

Rosen, B.S., Cook, K.S., Yaglom, J., et al. 1989. Adipsin and complement factor D activity: An immune-related defect in obesity. Science 244:1483–1487.

Ross, S.C., Densen, P. 1984. Complement deficiency states and infection: Epidemiology, pathogenesis and consequences of neisserial and other infections in an immune deficiency. Medicine (Baltimore) 63: 243–273.

Sachs, H., Omorokov, L. 1913. Über die Wirkung des Cobragiftes auf die Komplemente. II. Mitteilung. Z. Immun. Forsch. 11:710–724.

Schlesinger, M., Nave, Z., Levy, Y., Slater, P.E., Fishelson, Z. 1990. Prevalence of hereditary properdin, C7 and C8 deficiencies in patients with meningococcal infections. Clin. Exp. Immunol. 81:423–427.

Silverstein, A.M. 1960. Essential hypocomplementemia: Report of a case. Blood 16:1338–1341.

Sjoholm AG, Braconier JH, Soderstrom C. 1982. Properdin deficiency in a family with fulminant meningococcal infections. Clin Exp Immunol. 50, 291–297.

Sjoholm, A.G., Soderstrom, C., Nilsson, L.A. 1988. A second variant of properdin deficiency: The detection of properdin at low concentrations in affected males. Complement. 5:130–140.

Slingsby, J.H., Norsworthy, P., Pearce, G., et al. 1996. Homozygous hereditary C1q deficiency and systemic lupus erythematosus. A new family and the molecular basis of C1q deficiency in three families. Arthritis Rheum. 39:663–670.

Stengaard-Pedersen, K., Thiel, S., Gadjeva, M., et al. 2003. Inherited deficiency of mannan-binding lectin-associated serine protease 2. N. Engl. J. Med. 349: 554–560.

Thompson, R.A., Haeney, M., Reid, K.B., et al. 1980. A genetic defect of the C1q subcomponent of complement associated with childhood (immune complex) nephritis. N. Engl. J. Med. 303:22–24.

Topaloglu, R., Bakkaloglu, A., Slingsby, J.H., et al. 1996. Molecular basis of hereditary C1q deficiency associated with SLE and IgA nephropathy in a Turkish family. Kidney Int. 50:635–642.

van den Bogaard R., Fijen, C.A., Schipper, M.G., et al. 2000. Molecular characterisation of 10 Dutch properdin type I deficient families: Mutation analysis and X-inactivation studies. Eur. J. Hum. Genet. 8:513–518.

Volanakis J.E., Arlaud, G.J. 1998. Complement enzymes. In *The Human Complement System in Health and Disease*. Frank, M.M., and Volanakis, J.E., eds. Marcel Dekker, New York, pp. 49–82.

Walport, M.J., Davies, K.A., Botto, M. 1998. C1q and systemic lupus erythematosus. Immunobiology 199: 265–285.

Wank, R., Schendel, D.J., O'Neill, G.J., et al. 1984. Rare variant of complement C4 is seen in high frequency in patients with primary glomerulonephritis. Lancet 1:872–874.

Westberg, J., Fredrikson, G.N., Truedsson, L., Sjoholm, A.G., Uhlen, M. 1995. Sequence-based analysis of properdin deficiency: Identification of point mutations in two phenotypic forms of an X-linked immunodeficiency. Genomics 29:1–8.

Wetsel, R.A., Kulics, J., Lokki, M.L., et al. 1996. Type II human complement C2 deficiency. Allele-specific amino acid substitutions (Ser189 → Phe; Gly444 → Arg) cause impaired C2 secretion. J. Biol. Chem. 271:5824–5831.

Wilson, W.A., Perez, M.C. 1988. Complete C4B deficiency in black Americans with systemic lupus erythematosus. J. Rheumatol. 15:1855–1858.

Witzel-Schlomp, K., Spath, P.J., Hobart, M.J., et al. 1997. The human complement C9 gene: Identification of two mutations causing deficiency and revision of the gene structure. J. Immunol. 158:5043–5049.

Würzner, R. 2003. Deficiencies of the complement MAC II gene cluster (C6,C7,C9): Is subtotal C6 deficiency of particular evolutionary benefit? Clin. Exp. Immunol. 133:156–159.

Zhang, L., Rittner, C., Sodetz, J.M., Schneider, P.M., Kaufmann, T. 1995. The eighth component of human complement: Molecular basis of C8A (C81) polymorphism. Hum. Genet. 96:281–284.

Zhu, Z.B., Totemchokchyakarn, K., Atkinson, T.P., Volanakis, J.E. 1998. Molecular defects leading to human complement component C6 deficiency in an African-American family. Clin. Exp. Immunol. 111:91–96.

12

Toll-Like Receptor Genes

Bruce Beutler

The Protein Product(s) and Their Role in Infection

A total of 10 Toll-like receptors (TLRs) are encoded in the human genome, while 12 TLRs are encoded in the mouse genome, and perhaps different numbers in other mammalian genomes. These paralogous proteins (i.e., proteins that diverged from an ancestral sequence to form a clade within a single species) represent the principal sensors of microbial infections in the mammalian host. They discriminate between self and non-self and are ultimately responsible for most of the alterations in host physiology that occur during infection. Hence, fever, shock, metabolic disturbances, and indeed, most phenomena that occur during severe infections are ultimately traceable to the TLRs, but so are most beneficial aspects of the host immune response.

The TLRs evolved to promote a vigorous response to small, localized microbial inocula. When TLR signaling is globally absent, mammals are severely im-munocompromised, because most cellular immune "awareness" of infection is ablated. In the absence of TLR function, severe immunocompromise results.

The TLRs are named for their similarity to the *Drosophila* protein Toll, a plasma membrane receptor that was shown first to serve a developmental function and then to serve an immunologic function, as well. All of the TLRs are single-spanning transmembrane receptors that feature abundant leucine-rich repeat motifs in their ectodomains, and a single Toll/interleukin-1(IL-1) receptor/resistance (TIR) motif that comprises most of the cytoplasmic domain.

As the name suggests, the TIR motif is found in other receptors (members of the IL-1/IL-18 receptor family) and in plant disease resistance proteins. It is also a characteristic of specialized adapter proteins (discussed below) that mediate TLR signal transduction.

In mammals, the TLRs have no clear developmental function. Rather, they serve only to sense infection and do so through direct interaction with specific molecules of microbial origin. In this, they are distinct from their *Drosophila* namesake Toll, which engages a protein ligand, Spaetzle, which is generated from a precursor by proteolytic cleavage events triggered in the course of infection.

Pathogenesis

Specificity of Microbial Recognition by the TLRs

Each TLR recognizes a subset of molecules of microbial origin (table 12.1) and, in some instances, does so in conjunction with other TLRs and/or associated proteins. They have been described as "pattern recognition receptors." However, nothing in particular distinguishes them from other classes of plasma membrane receptor, and they do not recognize "patterns" per se, but discrete and definable molecular determinants. The term should probably be abandoned.

Receptors responsible for the recognition of molecular components of microbes had been widely believed to exist from the time their ligands were isolated in relatively pure form and chemically analyzed years ago (for review, see Beutler & Rietschel, 2003). However, the role of TLRs as the key mammalian sensors of microbial infection only recently became clear as a result of the positional cloning of the *Lps* locus in mice, a locus so named because mutations within it abolished all biologic responses to lipopolysaccharide (LPS). Mice of the C3H/HeJ strain, which are homozygous for the *Lps^d* allele at the *Lps* locus, are highly resistant to all cellular effects of LPS (Heppner & Weiss, 1965; Chiller et al., 1973; Skidmore et al., 1975a, 1975b, 1976, 1977; Weigle & Skidmore, 1975), yet highly susceptible to infection by authentic gram-negative bacteria (O'Brien et al., 1980; Rosenstreich et al., 1982; Hagberg et al., 1984), a fact that linked LPS sensing to host defense. This phenotype was ascribed to a missense mutation (P712H) that altered the cytoplasmic domain of the TLR4 protein (Poltorak et al., 1998).

Genetic complementation studies have indicated that TLR4 directly engages LPS in order to signal. In cells of C3H/HeJ origin (Poltorak et al., 2000), as in other transfected mammalian cells (Lien et al., 2000), the species origin of TLR4 was shown to determine receptor specificity.

Subsequently, gene knockout studies revealed that TLR2 is required for the sensing of numerous products of gram-positive bacteria, mycobacteria, fungi, and parasites (Takeuchi et al., 1999, 2000; Underhill et al., 1999; Maldonado et al., 2000; Campos et al., 2001). The knockout of other TLR genes has disclosed the

TABLE 12.1. The TLRs: their recognition properties, co-receptors, and adapters.

Gene ID	Aliases	Entrez Gene ID	Map Position	Active in	Associations	Adapter(s)	Ligand(s)
TLR 1	TIL1	7096	4p14	H/M	TLR2	MyD88, Mal	Triacyl lipopeptides
TLR 2	TIL4, CD282	7097	4q32	H/M	TLR1, TLR6, CD36, Dectin-1, CD14	MyD88, Mal	Di- and triacyl lipopeptides, zymosan, lipoteichoic acid, others
TLR 3	CD283	7098	4q35	H/M		Trif	dsRNA
TLR 4	hToll, CD284, Lps	7099	9q32-33	H/M	MD-2, CD14	MyD88, Mal, Trif, Tram,	LPS
TLR 5	TIL3	7100	1q32.3-q42	H/M		MyD88	Flagellin
TLR 6		10333	4p16.1	H/M	TLR2	MyD88, Mal	Diacyl lipopeptides
TLR 7		51284	Xp22.3	H/M		MyD88	ssRNA, imidazoquinolines
TLR 8		51311	Xp22	H		MyD88	ssRNA, imidazoquinolines
TLR 9	CD289	54106	3p21.3	H/M		MyD88	Unmethylated DNA
TLR 10		81793	4p14	H		Unknown	Unknown

function of each human paralog except TLR10, which has no mouse ortholog, and therefore cannot be deleted in the mouse. TLR2 has been shown to function both as a heteromer, in conjunction with TLR1 or TLR6 (Ozinsky et al., 2000). The TLR2:1 heteromer is responsible for sensing triacylated bacterial lipopeptides (Takeuchi et al., 2002); the TLR2:6 heteromer is responsible for sensing diacylated bacterial lipopeptides (Takeuchi et al., 2001). TLR3 senses double-stranded RNA (dsRNA) (Alexopoulou et al., 2001); TLR5 senses flagellin (Hayashi et al., 2001); TLRs 7 and 8 sense single-stranded RNA (ssRNA) (Diebold et al., 2004; Heil et al., 2004; Lund et al., 2004; Crozat & Beutler, 2004), as well as small nucleoside-based inflammatory drugs of the imidazoquinoline class (Hemmi et al., 2002; Jurk et al., 2002); and TLR9 senses DNA bearing unmethylated CpG motifs (Hemmi et al., 2000). TLR7 may have no function in humans, while in mice, its function is equivalent to that of human TLR8 (an ssRNA sensor).

The contribution of the *Lps* locus to defense against gram-negative bacteria was established in the 1980s, long before the identification of the relevant gene (O'Brien et al., 1980; Rosenstreich et al., 1982; Hagberg et al., 1984). With the identification of *Lps* as *Tlr4*, it became clear that TLR4 must protect against bacterial infection. The realization that other TLRs fulfilled similar functions with respect to gram-positive bacteria followed more recently (Takeuchi et al., 2000; Edelson & Unanue, 2002). Strikingly, while TLRs 1, 2, 4, 5, and 6 are important in antibacterial defense against bacteria, fungi, and protozoans, TLRs 3, 7 (in mice), 8 (in humans), and 9 are important in defense against viruses (Tabeta et al., 2004; Lund et al., 2003). The best studies of viral pathogenesis have been performed with mouse cytomegalovirus, and it has been observed that both the TLR3 → Trif signaling axis (Hoebe et al., 2003a) and the TLR9 → MyD88 signaling axis (Tabeta et al., 2004) are important for protection, which is ultimately mediated in large part by type I interferon-mediated activation of natural killer (NK) cells (the adapters MyD88 and Trif are described below).

TLRs 3, 7/8, and 9 are all located within the endosomal compartment and are not expressed on the cell surface. The ability of these TLRs to detect viral nucleic acids to the exclusion of host nucleic acids rests largely upon this compartmentalization. While it was appreciated some time ago that vertebrate nucleic acids can be distinguished from invertebrate nucleic acids by the methylation of cytosine residues in CpG dinucleotides, this distinction may be insufficient for discrimination in total, since host nucleic acids may help to sustain autoimmune reactions when access to the endosome is encouraged, for example, by anti-DNA antibodies (Leadbetter et al., 2002). TLRs 3, 7/8, and 9 all depend upon an intrinsic protein of the endoplasmic reticulum, UNC-93B, in order to signal. The means by which UNC-93B communicates with the endosomal compartment is not yet understood (Tabeta et al, 2006).

Not all TLRs act alone, but rather act in concert with other cell-surface proteins. For many years, it has been known that lipopolysaccharide binding protein (LBP) (Tobias et al., 1988) and CD14 (Wright et al., 1990; Haziot et al., 1996) concentrate the LPS signal, though they themselves are unable to signal in the absence of TLR4. MD-2, a small protein known to be tightly associated with the TLR4 ectodomain, is required for LPS sensing, as well, and to a large extent is required for surface expression of TLR4 (Nagai et al., 2002). TLR2:6 heteromers sense lipoteichoic acid as well as the diacylated lipopeptide MALP-2 in conjunction with CD36, a double-spanning member of the class B scavenger receptor family (Hoebe et al, 2005). These and other TLRs may also depend upon other carrier proteins; each TLR may sense microbial molecules in the context of a multisubunit protein complex.

The Essential Consequences of TLR Activation

The immediate containment of microbial pathogens in the mammalian host depends upon several events. First, immune cells that engulf pathogens must have a cell-autonomous means of destroying them. Second, the cytokine response elicited by infectious agents encourages the influx of "reinforcements": Circulating phagocytic cells (particularly neutrophils) are summoned to the site of an infection and help to eliminate it. Third, the adaptive immune response is activated and provides very specific and long-lived protection against the invader. Each of these events is initiated by TLR signaling, and the decipherment of TLR signaling pathways has stood as one of the major goals of research in the TLR field. The biochemistry of cytokine production and adaptive immune activation are now understood in broad outline, though some components of the signaling pathways may still be elusive.

Signaling Pathways

The TLRs all signal by way of cytoplasmic adapter proteins endowed with TIR domains homologous to those found in the receptors themselves. While the precise relationship between the adapters and the receptors is not known with certainty, it is assumed that they engage one another in a heterotypic fashion and, in this way, recruit other proteins to the TLR signaling complex. The receptors themselves may exist as homodimers (Schneider et al., 1991; Medzhitov et al., 1997) or heterodimers (Ozinsky et al., 2000), and the adapters may also exist as multimers, before or after receptor engagement.

The crystal structure of the TIR domains of TLRs 1 and 2 has been determined, as has the structure of TLR2 with the mutation equivalent to that specified by the Lps^d allele of TLR4 (Xu et al., 2000). These studies reveal that the critical proline modified in the TIR domain by this inactivating mutation exists on a protuberance (the BB loop) that is widely believed to interact with a docking site on the adapters. The precise nature of the interaction is unknown. However, the P → H substitution does not render the TIR domain insoluble or markedly change its shape.

The TIR adapter proteins include MyD88, Tirap (also known as Mal), Trif (also known as Ticam 1, or Lps2, after the mutation by which it was identified), Tram, and Sarm. Only the first four of these adapters are known to be required for signaling from the TLRs (figure 12.1). Moreover, compound homozygous mutations of the MyD88 and Trif genes are sufficient to abolish all TLR signaling, suggesting that in the absence of MyD88 and Trif, Tirap and Tram are unable to signal.

MyD88 is the most widely utilized TIR adapter protein, required entirely or in part by TLRs 1, 2, 4, 5, 6, 7, 8, and 9 for signal transduction. Trif is required by TLRs 3 and 4 (Hoebe et al., 2003a; Yamamoto et al., 2003a); Tram is required only by TLR4 (Yamamoto et al., 2003b), and Tirap is required by TLRs 2 and 4 (Yamamoto et al., 2002; Horng et al., 2002).

MyD88 signals by recruiting IRAK4, a serine kinase, though a death domain interaction (Suzuki et al., 2002). IRAK4 in turn phosphorylates IRAK (IRAK1), a homologous kinase that may serve a structural function

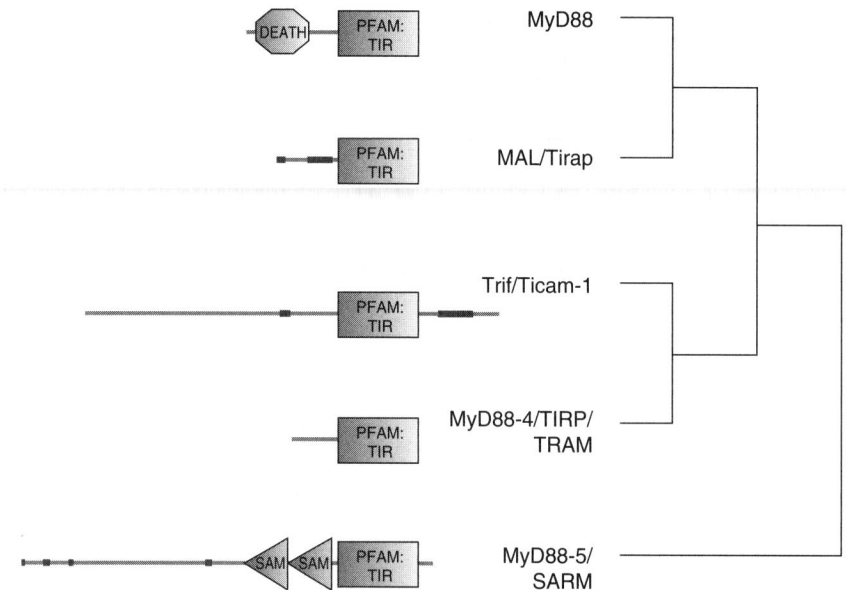

FIGURE 12.1. The TIR adapter proteins. Phylogenetic relationship (not to scale) is indicated by the dendrogram at the right. MyD88 and Tirap are most closely related, as are Trif and Tram. SARM is an outlier, characterized by sterile α-motifs (SAM) as well as a TIR domain. MyD88 alone possesses a death domain, by which it can interact with IRAK4.

as well as a catalytic function. The complete complex recruits TRAF6, another scaffold, which coordinates the phosphorylation of numerous protein kinases (JNK, p38 kinase, MAPK, and TAK-1) (Cao et al., 1996). TAK-1, and perhaps other kinases, as well, phosphorylates IκB kinase, which in turn triggers the nuclear translocation of the nuclear factor NF-κB as well as the phosphorylation and degradation of its inhibitor (IκB). This, together with the activation of the adaptor-related protein 1(AP-1), perhaps via JNK activation, leads to the transcription of numerous cytokine genes that generate the inflammatory response.

Trif, on the other hand, signals by activating a mitochondrial antiviral signaling protein (TBK-1) (Fitzgerald et al., 2003), which phosphorylates the transcription factor IRF-3. IRF-3 causes the production of type I interferons (especially interferon-β), which causes the induction of many other proteins. Among these other proteins are co-factors for adaptive immune activation: proteins such as CD80, CD86, and CD40, which are required for T-cell mitogenesis to proceed in the presence of a specific MHC-presented antigen. Hence, it has emerged that Trif signaling (and, more distally, type I interferon production) is of key importance to the adjuvant effect of microbial inducers such as LPS and dsRNA (Hoebe et al., 2003b). There is also intersection between the Trif- and MyD88-dependent pathways, occurring at the level of TRAF6, which is directly engaged by Trif and activated (Sato et al., 2003; Jiang et al., 2004).

Inhibition of TLR Signal Transduction

Feedback inhibition of signaling by TLRs is well known to occur and constitutes an important regulatory mechanism, in that unbounded responses to microbial inducers would be harmful to the host. Inhibitory loops have been best studied for LPS signaling, and the phenomenon of "endotoxin tolerance" has been known for some decades (Cross, 2002; Brint et al., 2004). IRAK-M, a member of the IRAK family of protein kinases, has an inhibitory effect on transduction through the MyD88 signaling pathway and is induced as an end point of signaling (Kobayashi et al., 2002). Suppressor of cytokine signaling 1 (SOCS-1) prevents type I interferon signal transduction via the signal transducer and activator protein (STAT-1) and thereby dampens the LPS response at an entirely different level (Kinjyo et al., 2002).

Gene Organization and Sequence

The 10 human TLR genes are scattered across the genome, although it is noteworthy that half of them are found on chromosome 4 and two of them are found on chromosome X (table 12.1). In mice, TLR10 does not exist as an intact gene. However, mice have TLRs 11, 12, and 13, as well (Tabeta et al., 2004), and these genes are not represented in humans. Moreover, they have no known ligands, though it has been reported that TLR11 (also separately reported as TLR12) somehow serves to recognize uropathogenic bacteria in mice (Zhang et al., 2004).

As is true for many receptors, the most conserved portion of the TLRs is the cytoplasmic domain, and in the case of the TLRs, the TIR domain represents most of the cytoplasmic sequence.

Polymorphisms and Populations

To date, only three of the human TLRs have been well studied for mutations and phenotypic correlates. These are *TLR2*, *TLR4*, and *TLR5*. Hypomorphic mutations affecting these receptors would be predicted to cause susceptibility to gram-positive and/or fungal infections, gram-negative infections, and infections with flagellated organisms, respectively.

TLR2 coding variants are known to exist (Lorenz et al., 2000; Smirnova et al., 2003) but are comparatively uncommon, and in no case have they been statistically associated with any form of disease.

TLR4 coding variation is somewhat more common, particularly in African populations (Smirnova et al., 2001). Among whites, a relatively common variant (the TLR4B allele) exists at a gene frequency of approximately 6%. It has been reported that this mutation creates hyporesponsiveness to LPS (Arbour et al., 2000); however, more recent analyses have challenged this assessment (Erridge et al., 2003). The mutation has a purported relationship to atherosclerotic disease (Kiechl et al., 2002). Here again, however, separate studies suggest that this may not be the case (Beutler & Beutler, 2002). Rare coding variants of *TLR4* are strongly linked to meningococcal disease, indicating that *TLR4* is one of the proteins required for effective protection against this organism (Smirnova et al., 2003). However, only a relatively small fraction of meningococcal sepsis can be ascribed to mutations at the *TLR4* locus.

A relatively common, codominant nonsense mutation in *TLR5* has been associated with enhanced risk of *Legionella* infection (Hawn et al., 2003), as determined by measuring the frequency of the mutation in infected and noninfected individuals in a population that was exposed to the organism. The work on both meningococcal disease and legionellosis suggest that codominance is not unusual in the TLR family of proteins, and therefore, even heterozygous coding variants can influence outcome during infection.

Mutations in *IRAK4* have been identified in human populations and show much more severe phenotypic effects than mutations in any of the individual TLRs (Picard et al., 2003). In these individuals, gram-positive (but not gram-negative) infections are common. Interestingly, the phenotype becomes less severe as patients mature, suggesting that adaptive immune protection may supervene to prevent infection.

Since, as described above, *IRAK4* mutations may, in part, be "bypassed" by the Trif → TRAF6 signaling pathway, it is plausible to think that some innate immune signals often reach the central response apparatus of the host, mitigating the effect of an IRAK4 lesion. Consistent with this interpretation, a far more severe immunodeficiency is observed with mutations that affect the inhibitor of IκB kinase IKKγ.

To date, no phenotypically significant mutations of *MYD88* or the gene for the toll-like receptor adaptor *TICAM1* have been reported in humans, and unpublished analyses of the coding region of the latter gene have shown only synonymous variation. It is known that mice with hypomorphic M*yd*88 mutations or null alleles are rather severely immunocompromised, that Trif mutant mice are moderately affected, and that double-mutant mice are more severely affected than either of the single mutants.

Conclusions and Prospects

The identification of the TLRs as the key sensors of the innate immune system has been a key advance in immunology, since TLRs are the heart of discrimination between self and nonself. Since activation of the innate immune system necessarily precedes activation of the adaptive immune system under most conditions, the TLRs are fundamental for normal immune function and for all consequences that follow from it. The TLRs may also be important in sterile inflammation, whether it is physiologic or pathologic. They ulti-

mately mediate the adjuvant effects that microbes are well known to exert.

The practical consequences of our understanding of the TLRs will likely flow in three directions. First, on occasion, it may be desirable to block TLR signaling under some circumstances (e.g., when it drives sterile inflammation, or when it drives septic shock). LPS antagonists, such as E5531 (Su et al., 2003; Akashi et al., 2003) and its successors, are already being considered for clinical application with this in mind. Second, it may be important to utilize TLR signaling for therapeutic purposes. Drugs such as imiquimod, which stimulates TLR7 and is now widely used for the treatment of papillomavirus infection and basal cell carcinoma (Hemmi et al., 2002), may be the first of a new class of agents that can actually cure infections and tumors. The use of CpG oligodeoxynucleotides as adjuvants presents another example. Third, the inheritance of susceptibility to infectious disease has been very well documented (Sorensen et al., 1988). Since the preponderance of resistance to infection is provided by innate immunity (which might equally be called inherited immunity), mutations that affect structural components of the innate immune system are almost certainly the cause of much of inherited susceptibility.

The TLRs and their signaling partners (the cofactors for ligand recognition, adapter proteins, kinases, transcription factors, and both primary and secondary effector molecules) form a framework for understanding innate immunity and also present likely candidates for the identification of mutations that cause immunocompromise. As techniques for resequencing (including, perhaps, the use of sequencing chips) improve, it is likely that a global assessment of the structural substrate for innate immune defense might be made in human patients. Such an assessment would likely have predictive value, permitting a reasoned declaration of which individuals are at risk for catastrophic infections, and perhaps for sterile inflammatory (i.e., autoimmune) diseases, as well.

References

Akashi, S., Saitoh, S., Wakabayashi, Y., Kikuchi, T., Takamura, N., Nagai, Y., Kusumoto, Y., Fukase, K., Kusumoto, S., Adachi, Y., Kosugi, A., & Miyake, K. (2003) Lipopolysaccharide interaction with cell surface Toll-like receptor 4-MD-2: Higher affinity than that with MD-2 or CD14. Journal of Experimental Medicine, 198, 1035–1042.

Alexopoulou, L., Holt, A.C., Medzhitov, R., & Flavell, R.A. (2001) Recognition of double-stranded RNA and activation of NF-kappaB by Toll-like receptor 3. Nature, 413, 732–738.

Arbour, N.C., Lorenz, E., Schutte, B.C., Zabner, J., Kline, J.N., Jones, M., Frees, K., Watt, J.I., & Schwartz, D.A. (2000) TLR4 mutations are associated with endotoxin hyporesponsiveness in humans. Nature Genetics, 25, 187–192.

Beutler, B., & Beutler, E. (2002) Toll-like receptor 4 polymorphisms and atherogenesis. New England Journal of Medicine, 347, 1978–1980.

Beutler, B., & Rietschel, E.T. (2003) Timeline: Innate immune sensing and its roots: The story of endotoxin. Nature Reviews Immunology, 3, 169–176.

Brint, E.K., Xu, D., Liu, H., Dunne, A., McKenzie, A.N., O'Neill, L.A., & Liew, F.Y. (2004) ST2 is an inhibitor of interleukin 1 receptor and Toll-like receptor 4 signaling and maintains endotoxin tolerance. Nature Immunology, 5, 373–379.

Campos, M.A., Almeida, I.C., Takeuchi, O., Akira, S., Valente, E.P., Procopio, D.O., Travassos, L.R., Smith, J.A., Golenbock, D.T., & Gazzinelli, R.T. (2001) Activation of Toll-like receptor-2 by glycosylphosphatidylinositol anchors from a protozoan parasite. Journal of Immunology, 167, 416–423.

Cao, Z., Xiong, J., Takeuchi, M., Kurama, T., & Goeddel, D.V. (1996) TRAF6 is a signal transducer for interleukin-1. Nature, 383, 443–446.

Chiller, J.M., Skidmore, B.J., Morrison, D.C., & Weigle, W.O. (1973) Relationship of the structure of bacterial lipopolysaccharides to its function in mitogenesis and adjuvanticity. Proceedings of the National Academy of Sciences of the United States of America, 70, 2129–2133.

Cross, A.S. (2002) Endotoxin tolerance—current concepts in historical perspective. Journal of Endotoxin Research, 8, 83–98.

Crozat, K., & Beutler, B. (2004) TLR7: A new sensor of viral infection. Proceedings of the National Academy of Sciences of the United States of America, 101, 6835–6836.

Diebold, S.S., Kaisho, T., Hemmi, H., Akira, S., & Reis e Sousa, C. (2004) Innate antiviral responses by means of TLR7-mediated recognition of single-stranded RNA. Science, 303, 1529–1531.

Edelson, B.T., & Unanue, E.R. (2002) MyD88-dependent but Toll-like receptor 2-independent innate immunity to Listeria: No role for either in macrophage listericidal activity. Journal of Immunology, 169, 3869–3875.

Erridge, C., Stewart, J., & Poxton, I.R. (2003) Monocytes heterozygous for the Asp299Gly and Thr399Ile mutations in the Toll-like receptor 4 gene show no deficit in lipopolysaccharide signalling. Journal of Experimental Medicine, 197, 1787–1791.

Fitzgerald, K.A., McWhirter, S.M., Faia, K.L., Rowe, D.C., Latz, E., Golenbock, D.T., Coyle, A.J., Liao, S.M., & Maniatis, T. (2003) IKKepsilon and TBK1 are essential components of the IRF3 signaling pathway. Nature Immunology, 4, 491–496.

Hagberg, L., Hull, R., Hull, S., McGhee, J.R., Michalek, S.M., & Svanborg Eden, C. (1984) Difference in susceptibility to gram-negative urinary tract infection between C3H/HeJ and C3H/HeN mice. Infection and Immunity, 46, 839–844.

Hawn, T.R., Verbon, A., Lettinga, K.D., Zhao, L.P., Li, S.S., Laws, R.J., Skerrett, S.J., Beutler, B., Schroeder, L., Nachman, A., Ozinsky, A., Smith, K.D., & Aderem, A. (2003) A common dominant TLR5 stop codon polymorphism abolishes flagellin signaling and is associated with susceptibility to Legionnaires' disease. Journal of Experimental Medicine, 198, 1563–1572.

Hayashi, F., Smith, K.D., Ozinsky, A., Hawn, T.R., Yi, E.C., Goodlett, D.R., Eng, J.K., Akira, S., Underhill, D.M., & Aderem, A. (2001) The innate immune response to bacterial flagellin is mediated by Toll-like receptor 5. Nature, 410, 1099–1103.

Haziot, A., Ferrero, E., Kontgen, F., Hijiya, N., Yamamoto, S., Silver, J., Stewart, C.L., & Goyert, S.M. (1996) Resistance to endotoxin shock and reduced dissemination of gram-negative bacteria in CD14-deficient mice. Immunity, 4, 407–414.

Heil, F., Hemmi, H., Hochrein, H., Ampenberger, F., Kirschning, C., Akira, S., Lipford, G., Wagner, H., & Bauer, S. (2004) Species-specific recognition of single-stranded RNA via Toll-like receptor 7 and 8. Science, 303, 1526–1529.

Hemmi, H., Kaisho, T., Takeuchi, O., Sato, S., Sanjo, H., Hoshino, K., Horiuchi, T., Tomizawa, H., Takeda, K., & Akira, S. (2002) Small anti-viral compounds activate immune cells via the TLR7 MyD88-dependent signaling pathway. Nature Immunology, 3, 196–200.

Hemmi, H., Takeuchi, O., Kawai, T., Kaisho, T., Sato, S., Sanjo, H., Matsumoto, M., Hoshino, K., Wagner, H., Takeda, K., & Akira, S. (2000) A Toll-like receptor recognizes bacterial DNA. Nature, 408, 740–745.

Heppner, G., & Weiss, D.W. (1965) High susceptibility of strain A mice to endotoxin and endotoxin-red blood cell mixtures. Journal of Bacteriology, 90, 696–703.

Hoebe, K., Du, X., Georgel, P., Janssen, E., Tabeta, K., Kim, S.O., Goode, J., Lin, P., Mann, N., Mudd, S., Crozat, K., Sovath, S., Han, J., & Beutler, B. (2003a) Identification of Lps2 as a key transducer of MyD88-independent TIR signaling. Nature, 424, 743–748.

Hoebe, K., Georgel, P., Rutschmann, S., Du, X., Mudd, S., Crozat, K., Sovath, S., Shamel, L., Hartung, T., Zahringer, U., & Beutler, B. (2005) CD36 is a sensor of diacylglycerides. Nature, 433, 523–527.

Hoebe, K., Jannsen, E.M., Kim, S.O., Alexopoulou, L., Flavell, R.A., Han, J., & Beutler, B. (2003b) Upregulation of costimulatory molecules induced by lipopolysaccharide and double-stranded RNA occurs by Trif-dependent and Trif-independent pathways. Nature Immunology, 4, 1223–1229.

Horng, T., Barton, G.M., Flavell, R.A., & Medzhitov, R. (2002) The adaptor molecule TIRAP provides signalling specificity for Toll-like receptors. Nature, 420, 329–333.

Jiang, Z., Mak, T.W., Sen, G., & Li, X. (2004) Toll-like receptor 3-mediated activation of NF-kappaB and IRF3 diverges at Toll-IL-1 receptor domain-containing adapter inducing IFN-beta. Proceedings of the National Academy of Sciences of the United States of America, 101, 3533–3538.

Jurk, M., Heil, F., Vollmer, J., Schetter, C., Krieg, A.M., Wagner, H., Lipford, G., & Bauer, S. (2002) Human TLR7 or TLR8 independently confer responsiveness to the antiviral compound R-848. Nature Immunology, 3, 499.

Kiechl, S., Lorenz, E., Reindl, M., Wiedermann, C.J., Oberhollenzer, F., Bonora, E., Willeit, J., & Schwartz, D.A. (2002) Toll-like receptor 4 polymorphisms and atherogenesis. New England Journal of Medicine, 347, 185–192.

Kinjyo, I., Hanada, T., Inagaki-Ohara, K., Mori, H., Aki, D., Ohishi, M., Yoshida, H., Kubo, M., & Yoshimura, A. (2002) SOCS1/JAB is a negative regulator of LPS-induced macrophage activation. Immunity, 17, 583–591.

Kobayashi, K., Hernandez, L.D., Galan, J.E., Janeway, C.A., Jr., Medzhitov, R., & Flavell, R.A. (2002) IRAK-M is a negative regulator of Toll-like receptor signaling. Cell, 110, 191–202.

Leadbetter, E.A., Rifkin, I.R., Hohlbaum, A.M., Beaudette, B.C., Shlomchik, M.J., & Marshak-Rothstein, A. (2002) Chromatin-IgG complexes activate B cells by dual engagement of IgM and Toll-like receptors. Nature, 416, 603–607.

Lien, E., Means, T.K., Heine, H., Yoshimura, A., Kusumoto, S., Fukase, K., Fenton, M.J., Oikawa, M., Qureshi, N., Monks, B., Finberg, R.W., Ingalls, R.R., & Golenbock, D.T. (2000) Toll-like receptor 4 imparts ligand-specific recognition of bacterial lipopolysaccharide. Journal of Clinical Investigation, 105, 497–504.

Lorenz, E., Mira, J.P., Cornish, K.L., Arbour, N.C., & Schwartz, D.A. (2000) A novel polymorphism in the toll-like receptor 2 gene and its potential association with staphylococcal infection. Infection and Immunity, 68, 6398–6401.

Lund, J., Sato, A., Akira, S., Medzhitov, R., & Iwasaki, A. (2003) Toll-like receptor 9-mediated recognition of Herpes simplex virus-2 by plasmacytoid dendritic cells. Journal of Experimental Medicine, 198, 513–520.

Lund, J.M., Alexopoulou, L., Sato, A., Karow, M., Adams, N.C., Gale, N.W., Iwasaki, A., & Flavell, R.A. (2004) Recognition of single-stranded RNA viruses by Toll-like receptor 7. Proceedings of the National Academy of Sciences of the United States of America, 101, 5598–5603.

Maldonado, C., Trejo, W., Ramirez, A., Carrera, M., Sanchez, J., Lopez-Macias, C., & Isibasi, A. (2000) Lipophosphopeptidoglycan of Entamoeba histolytica induces an antiinflammatory innate immune response and downregulation of Toll-like receptor 2 (TLR-2) gene expression in human monocytes. Archives of Medical Research, 31, S71-S73.

Medzhitov, R., Preston-Hurlburt, P., & Janeway, C.A., Jr. (1997) A human homologue of the Drosophila Toll protein signals activation of adaptive immunity. Nature, 388, 394–397.

Nagai, Y., Akashi, S., Nagafuku, M., Ogata, M., Iwakura, Y., Akira, S., Kitamura, T., Kosugi, A., Kimoto, M., & Miyake, K. (2002) Essential role of MD-2 in LPS responsiveness and TLR4 distribution. Nature Immunology, 3, 667–672.

O'Brien, A.D., Rosenstreich, D.L., Scher, I., Campbell, G.H., MacDermott, R.P., & Formal, S.B. (1980) Genetic control of susceptibility to Salmonella typhimurium in mice: Role of the LPS gene. Journal of Immunology, 124, 20–24.

Ozinsky, A., Underhill, D.M., Fontenot, J.D., Hajjar, A.M., Smith, K.D., Wilson, C.B., Schroeder, L., & Aderem, A. (2000) The repertoire for pattern recognition of pathogens by the innate immune system is defined by cooperation between toll-like receptors. Proceedings of the National Academy of Sciences of the United States of America, 97, 13766–13771.

Picard, C., Puel, A., Bonnet, M., Ku, C.L., Bustamante, J., Yang, K., Soudais, C., Dupuis, S., Feinberg, J., Fieschi, C., Elbim, C., Hitchcock, R., Lammas, D., Davies, G., Al Ghonaium, A., Al Rayes, H., Al Jumaah, S., Al Hajjar, S., Al Mohsen, I.Z., Frayha, H.H., Rucker, R., Hawn, T.R., Aderem, A., Tufenkeji, H., Haraguchi, S., Day, N.K., Good, R.A., Gougerot-Pocidalo, M.A., Ozinsky, A., & Casanova, J.L. (2003) Pyogenic bacterial infections in humans with IRAK-4 deficiency. Science, 299, 2076–2079.

Poltorak, A., He, X., Smirnova, I., Liu, M.-Y., Van Huffel, C., Du, X., Birdwell, D., Alejos, E., Silva,

M., Galanos, C., Freudenberg, M.A., Ricciardi-Castagnoli, P., Layton, B., & Beutler, B. (1998) Defective LPS signaling in C3H/HeJ and C57BL/10ScCr mice: Mutations in Tlr4 gene. Science, 282, 2085–2088.

Poltorak, A., Ricciardi-Castagnoli, P., Citterio, A., & Beutler, B. (2000) Physical contact between LPS and Tlr4 revealed by genetic complementation. Proceedings of the National Academy of Sciences of the United States of America, 97, 2163–2167.

Rosenstreich, D.L., Weinblatt, A.C., & O'Brien, A.D. (1982) Genetic control of resistance to infection in mice. CRC Critical Reviews in Immunology, 3, 263–330.

Sato, S., Sugiyama, M., Yamamoto, M., Watanabe, Y., Kawai, T., Takeda, K., & Akira, S. (2003) Toll/IL-1 receptor domain-containing adaptor inducing IFN-beta (TRIF) associates with TNF receptor-associated factor 6 and TANK-binding kinase 1, and activates two distinct transcription factors, NF-kappa B and IFN-regulatory factor-3, in the Toll-like receptor signaling. Journal of Immunology, 171, 4304–4310.

Schneider, D.S., Hudson, K.L., Lin, T.Y., & Anderson, K.V. (1991) Dominant and recessive mutations define functional domains of Toll, a transmembrane protein required for dorsal-ventral polarity in the Drosophila embryo. Genes and Development, 5, 797–807.

Skidmore, B.J., Chiller, J.M., Morrison, D.C., & Weigle, W.O. (1975a) Immunologic properties of bacterial lipopolysaccharide (LPS): Correlation between the mitogenic, adjuvant, and immunogenic activities. Journal of Immunology, 114, 770–775.

Skidmore, B.J., Chiller, J.M., & Weigle, W.O. (1977) Immunologic properties of bacterial lipopolysaccharide (LPS). IV. Cellular basis of the unresponsiveness of C3H/HeJ mouse spleen cells to LPS-induced mitogenesis. Journal of Immunology, 118, 274–281.

Skidmore, B.J., Chiller, J.M., Weigle, W.O., Riblet, R., & Watson, J. (1976) Immunologic properties of bacterial lipopolysaccharide (LPS). III. Genetic linkage between the in vitro mitogenic and in vivo adjuvant properties of LPS. Journal of Experimental Medicine, 143, 143–150.

Skidmore, B.J., Morrison, D.C., Chiller, J.M., & Weigle, W.O. (1975b) Immunologic properties of bacterial lipopolysaccharide (LPS). II. The unresponsiveness of C3H/HeJ mouse spleen cells to LPS-induced mitogenesis is dependent on the method used to extract LPS. Journal of Experimental Medicine, 142, 1488–1508.

Smirnova, I., Hamblin, M., McBride, C., Beutler, B., & Di Rienzo, A. (2001) Excess of rare amino acid polymorphisms in the Toll-like receptor 4 in humans. Genetics, 158, 1657–1664.

Smirnova, I., Mann, N., Dols, A., Derkx, H.H., Hibberd, M.L., Levin, M., & Beutler, B. (2003) Assay of locus-specific genetic load implicates rare Toll-like receptor 4 mutations in meningococcal susceptibility. Proceedings of the National Academy of Sciences of the United States of America, 100, 6075–6080.

Sorensen, T.I., Nielsen, G.G., Andersen, P.K., & Teasdale, T.W. (1988) Genetic and environmental influences on premature death in adult adoptees. New England Journal of Medicine, 318, 727–732.

Su, Z., Dannull, J., Heiser, A., Yancey, D., Pruitt, S., Madden, J., Coleman, D., Niedzwiecki, D., Gilboa, E., & Vieweg, J. (2003) Immunological and clinical responses in metastatic renal cancer patients vaccinated with tumor RNA-transfected dendritic cells. Cancer Research, 63, 2127–2133.

Suzuki, N., Suzuki, S., Duncan, G.S., Millar, D.G., Wada, T., Mirtsos, C., Takada, H., Wakeham, A., Itie, A., Li, S., Penninger, J.M., Wesche, H., Ohashi, P.S., Mak, T.W., & Yeh, W.C. (2002) Severe impairment of interleukin-1 and Toll-like receptor signalling in mice lacking IRAK-4. Nature, 416, 750–756.

Tabeta, K., Georgel, P., Janssen, E., Du, X., Hoebe, K., Crozat, K., Mudd, S., Shamel, L., Sovath, S., Goode, J., Alexopoulou, L., Flavell, R., & Beutler, B. (2004) TLR9 and TLR3 as essential components of innate immune defense against mouse cytomegalovirus. Proceedings of the National Academy of Sciences of the United States of America, 101, 3516–3521.

Tabeta, K., Hoebe, K. Janssen, E.M., Du, X., Georgel, P., Crozat, K., Mudd, S., Mann, N., Sovath, S., Goode, J., Shamel, L., Herskovits, A., Portnoy, D., Cooke, M., Tarantion, L.M., Wiltshire, T., Steinberg, B.E., Grinstein, S., & Beutler, B. (2006) The Unc93b1 mutation 3d disrupts exogenous antigen presentation signaling via Toll-like receptors 3, 7 and 9. Nature Immunology, 7, 156–164.

Takeuchi, O., Hoshino, K., & Akira, S. (2000) Cutting edge: TLR2-deficient and MyD88-deficient mice are highly susceptible to Staphylococcus aureus infection. Journal of Immunology, 165, 5392–5396.

Takeuchi, O., Hoshino, K., Kawai, T., Sanjo, H., Takada, H., Ogawa, T., Takeda, K., & Akira, S. (1999) Differential roles of TLR2 and TLR4 in recognition of gram-negative and gram-positive bacterial cell wall components. Immunity, 11, 443–451.

Takeuchi, O., Kawai, T., Muhlradt, P.F., Morr, M., Radolf, J.D., Zychlinsky, A., Takeda, K., & Akira, S. (2001) Discrimination of bacterial lipoproteins by Toll-like receptor 6. International Immunology, 13, 933–940.

Takeuchi, O., Sato, S., Horiuchi, T., Hoshino, K., Takeda, K., Dong, Z., Modlin, R.L., & Akira, S. (2002) Cutting edge: Role of Toll-like receptor 1 in mediating immune response to microbial lipoproteins. Journal of Immunology, 169, 10–14.

Tobias, P.S., Mathison, J.C., & Ulevitch, R.J. (1988) A family of lipopolysaccharide binding proteins involved in responses to gram-negative sepsis. Journal of Biological Chemistry, 263, 13479–13481.

Underhill, D.M., Ozinsky, A., Smith, K.D., & Aderem, A. (1999) Toll-like receptor-2 mediates mycobacteria-induced proinflammatory signaling in macrophages. Proceedings of the National Academy of Sciences of the United States of America, 96, 14459–14463.

Weigle, W.O., & Skidmore, B.J. (1975) Mechanism of activation and tolerance induction in B lymphocytes. Transplantation Reviews, 23, 250–257.

Wright, S.D., Ramos, R.A., Tobias, P.S., Ulevitch, R.J., & Mathison, J.C. (1990) CD14, a receptor for complexes of lipopolysaccharide (LPS) and LPS binding protein. Science, 249, 1431–1433.

Xu, Y., Tao, X., Shen, B., Horng, T., Medzhitov, R., Manley, J.L., & Tong, L. (2000) Structural basis for signal transduction by the Toll/interleukin-1 receptor domains. Nature, 408, 111–115.

Yamamoto, M., Sato, S., Hemmi, H., Hoshino, K., Kaisho, T., Sanjo, H., Takeuchi, O., Sugiyama, M., Okabe, M., Takeda, K., & Akira, S. (2003a) Role of adapter TRIF in the MyD88-independent Toll-like receptor signaling pathway. Science, 301, 640–643.

Yamamoto, M., Sato, S., Hemmi, H., Sanjo, H., Uematsu, S., Kaisho, T., Hoshino, K., Takeuchi, O., Kobayashi, M., Fujita, T., Takeda, K., & Akira, S. (2002) Essential role for TIRAP in activation of the signalling cascade shared by TLR2 and TLR4. Nature, 420, 324–329.

Yamamoto, M., Sato, S., Hemmi, H., Uematsu, S., Hoshino, K., Kaisho, T., Takeuchi, O., Takeda, K., & Akira, S. (2003b) TRAM is specifically involved in the Toll-like receptor 4-mediated MyD88-independent signaling pathway. Nature Immunology, 4, 1144–1150.

Zhang, D., Zhang, G., Hayden, M.S., Greenblatt, M.B., Bussey, C., Flavell, R.A., & Ghosh, S. (2004) A toll-like receptor that prevents infection by uropathogenic bacteria. Science, 303, 1522–1152.

13

Metal Transport Genes

Jean-François Marquis, John R. Forbes, François Canonne-Hergaux,
Cynthia Horth, & Philippe Gros

Susceptibility to infections, with respect to initial onset, progression, and ultimate outcome of disease, is influenced by a number of factors, including pathogen-encoded virulence determinants, the genetic makeup of the host, and environmental factors that can modulate the expression of both. The laboratory mouse has been a valuable model for the genetic analysis of host susceptibility determinants and pathogen-encoded virulence factors. The discovery of a mutation in a macrophage-specific metal transporter that causes susceptibility to infection by several unrelated intracellular pathogens has suggested that metal deprivation is a critical mechanism by which macrophages restrict replication of intracellular pathogens. Likewise, the observation that pathogens possess a number of metal acquisition systems, some of which are essential for virulence *in vivo*, has confirmed the critical importance of divalent metals in the outcome of host–pathogen interaction. Metals may be required for the basic metabolic activity necessary for expression of intracellular survival strategies, including the modulation of phagosome maturation,

and/or may be required for the activity of microbial enzymes essential for detoxification of the phagosomal environment. This review discusses two families of mammalian metal transporters expressed in macrophages, Nramp (Slc11a1, Slc11a2) and ferroportin (Slc40a1), and the possible roles these proteins play in the antimicrobial properties of these cells. Recent studies characterizing the biochemical content of bacterial phagosomes formed in macrophages, and the transcriptional responses of bacteria exposed to this environment are also reviewed.

The Nramp Protein Family and Evolutionary Relationships

Susceptibility to infection by a broad spectrum of intracellular pathogens, including *Mycobacterium*, *Leishmania*, and *Salmonella*, is controlled in mice by a single locus known as *Ity*, *Lsh*, or *Bcg* (Skamene et al., 1998). Characterization of the *Bcg/Ity/Lsh* locus identified the *Nramp1* gene (natural resistance associated macrophage protein 1; recently renamed solute carrier family 11 member 1, *Slc11a1*: Online Mendelian Inheritance in Man [OMIM] ID 600266) as a positional candidate whose mRNA expression was limited to macrophages and polymorphonuclear leukocytes (Govoni et al., 1997; Vidal et al., 1993). A second mammalian Nramp gene was identified, *Nramp2* (OMIM ID 600523; also known as *DMT1*, *DCT1*, and now designated *Slc11a2*), whose product shares 64% amino acid identity (78% overall similarity) with Nramp1 (Gruenheid et al., 1995).

Large-scale genome sequencing projects have shown that mammalian Nramp is part of a very ancient family of membrane proteins with orthologs described in mammals, birds, insects, plants, fish, yeast, and bacteria (Forbes and Gros, 2001; Lam-Yuk-Tseung and Gros, 2003). For example, the yeast *Saccharomyces cerevisiae* expresses three members of the *Nramp* family, *SMF1*, -2, and -3 (Portnoy et al., 2000). Studies in yeast (Portnoy et al., 2000; Supek et al., 1997) and in *Xenopus laevis* oocytes (Chen et al., 1999; Sacher et al., 2001) have revealed that all three proteins function as pH-dependent, divalent-metal transporters with a broad substrate specificity (Fe^{2+}, Mn^{2+}, Cd^{2+}, Cu^{2+}), with Smf3p being more selective for Fe^{2+}. Similarly, bacterial members of this family (designated MntH) from *Escherichia coli*, *Salmonella typhimurium*, and *Mycobacterium tuberculosis* have been shown to be multispecific, pH-dependent, divalent-metal uptake transporters exhibiting a preference for Mn^{2+} ions (Agranoff et al., 1999; Kehres et al., 2000; Makui et al., 2000). Complementation studies using model organisms such as *Drosophila melanogaster* and *S. cerevisiae* have shown that within the *Nramp* family, sequence conservation is directly translated into functional conservation as mammalian Nramp2 can complement loss-of-function mutants at both corresponding fly and yeast loci (Forbes and Gros, 2001; Lam-Yuk-Tseung and Gros, 2003).

NRAMP1-induced Metal Deprivation and Susceptibility to Infections

NRAMP1 Gene (Now Designated *SLC11A1*) in Infection

The murine *Nramp1* gene (now *Slc11a1*) controls susceptibility to infection by a broad spectrum of intracellular bacteria/parasites, including *Mycobacterium*, *Leishmania*, and *Salmonella* (Skamene et al., 1998). Susceptible mice (*Bcg^s*) exhibit rapid microbial replication within the reticuloendothelial organs, whereas resistant (*Bcg^r*) animals do not. Experiments *in vivo* and with explanted cell populations have demonstrated that macrophages are responsible for the phenotypic expression of infection resistance/susceptibility in mice (Gros et al., 1983). The critical role of Nramp1 in susceptibility to infection in mice was confirmed by the creation and characterization of gain-of-function and loss-of-function mutations in transgenic mice (Govoni et al., 1996; Vidal et al., 1995b).

In macrophages, Nramp1 is synthesized as a 56-kDa precursor (Cellier et al., 1995) and is modified to a 90- to 100-kDa phosphoglycoprotein expressed in the membrane fraction of macrophages (Vidal et al., 1996). Nramp1 is localized to the membrane of Lamp-1–positive lysosomes/late-endosomes in primary macrophages and macrophage-derived cell lines (Gruenheid et al., 1997). During phagocytosis by macrophages, Nramp1 is rapidly recruited from late endosomes/lysosomes to the membrane of phagosomes containing either inert particles (Gruenheid et al., 1997) or live pathogens, including *Salmonella*, *Leishmania*, *Mycobacterium*, and *Yersinia* (Cuellar-Mata et al., 2002; Govoni et al., 1999; et al., 1998) (figure 13.1).

Using microfluorescence imaging with metal-sensitive fluorescent dyes to monitor divalent-metal fluxes across the membrane of phagosomes in primary murine *Nramp1$^{+/+}$* or *Nramp1$^{-/-}$* macrophages (Jabado et al., 2000), we observed that *Nramp1$^{+/+}$* phagosomes show reduced accumulation of Mn^{2+} ions at steady state. In addition, *Nramp1$^{+/+}$* phagosomes showed increased release of Mn^{2+} from preloaded phagosomes together demonstrating that Nramp1 functions in a pH-dependent fashion to efflux Mn^{2+} ions from acidified phagosomes down the proton gradient. Independent biochemical studies (Atkinson and Barton, 1998, 1999) support the notion that this transport mechanism resembles iron transport by Nramp2 at the membrane of acidified endosomes.

Mycobacterial Infections

Many studies of Nramp1 and its role in mycobacterial infections have been performed. Mycobacteria survive within macrophages by inhibiting the maturation of phagosomes into fully bactericidal phagolysosomes (Clemens and Horwitz, 1995; Clemens et al., 2000a, 2000b; Russell et al., 1996; Schaible et al., 1998;

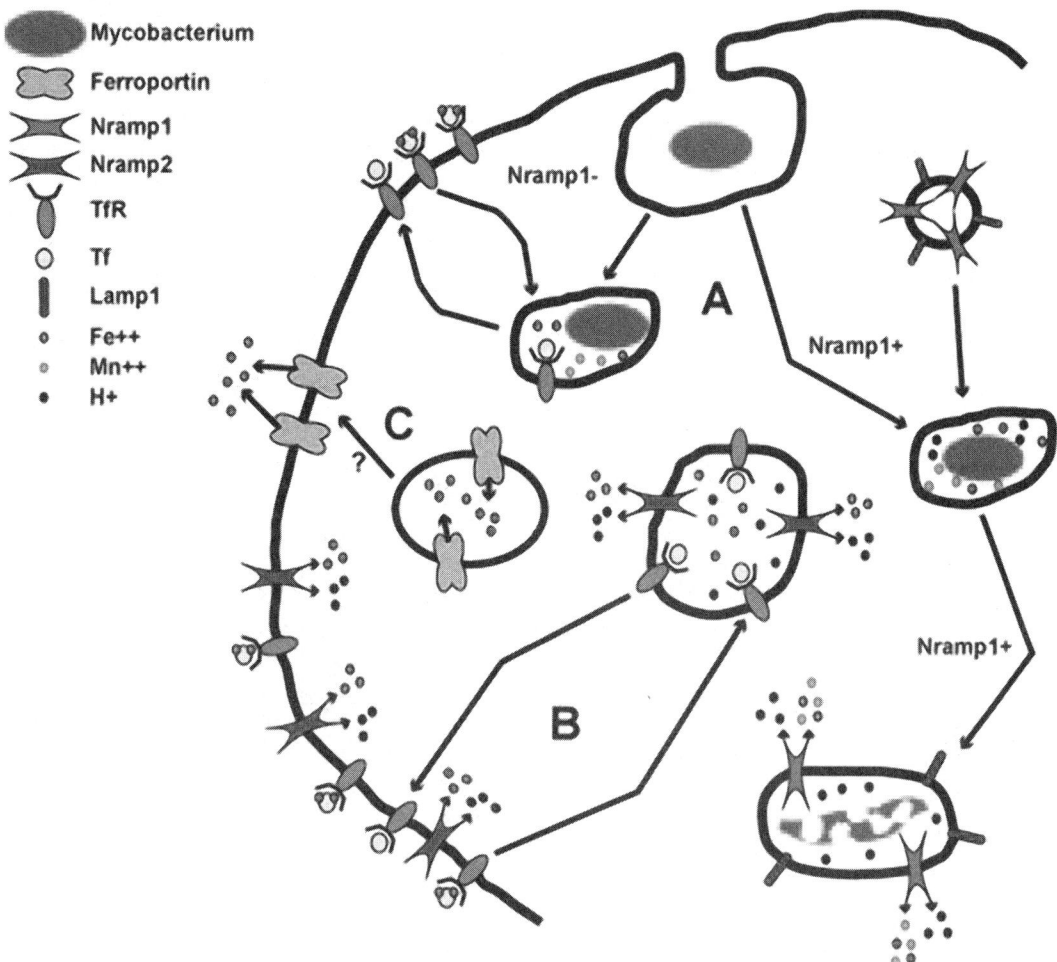

FIGURE 13.1. Model for metal transport by Nramp1 and ferroportin in macrophages. (A) Mycobacteria phagocytosed by macrophages are initially enclosed within a PM-derived phagosome. In $Nramp1^{-/-}$ macrophages, these phagosomes remain immature, displaying characteristics of recycling endosomes and are positive for transferrin receptor (TfR). Such phagosomes are permissive for bacterial replication. In $Nramp1^{+/+}$ macrophages, mycobacterial phagosomes fuse with Lamp-1–positive and Nramp1-positive late endosomes/ lysosomes and mature to acidified phagolysosomes. Such phagosomes are nonpermissive for bacterial replication, and mycobacteria internalized under these conditions are destroyed (Frehel et al, 2002). Mycobacterial inhibition of phagosome maturation is an active, metal-dependent process. Nramp1-mediated efflux of divalent metals such as iron and manganese from the phagosomal lumen would antagonize this process. (B) Nramp2 expressed at the duodenum brush border is responsible for transferrin-independent uptake of dietary iron. In peripheral cells, including macrophages, the majority of Nramp2 is found in TfR-positive recycling endosomes (and late endosomes), where it acts to efflux transferrin-delivered iron into the cytosol down a pH gradient generated by the vacuolar H^+-ATPase. The endomembrane Nramp2 pool is in dynamic equilibrium with a smaller PM pool, and Nramp2 cycles between the two using phosphatidyl inositol-3-kinase–regulated exocytosis and clathrin-dependent endocytosis pathways. (C) Ferroportin is inducible by iron and copper and in macrophages stimulates iron efflux from phagocytosed red blood cells (erythrophagocytosis). Since ferroportin has not been detected at the PM, it has been proposed that metal efflux may occur by redistribution of the protein to the PM in response to intracellular iron (Knutson et al., 2003) or by transport into an endomembrane compartment followed by exocytosis.

Sturgill-Koszycki et al., 1994, 1996). Electron micros-copy studies show that recruitment of Nramp1 to the membrane of *M. avium* containing phagosomes causes bacteriostasis, increased bacterial damage, increased acidification and increased fusion to lysosomes when compared to $Nramp1^{-/-}$ phagosomes (Frehel et al., 2002; Hackam et al., 1998). A simple explanation of these results is that inhibition of phagosome maturation by mycobacteria requires a metal-dependent, active process that can be antagonized by Nramp1-mediated metal efflux from the phagosomal lumen.

Infection of human macrophages or mice with *M. tuberculosis* results in induction of several mycobacte-rial genes required for siderophore-mediated iron up-take, and mutations of some of these genes attenuate virulence *in vivo* (De Voss et al., 2000; Gold et al., 2001; Timm et al., 2003). This suggests that iron is li-miting during mycobacterial infection, including with-in the macrophage-specific phagosomal stage. Indeed, iron enhances mycobacterial growth in $Nramp1^{+/+}$ mice and promotes development of active tuberculosis (and growth of other pathogens) in humans (Gomes and Appelberg, 1998; Ratledge, 2004). The ability of mycobacteria to modulate phagosomal maturation and the capacity of Nramp1 to antagonize this phenome-non have now been linked to iron (Kelley and Schorey, 2003). Rab5 is a cytosolic GTPase involved in regu-lating fusion of endosomes with phagosomes that may be targeted for inhibition by mycobacteria-dependent arrest of phagosome maturation at the immature en-dosomal stage (Clemens et al., 2000a; Kelley and Schorey, 2003). Expression of a dominant-negative Rab5 mutant into $Nramp1^{-/-}$ bone marrow macro-phages was shown to stimulate maturation of *M. avium*-containing phagosomes toward mature, Lamp-1–positive, phagolysosomes, causing increased bacte-riostatic activity (Kelley and Schorey, 2003). Rab5-forced maturation could be inhibited by preloading the macrophage with iron citrate. These results suggest that an adequate supply of iron within the phagosome is required by mycobacteria to maintain the block of phagosomal maturation and therefore survive intra-cellularly. Thus, Nramp1-induced depletion of pha-gosomal iron could impair the ability of mycobacteria to modulate phagolysosomal fusion.

Salmonella Infections

As with mycobacteria, *Salmonella* survive within mac-rophages by interfering with phagosome maturation

and reside in specialized *Salmonella*-containing vac-uoles (SCVs) (Knodler and Steele-Mortimer, 2003). $Nramp1^{-/-}$ SCVs exhibit reduced incorporation of the lysosomal M6PR (marker mannose 6 phosphate receptor) and become inaccessible to endosomal ves-icles loaded with extracellular fluid-phase tracers after invasion, both of which occur robustly in $Nramp1^{+/+}$ SCVs. Nramp1 is able to counteract the ability of *Salmonella* to become secluded from the degradative pathways of macrophage (Cuellar-Mata et al., 2002). As opposed to mycobacteria, SCVs formed in both $Nramp1^{+/+}$ and $Nramp1^{-/-}$ macrophages acidify fully and recruit the lysosomal marker Lamp-1. The phagosomal bacteria reacted to the presence of Nramp1 by the transcriptional induction of a number of viru-lence genes, including *ssrA* and *sseJ* that map within *Salmonella* pathogenicity island 2 (*SPI2*) (Zaharik et al., 2002). Thus, presence of Nramp1 at the mem-brane of SCV is associated with changes in biochem-ical and fusogenic properties of these vesicles, resulting in increased bacteriostatic activity of macrophages.

An adequate supply of iron and manganese is es-sential for *Salmonella* virulence *in vivo*, and for intra-cellular replication in macrophages *in vitro* (Kehres and Maguire, 2003; Ratledge, 2004). *Salmonella* pos-sesses several high- or low-affinity, ATP-dependent or proton-coupled (*tonB* dependent) iron transporters, such as *fepBCDG*, *sitA-D*, *FeoABC*, *CorAD*, and the *Nramp* homolog *MntH* (Hantke, 1997; Kammler et al., 1993; Kehres et al., 2002; Tsolis et al., 1996; Zhou et al., 1999). Many of these transporters have been shown to be essential for *Salmonella* virulence *in vivo* (Bearden and Perry, 1999; Boyer et al., 2002; Jana-kiraman and Slauch, 2000; Tsolis et al., 1996). Single mutations at *feoB* or *sitA-D* reduced virulence, while double mutations at *mntH*, *sitA-D*, or *feoB* completely abrogated *Salmonella* virulence in $Nramp1^{-/-}$ mu-tant 129sv mice *in vivo*.

Pathogenesis

In humans, NRAMP1 mRNA is expressed in spleen and lung and at high levels in peripheral blood leu-kocytes (Cellier et al., 1997). Studies in primary cells as well as in model cell lines (HL-60) established that NRAMP1 mRNA expression in monocytes is increased upon migration of these cells to tissues and is partic-ularly abundant in neutrophils (Cellier et al., 1997). The cellular and subcellular localization of the human NRAMP1 protein was studied in primary neutrophils

(Canonne-Hergaux et al., 2002). Subcellular fractionation of granule populations together with immunoblotting studies with granule-specific markers showed that NRAMP1 is primarily in tertiary granules that are positive for the matrix enzyme gelatinase and membrane subunits of the vacuolar H^+-ATPase. Immunofluorescence studies of *Candida albicans*–containing phagosomes formed in neutrophils indicate that NRAMP1 is recruited from tertiary granules to the phagosomal membrane upon phagocytosis (Canonne-Hergaux et al., 2002). These results suggest that, as in mouse macrophages, human NRAMP1 may play an important role in the antimicrobial and inflammatory activity of neutrophils.

Gene Organization and Regulation

The human *SLC11A1* gene for NRAMP1 maps to chromosomal region 2q35 (table 13.1) in close proximity to the interleukin-8 (IL-8) receptor gene (Cellier et al., 1994). The gene is composed of 15 exons, including one that is alternatively spliced. Comparison of the human (locus link 6556) and mouse (locus link 18173) predicted NRAMP protein sequences revealed a remarkable degree of conservation between the two polypeptides, with 88% identical residues and 93% overall sequence similarity (Cellier et al., 1994). *SLC11A1* gene expression has been shown to be induced in HL-60 cells treated with the active form of vitamin D [VD; 1α, 25-$(OH)_2D_3$1α,25-dihydroxyvitamin D_3], a steroid hormone known to stimulate the production and terminal maturation of bactericidal macrophages. Indeed, VD genomic effects stimulate NRAMP1 transcription and protein expression in maturing phagocytes (Roig et al., 2002).

Nramp1 mRNA is transcribed from a TATA-less promoter that contains consensus binding sequences for the macrophage and B-cell–specific transcription factor PU.1, response elements for lipopolysaccharide (LPS) and interferon-γ (IFN-γ), and *cis*-acting

TABLE 13.1. Human *Nramp* and *Ferroportin* genes.

Gene ID	Common Name(s)	Locus Link	OMIM ID	Map Position	Single Nucleotide Polymorphisms, Indels, Truncations	References
SLC11A1	NRAMP1 ITY LSH BCG	6556 *18173*[a]	600266	2q35	Two in promoter region [1 $(CA)_n$ repeat, −236C/T], four in the coding portion [A318V (exon 9), D543N (exon 15); 2 silent], one in introns 4 (469 + 14G/C), 5 (577−18G/A), and 13 (1465−85G/A), and two insertion/deletion polymorphisms in the 3′ UTR (1729 + 55delTGTG and 276insCAAA280)	(Blackwell et al, 1995; Buu et al, 1995; Lewis et al, 1996; Liu et al, 1995)
SLC11A2	NRAMP2D CT1 DMT1	4891 *18174*[a]	600523	12q13	One mutation in exon 12 of *DMT1* (1285G > C; E399D), a 3-bp deletion (del CTT) in intron 4, and an amino acid substitution in exon 13 ($DMT1^{C1246T}$, R416C)	(Gunshin et al, 2005b; Iolascon et al, 2006; Lam-Yuk-Tseung et al, 2005, 2006; Priwitzerova et al, 2004, 2005)
SLC40A1	FPN1 (ferroportin) SLC11A3IR EG1 MTP1 HFE4	30061 *53945*[a]	604653	2q32	Y64N, A77D, N144X, D157G, Δ162, Q182H, Q248H, G323V, C326Y, G490D	(Wessling-Resnick, 2006)

[a]Mouse locus link.

elements for binding transcription factors AP1 through AP3 and the Sp1 binding motif (Govoni et al., 1995). Nramp1 mRNA expression in macrophages can be stimulated by LPS, IFN γ, or inflammatory stimuli *in vivo* (Govoni et al., 1995, 1997). This positive regulation occurs via synergistic binding of the transcription factors IRF-8, Miz-1, and PU.1 to the *Nramp1* promoter (Alter-Koltunoff et al., 2003; Bowen et al., 2002et al., 2003). c-Myc represses Nramp1 transcription through competitive inhibition of Miz-1 binding (Bowen et al., 2002et al., 2003). IRF-8 is also involved in regulating the expression of inflammatory cytokines IL-12, IL-18, and IL-1β and plays a role in controlling the macrophage reactive oxygen (*phox*) and nitrogen (*iNOS*) production pathways, thereby linking Nramp1 expression to the inflammatory response of mature macrophages against microbial pathogens (Alter-Koltunoff et al., 2003).

Polymorphisms and Populations

In mice, susceptibility to bacterial/parasitic infection is caused by a single Gly169Asp amino acid substitution in the predicted TM4 of Nramp1 that leads to a loss of protein expression in macrophage (Vidal et al., 1993, 1996).

In humans, a total of 11 sequence polymorphisms have been so far identified in *SLC11A1*, with two located in the promoter region [1 (CA)$_n$ repeat, −236C/T], four in the coding portion (A318V, D543N; two silent), three in introns 4, 5, and 13, and two insertion/deletion polymorphisms in the 3′ region of the gene (Blackwell et al., 1995; Buu et al., 1995; Lewis et al., 1996; Liu et al., 1995) (table 13.1). Of particular interest is the 5′ (CA)$_n$ polymorphism, for which several informative alleles have been identified. This polymorphism was shown to be functional as several alleles drive different levels of expression of a reporter luciferase gene (Searle and Blackwell, 1999) following transfection into U937 cells. Over the past years, a number of these polymorphic variants have been used in linkage or in association studies to investigate the possible association of *SLC11A1* with disease. Table 13.2 summarizes reports showing positive association of *SLC11A1* polymorphisms with infectious diseases such as tuberculosis and leprosy, and also with inflammatory conditions such as rheumatoid arthritis and inflammatory bowel diseases. In many instances, both positive associations and a lack of association in different populations and in different

study designs have been reported, and the reader is referred to chapter 22 and to excellent recent reviews for a more complete description of the relationship between *SLC11A1* and these diseases (Blackwell et al., 2004; Poon and Schurr, 2004).

SLC11A2 (Encoding NRAMP2)

Pathogenesis

Transport studies in *Xenopus* oocytes and mammalian cells (Forbes and Gros, 2003; Gunshin et al., 1997; Lam-Yuk-Tseung et al., 2003; Picard et al., 2000; Tandy et al., 2000) have shown that Nramp2 transports many divalent metals, including iron. Metal transport was saturable and pH dependent (Forbes and Gros, 2003; Gunshin et al., 1997; Picard et al., 2000; Tandy et al., 2000). It has been shown that Nramp2 is an active, proton/divalent-metal cotransporter (Gunshin et al., 1997). In mice, Nramp2 is ubiquitously expressed but is most abundant in the kidney and intestine (Canonne-Hergaux et al., 2000; Canonne-Hergaux and Gros, 2002; Gruenheid et al., 1995). The Nramp2 protein is expressed at the duodenum brush border, where it is regulated by dietary iron and is responsible for transferrin-independent uptake of dietary iron from the intestinal lumen (Canonne-Hergaux et al., 1999). Subcellular localization studies in reticulocytes and transfected epithelial cells showed that the majority of Nramp2 is found within an acidic endomembrane compartment positive for the transferrin receptor that corresponds to recycling endosomes (Canonne-Hergaux et al., 2001; Touret et al., 2003). Nramp2 transports transferrin-delivered iron from the lumen of acidified endosomes into the cytoplasm, down a proton gradient generated by vacuolar H^+-ATPase (Canonne-Hergaux et al., 2001; Fleming et al., 1998; Gruenheid et al., 1999; Touret et al., 2003). The endomembrane Nramp2 pool is in dynamic equilibrium with a smaller plasma membrane (PM) pool and Nramp2 cycles between the two using phosphatidylinositol-3-kinase–regulated exocytosis and clathrin-dependent endocytosis pathways (Touret et al., 2003). Nramp2 has been shown to associate with latex-bead– or red-blood-cell–containing phagosomes formed in J774 or Raw264.7 macrophage cell lines, and with spermatozoid-containing phagosomes formed in Sertoli cells (Sertoli cell line TM4) (Gruenheid et al., 1999; Jabado et al., 2002). Thus, Nramp2 may be involved in the recycling

TABLE 13.2. The association of *NRAMP1* polymorphisms with infectious diseases, autoimmune diseases, or inflammatory conditions.

Phenotype/Disease	Populations	$(GT)_n$ Allele[a] Associated	References
Tuberculosis	Canada	Not done	Greenwood et al (2000)
	Gambia	Allele 2	Bellamy et al (1998)
	Japan	Allele 2	Gao et al (2000)
	Guinea-Conakry	$(GT)_n$ not associated	Cervino et al (2000)
	Denmark	$(GT)_n$ not associated	Soborg et al (2002)
Pediatric tuberculosis	USA (Houston)	Allele 3	Malik et al (2005)
Leprosy	Vietnam	Not done	Abel et al (1998)
Leprosy (Mitsuda)	Vietnam	Not done	Alcais et al (2000)
HIV	Colombia	Allele 3	Marquet et al (1999)
Kawasaki disease	Japan	Allele 1	Ouchi et al (2003)
Leishmaniasis	Sudan	$(GT)_n$ not associated	Bucheton et al (2003)
Rheumatoid arthritis	UK	Allele 3	Shaw et al (1996)
	Canada	$(GT)_n$ not associated	Singal et al (2000)
	Korea	$(GT)_n$ not associated	Yang et al (2000)
	Latvia	Allele 3	Sanjeevi et al (2000)
	Spain	Allele 2	Rodriguez et al (2002)
Type 1 diabetes	United Kingdom	Allele 3	Esposito et al (1998)
	Japan	Allele 2 (lower in patients)	Bassuny et al (2002)
Inflammatory bowel disease, Crohn's disease, ulcerative colitis	United States	Not done	Hofmeister et al (1997)
	Japan	Allele 7	Kojima et al (2001)
Primary biliary cirrhosis	United Kingdom	Allele 5	Graham et al (2000)
Multiple sclerosis	South Africa	Allele 3 and 5	Kotze et al (2001)

[a]Associations with the major alleles at the functional $(GT)_n$ promoter region polymorphism are shown. Not done indicates that this particular polymorphism was not examined, but associations with other polymorphisms across the locus were demonstrated. Allele 1 = t(GT)5ac(GT)5ac (GT)11g; Allele 2 = /t(GT)5ac(GT)5ac(GT)10g; Allele 3 = /t(GT)5ac(GT)5ac(GT)9g; Allele 5 = /t(GT)4ac(GT)5ac(GT)10g; Allele 7 = /t(GT)5ac(GT)5at(GT)11g.

of iron from effete red blood cells or from degenerating sperm cells after phagocytosis by splenic macrophages or Sertoli cells, respectively. However, Nramp2 function at the phagosomal membrane remains to be confirmed. Based on previous observations (Breuer et al., 1995; Cellier et al., 1995; Chen et al., 1999; Courville et al., 2004; Forbes and Gros, 2003; Gunshin et al., 1997; Keen et al., 2000; Kehres et al., 2000; Lam-Yuk-Tseung et al., 2003; Picard et al., 2000; Sacher et al., 2001; Tandy et al., 2000), Nramp1 and Nramp2 function identically but transport metals in different cell types and, more important, across different cellular membranes and compartments, namely, the PM and recycling endosomes for Nramp2, and the membrane of phagosomes in macrophages for Nramp1 (figure 13.1). The reader is referred to a recent excellent review (Mackenzie and Hediger, 2004) for additional discussion of transport properties of Nramp1/2, with respect to substrate specificity, proton cotransport, and pH dependence.

Gene Organization and Sequence

The human *SLC11A2* gene maps to chromosome 12q13 (Vidal et al., 1995a). The *SLC11A2* (locus link 4891) coding nucleotide sequence is 64% identical to *SLC11A1* (Kishi and Tabuchi, 1997). However, the *SLC11A2* gene contains one additional 5′ exon and one additional alternative spliced 3′ exon (Lee et al., 1998). Alternate splicing at the 3′ end of *SLC11A2* gives rise to two mRNAs distinguished by the presence (isoform I) or absence (isoform II) of an iron-responsive element in the 3′ untranslated region and by different sequences of the carboxy terminus. While isoform I is expressed mainly in epithelial cells, isoform II is expressed abundantly in the erythroid system (Canonne-Hergaux et al., 1999, 2000; Canonne-Hergaux and Gros, 2002).

Polymorphisms and Populations

A Gly185Arg amino acid substitution in Nramp2 causes microcytic anemia in *mk* mice and *Belgrade* rats (Fleming et al., 1997, 1998). This mutation is associated with reduced Nramp2 transport function (Lam-Yuk-Tseung et al., 2003; Su et al., 1998) and defective intracellular targeting (Canonne-Hergaux et al., 2000), thereby impairing both intestinal iron absorption and endosomal iron efflux (Canonne-Hergaux et al., 2001). A similar but more severe phenotype has recently been reported for a mouse mutant with a complete inactivation of *DMT1* ($DMT1^{-/-}$) (Gunshin et al., 2005a).

In humans, a single patient with severe microcytic anemia and iron overload has been reported to carry a mutation in exon 12 of *DMT1* (1285G → C). The mutation has two effects. In a single patient, it severely impaired splicing, caused skipping of exon 12 and introduced an amino acid polymorphism (E399D) in the protein encoded by the remaining properly spliced transcript found in the patient (Priwitzerova et al., 2004). The E399D mutation does not in itself affect expression, function, or targeting of the DMT1 protein (Gunshin et al., 2005b; Lam-Yuk-Tseung et al., 2005; Priwitzerova et al., 2005), and reduced DMT1 function in this patient was likely caused by a quantitative reduction in *DMT1* mRNA levels due to improper splicing. Another patient suffering from microcytic anemia and hepatic iron overload was found to be compound heterozygote for polymorphisms in the iron transporter *DMT1* (Iolascon et al., 2006). The patient possesses two novel mutations in *DMT1*: a 3-bp deletion (del CTT) in intron 4 that partially impairs splicing, and an amino acid substitution in exon 13 ($DMT1^{C1246T}$, R416C) at a conserved residue in transmembrane domain 9 of the protein. $DMT1^{C1246T}$ (R416C) may represent a complete loss-of-function, and a quantitative reduction in DMT1 expression may cause the microcytic anemia and iron overload (Lam-Yuk-Tseung et al., 2006).

The role of NRAMP2/DMT1, if any, in susceptibility to infections in humans (or mice) has not been established. However, the demonstrated expression of this protein in macrophages, the critical role that macrophages play in iron recycling, the noted association of Nramp2 with phagosomes, and the noted effect of overall iron homeostasis on susceptibility to infections (including tuberculosis) suggest that NRAMP2/DMT1 is not unlikely to affect susceptibility.

SLC40A1 (Encoding Ferroportin)

Macrophages express abundant levels of another iron transporter, ferroportin. While not a member of the Nramp family, ferroportin (also called Fpn1, Ireg1, Mtp1) shares some structural similarity with Nramp proteins and has been classified into the solute carrier family in mouse as well as humans, where it is encoded by *SLC40A1* (formerly FPN1).

Pathogenesis

Ferroportin is an integral membrane protein composed of 10 putative transmembrane domains and is expressed in liver, spleen, and bone marrow macrophages (Abboud and Haile, 2000; Donovan et al., 2000; Yang et al., 2002). Ferroportin was originally localized to the basolateral pole of duodenum mucosal cells, where it transports dietary iron across the basal membrane and into the circulation, presumably following uptake of iron at the apical pole by Nramp2 (Abboud and Haile, 2000; Donovan et al., 2000; McKie et al., 2000). In bone marrow macrophages, the ferroportin protein is expressed as a 62-kDa polypeptide (Delaby et al., 2005). Immunofluorescence experiments show that ferroportin is not present at the PM but is found instead in intracellular vesicles (Abboud and Haile, 2000; Yang et al., 2002). In Kupffer cells, these vesicles are positive for both ferroportin and hemosiderin (Abboud and Haile, 2000), suggesting a possible role for ferroportin in intracellular iron trafficking.

In several mouse models of iron deficiency and anemia, expression of ferroportin protein in the spleen is greatly enhanced (F. Canonne-Hergaux, unpublished data), suggesting negative regulation by the body iron store. In LPS-stimulated or *Leishmania donovani* infected mice, ferroportin expression in macrophages was shown to be down-regulated (Yang et al., 2002). Additionally, *in vitro* studies show that IFN-γ and LPS treatment down-regulates expression of ferroportin mRNA in monocytes (Ludwiczek et al., 2003) and macrophages (Delaby 2005). These studies suggest that inflammatory cytokines may regulate iron metabolism in macrophages through modulation of ferro-portin activity, thereby influencing microbial patho-genesis and susceptibility to infections.

Gene Organization, Sequence, and Polymorphisms

Ferroportin is a highly conserved 571 amino acid protein with human, mouse, and rat clones being 90–95% homologous at the protein level. Patients with mutations (see table 13.1) in the *SLC40A1* (ferro-portin) gene (locus link 30061) develop an autosomal-dominant form of iron overload with iron accumula-tion in the reticuloendothelial system (Devalia et al., 2002; Montosi et al., 2001; Njajou et al., 2001; Pie-trangelo, 2004; Wallace et al., 2002; Wessling-Resnick, 2006).

Mutant mice bearing a conditional deletion of the *Slc40a1* gene in macrophages show retention of iron by hepatic Kupffer cells and splenic macrophages (Do-novan et al., 2003), strongly suggesting that ferroportin participates in iron metabolism in macrophages.

Conclusions and Prospects/Needs

The ability to analyze transcription of whole microbial genomes using microarrays has provided a fresh oppor-tunity to gain insight into the nature of the biochem-ical environment pathogens face while inside macro-phages and the type of adaptive response they develop in response to insults from the host, and has allowed the identification of new pathways or targets for phar-macological intervention. Of particular interest are two studies where the transcript profiles of *M. tuber-culosis* (Schnappinger et al., 2003) and *Salmonella* (Eriksson et al., 2003) isolated from macrophage pha-gosomes have been determined.

Since IFN-γ activation of *Nramp1*$^{-/-}$ macrophage stimulates phagolysosomal maturation (Schaible et al., 1998), it is tempting to speculate that IFN-γ–induced conditions may mimic those found in *Nramp1*$^{+/+}$ phagosomes. Indeed, one of the key bacterial responses following macrophage activation was up-regulation of mycobacterial genes involved in metal acquisition (Schnappinger et al., 2003). These accounted for more than half of IFN-γ–responsive genes, suggestive of low metal availability within mycobacterial phagosomes and further emphasizing the critical role of metals in mycobacterial infection. In an *Nramp1*$^{-/-}$ phago-some, metal limitation may have been the result of

activation-dependent phagosomal maturation, decreas-ing the accessibility of phagosomes to transferrin and thereby reducing iron availability (Olakanmi et al., 2002; Schaible et al., 1998).

In contrast to observations in the *Mycobacterium*-containing phagosome, expression profiling of intra-cellular *Salmonella* have suggested an environment replete with oxygen, iron, and amino while deficient in magnesium and phosphate ions. It is possible that this iron-rich environment may be linked in part to the absence of functional Nramp1 in J774 macrophage. One might predict that Nramp1 expression would re-sult in the up-regulation of *Salmonella* metal acquisi-tion systems by depletion of intraphagosomal divalent metals and place the bacteria in a much harsher in-tracellular environment by promoting formation of mature phagolysosomes (Cuellar-Mata et al., 2002; Zaharik et al., 2002).

Current evidence suggests a model in which Nramp1 and possibly ferroportin may compete with bacterially encoded bacterial divalent-metal transport systems for the acquisition of divalent metals within the phagosomal space (Forbes and Gros, 2001). The ultimate outcome of this competitive interaction may determine the success with which intracellular or-ganisms survive and replicate. Divalent metals such as Zn^{2+}, Cu^{2+}, Fe^{2+}, and Mn^{2+} are all essential bacterial micronutrients acting as co-factors in many enzymatic reactions. Therefore, depletion of one or more of these divalent metals from the phagosome by Nramp1 may have a simple and direct bacteriostatic effect by re-moving a rate-limiting nutrient from the ecological niche of intracellular pathogens. Metal depletion of bacteria contained within phagosomes may also en-hance the bactericidal mechanisms of the macrophage by rendering the pathogen more sensitive to killing by reactive nitrogen and/or oxygen species since bacterial antioxidant defense relies in part on the presence of iron or manganese dependent catalase and superoxide-dismutase enzymes. Additionally, Nramp1-mediated depletion of divalent metals from the phagosomal space, either during or prior to phagocytosis, could affect the expression and/or function of secreted bac-terial effector proteins or lipids involved in the mod-ulation of phagosome maturation, thereby having an indirect effect on pathogen survival by promoting the formation of mature bacteriocidal phagolysosomes. Thus, prokaryotic and mammalian divalent-metal transporters appear to be key determinants of bacte-rial virulence and host defenses during intracellular parasitism. Pharmacological modulation of this interaction may represent an appropriate means for the treatment of infections.

References

Abboud, S., & Haile, D.J. (2000) A novel mammalian iron-regulated protein involved in intracellular iron metabolism. *J Biol Chem*, **275**, 19906–19912.

Abel, L., Sanchez, F.O., Oberti, J., Thuc, N.V., Hoa, L.V., Lap, V.D., Skamene, E., Lagrange, P.H., & Schurr, E. (1998) Susceptibility to leprosy is linked to the human NRAMP1 gene. *J Infect Dis*, **177**, 133–145.

Agranoff, D., Monahan, I.M., Mangan, J.A., Butcher, P.D., & Krishna, S. (1999) *Mycobacterium tuberculosis* expresses a novel pH-dependent divalent cation transporter belonging to the Nramp family. *J Exp Med*, **190**, 717–724.

Alcais, A., Sanchez, F.O., Thuc, N.V., Lap, V.D., Oberti, J., Lagrange, P.H., Schurr, E., & Abel, L. (2000) Granulomatous reaction to intradermal injection of lepromin (Mitsuda reaction) is linked to the human NRAMP1 gene in Vietnamese leprosy sibships. *J Infect Dis*, **181**, 302–308.

Alter-Koltunoff, M., Ehrlich, S., Dror, N., Azriel, A., Eilers, M., Hauser, H., Bowen, H., Barton, C.H., Tamura, T., Ozato, K., & Levi, B.Z. (2003) Nramp1-mediated innate resistance to intraphagosomal pathogens is regulated by IRF-8, PU.1, and Miz-1. *J Biol Chem*, **278**, 44025–44032.

Atkinson, P.G., & Barton, C.H. (1998) Ectopic expression of Nramp1 in COS-1 cells modulates iron accumulation. *FEBS Lett*, **425**, 239–242.

Atkinson, P.G., & Barton, C.H. (1999) High level expression of Nramp1G169 in RAW264.7 cell transfectants: Analysis of intracellular iron transport. *Immunology*, **96**, 656–662.

Bassuny, W.M., Ihara, K., Matsuura, N., Ahmed, S., Kohno, H., Kuromaru, R., Miyako, K., & Hara, T. (2002) Association study of the NRAMP1 gene promoter polymorphism and early-onset type 1 diabetes. *Immunogenetics*, **54**, 282–285.

Bearden, S.W., & Perry, R.D. (1999) The Yfe system of *Yersinia pestis* transports iron and manganese and is required for full virulence of plague. *Mol Microbiol*, **32**, 403–414.

Bellamy, R., Ruwende, C., Corrah, T., McAdam, K.P., Whittle, H.C., & Hill, A.V. (1998) Variations in the NRAMP1 gene and susceptibility to tuberculosis in West Africans. *N Engl J Med*, **338**, 640–644.

Blackwell, J.M., Barton, C.H., White, J.K., Searle, S., Baker, A.M., Williams, H., & Shaw, M.A. (1995) Genomic organization and sequence of the human NRAMP gene: Identification and mapping of a promoter region polymorphism. *Mol Med*, **1**, 194–205.

Blackwell, J.M., Jiang, H. R., & White, J.K. (2004) Role of Nramp family in pro-inflammatory diseases. In: *The Nramp Family* (M. Cellier & P. Gros, eds.), pp. 53–64. Eurekah.com and Kluwer Academic/Plenum Publishers, New York.

Bowen, H., Biggs, T.E., Phillips, E., Baker, S.T., Perry, V.H., Mann, D.A., & Barton, C.H. (2002) c-Myc represses and Miz-1 activates the murine natural resistance-associated protein 1 promoter. *J Biol Chem*, **277**, 34997–35006.

Bowen, H., Lapham, A., Phillips, E., Yeung, I., Alter-Koltunoff, M., Levi, B.Z., Perry, V.H., Mann, D.A., & Barton, C.H. (2003) Characterization of the murine Nramp1 promoter: Requirements for transactivation by Miz-1. *J Biol Chem*, **278**, 36017–36026.

Boyer, E., Bergevin, I., Malo, D., Gros, P., & Cellier, M.F. (2002) Acquisition of Mn(II) in addition to Fe(II) is required for full virulence of *Salmonella enterica* serovar *typhimurium*. *Infect Immun*, **70**, 6032–6042.

Breuer, W., Epsztejn, S., & Cabantchik, Z.I. (1995) Iron acquired from transferrin by K562 cells is delivered into a cytoplasmic pool of chelatable iron(II). *J Biol Chem*, **270**, 24209–24215.

Bucheton, B., Abel, L., Kheir, M.M., Mirgani, A., El-Safi, S.H., Chevillard, C., & Dessein, A. (2003) Genetic control of visceral leishmaniasis in a Sudanese population: Candidate gene testing indicates a linkage to the NRAMP1 region. *Genes Immun*, **4**, 104–109.

Buu, N.T., Cellier, M., Gros, P., & Schurr, E. (1995) Identification of a highly polymorphic length variant in the 3'UTR of NRAMP1. *Immunogenetics*, **42**, 428–429.

Canonne-Hergaux, F., Calafat, J., Richer, E., Cellier, M., Grinstein, S., Borregaard, N., & Gros, P. (2002) Expression and subcellular localization of NRAMP1 in human neutrophil granules. *Blood*, **100**, 268–275.

Canonne-Hergaux, F., Fleming, M.D., Levy, J.E., Gauthier, S., Ralph, T., Picard, V., Andrews, N.C., & Gros, P. (2000) The Nramp2/DMT1 iron transporter is induced in the duodenum of microcytic anemia mk mice but is not properly targeted to the intestinal brush border. *Blood*, **96**, 3964–3970.

Canonne-Hergaux, F., & Gros, P. (2002) Expression of the iron transporter DMT1 in kidney from normal and anemic *mk* mice. *Kidney Int*, **62**, 147–156.

Canonne-Hergaux, F., Gruenheid, S., Ponka, P., & Gros, P. (1999) Cellular and subcellular localization of the Nramp2 iron transporter in the intestinal brush border and regulation by dietary iron. *Blood*, **93**, 4406–4417.

Canonne-Hergaux, F., Zhang, A.S., Ponka, P., & Gros, P. (2001) Characterization of the iron transporter DMT1 (NRAMP2/DCT1) in red blood cells of normal and anemic mk/mk mice. *Blood*, **98**, 3823–3830.

Cellier, M., Govoni, G., Vidal, S., Kwan, T., Groulx, N., Liu, J., Sanchez, F., Skamene, E., Schurr, E., & Gros, P. (1994) Human natural resistance-associated macrophage protein: CDNA cloning, chromosomal mapping, genomic organization, and tissue-specific expression. *J Exp Med*, **180**, 1741–1752.

Cellier, M., Prive, G., Belouchi, A., Kwan, T., Rodrigues, V., Chia, W., & Gros, P. (1995) Nramp defines a family of membrane proteins. *Proc Natl Acad Sci USA*, **92**, 10089–10093.

Cellier, M., Shustik, C., Dalton, W., Rich, E., Hu, J., Malo, D., Schurr, E., & Gros, P. (1997) Expression of the human NRAMP1 gene in professional primary phagocytes: Studies in blood cells and in HL-60 promyelocytic leukemia. *J Leukoc Biol*, **61**, 96–105.

Cervino, A.C., Lakiss, S., Sow, O., & Hill, A.V. (2000) Allelic association between the NRAMP1 gene and susceptibility to tuberculosis in Guinea-Conakry. *Ann Hum Genet*, **64**, 507–512.

Chen, X.Z., Peng, J.B., Cohen, A., Nelson, H., Nelson, N., & Hediger, M.A. (1999) Yeast SMF1 mediates H(+)-coupled iron uptake with concomitant uncoupled cation currents. *J Biol Chem*, **274**, 35089–35094.

Clemens, D.L., & Horwitz, M.A. (1995) Characterization of the *Mycobacterium tuberculosis* phagosome and evidence that phagosomal maturation is inhibited. *J Exp Med*, **181**, 257–270.

Clemens, D.L., Lee, B.Y., & Horwitz, M.A. (2000a) Deviant expression of Rab5 on phagosomes containing the intracellular pathogens *Mycobacterium tuberculosis* and *Legionella pneumophila* is associated with altered phagosomal fate. *Infect Immun*, **68**, 2671–2684.

Clemens, D.L., Lee, B.Y., & Horwitz, M.A. (2000b) *Mycobacterium tuberculosis* and *Legionella pneumophila* phagosomes exhibit arrested maturation despite acquisition of Rab7. *Infect Immun*, **68**, 5154–5166.

Courville, P., Chaloupka, R., Veyrier, F., & Cellier, M.F. (2004) Determination of transmembrane topology of the *Escherichia coli* natural resistance-associated macrophage protein (Nramp) ortholog. *J Biol Chem*, **279**, 3318–3326.

Cuellar-Mata, P., Jabado, N., Liu, J., Furuya, W., Finlay, B.B., Gros, P., & Grinstein, S. (2002) Nramp1 modifies the fusion of *Salmonella typhimurium*-containing vacuoles with cellular endomembranes in macrophages. *J Biol Chem*, **277**, 2258–2265.

Delaby, C., Pilard, N., Hetet, G., Driss, F., Grandchamp, B., Beaumont, C. & Canonne-Hergaux, F. (2005) A physiological model to study iron recycling in macrophages. *Exp Cell Res*, **310**, 43–53.

Devalia, V., Carter, K., Walker, A.P., Perkins, S.J., Worwood, M., May, A., & Dooley, J.S. (2002) Autosomal dominant reticuloendothelial iron overload associated with a 3-base pair deletion in the ferroportin 1 gene (SLC11A3). *Blood*, **100**, 695–697.

De Voss, J.J., Rutter, K., Schroeder, B.G., Su, H., Zhu, Y., & Barry, C.E., 3rd (2000) The salicylate-derived mycobactin siderophores of *Mycobacterium tuberculosis* are essential for growth in macrophages. *Proc Natl Acad Sci USA*, **97**, 1252–1257.

Donovan, A., Brownlie, A., Zhou, Y., Shepard, J., Pratt, S.J., Moynihan, J., Paw, B.H., Drejer, A., Barut, B., Zapata, A., Law, T.C., Brugnara, C., Lux, S.E., Pinkus, G.S., Pinkus, J.L., Kingsley, P.D., Palis, J., Fleming, M.D., Andrews, N.C., & Zon, L.I. (2000) Positional cloning of zebrafish ferroportin1 identifies a conserved vertebrate iron exporter. *Nature*, **403**, 776–781.

Donovan, A., Lima, C., & Andrews, N.C. (2003) Analysis of iron homeostasis in mice with a targeted deletion of the gene encoding the iron exporter ferroportin 1 (Fpn1). *Blood*, **102**, abstract 540.

Eriksson, S., Lucchini, S., Thompson, A., Rhen, M., & Hinton, J.C. (2003) Unravelling the biology of macrophage infection by gene expression profiling of intracellular *Salmonella enterica*. *Mol Microbiol*, **47**, 103–118.

Esposito, L., Hill, N.J., Pritchard, L.E., Cucca, F., Muxworthy, C., Merriman, M.E., Wilson, A., Julier, C., Delepine, M., Tuomilehto, J., Tuomilehto-Wolf, E., Ionesco-Tirgoviste, C., Nistico, L., Buzzetti, R., Pozzilli, P., Ferrari, M., Bosi, E., Pociot, F., Nerup, J., Bain, S.C., & Todd, J.A. (1998) Genetic analysis of chromosome 2 in type 1 diabetes: Analysis of putative loci IDDM7, IDDM12, and IDDM13 and candidate genes NRAMP1 and IA-2 and the interleukin-1 gene cluster. IMDIAB Group. *Diabetes*, **47**, 1797–1799.

Fleming, M.D., Romano, M.A., Su, M.A., Garrick, L.M., Garrick, M.D., & Andrews, N.C. (1998) Nramp2 is mutated in the anemic Belgrade (b) rat: Evidence of a role for Nramp2 in endosomal iron transport. *Proc Natl Acad Sci USA*, **95**, 1148–1153.

Fleming, M.D., Trenor, C.C., 3rd, Su, M.A., Foernzler, D., Beier, D.R., Dietrich, W.F. & Andrews, N.C. (1997) Microcytic anaemia mice have a mutation in Nramp2, a candidate iron transporter gene. *Nat Genet*, **16**, 383–386.

Forbes, J.R., & Gros, P. (2001) Divalent-metal transport by NRAMP proteins at the interface of host-pathogen interactions. *Trends Microbiol*, **9**, 397–403.

Forbes, J.R., & Gros, P. (2003) Iron, manganese, and cobalt transport by Nramp1 (Slc11a1) and Nramp2

(Slc11a2) expressed at the plasma membrane. *Blood*, **102**, 1884–1892.

Frehel, C., Canonne-Hergaux, F., Gros, P., & De Chastellier, C. (2002) Effect of Nramp1 on bacterial replication and on maturation of *Mycobacterium avium*-containing phagosomes in bone marrow-derived mouse macrophages. *Cell Microbiol*, **4**, 541–556.

Gao, P.S., Fujishima, S., Mao, X.Q., Remus, N., Kanda, M., Enomoto, T., Dake, Y., Bottini, N., Tabuchi, M., Hasegawa, N., Yamaguchi, K., Tiemessen, C., Hopkin, J.M., Shirakawa, T., & Kishi, F. (2000) Genetic variants of NRAMP1 and active tuberculosis in Japanese populations. International Tuberculosis Genetics Team. *Clin Genet*, **58**, 74–76.

Gold, B., Rodriguez, G.M., Marras, S.A., Pentecost, M., & Smith, I. (2001) The *Mycobacterium tuberculosis* IdeR is a dual functional regulator that controls transcription of genes involved in iron acquisition, iron storage and survival in macrophages. *Mol Microbiol*, **42**, 851–865.

Gomes, M.S., & Appelberg, R. (1998) Evidence for a link between iron metabolism and Nramp1 gene function in innate resistance against *Mycobacterium avium*. *Immunology*, **95**, 165–168.

Govoni, G., Canonne-Hergaux, F., Pfeifer, C.G., Marcus, S.L., Mills, S.D., Hackam, D.J., Grinstein, S., Malo, D., Finlay, B.B. & Gros, P. (1999) Functional expression of Nramp1 in vitro in the murine macrophage line RAW264.7. *Infect Immun*, **67**, 2225–2232.

Govoni, G., Gauthier, S., Billia, F., Iscove, N.N. & Gros, P. (1997) Cell-specific and inducible Nramp1 gene expression in mouse macrophages in vitro and in vivo. *J Leukoc Biol*, **62**, 277–286.

Govoni, G., Vidal, S., Cellier, M., Lepage, P., Malo, D., & Gros, P. (1995) Genomic structure, promoter sequence, and induction of expression of the mouse Nramp1 gene in macrophages. *Genomics*, **27**, 9–19.

Govoni, G., Vidal, S., Gauthier, S., Skamene, E., Malo, D., & Gros, P. (1996) The Bcg/Ity/Lsh locus: Genetic transfer of resistance to infections in C57BL/6J mice transgenic for the Nramp1 Gly169 allele. *Infect Immun*, **64**, 2923–2929.

Graham, A.M., Dollinger, M.M., Howie, S.E., & Harrison, D.J. (2000) Identification of novel alleles at a polymorphic microsatellite repeat region in the human NRAMP1 gene promoter: Analysis of allele frequencies in primary biliary cirrhosis. *J Med Genet*, **37**, 150–152.

Greenwood, C.M., Fujiwara, T.M., Boothroyd, L.J., Miller, M.A., Frappier, D., Fanning, E.A., Schurr, E., & Morgan, K. (2000) Linkage of tuberculosis to chromosome 2q35 loci, including NRAMP1, in a large aboriginal Canadian family. *Am J Hum Genet*, **67**, 405–416.

Gros, P., Skamene, E., & Forget, A. (1983) Cellular mechanisms of genetically controlled host resistance to Mycobacterium bovis (BCG). *J Immunol*, **131**, 1966–1972.

Gruenheid, S., Canonne-Hergaux, F., Gauthier, S., Hackam, D.J., Grinstein, S. & Gros, P. (1999) The iron transport protein NRAMP2 is an integral membrane glycoprotein that colocalizes with transferrin in recycling endosomes. *J Exp Med*, **189**, 831–841.

Gruenheid, S., Cellier, M., Vidal, S., & Gros, P. (1995) Identification and characterization of a second mouse Nramp gene. *Genomics*, **25**, 514–525.

Gruenheid, S., Pinner, E., Desjardins, M., & Gros, P. (1997) Natural resistance to infection with intracellular pathogens: The Nramp1 protein is recruited to the membrane of the phagosome. *J Exp Med*, **185**, 717–730.

Gunshin, H., Fujiwara, Y., Custodio, A.O., Direnzo, C., Robine, S., & Andrews, N.C. (2005a) Slc11a2 is required for intestinal iron absorption and erythropoiesis but dispensable in placenta and liver. *J Clin Invest*, **115**, 1258–1266.

Gunshin, H., Jin, J., Fujiwara, Y., Andrews, N.C., Mims, M., & Prchal, J. (2005b) Analysis of the E399D mutation in SLC11A2. *Blood*, **106**, 2221; author reply 2221–2222.

Gunshin, H., Mackenzie, B., Berger, U.V., Gunshin, Y., Romero, M.F., Boron, W.F., Nussberger, S., Gollan, J.L. & Hediger, M.A. (1997) Cloning and characterization of a mammalian proton-coupled metal-ion transporter. *Nature*, **388**, 482–488.

Hackam, D.J., Rotstein, O.D., Zhang, W., Gruenheid, S., Gros, P., & Grinstein, S. (1998) Host resistance to intracellular infection: Mutation of natural resistance-associated macrophage protein 1 (Nramp1) impairs phagosomal acidification. *J Exp Med*, **188**, 351–364.

Hantke, K. (1997) Ferrous iron uptake by a magnesium transport system is toxic for *Escherichia coli* and *Salmonella typhimurium*. *J Bacteriol*, **179**, 6201–6204.

Hofmeister, A., Neibergs, H.L., Pokorny, R.M., & Galandiuk, S. (1997) The natural resistance-associated macrophage protein gene is associated with Crohn's disease. *Surgery*, **122**, 173–178; discussion 178–179.

Hubert, N., & Hentze, M.W. (2002) Previously uncharacterized isoforms of divalent metal transporter (DMT)-1: Implications for regulation and cellular function. *Proc Natl Acad Sci USA*, **99**, 12345–12350.

Iolascon, A., d'Apolito, M., Servedio, V., Cimmino, F., Piga, A., & Camaschella, C. (2006) Microcytic anemia and hepatic iron overload in a child with compound heterozygous mutations in DMT1 (SCL11A2). *Blood*, **107**, 349–354.

Jabado, N., Canonne-Hergaux, F., Gruenheid, S., Picard, V. & Gros, P. (2002) Iron transporter Nramp2/DMT-1 is associated with the membrane of phagosomes in macrophages and Sertoli cells. *Blood*, **100**, 2617–2622.

Jabado, N., Jankowski, A., Dougaparsad, S., Picard, V., Grinstein, S., & Gros, P. (2000) Natural resistance to intracellular infections: Natural resistance-associated macrophage protein 1 (Nramp1) functions as a pH-dependent manganese transporter at the phagosomal membrane. *J Exp Med*, **192**, 1237–1248.

Janakiraman, A., & Slauch, J.M. (2000) The putative iron transport system SitABCD encoded on SPI1 is required for full virulence of *Salmonella typhimurium*. *Mol Microbiol*, **35**, 1146–1155.

Kammler, M., Schon, C., & Hantke, K. (1993) Characterization of the ferrous iron uptake system of *Escherichia coli*. *J Bacteriol*, **175**, 6212–6219.

Keen, C.L., Ensunsa, J.L., Clegg, M.S. (2000) Manganese metabolism in animals and humans including the toxicity of manganese. In: *Manganese and its role in biological processes*, vol. 37 (A. Sigel & H. Sigel, eds.), pp. 89–121. Marcel Dekker, Inc.

Kehres, D.G., Janakiraman, A., Slauch, J.M., & Maguire, M.E. (2002) SitABCD is the alkaline Mn(2+) transporter of *Salmonella enterica* serovar *typhimurium*. *J Bacteriol*, **184**, 3159–3166.

Kehres, D.G., & Maguire, M.E. (2003) Emerging themes in manganese transport, biochemistry and pathogenesis in bacteria. *FEMS Microbiol Rev*, **27**, 263–290.

Kehres, D.G., Zaharik, M.L., Finlay, B.B., & Maguire, M.E. (2000) The NRAMP proteins of *Salmonella typhimurium* and *Escherichia coli* are selective manganese transporters involved in the response to reactive oxygen. *Mol Microbiol*, **36**, 1085–1100.

Kelley, V.A., & Schorey, J.S. (2003) Mycobacterium's arrest of phagosome maturation in macrophages requires Rab5 activity and accessibility to iron. *Mol Biol Cell*, **14**, 3366–3377.

Kishi, F., & Tabuchi, M. (1997) Complete nucleotide sequence of human NRAMP2 cDNA. *Mol Immunol*, **34**, 839–842.

Knodler, L.A., & Steele-Mortimer, O. (2003) Taking possession: Biogenesis of the *Salmonella*-containing vacuole. *Traffic*, **4**, 587–599.

Knutson, M.D., Vafa, M.R., Haile, D.J., & Wessling-Resnick, M. (2003) Iron loading and erythrophagocytosis increase ferroportin 1 (FPN1) expression in J774 macrophages. *Blood*, **102**, 4191–4197.

Kojima, Y., Kinouchi, Y., Takahashi, S., Negoro, K., Hiwatashi, N., & Shimosegawa, T. (2001) Inflammatory bowel disease is associated with a novel promoter polymorphism of natural resistance-associated macrophage protein 1 (NRAMP1) gene. *Tissue Antigens*, **58**, 379–384.

Kotze, M.J., de Villiers, J.N., Rooney, R.N., Grobbelaar, J.J., Mansvelt, E.P., Bouwens, C.S., Carr, J., Stander, I., & du Plessis, L. (2001) Analysis of the NRAMP1 gene implicated in iron transport: Association with multiple sclerosis and age effects. *Blood Cells Mol Dis*, **27**, 44–53.

Lam-Yuk-Tseung, S., Camaschella, C., Iolascon, A., & Gros, P. (2006) A novel R416C mutation in human DMT1 (SLC11A2) displays pleiotropic effects on function and causes microcytic anemia and hepatic iron overload. *Blood Cells Mol Dis*, **36**, 347–354.

Lam-Yuk-Tseung, S., Govoni, G., Forbes, J., & Gros, P. (2003) Iron transport by NRAMP2/DMT1: pH regulation of transport by two histidines in transmembrane domain 6. *Blood*, **101**, 3699–3707.

Lam-Yuk-Tseung, S., & Gros, P. (2003) Genetic control of susceptibility to bacterial infections in mouse models. *Cell Microbiol*, **5**, 299–313.

Lam-Yuk-Tseung, S., Mathieu, M., & Gros, P. (2005) Functional characterization of the E399D DMT1/NRAMP2/SLC11A2 protein produced by an exon 12 mutation in a patient with microcytic anemia and iron overload. *Blood Cells Mol Dis*, **35**, 212–216.

Lee, P.L., Gelbart, T., West, C., Halloran, C., & Beutler, E. (1998) The human Nramp2 gene: Characterization of the gene structure, alternative splicing, promoter region and polymorphisms. *Blood Cells Mol Dis*, **24**, 199–215.

Lewis, L.A., Victor, T.C., Helden, E.G., Blackwell, J.M., da Silva-Tatley, F., Tullett, S., Ehlers, M., Beyers, N., Donald, P.R., & van Helden, P.D. (1996) Identification of C to T mutation at position −236 bp in the human NRAMP1 gene promoter. *Immunogenetics*, **44**, 309–311.

Liu, J., Fujiwara, T.M., Buu, N.T., Sanchez, F.O., Cellier, M., Paradis, A.J., Frappier, D., Skamene, E., Gros, P., Morgan, K., & et al. (1995) Identification of polymorphisms and sequence variants in the human homologue of the mouse natural resistance-associated macrophage protein gene. *Am J Hum Genet*, **56**, 845–853.

Ludwiczek, S., Aigner, E., Theurl, I., & Weiss, G. (2003) Cytokine-mediated regulation of iron transport in human monocytic cells. *Blood*, **101**, 4148–4154.

Mackenzie, B., & Hediger, M.A. (2004) SLC11 family of H(+)-coupled metal-ion transporters NRAMP1 and DMT1. *Pflugers Arch*, **447**, 571–579.

Makui, H., Roig, E., Cole, S.T., Helmann, J.D., Gros, P., & Cellier, M.F. (2000) Identification of the *Escherichia coli* K-12 Nramp orthologue (MntH) as a selective divalent metal ion transporter. *Mol Microbiol*, **35**, 1065–1078.

Malik, S., Abel, L., Tooker, H., Poon, A., Simkin, L., Girard, M., Adams, G.J., Starke, J.R., Smith, K.C., Graviss, E.A., Musser, J.M., & Schurr, E. (2005) Alleles of the NRAMP1 gene are risk factors for pediatric tuberculosis disease. *Proc Natl Acad Sci U S A*, **102**, 12183–12188.

Marquet, S., Sanchez, F.O., Arias, M., Rodriguez, J., Paris, S.C., Skamene, E., Schurr, E., & Garcia, L.F. (1999) Variants of the human NRAMP1 gene and altered human immunodeficiency virus infection susceptibility. *J Infect Dis*, **180**, 1521–1525.

McKie, A.T., Marciani, P., Rolfs, A., Brennan, K., Wehr, K., Barrow, D., Miret, S., Bomford, A., Peters, T.J., Farzaneh, F., Hediger, M.A., Hentze, M.W., & Simpson, R.J. (2000) A novel duodenal iron-regulated transporter, IREG1, implicated in the basolateral transfer of iron to the circulation. *Mol Cell*, **5**, 299–309.

Montosi, G., Donovan, A., Totaro, A., Garuti, C., Pignatti, E., Cassanelli, S., Trenor, C.C., Gasparini, P., Andrews, N.C., & Pietrangelo, A. (2001) Autosomal-dominant hemochromatosis is associated with a mutation in the ferroportin (SLC11A3) gene. *J Clin Invest*, **108**, 619–623.

Njajou, O.T., Vaessen, N., Joosse, M., Berghuis, B., van Dongen, J.W., Breuning, M.H., Snijders, P.J., Rutten, W.P., Sandkuijl, L.A., Oostra, B.A., van Duijn, C.M., & Heutink, P. (2001) A mutation in SLC11A3 is associated with autosomal dominant hemochromatosis. *Nat Genet*, **28**, 213–214.

Olakanmi, O., Schlesinger, L.S., Ahmed, A., & Britigan, B.E. (2002) Intraphagosomal *Mycobacterium tuberculosis* acquires iron from both extracellular transferrin and intracellular iron pools. Impact of interferon-gamma and hemochromatosis. *J Biol Chem*, **277**, 49727–49734.

Ouchi, K., Suzuki, Y., Shirakawa, T., & Kishi, F. (2003) Polymorphism of SLC11A1 (formerly NRAMP1) gene confers susceptibility to Kawasaki disease. *J Infect Dis*, **187**, 326–329.

Picard, V., Govoni, G., Jabado, N., & Gros, P. (2000) Nramp 2 (DCT1/DMT1) expressed at the plasma membrane transports iron and other divalent cations into a calcein-accessible cytoplasmic pool. *J Biol Chem*, **275**, 35738–35745.

Pietrangelo, A. (2004) The ferroportin disease. *Blood Cells Mol Dis*, **32**, 131–138.

Poon, A., & Schurr, E. (2004) The NRAMP genes and human susceptibility to common diseases. In: *The Nramp Family* (M. Cellier & P. Gros, eds.), pp. 29–43. Eurekah.com and Kluwer Academic/Plenum Publishers.

Portnoy, M.E., Liu, X.F., & Culotta, V.C. (2000) Saccharomyces cerevisiae expresses three functionally distinct homologues of the nramp family of metal transporters. *Mol Cell Biol*, **20**, 7893–7902.

Priwitzerova, M., Nie, G., Sheftel, A.D., Pospisilova, D., Divoky, V., & Ponka, P. (2005) Functional consequences of the human DMT1 (SLC11A2) mutation on protein expression and iron uptake. *Blood*, **106**, 3985–3987.

Priwitzerova, M., Pospisilova, D., Prchal, J.T., Indrak, K., Hlobilkova, A., Mihal, V., Ponka, P., & Divoky, V. (2004) Severe hypochromic microcytic anemia caused by a congenital defect of the iron transport pathway in erythroid cells. *Blood*, **103**, 3991–3992.

Ratledge, C. (2004) Iron, mycobacteria and tuberculosis. *Tuberculosis (Edinb)*, **84**, 110–130.

Rodriguez, M.R., Gonzalez-Escribano, M.F., Aguilar, F., Valenzuela, A., Garcia, A., & Nunez-Roldan, A. (2002) Association of NRAMP1 promoter gene polymorphism with the susceptibility and radiological severity of rheumatoid arthritis. *Tissue Antigens*, **59**, 311–315.

Roig, E.A., Richer, E., Canonne-Hergaux, F., Gros, P., & Cellier, M.F. (2002) Regulation of NRAMP1 gene expression by 1alpha,25-dihydroxy-vitamin D(3) in HL-60 phagocytes. *J Leukoc Biol*, **71**, 890–904.

Russell, D.G., Dant, J., & Sturgill-Koszycki, S. (1996) *Mycobacterium avium*- and *Mycobacterium tuberculosis*-containing vacuoles are dynamic, fusion-competent vesicles that are accessible to glycosphingolipids from the host cell plasmalemma. *J Immunol*, **156**, 4764–4773.

Sacher, A., Cohen, A., & Nelson, N. (2001) Properties of the mammalian and yeast metal-ion transporters DCT1 and Smf1p expressed in *Xenopus laevis* oocytes. *J Exp Biol*, **204**, 1053–1061.

Sanjeevi, C.B., Miller, E.N., Dabadghao, P., Rumba, I., Shtauvere, A., Denisova, A., Clayton, D., & Blackwell, J.M. (2000) Polymorphism at NRAMP1 and D2S1471 loci associated with juvenile rheumatoid arthritis. *Arthritis Rheum*, **43**, 1397–1404.

Schaible, U.E., Sturgill-Koszycki, S., Schlesinger, P.H., & Russell, D.G. (1998) Cytokine activation leads to acidification and increases maturation of *Mycobacterium avium*-containing phagosomes in murine macrophages. *J Immunol*, **160**, 1290–1296.

Schnappinger, D., Ehrt, S., Voskuil, M.I., Liu, Y., Mangan, J.A., Monahan, I.M., Dolganov, G., Efron, B., Butcher, P.D., Nathan, C., & Schoolnik, G.K. (2003) Transcriptional adaptation of *Mycobacterium tuberculosis* within macrophages: Insights into the phagosomal environment. *J Exp Med*, **198**, 693–704.

Searle, S., & Blackwell, J.M. (1999) Evidence for a functional repeat polymorphism in the promoter of the human NRAMP1 gene that correlates with autoimmune versus infectious disease susceptibility. *J Med Genet*, **36**, 295–299.

Searle, S., Bright, N.A., Roach, T.I., Atkinson, P.G., Barton, C.H., Meloen, R.H., & Blackwell, J.M. (1998) Localisation of Nramp1 in macrophages: Modulation with activation and infection. *J Cell Sci*, **111** (Pt 19), 2855–2866.

Shaw, M.A., Clayton, D., Atkinson, S.E., Williams, H., Miller, N., Sibthorpe, D., & Blackwell, J.M. (1996) Linkage of rheumatoid arthritis to the candidate gene NRAMP1 on 2q35. *J Med Genet*, **33**, 672–677.

Singal, D.P., Li, J., Zhu, Y., & Zhang, G. (2000) NRAMP1 gene polymorphisms in patients with rheumatoid arthritis. *Tissue Antigens*, **55**, 44–47.

Skamene, E., Schurr, E., & Gros, P. (1998) Infection genomics: Nramp1 as a major determinant of natural resistance to intracellular infections. *Annu Rev Med*, **49**, 275–287.

Soborg, C., Andersen, A.B., Madsen, H.O., Kok-Jensen, A., Skinhoj, P., & Garred, P. (2002) Natural resistance-associated macrophage protein 1 polymorphisms are associated with microscopy-positive tuberculosis. *J Infect Dis*, **186**, 517–521.

Sturgill-Koszycki, S., Schaible, U.E., & Russell, D.G. (1996) Mycobacterium-containing phagosomes are accessible to early endosomes and reflect a transitional state in normal phagosome biogenesis. *Embo J*, **15**, 6960–6968.

Sturgill-Koszycki, S., Schlesinger, P.H., Chakraborty, P., Haddix, P.L., Collins, H.L., Fok, A.K., Allen, R.D., Gluck, S.L., Heuser, J., & Russell, D.G. (1994) Lack of acidification in Mycobacterium phagosomes produced by exclusion of the vesicular proton-ATPase. *Science*, **263**, 678–681.

Su, M.A., Trenor, C.C., Fleming, J.C., Fleming, M.D., & Andrews, N.C. (1998) The G185R mutation disrupts function of the iron transporter Nramp2. *Blood*, **92**, 2157–2163.

Supek, F., Supekova, L., Nelson, H., & Nelson, N. (1997) Function of metal-ion homeostasis in the cell division cycle, mitochondrial protein processing, sensitivity to mycobacterial infection and brain function. *J Exp Biol*, **200** (**Pt 2**), 321–330.

Tandy, S., Williams, M., Leggett, A., Lopez-Jimenez, M., Dedes, M., Ramesh, B., Srai, S.K., & Sharp, P. (2000) Nramp2 expression is associated with pH-dependent iron uptake across the apical membrane of human intestinal Caco-2 cells. *J Biol Chem*, **275**, 1023–1029.

Tchernitchko, D., Bourgeois, M., Martin, M.E., & Beaumont, C. (2002) Expression of the two mRNA isoforms of the iron transporter Nrmap2/DMTI in mice and function of the iron responsive element. *Biochem J*, **363**, 449–455.

Timm, J., Post, F.A., Bekker, L.G., Walther, G.B., Wainwright, H.C., Manganelli, R., Chan, W.T., Tsenova, L., Gold, B., Smith, I., Kaplan, G., & McKinney, J.D. (2003) Differential expression of iron-, carbon-, and oxygen-responsive mycobacterial genes in the lungs of chronically infected mice and tuberculosis patients. *Proc Natl Acad Sci USA*, **100**, 14321–14326.

Touret, N., Furuya, W., Forbes, J., Gros, P., & Grinstein, S. (2003) Dynamic traffic through the recycling compartment couples the metal transporter Nramp2 (DMT1) with the transferrin receptor. *J Biol Chem*, **278**, 25548–25557.

Tsolis, R.M., Baumler, A.J., Heffron, F., & Stojiljkovic, I. (1996) Contribution of TonB- and Feo-mediated iron uptake to growth of *Salmonella typhimurium* in the mouse. *Infect Immun*, **64**, 4549–4556.

Vidal, S., Belouchi, A.M., Cellier, M., Beatty, B., & Gros, P. (1995a) Cloning and characterization of a second human NRAMP gene on chromosome 12q13. *Mamm Genome*, **6**, 224–230.

Vidal, S.M., Malo, D., Vogan, K., Skamene, E., & Gros, P. (1993) Natural resistance to infection with intracellular parasites: Isolation of a candidate for Bcg. *Cell*, **73**, 469–485.

Vidal, S.M., Pinner, E., Lepage, P., Gauthier, S., & Gros, P. (1996) Natural resistance to intracellular infections: Nramp1 encodes a membrane phosphoglycoprotein absent in macrophages from susceptible (Nramp1 D169) mouse strains. *J Immunol*, **157**, 3559–3568.

Vidal, S., Tremblay, M.L., Govoni, G., Gauthier, S., Sebastiani, G., Malo, D., Skamene, E., Olivier, M., Jothy, S., & Gros, P. (1995b) The Ity/Lsh/Bcg locus: Natural resistance to infection with intracellular parasites is abrogated by disruption of the Nramp1 gene. *J Exp Med*, **182**, 655–666.

Wallace, D.F., Pedersen, P., Dixon, J.L., Stephenson, P., Searle, J.W., Powell, L.W., & Subramaniam, V.N. (2002) Novel mutation in ferroportin1 is associated with autosomal dominant hemochromatosis. *Blood*, **100**, 692–694.

Wessling-Resnick, M. (2006) Iron imports. III. Transfer of iron from the mucosa into circulation. *Am J Physiol Gastrointest Liver Physiol*, **290**, G1–6.

Yang, Y.S., Kim, S.J., Kim, J.W., & Koh, E.M. (2000) NRAMP1 gene polymorphisms in patients with rheumatoid arthritis in Koreans. *J Korean Med Sci*, **15**, 83–87.

Yang, F., Liu, X.B., Quinones, M., Melby, P.C., Ghio, A., & Haile, D.J. (2002) Regulation of reticuloendothelial iron transporter MTP1 (Slc11a3) by inflammation. *J Biol Chem*, **277**, 39786–39791.

Zaharik, M.L., Vallance, B.A., Puente, J.L., Gros, P., & Finlay, B.B. (2002) Host-pathogen interactions: Host resistance factor Nramp1 up-regulates the expression of Salmonella pathogenicity island-2 virulence genes. *Proc Natl Acad Sci USA*, **99**, 15705–15710.

Zhou, D., Hardt, W.D., & Galan, J.E. (1999) *Salmonella typhimurium* encodes a putative iron transport system within the centisome 63 pathogenicity island. *Infect Immun*, **67**, 1974–1981.

14

Tumor Necrosis Factor and Related Genes

Grant Gallagher, Milton O. Moraes, & Juan-Manuel Anaya

The tumor necrosis factor (TNF) region spans four loci: lymphotoxin α (*LTA*), lymphotoxin β (*LTB*), tumor necrosis factor (*TNF*), and leukocyte-specific transcript 1 (*LST1*). Much is known about the functions of the products of three of these genes—LTα, LTβ, and TNF. The fourth gene has been relatively ignored since its discovery in the early 1990s. The most studied gene product is the cytokine is TNF (also known as TNF-α), which is produced largely by monocytes, macrophages, and T cells (Correa & Anaya, 2001). TNF is synthesized as a 26-kDa membrane protein, which is cleaved to produce its soluble 17-kDa form. TNF is a pleiotropic and proinflammatory cytokine that displays a wide range of biological activities regulating normal functions such as hematopoiesis, morphogenesis, lipid metabolism, and endothelial function and has several local effects, including protection against infections. However, TNF overproduction can lead to severe tissue damage, organ failure, and occasionally death.

Both LTα (formerly known as TNF-β) and LTβ exhibit significant homology with TNF and exert similar biological effects although production is restricted largely to lymphocytes. Both TNF and the LTα homotrimer bind to both TNF receptor I and II. LTβ, which binds exclusively LTβ receptors, is a membrane protein that forms heterotrimers with LTα, anchoring LTα to the membrane. LST1 is an interferon-γ (IFN-γ)–inducible gene expressed mostly in T cells and macrophages. It shows several alternative splice forms and affects immune cell function (de Baey et al., 1995, 1997; Holzinger et al., 1995; Rollinger-Holzinger et al., 2000).

Information about the genetics of LTβ and LST1 is scarce, whereas LTα has often been studied in conjunction with TNF-α. There is considerable evidence that differential levels of secreted TNF can be genetically controlled. This review concentrates on epidemiological and biological studies of genetic markers in genes for TNF and LTα performed in population-based studies (generally of case–control design) or in functional analysis. These relationships are also well documented in the periodically updated list of cytokine genetic studies (Bidwell et al., 1999, 2001; Haukim et al., 2002; Hollegaard and Bidwell, 2006).

TNF and *LTA* Genes

The *TNF* Gene Product in Infection

TNF exerts a range of inflammatory and immuno-modulatory activities that are important in host defense. The following illustrative examples speak to the central role of TNF-α in host defense and general im-munohomeostasis and how a disruption of its function and/or regulation can be damaging. TNF has been implicated in the pathogenesis of different diseases. These include autoimmune diseases such as rheuma-toid arthritis (RA) (Feldmann et al., 1996), Crohn's disease (Plevy et al., 1996), systemic lupus erythema-tosus (SLE) (Gomez et al., 2004), and primary Sjög-ren's syndrome (Fox et al., 1994). Indeed, anti-TNF therapy has been a breakthrough in the management of RA (Feldmann, 2002) and inflammatory bowel disease (Suryaprasad & Prindiville, 2003); however, the use of TNF-α blockers (e.g., etanercept, infliximab) appears to promote reactivation and/or acquisition of tuberculosis (TB) in certain individuals (Dinarello, 2003). This can be explained by the fact that TNF is a key cytokine in the resistance to intracellular patho-gens associated with several infectious diseases such as TB, leprosy, Chagas' disease, and leishmaniasis, where this cytokine plays a very important role in the for-mation and maintenance of the granulomas and acti-vation of microbicidal function in macrophages (Flynn & Chan, 2001). However, TNF-α overproduction has been shown to be deleterious for the host, leading to irreversible organ failure and death (Aggarwal, 2003). The best examples of TNF damaging effects as a result of its overproduction associated with infectious dis-eases are cerebral malaria (chapter 24), erythema no-dosum leprosum in leprosy patients (chapter 22), and mucosal leishmaniasis (chapter 25). TNF also has been implicated in the development of cardiac pathol-ogy such as that seen in chronic chagasic cardiopathy. It has been shown to stimulate the release of endo-thelial cytokines and nitric oxide, increase vascular per-meability, decrease contractility, and induce a pro-thrombotic state (Vadlamani & Iyengar, 2004). The increase of vascular permeability and its proinflam-matory properties has been studied in the physiopa-thology of sepsis (Bochud & Calandra, 2003).

Pathogenesis

TNF and its counterpart, interleukin-10 (IL-10), have often been studied together. A range of experiments in murine models (see below), together with *in vitro* and *ex vivo* studies in humans, demonstrate that variation in TNF production can profoundly alter the response to and outcome of infection. Studies on TNF and IL-10 (see chapter 15) are complementary to each other and worth considering together.

Experimental studies show clearly that levels of TNF are important in determining the course and outcome of infectious disease, and studies in human infection have supported this concept. Westendorp and colleagues (Westendorp et al., 1997a, 1997b; van Dissel et al., 1998) have shown that low TNF pro-duction was associated with a 10-fold increased risk of fatality from meningococcal meningitis, while high IL-10 levels were associated with a 20-fold higher risk. Despite the recognized ability of TNF to induce IL-10 levels from monocytes and IL-10 to down-regulate TNF, these two factors appeared independent; that is, the levels of one cytokine were not dependent upon those of the other.

Organization and Sequence of the Human *TNF* Locus

Primarily because the protein encoded by human *TNF* locus plays a key role in inflammatory responses and contributes in a fundamental way to many human dis-eases and disorders, it has been the subject of more ge-netic studies than any other immune response gene out-side of the major histocompatibility complex (MHC) (table 14.1). This phrase "outside of" the MHC is in itself ambiguous because physically the *TNF* locus sits squarely within the wider MHC region, trapped in linkage disequilibrium between the *HLA-B* and *HLA-DRB1* loci (e.g., Abraham et al., 1993; Dawkins et al., 1989; Jongeneel et al., 1991; Nedospasov et al., 1991). On the other hand, a careful look at certain disease associations ties them, often inseparably, to the *TNF* locus and its molecular product but in the context of different MHC backgrounds (see below). Thus, further work on disease susceptibility and severity associated with the small four-gene TNF region will need to con-sider how it functions both in a "life of its own" and against the background of nearby MHC genes.

The *TNF* gene itself is located within the class III (occasionally distinguished as "class IV") region of the

TABLE 14.1. TNF gene summary.

Gene ID (NCBI)	Common Name(s)	Entrez Gene ID (Locus Link)	Map Position	Notes on Important SNPs, Indels, Truncations (Region, Reference Sequence [rs] Number)	References
TNF	TNF TNF-α Cachectin	7124	6p21.3	At least 10 SNPs in the promoter region; very little coding region diversity	Iida et al. (2003) NIH, NHLBI Programs for Genomic Applications (PGA)
LTA	LTα	4049	6p21.3	At least three nonsynonymous SNPs in the coding region; additional variation in promoter and untranslated region	NIH, NHLBI Programs for Genomic Applications (PGA)[a]

[a]The National Heart, Lung, and Blood Institute Programs for Genomic Applications can be accessed at pga.gs.washington.edu/.

MHC on chromosome 6 and is highly polymorphic (figure 14.1; Hajeer & Hutchinson, 2001). The boundaries of the "TNF locus" under study have not always been carefully defined by investigators. One definition represents them as shown in figure 14.1a— lying between the TNFa/b microsatellite, telomeric of the LTA gene, and the TNFd/e microsatellite close to the end of the LST1 gene. Five microsatellites (TNFa– TNFe; Udalova et al., 1993) and the closely associated BAT2 (Gallagher et al., 1997a) microsatellite (figure 14.1a) have been described; there are also numerous single nucleotide polymorphisms (SNPs) concentrated in the promoter. Two of these SNPs representing a G/A transition at promoter positions, usually designated −238 and −308, have been examined extensively in both autoimmune and infectious diseases with diverse results (sometimes associated, sometimes not). Apparent discrepancies are most likely due to differences in the origin of the studied populations, linkage disequilibrium with other MHC genes, or insufficient sample size (Bayley et al., 2004; Hajeer & Hutchinson, 2001). Indeed, most case–control studies that have tested associations of TNF promoter SNPs with infectious diseases have been underpowered (see below). Some studies have also suggested that these variants may not be functional in altering transcription (Stuber et al., 1995). Uncertainty about the true structural nature of the TNF locus itself may have also contributed to the contradictory findings. There are many SNPs within the TNF gene (e.g., figure 14.1b). In the promoter, these are at positions −1031 (T/C), −863 (C/A), −857 (C/A), −851 (C/T), −419 (G/C), −376 (G/A), −308 (G/A), −238 (G/A), −162 (G/A), and −49 (G/A), although those at positions −419, −163, and −49 are rare in Caucasians (Mira et al., 1999). New polymorphisms in this region continue to be discovered (Iida

et al., 2003). In addition, there is an insertion of a cytosine at position 70 in the first exon, a G/A substitution at position 488 in the first intron (D'Alfonso and Richiardi, 1996) that confers a difference in TNF expression (van Krugten et al., 1999), and a deletion of a G at position 691 in the first intron (Azmy et al., 1999). Consequently, the 5′ region of the TNF gene is highly polymorphic. By contrast, the 3′ region of the TNF gene appears to be highly conserved (Becker et al., 1995; Waldron-Lynch et al., 1999). This sequence information is continuously updated, and most of the SNPs can be found at any of several Web sites (e.g., dbSNP database available via www.ncbi.nlm.nih.gov or the International HapMap Project available via snp.cshl.org).

Polymorphism, Populations, and Disease Associations

As noted above, the −308A allele in the TNF promoter (also known as TNF2) is a G/A transition and the most studied SNP in this gene. Several other SNPs in the promoter have been mapped (figure 14.1b). Numerous publications describe SNPs, and associate them with diseases. Most of these studies are case–control studies comparing the frequencies of specific SNPs in two groups of individuals and analyzing their association with disease (or other phenotypes). Table 14.2 summarizes studies on these TNF SNPs in infectious diseases.

A good example of the many discrepancies obtained in various studies on TNF is observed in leprosy. Table 14.2 shows different populations (Indian, Brazilian, Vietnamese, and Malawi) tested using population or family-based approaches in leprosy. Associations of TNF −308A were opposite in direction in cases

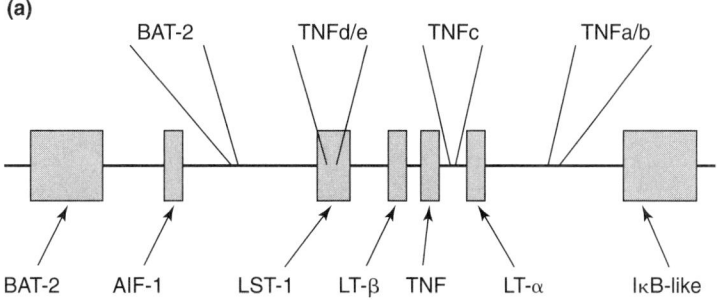

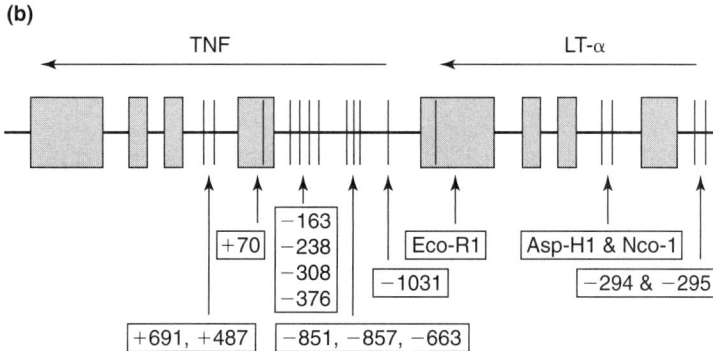

FIGURE 14.1. Polymorphic elements in the human *TNF* locus. The human *TNF* locus is situated in the MHC, at 6p21.3. There are many polymorphic elements. (a) The positions of the 6 microsatellites referred to in the text are shown relative to the genes present. (b) Positions of many single nucleotide polymorphisms (SNPs) in the *TNF* and *LTA* genes. This list is not exhaustive but illustrative of the heavy evolutionary pressure on this region of the genome.

and controls from India and Brazil. The Brazilian study (Santos et al., 2000, 2002) suggested that −308A is associated with resistance to leprosy, while the Indians showed increased frequency of that allele among the severe or lepromatous type of the disease (Roy et al., 1997). A later study in another Brazilian population (northern Brazil) confirmed the association of −308A with resistance using a different approach (Shaw et al., 2001). On the other hand, Fitness et al. (2004) working in Malawi failed to replicate either finding, and no association was found with −238, −308, −376, or −863 SNPs, although a microsatellite in *LTA* was associated with susceptibility to leprosy. Shaw et al. (2001) also found an intronic SNP in *LTA* (at +252) associated with leprosy.

Interestingly, family-based studies in leprosy contribute to this discussion. Mira et al. (2003) using a genomewide scan also found the 6p21 region, including human leukocyte antigen (HLA) and *TNF*, linked to leprosy per se. Thus, it is likely that *TNF* or a closely linked gene contributes to leprosy resistance/susceptibility and/or severity. The presence of other markers in the surrounding TNF/HLA loci (e.g., HSP, the family of genes for heat-shock protein molecules, or genes for TAP, transporters associated with antigen processing) obviously may also contribute to leprosy susceptibility or severity (Fitness et al., 2002).

Table 14.2 also shows studies in TB suggesting the absence of associations between variations in the TNF region and disease, although some data are controversial (see "Infectious disease and autoimmunity: reciprocal genetics?" below).

The −308A allele has been associated with severity of inflammatory reactions in viral diseases such as

TABLE 14.2. Association of TNF locus SNPs and microsatellites with infectious diseases.

Study Design (Population)	SNP/Haplotypes	Phenotype	Reference
Case–control (India)	−308A	Susceptibility to lepromatous form of leprosy	Roy et al (1997)
Case–control (Brazil)	−308A	Resistance to leprosy per se	Santos et al (2002)
TdT (Brazil)	−308A	Resistance to leprosy per se	Shaw et al (2001)
Linkage (Vietnam)	STRs	No association with leprosy	Mira et al (2003)
Case–control (Malawi)	LTA STR	Susceptibility to leprosy per se	Fitness et al (2004)
Case–control (India)	−308	No association with TB	Selvaraj et al (2001)
Case–control (Cambodia)	−308	No association with TB	Delgado et al (2002)
Case–control (Colombia)	−308A/−238G	Susceptibility to TB	Correa et al (2005)
Case–control (Finland)	−308A	Severity in renal syndrome hantavirus infection	Makela et al (2001)
Case–control (Venezuela)	−308A	Severity in hemorrhagic fever of dengue infection	Fernandez-Mestre et al (2004)
Case–control (Korea)	−308A and −863C	Significant association with resolution of HBV infection	Kim et al (2003)
Case–control (Germany)	−238A	Susceptibility to chronic HBV infection	Hoeler et al (1998)
Case–control (China)	−238 (GG)	Protection against chronic HBV infection	Li et al (2005)
Case–control (USA)	−863C/−308G	Viral persistence in HCV infection (African Americans)	Thio et al (2004)
Case–control (Japanese)	−238 and −308	No association in HCV infection	Kusumoto et al (2006)
Case–control (France)	−308A	Susceptibility to septic shock and death due to septic shock	Mira et al (1999)
Case–control (USA)	−308A	Association with mortality in septic patients	Hedberg et al (2004)
Case–control (Japanese)	−308A	Susceptibility to sepsis in critically ill patients	Nakada et al (2005)
Case–control (USA)	−308A	Susceptibility to severe sepsis after burn injury	Barber et al (2004)
Case–control (Holland)	+252A/−308A	Protection to severe sepsis	Majetschak et al (2002)
Case–control (Germany)	+252	No association in critically ill patients	Rauchschwalbe et al (2004)
Case–control (Germany)	−308GG	Susceptibility of duodenal ulcer in patients infected with Helicobacter pylori	Kunstmann et al (1999)
Case–control (Korean)	−308A	Susceptibility to gastric ulcer in patients infected with H. pylori (cagA subtype)	Yea et al (2001)

TABLE 14.2. (continued)

Study Design (Population)	SNP/Haplotypes	Phenotype	Reference
Case–control (Portugal)	−308A	Susceptibility to gastric carcinoma in *H. pylori*–positive patients	Machado et al (2003)
Case–control (Taiwan)	−857T	Protection against gastric carcinoma (maltoma) in *H. pylori*–positive patients	Wu et al (2004)
Case–control (Italian)	−857 (TT)	Susceptibility to duodenal ulcer in *H. pylori*–positive patients	Zambon et al (2005)
Case–control (Taiwan)	−1031C or −863A	Susceptibility to ulcer after *H. pylori* infection	Lu et al (2005)
Case–control (Venezuela)	−308A	Severity (mucosal form) of tegumentary leishmaniasis	Cabrera et al (1995)
TdT (Brazil)	−308A	Association of symptomatic VL	Karplus et al (2002)
Case–control (Tunisia)	+252LTA and −308	No association with VL	Meddeb-Garnaoui et al (2001)
Case–control (Peru)	−238, −244, −308	No association with Chagas' disease per se or chronic cardiopathic	Beraun et al (1998)
Case–control (Mexico)	−308A	Association with susceptibility of Chagas' disease per se or chronic phase	Rodriguez-Perez et al (2005)
Case–control (Brazil)	−308A	Association with severity in chronic chagasic cardiopathy and mortality	Drigo et al (2006)
Case–control (Gambia)	−308A	Association of severity in cerebral malaria (risk of death)	McGuire et al (1994)
Case–control (Gambia)	−376A	Susceptibility to cerebral malaria	Knight et al (1999)
Case–control (Sri Lanka)	−308A	Susceptibility to severe malaria	Wattavidanage et al (1999)
Case–control (Kenya)	−308A	Association with high density *P. falciparum* parasitemia and increased risk for severe malaria anemia	Aidoo et al (2001)
Family-based (Burkina-Faso)	−238, +1304, and +851	Association with maximum malaria parasitemia	Flori et al (2005)

nephropathy caused by Puumala hantavirus infection (Makela et al., 2001) and hemorrhagic fever caused by dengue virus infection (Fernandez-Mestre et al., 2004). In infection with hepatitis B virus (HBV) (see chapter 21), the presence of −308A and −863C was associated with viral clearance (Kim et al., 2003). On the other hand, studies in Germans and Chinese implicated other SNP (−238) with chronic HBV infection, where −238G was associated with protection against chronic hepatitis (Hohler et al., 1998; Li et al.,

2005). In hepatitis C virus (HCV) infection, the haplotype −863C/−308G was associated with viral persistence in African Americans (Thio et al., 2004), although no differences were observed for this infection in a Japanese study (Kusumoto et al., 2006).

In sepsis, genetic epidemiological studies in adult French patients as well as in American children documented an association of −308A with susceptibility to sepsis, shock, and death (Mira et al., 1999; Hedberg et al., 2004). Nakada et al. (2005) studying a group of critically ill patients showed that the frequency of the −308G/A genotype was significantly higher in the septic than in the control group and was also associated with poor outcome of sepsis. In burn trauma patients exhibiting severe sepsis, an increased risk was observed for patients carrying −308A allele (Barber et al., 2004). On the other hand, an extended haplotype combining +252A and −308A appeared to protect against the development of sepsis (Majetschak et al., 2002), while no association was detected in critically ill patients (Rauchschwalbe et al., 2004).

Studies evaluating patients infected with *Helicobacter pylori* in association with development of cancer or ulcer suggests that TNF polymorphisms are not associated with susceptibility to the bacterial infection per se, but with complications such as gastric ulcers or carcinoma associated with the infection. The severity of the disease analyzed in *H. pylori*–infected patients demonstrated that women with the −308G/G genotype have an increased risk for duodenal ulcer (Kunstmann et al., 1999). Among Korean patients with *H. pylori* infection, −238 and −308 SNPs were not correlated with the severity of disease, but −308A was significantly associated with the *H. pylori* cagA subtype infection with gastric disease (Yea et al., 2001). In a Portuguese study with *H. pylori*–infected individuals carrying the −308A allele had an increased risk for gastric carcinoma (Machado et al., 2003). On the other hand, the analysis of another SNP in *TNF* promoter generated opposite results in Taiwanese and Italian populations. In the first population (Wu et al., 2004), the −857T SNP was associated with protection against a gastric carcinoma (maltoma). In the second, the −857T/T genotype was associated with susceptibility gastric ulcer (Zambon et al., 2005). In an investigation of other *TNF* promoter positions, −1031C and −863A were risk factors for gastric inflammation and peptic ulceration upon *H. pylori* infection (Lu et al., 2005).

In parasitic diseases, TNF SNPs were studied in leishmaniasis (see also chapter 25), where the intronic LTA +252G and the TNF −308A were observed in a higher frequency in patients exhibiting the severe mucosal form (Cabrera et al., 1995). The outcome and development of visceral leishmaniasis (VL) were assessed in a family-based study of asymptomatic and symptomatic Brazilian VL patients. TNF −308G was associated with asymptomatic, while TNF −308A was associated with symptomatic VL (Karplus et al., 2002). In contrast, in Tunisia, no association was found between VL and either SNP (at LTA +252 or TNF −308) (Meddeb-Garnaoui et al., 2001). Severity of Chagas' disease was tested in a population-based study comparing asymptomatic and chronic cardiopathic chagasic (CCC) Peruvian patients. The investigation of SNPs at −308, −244, and −238 yielded no association). In a Mexican population the frequency of TNF −308A was higher in CCC patients than in asymptomatic patients (Rodriguez-Perez et al., 2005). Drigo et al. (2006) observed that −308A was a predictor for mortality among CCC patients. With malaria (see also chapter 24), −308A has been associated with severity in cerebral malaria in Gambians and Sri Lankans (McGuire et al., 1994; Wattavidanage et al., 1999). The −376A SNP was also associated with cerebral malaria in a different study (Knight et al., 1999). In Kenyans, the −308A was associated with high density parasitemia and severe anemia (Aidoo et al., 2001), while in Burkina-Faso, highest parasitemia was linked to −238, +1304, and +851 SNPs (Flori et al., 2005).

The ambiguous and at times conflicting results summarized above, particularly for the TNF −308A allele, have several possible explanations. In some case–control studies, low numbers of subjects could have led to an unstable estimation of an effect and chance association of a marker with the condition under study or, more likely, a negative result due to insufficient statistical power. Appropriate selection of controls is also a problem for infectious diseases. Healthy individuals enrolled in a study as controls should have the potential to become cases. Subjects not chosen for exposure comparable to that of cases (e.g., with infection that is less well defined, intense, or continuous) do not represent optimal controls. Discrepancy between populations may also be ascribed to association with polymorphisms of other genes in the region (including those in the HLA or the HSP family, *LTA, LTB, LST1,* or *TAP1*), which may follow different patterns of linkage disequilibrium with the −308A allele in different populations. A third possibility is that differential selective pressures on populations have evolved ethnic-specific host genetic factors. Thus, meta-analysis of published associations of this TNF allele with SLE revealed discrepancies consistent with ethnic origin of the studied population. Reanalysis of the associations of −308A with SLE in European, Asian, African, and Mexican populations demonstrated significant results restricted to the European populations (Lee et al., 2006). Similar meta-analysis in asthma showed an increased risk for −308A carriers (Gao et al.,

2006) and further argues for exploring that strategy to improve our understanding of the role of such prominent candidate SNPs in infectious disease susceptibility.

Infectious Disease and Autoimmunity: Reciprocal Genetics?

TNF is a pluripotent molecule, and its role in different immunologically mediated diseases may well vary. With autoimmune disorders, while there is compelling evidence indicating a pathogenic role of this cytokine in RA (Feldmann et al., 1996; Vassalli, 1992), a protective role has been suggested in SLE (Aringer & Smolen, 2003), and incomplete knowledge exists concerning its function in progressive systemic sclerosis (PSS). Studies of TNF promoter SNPs have proceeded on the assumption that discoveries about gene variants with a significant role in pathology will lead to a greater understanding of the regulatory mechanisms involved in both health and disease and may provide useful knowledge for identifying and enhancing early interventions in at-risk individuals (Cardon & Bell, 2001).

Autoimmune diseases frequently occur in genetically susceptible individuals in whom the clinical expression of the disease is modulated by permissive and protective environments. These are genetically complex diseases, that is, polygenic rather than following a single-gene dominant or recessive Mendelian law. A number of studies have indicated that the TNF −308A/−238G haplotype constitutes a common susceptibility marker for autoimmune diseases (RA, SLE, and PSS). They support the common variants/multimultiple disease hypothesis, which emphasizes that many genes are unlikely to be disease specific and that similar immunogenetic mechanisms may underlie related diseases (Anaya & Talal, 1999; Heward & Gough, 1997; Becker et al., 1998; Becker, 2004).

In contrast to the role of the TNF −308A/−238G haplotype in autoimmunity, it has appeared protective in the context of infection. For example, in the same study demonstrating its association with susceptibility to SLE, RA, and PSS in Colombians (Correa et al. 2005), this haplotype was associated with protection against TB. The data suggested the occurrence of overdominant selection (heterozygote advantage) in this population, in which the heterozygotes for a particular allele (−308A) were resistant to one condition (TB) but susceptible to another (autoimmunity). There are other examples of this inverse relationship between occurrence of TB and autoimmune diseases (Mobley, 2004; Rothschild et al., 2003). Natural selection for resistance to a pathogen can lead to the increase in frequency of alleles that are otherwise deleterious (Dean et al., 2002). A higher level of TNF was found to be a risk factor for death from cardiovascular disease in a group of elderly women (Van Den Biggelaar et al., 2004). Caucasians may have experienced very strong natural selection during millennia of continuous exposure viral and bacterial pathogens with successive epidemics. These selective pressures might have generated a genetic background that is broadly protective through strong immune responses upon challenge with infectious agents. On the other hand, a much higher degree of susceptibility may have accumulated in isolated, long-unexposed (e.g., aboriginal) populations, who evolved in environments with different selective pressure exerted by diverse infectious agents (Greenwood et al., 2000).

If protection from infection is a stronger selective force than the negatively selected phenotype, the "deleterious" allele will accumulate in the population as long as the infectious agent remains prevalent. This may be particularly true if that allele does not exert its disadvantage until after the normal age of reproduction or if its effects are not rapidly fatal, as expected with the autoimmune diseases. However, the heterozygote advantage seen in Colombia (Correa et al., 2005) has not been observed uniformly in all settings: Two previous studies performed in Asia did not find an association between the −238 and −308 SNPs and pulmonary TB (Delgado et al., 2002; Selvaraj et al., 2001). Such inconsistency could signify variability in TNF polymorphism among populations (Baena et al., 2002) so great that studies of this polymorphism in infection could help elucidate the history of human populations.

Functional Relationships with TNF

The great variability in levels of TNF among individuals has led to intensive effort to identify the most informative genetic markers with which to interrogate the heritable basis of this variability. At the TNF locus, a complex pattern of linkage disequilibrium across microsatellite and SNP alleles defines three families of haplotypes, which are associated with differential TNF secretion. Although there are clearly relationships between *TNF* variants and the class I and class II MHC alleles, and TNF secretion does appear to vary with MHC genotype, the differences are not due merely to more extensive linkage disequilibrium between the two regions. (Gallagher et al., 1997b). Several studies have shown an association between *HLA-DRB1* alleles and the *in vitro* production of TNF. The DR3, DR1, DR4, and DR7 allele groups have been associated with higher TNF production (Bendtzen et al., 1988; Jacob et al., 1990; Pociot et al., 1993), whereas DR2 and DR5 groups have been associated with lower TNF responses (Molvig et al., 1990). The ability of DR molecules to confer differential cell activation and cytokine secretion has been localized to their intracellular elements (Fleury et al., 1995). Interestingly, differential IFN-γ production has also been associated with particular MHC molecules (Petrovsky & Harrison, 1997). Linkage disequilibrium between TNF polymorphisms and DR types may explain a portion of this phenomenon. However, TNF secretion following lipopolysaccharide (LPS) stimulation (see below) has been shown to vary independently of the MHC allelic variation (Pociot et al., 1993), and some disease associations with the *TNF* locus are independent of (although complementary to) those with the MHC (Caballero et al., 2000; Rood et al., 2000).

More work is in order to define the gene variation–function relationships. Microsatellite markers and SNPs can be arranged to form haplotypes that are likely to mediate this regulatory action on TNF-α secretion, although few studies have provided information of these combinations affecting TNF-α expression. Observation of a functional promoter can be obtained by the detection of either mRNA or protein. Analysis of promoter functions can also be achieved with gene reporter assays, that is, by assessing promoter inducibility in transfected cells or by applying the electrophoretic mobility shift assay (EMSA) that measures the ability of double-strand oligonucleotides to bind to transcription factors.

The −308A allele was assumed to be associated with high TNF-α production in studies using mRNA/protein detection or gene-reporter assays, but contrasting results of studies to date have left unclear whether this variation in the promoter region was responsible for observed differences in TNF-α production. A summary of studies concerning the production of mRNA and protein secretion is presented in table 14.3. These studies have been performed in order to try to link the genetic variability within the promoter with

functional activity. The experimental design is variable and almost certainly has further confounded the data. Six of 20 studies selected here used healthy donor cells, while other studies used samples from patients from different infectious or other diseases. Four studies measured TNF-α in the serum/plasma directly whereas 10 used peripheral blood morphonuclear cells (PBMCs) or whole blood stimulated mainly by LPS (ranging from 1 to 1,000 ng/ml, including different periods of incubation). Eight studies demonstrated that TNF-α promoter polymorphism −308G/A or −238G/A was associated with levels of TNF-α message or protein, while the remainder either failed to detect such differences or implicated other polymorphisms (−863 and −857) as responsible for high versus low TNF-α production, respectively. In short, the studies on which, if any, TNF-α promoter polymorphisms affect TNF-α production have been inconclusive.

Another approach to testing the functionality of *TNF* promoter polymorphisms has been measurement of clinical or biological parameters believed to be influenced by TNF-α concentrations. For example, the injection of heat-killed *Mycobacterium leprae* in the forearm induces a delayed-type immune response approximately 28 days after the injection. The −308A allele was found to be associated with a stronger response to heat-killed *M. leprae* in borderline tuberculoid leprosy patients (Moraes et al., 2001). In leprosy, slit skin smears are used as an alternative for *in vivo* determination of the bacterial load. Vanderborght et al. (2004) demonstrated that TNF −308A had an impact on the burden of bacilli carried by a patient: Carriers of that allele had lower bacteriological index than did noncarriers. This work offered indirect evidence that the −308A allele augmented TNF production, but another functional polymorphism in linkage disequilibrium with the TNF −308A allele may have equally well accounted for these findings. Whether the promoter polymorphisms are functional has not been resolved.

The results of gene reporter assays have also been ambiguous where the transfected −308A allele did (and sometimes did not) alter the levels of the inducible reporter gene using different cell types such as Raji B cells, U937, HeLa, Jurkat, and HepG2 (Brinkman et al., 1995–1996; Stuber et al., 1995; Wilson et al., 1997; Kroeger et al., 1997; Bayley et al., 2001). Numerous other studies have analyzed the effect of SNPs on promoter activity with inconsistent and even conflicting results. In short, all of this work has not settled the role of −308A.

TABLE 14.3. TNF promoter functionality as analyzed by detection of protein and mRNA.

Cell Type	Sampling	Stimulation (Time)	SNP or Allele	TNF Production (↑ = High or ↓ = Low)	References
Monocytes	72 and 32 healthy donors	LPS allogeneic	−238A	Protein: no difference	Pociot et al (1993)
PBMC	30 irritable bowel disease patients	1 μg/ml anti-CD3 + 1 μg/ml anti-CD28 (48 h)	−308A	↑ protein	Bouma et al (1996)
Whole blood	62 healthy donors	1 ng/ml LPS (3 h)	−308A	↑ protein	Louis et al (1998)
Oral PMN	32 patients	—	−308A	↑ protein	Galbraith et al (1998)
BAL	44 sarcoidosis	None	−308A	Protein: no difference	Somoskovi et al (1999)
Serum	156 healthy men	—	−863A −308A	↓ protein No difference	Skoog et al (1999)
PBMC	47 psoriasis patients	50 ng/ml PMA[1] 1 μg/ml + ionomycin (8 h, 15 h)	−308 −238A	No difference ↓ protein	Kaluza et al (2000)
Whole blood	Ulcerative colitis	LPS	−308A	↑ protein	Koss et al (2000)
Serum	57 leprosy patients	—	−308A	Protein: no differences	Sarno et al (2000)
Adipose tissue	24 nonobese 56 obese		−863A −857A	↓ protein (nonobese), no difference (obese) ↑ protein (nonobese)	Skoog et al (2001)
PBMC	21 non-Hodgkin's lymphoma patients	1 μg/ml LPS (30 min)	−308A	↑ RNA Protein: no difference	Baseggio et al (2002)
PBMC	Healthy donors	LPS, PMA, anti-CD3, anti-CD28 Different time periods	−1031; −863 −857; −308	RNA: No differences	Kaijzel et al (2001)
Plasma	35 antiphospholipid syndrome patients	—	−308 −238	Protein: no differences	Bertolaccini et al (2001)
BAL	20 chronic beryllium disease patients	Beryllium antigen	−308A	↑ protein	Maier et al (2001)
Whole blood	59 typhoid fever patients	1 μg/ml LPS (24h)	−308	Protein: no difference	House et al (2002)
Whole blood	129 healthy	LPS	−376 −308 −238 +489	Protein: no difference	de Jong et al (2002)
Whole blood	92 RA and 42 healthy	LPS	−308	Protein: no difference	Cuenca et al (2003)
PBMC	41 liver transplant recipients	10 μg/mL con-A 1 and 2 days	−308A	Protein: no difference	Warle et al (2003)
Serum	50 patients (Crohn's disease)	—	−308A	↑ ($p < 0.05$)	Gonzalez et al (2003)
Plasma	208 patients (pancreatitis)	—	−308	No differences	Dianliang et al (2003)

[1]PMA, phorbol myristic acetate

More recently, an elegant characterization of the TNF-α region has shed new light on the debate by suggesting that TNF −308 itself may not be a functional polymorphism (Knight et al., 2003): The study revealed that −308A was not loaded with increased amount phosphorylated (activated) RNA polymerase II, implying that both alleles (−308G and −308A) have similar transcriptional activity. Even more important, the investigators found that the LTA +252G, linked in a haplotype with TNF −308A, showed enhanced loading by phosphorylated polymerase II when compared with the contribution of the +252A allele. A recent (Ozaki et al., 2002) genomewide case–control study implicated this same variation (+252G) in myocardial infarction. Functional analyses demonstrated that the G allele had an increased binding capacity to an unknown transcription factor in Jurkat T cells and also exhibited greater (1.5-fold) transcriptional activity.

Taken together, the many studies of the TNF −308 SNP suggest that the design (plasmid constructs, stimuli, oligonucleotide design, etc.) may have drastically modified the results obtained in experimental studies. Moreover, it now appears that, as always with an isolated marker like this SNP, failure to consider linkage disequilibrium in population studies may have accounted for at least some of the discrepancy. The upstream LTA SNP +252G, that has also been designated −3025 in relation to the TNF-α transcript start site, exhibits relevant and differential activity on both LTα and TNF-α. Specifically, healthy donors carrying +252G produce more TNF-α in cultures of whole blood cells stimulated with LPS (Heesen et al., 2003). Temple et al. (2003) obtained similar results at the mRNA level.

It is increasingly clear that high and low TNF-α producers exist and that production level is at least partially inherited, although the genetic regulatory determinants have not been precisely defined. Comprehensive examination of the SNPs and microsatellite alleles described above should define the genetic factors more accurately and completely. As an alternative to examining the multiple SNPs identified above, the microsatellite loci TNFd4 and TNFa2 (Weissensteiner & Lanchbury, 1997; Pociot et al., 1993) offer excellent resolution of the bewildering array of SNP allelic combinations. Indeed, the TNF2-d4 haplotype has been associated with a range of chronic inflammatory disorders against disparate MHC backgrounds (Mattey et al., 1999; Plevy et al., 1996). A clearer understanding of genetic regulation of TNF production and the effects of its variation should finally emerge when the entire TNF gene cluster is described and examined in an orderly manner, taking full account of the MHC haplotypes in which it resides.

Animal Studies

TNF is an important mediator of protection from parasitic, bacterial, and viral infection (Vassalli, 1992). With Listeria monocytogenes as a model organism, it has been shown that neutralizing TNF with monoclonal antibodies is extremely detrimental (Havell, 1989). However, the effects of high or low TNF are not entirely uniform or clear cut and appear to vary with the infection. For example, withdrawing TNF protects mice from endotoxemic death (Beutler et al., 1985), in contrast to the association of elevated TNF levels with a much poorer outcome in human malaria (Kwiatkowski et al., 1990). Conversely, anti–TNF-α administration in experimental models leads to the absence of mature granulomas and increased numbers of mycobacteria (Kindler et al., 1989). Similar results were obtained with thalidomide, a selective inhibitor of TNF-α, in BCG-infected mice (Aarestrup et al., 1995). In fact, TNF knockout mice are completely susceptible to mycobacterial infections; the animals develop uncontrolled, fatal infections (Jacobs et al., 2000; Douni et al., 1995–1996).

Conclusion

The human TNF locus is a structural part of the region of chromosome 6 containing the MHC. It exhibits substantial polymorphism and has a complex evolutionary history. While its role in the etiology of human disease has now been studied quite extensively, the precise consequences of its heritable genetic variation are still uncertain. Certain TNF polymorphisms have been rather convincingly associated with autoimmune diseases but more tentatively with infectious diseases. New knowledge about structure and variation of the TNF gene and its related neighbors should help resolve the complexity and lead to clearer understanding of functional associations.

Acknowledgments

We thank all of the members of our laboratories who contributed to this work: David A. Campbell, Paula A.

Correa, Joyce Eskdale, Hui-Hui Oh, Leigh McCauley, Susan Richards, and Gabriel J. Tabon. We are also indebted to colleagues for helpful discussions: Tevfik Dorak, Max Field, Michael McDermott, Janet McNicholl, Sergei Nedospasov, Cynthia Chester Cardoso, Tom Huizinga, and Tom Ottenhoff.

References

Aarestrup, F.M., Goncalves-da-Costa, S.C., & Sarno, E.N. (1995) The effect of thalidomide on BCG-induced granulomas in mice. *Brazilian Journal of Medical and Biological Research*, 28, 1069–1076.

Abraham, L.J., Marley, J.V., Nedospasov, S.A., Cambon-Thomsen, A., Crouau-Roy, B., Dawkins, R.L., & Giphart, M.J. (1993) Microsatellite, restriction fragment-length polymorphism, and sequence-specific oligonucleotide typing of the tumor necrosis factor region. Comparisons of the 4AOHW cell panel. *Human Immunology*, 38, 17–23.

Aggarwal, B.B. (2003) Signalling pathways of the TNF superfamily: a double-edged sword. *Nature Reviews Immunology*, 3, 745–756.

Aidoo, M., McElroy, P.D., Kolczak, M.S., Terlouw, D.J., ter Kuile, F.O., Nahlen, B., Lal, A.A., & Udhayakumar, V. (2001) Tumor necrosis factor-alpha promoter variant 2 (TNF2) is associated with pre-term delivery, infant mortality, and malaria morbidity in western Kenya: Asembo Bay Cohort Project IX. *Genetic Epidemiology*, 21, 201–211.

Anaya, J.M., & Talal, N. (1999) Sjögren's syndrome comes of age. *Seminars in Arthritis and Rheumatism*, 28, 355–359.

Aringer, M., & Smolen, J.S. (2003) Complex cytokine effects in a complex autoimmune disease: tumor necrosis factor in systemic lupus erythematosus. *Arthritis Research and Therapy*, 5, 172–177.

Azmy, I., Hajeer, A., Ollier, W.E.R., & Wilson, A.G. (1999) Association between an intronic TNFA polymorphism (-691) and TNF locus microsatellites. *Annals of Rheumatic Diseases*, 58 (abstr. suppl.), 41.

Baena, A., Leung, J.Y., Sullivan, A.D., Landires, I., Vasquez-Luna, N., Quinones-Berrocal, J., Fraser, P.A., Uko, G.P., Delgado, J.C., Clavijo, O.P., Thim, S., Meshnick, S.R., Nyirenda, T., Yunis, E.J., & Goldfeld, A.E. (2002) TNF-alpha promoter single nucleotide polymorphisms are markers of human ancestry. *Genes and Immunity*, 3, 482–487.

Barber, R.C., Aragaki, C.C., Rivera-Chavez, F.A., Purdue, G.F., Hunt, J.L., & Horton, J.W. (2004) TLR4 and TNF-alpha polymorphisms are associated with an increased risk for severe sepsis following burn injury. *Journal of Medical Genetics*, 41, 808–813.

Baseggio, L., Charlot, C., Bienvenu, J., Felman, P., & Salles, G. (2002) Tumor necrosis factor-alpha mRNA stability in human peripheral blood cells after lipopolysaccharide stimulation. *European Cytokine Network*, 13, 92–98.

Bayley, J.-P., de Rooij, H., van den Elsen, P.J., Huizinga, T.W., & Verweij, C.L. (2001) Functional analysis of linker-scan mutants spanning the −376, −308, −244, and −238 polymorphic sites of the TNF-alpha promoter. *Cytokine*, 14, 316–323.

Bayley, J.-P, Ottenhoff, T.H., & Verweij, C.L. (2004) Is there a future for TNF promoter polymorphisms? *Genes and Immunity*, 5, 1–15.

Becker, K.G. (2004) The common variants/multiple disease hypothesis of common complex genetic disorders. *Medical Hypotheses*, 62, 309–317.

Becker, K.G., Simon, R.M., Bailey-Wilson, J.E., Freidlin, B., Biddison, W.E., McFarland, H.F., & Trent, J.M. (1998) Clustering of non-major histocompatibility complex susceptibility candidate loci in human autoimmune diseases. *Proceedings of the National Academy of Sciences of the United States of America*, 95, 9979–9984.

Becker, L., Brown, T., Fink, C., Marks, J., Lavandosky, G. & Giroir, B.P. (1995) Sequence analysis of the tumor necrosis factor gene in pediatric patients with autoimmunity. *Pediatric Research*, 37, 165–168.

Bendtzen, K., Morling, N., Fomsgaard. A, Svenson, M., Jakobsen, B., Odum, N., & Svejgaard A. (1988) Association between HLA-DR2 and production of tumour necrosis factor alpha and interleukin 1 by mononuclear cells activated by lipopolysaccharide. *Scandinavian Journal of Immunology*, 28, 599–606.

Beraun, Y. Nieto, A., Collado, M.D., Gonzalez, A., & Martin, J. (1998) Polymorphisms at tumor necrosis factor (TNF) loci are not associated with Chagas' disease, *Tissue Antigens*, 52, 81–83.

Bertolaccini, M.L., Atsumi, T., Lanchbury, J.S., Caliz, A.R., Katsumata, K., Vaughan, R.W., Kondeatis, E., Khamashta, M.A., Koike, T., & Hughes, G.R. (2001) Plasma tumor necrosis factor alpha levels and the −238*A promoter polymorphism in patients with antiphospholipid syndrome. *Thrombosis and Haemostasis*, 85, 198–203.

Beutler, B., Milsark, I.W., & Cerami, A.C. (1985) Passive immunisation against cachectin/tumor necrosis factor protects mice from the lethal effects of endotoxin. *Science*, 229, 869–871.

Bidwell, J., Keen, L., Gallagher, G., Kimberly, R., Huizinga, T., McDermott, M.F., Oksenberg, J., McNicholl, J., Pociot, F., Hardt, C., & D'Alfonso, S. (1999) Cytokine gene polymorphism in human disease: on-line databases. *Genes and Immunity*, 1, 3–19.

Bidwell, J., Keen, L., Gallagher, G., Kimberly, R., Huizinga, T., McDermott, M.F., Oksenberg, J., McNicholl, J., Pociot, F., Hardt, C., & D'Alfonso, S. (2001)
Cytokine gene polymorphism in human disease: on-
line databases, supplement 1. Genes and Immunity,
2, 61–70.

Bochud, P.Y., & Calandra, T. (2003) Science, medicine,
and the future: pathogenesis of sepsis: new concepts
and implications for future treatment. British Medical Journal, 326, 262–266.

Bouma, G., Crusius, J.B., Oudkerk Pool, M., Kolkman,
J.J., von Blomberg, B.M., Kostense, P.J., Giphart,
M.J., Schreuder, G.M., Meuwissen, S.G., & Pena,
A.S. (1996) Secretion of tumour necrosis factor alpha
and lymphotoxin alpha in relation to polymorphisms
in the TNF genes and HLA-DR alleles. Relevance
for inflammatory bowel disease. Scandinavian Journal of Immunology, 43, 456– 463.

Brinkman, B.M., Zuijdeest, D., Kaijzel, E.L., Breedveld,
F.C., & Verweij, C.L. (1995–1996) Relevance of the
tumor necrosis factor alpha (TNF alpha) −308 pro-
hism in TNF alpha gene regulation. Journal of
Inflammation, 46, 32– 41.

Caballero, A., Bravo, M.J., Nieto, A., Colmenero, J.D.,
ALonso, A., & Martin, J. (2000) TNF-A promoter
polymorphism and susceptibility to brucellosis. Clinical and Experimental Immunology, 121, 480– 483.

Cabrera, M. Shaw, M.A., Sharples, C., Williams, H.,
Castes, M., Convit, J., & Blackwell, J.M. (1995)
Polymorphism in tumor necrosis factor genes asso-
ciated with mucocutaneous leishmaniasis, Journal of
Experimental Medicine, 182, 1259–1264,

Cardon, L.R., & Bell, J. (2001) Association study designs
for complex diseases. Nature Reviews Genetics, 2,
91–99

Correa, P.A., & Anaya, J.M. (2001) Molecular understanding of TNF alpha in rheumatoid arthritis. Re-
vista Colombiana de Reumatologia, 8, 236–520.

Correa, P.A., Gomez, L.M., Cadena, J., & Anaya, J.M.
(2005) Tumor necrosis factor alpha polymorphism
in autoimmune rheumatic diseases and tuberculosis.
Journal of Rheumatology, 32, 219–224.

Cuenca, J., Cuchacovich, M., Perez, C., Ferreira, L.,
Aguirre, A., Schiattino, I., Soto, L., Cruzat, A.,
Salazar-Onfray, F., & Aguillon, J.C. (2003) The
−308 polymorphism in the tumour necrosis factor
(TNF) gene promoter region and ex vivo lipopolysaccharide-induced TNF expression and cytotoxic
activity in Chilean patients with rheumatoid arthritis. Rheumatology (Oxford), 42, 308–313.

D'Alfonso, S., & Richiardi, P.M. (1996) An intragenic
polymorphism in the human tumor necrosis factor
alpha (TNFA) chain encoding gene. Immunogenetics, 44, 321–322.

Dawkins, R.L., Leaver, A., Cameron, P.U., Martin, E.,
Kay, P.H., & Christiansen, F.T. (1989) Some
disease-associated ancestral haplotypes carry a polymorphism of TNF. Human Immunology, 26, 91–97.

Dean, M., Carrington, M., & O'Brien, S.J. (2002) Balanced polymorphism selected by genetic versus infectious human disease. Annual Reviews in Genomics and Human Genetics, 3, 263–292.

de Baey, A., Holzinger, I., Scholz, S., Keller, E., Weiss,
E.H., & Albert E. (1995) Pvu II polymorphism in the
primate homologue of the mouse B144 (LST-1): a
novel marker gene within the tumor necrosis factor
region. Human Immunology, 42, 9–14.

de Baey, A., Fellerhoff, B., Maier, S., Martinozzi, S.,
Weidle, U., & Weiss, E.H. (1997) Complex expression pattern of the TNF region gene LST1 through
differential regulation, initiation, and alternative
splicing. Genomics, 45, 591–600.

de Jong, B.A., Westendorp, R.G., Bakker, A.M., & Huizinga, T.W. (2002) Polymorphisms in or near tumour necrosis factor (TNF)-gene do not determine
levels of endotoxin-induced TNF production. Genes
and Immunity, 3: 25–29.

Delgado, J.C., Baena, A., Thim, S., & Goldfeld, A.E.
(2002) Ethnic-specific genetic associations with
pulmonary tuberculosis. Journal of Infectious Diseases, 186, 1463–1468.

Dianliang, Z., Jieshou, L., Zhiwei, J., & Baojun, Y. (2003)
Association of plasma levels of tumor necrosis factor
(TNF)-alpha and its soluble receptors, two polymorphisms of the TNF gene, with acute severe pancre-
atitis and early septic shock due to it. Pancreas, 26,
339–343.

Dinarello, C.A. (2003) Anti-cytokine therapeutics and
infections. Vaccine, 21 (Suppl. 2), S24–S34.

Douni, E., Akassoglou, K., Alexopoulou, L., Georgopou-
los, S., Haralambous, S., Hill, S., Kassiotis, G.,
Kontoyiannis, D., Pasparakis, M., Plows, D., Probert,
L., Kollias, G. (1995–1996) Transgenic and knockout analyses of the role of TNF in immune regulation and disease pathogenesis. Journal of Inflammation, 47, 27–38.

Drigo, S.A., Cunha-Neto, E., Ianni, B., Cardoso, M.R.,
Braga, P.E., Fae, K.C., Nunes, V.L., Buck, P., Mady,
C., Kalil, J., & Goldberg, A.C. (2006) TNF gene
polymorphisms are associated with reduced survival
in severe Chagas' disease cardiomyopathy patients.
Microbes and Infection, 8, 598–603.

Feldmann, M. (2002) Development of anti-TNF therapy
for rheumatoid arthritis. Nature Reviews Immunology,
2, 364–371.

Feldmann, M., Brennan, F.M., & Maini, R.N. (1996)
Role of cytokines in rheumatoid arthritis. Annual
Review of Immunology, 14, 397– 440.

Fernandez-Mestre, M.T., Gendzekhadze, K., Rivas-Vetencourt, P., & Layrisse, Z. (2004) TNF-alpha-308A allele, a possible severity risk factor of hemorrhagic manifestation in dengue fever patients. *Tissue Antigens*, 64, 469–472.

Fitness, J., Floyd, S., Warndorff, D.K., Sichali, L., Mwaungulu, L., Crampin, A.C., Fine, P.E., & Hill, A.V. (2004) Large-scale candidate gene study of leprosy susceptibility in the Karonga district of northern Malawi. *American Journal of Tropical Medicine and Hygiene*, 71, 330–340.

Fitness, J., Tosh, K., & Hill, A.V. (2002) Genetics of susceptibility to leprosy. *Genes and Immunity*, 3, 441–453.

Fleury, S., Thibodeau, J., Croteau, G., Labrecque, N., Aronson, H.E., Cantin, C., Long, E.O., & Sekaly, R.P. (1995) HLA-DR polymorphism affects the interaction with CD4. *Journal of Experimental Medicine*, 182, 733–741.

Flori, L., Delahaye, N.F., Iraqi, F.A., Hernadez-Valladares, M., Fumoux, F., & Rihet, P. (2005) TNF as a malaria candidate gene: polymorphism-screening and family-based association analysis of mild malaria attack and parasitemia in Burkina Faso. *Genes and Immunity*, 6, 472–480.

Flynn, J.L., & Chan, J. (2001) Immunology of tuberculosis. *Annual Reviews of Immunology*, 19, 93–129.

Fox, R.I., Kang, H.I., Ando, D., Abrams, J., & Pisa, E. (1994) Cytokine mRNA expression in salivary gland biopsies of Sjogren's syndrome. *Journal of Immunology*, 152, 5532–5539.

Galbraith, G.M., Steed, R.B., Sanders, J.J., & Pandey, J.P. (1998) Tumor necrosis factor alpha production by oral leukocytes: influence of tumor necrosis factor genotype. *Journal of Periodontology*, 69, 428–433.

Gallagher, G., Eskdale, J., & Miller, S. (1997a) A highly polymorphic microsatellite marker in the human MHC class III region, close to the BAT2 gene. *Immunogenetics*, 46, 357–358.

Gallagher, G., Eskdale, J., Oh, H.H., Richards, S.D., Campbell, D.A., Field, M. (1997b) Polymorphisms in the TNF gene cluster and MHC serotypes in the west of Scotland. *Immunogenetics*, 45, 188–194.

Gao, J., Shan, G., Sun, B., Thompson, P.J., & Gao, X. (2006) Association between polymorphism of tumour necrosis factor α-308 gene promoter and asthma: a meta-analysis. *Thorax*, 61, 466–471.

Gomez, D., Correa, P.A., Gomez, L.M., Cadena, J., Molina, J.F., & Anaya, J.M. (2004) Th1/Th2 cytokines in patients with systemic lupus erythematosus: is tumor necrosis factor alpha protective? *Seminars in Arthritis and Rheumatism*, 33, 404–413.

Gonzalez, S., Rodrigo, L., Martinez-Borra, J., Lopez-Vazquez, A., Fuentes, D., Nino, P., Cadahia, V., Saro, C., Dieguez, M.A., & Lopez-Larrea, C. (2003) TNF-alpha −308A promoter polymorphism is associated with enhanced TNF-alpha production and inflammatory activity in Crohn's patients with fistulizing disease. *American Journal of Gastroenterology*, 98, 1101–1006.

Greenwood, C.M., Fujiwara, T.M., Boothroyd, L.J., Miller, M.A., Frappier, D., Fanning, E.A., Schurr, E., & Morgan, K. (2000) Linkage of tuberculosis to chromosome 2q35 loci, including NRAMP1, in a large aboriginal Canadian family. *American Journal of Human Genetics*, 67, 405–416.

Hajeer, A.H., & Hutchinson, I.V. (2001) Influence of TNFα gene polymorphisms on TNFα production and disease. *Human Immunology*, 62, 1191–1199.

Haukim, N., Bidwell, J.L., Smith, A.J., Keen, L.J., Gallagher, G., Kimberly, R., Huizinga, T., McDermott, M.F., Oksenberg, J., McNicholl, J., Pociot, F., Hardt, C., & D'Alfonso, S. (2002) Cytokine gene polymorphism in human disease: on-line databases, supplement 2. *Genes Immunity*, 3, 313–330.

Havell, E.A. (1989) Evidence that tumor necrosis factor has an important role in antibacterial resistance. *Journal of Immunology*, 143, 2894–2899.

Heesen, M., Kunz, D., Bachmann-Mennenga, B., Merk, H.F., & Bloemeke, B. (2003) Linkage disequilibrium between tumor necrosis factor (TNF)-alpha-308 G/A promoter and TNF-beta NcoI polymorphisms: Association with TNF-alpha response of granulocytes to endotoxin stimulation. *Critical Care Medicine*, 31, 211–214.

Heward, J., & Gough, S.C.L. (1997) Genetic susceptibility to the development of autoimmune disease. *Clinical Science*, 93, 479–491.

Hohler, T., Kruger, A., Gerken, G., Schneider, P.M., Meyer zum Buschnefelde, K.H., & Rittner, C. (1998) A tumor necrosis factor-alpha (TNF-alpha) promoter polymorphism is associated with chronic hepatitis B infection. *Clinical Experimental Immunology*, 111, 579–582.

Hollegaard, M.V., & Bidwell, J.L. (2006) Cytokine gene polymorphism in human disease: on-line databases, supplement 3. *Genes and Immunity*, 7, 269–276.

Holzinger, I., de Baey, A., Messer, G., Kick, G., Zwierzina, H., & Weiss, E.H. (1995) Cloning and genomic characterization of LST1: a new gene in the human TNF region. *Immunogenetics*, 42, 315–322.

House, D., Chinh, N.T., Hien, T.T., Parry, C.P., Ly, N.T., Diep, T.S., Wain, J., Dunstan, S., White, N.J., Dougan, G., & Farrar, J.J. (2002) Cytokine release by lipopolysaccharide-stimulated whole blood from patients with typhoid fever. *Journal of Infectious Diseases*, 186, 240–245.

Iida, A., Ozaki, K., Ohnishi, Y., Tanaka, T., & Nakamura, Y. (2003) Identification of 46 novel SNPs in the 130-kb region containing a myocardial infarction susceptibility gene on chromosomal band 6p21. *Journal of Human Genetics*, 48, 476–479.

Jacob, C.O., Fronek, Z., Lewis, G.D., Koo, M., Hansen, J.A., & McDevitt, H.O. (1990) Heritable major histocompatibility complex class II-associated differences in production of tumor necrosis factor alpha: relevance to genetic predisposition to systemic lupus erythematosus. *Proceedings of the National Academy of Sciences of the United States of America*, 87, 1233–1237.

Jacobs, M., Brown, N., Allie, N., & Ryffel B. (2000) Fatal *Mycobacterium bovis* BCG infection in TNF-LT-alpha-deficient mice. *Clinical Immunology*, 94, 192–199.

Jongeneel, C.V., Briant, L., Udalova, I.A., Sevin, A., Nedospasov, S.A., & Cambon-Thomsen, A. (1991) Extensive genetic polymorphism in the human tumor necrosis factor region and relation to extended HLA haplotypes. *Proceedings of the National Academy of Sciences of the United States of America*, 88, 9717–9721.

Kaijzel, E.L., Bayley, J.P., van Krugten, M.V., Smith, L., van de Linde, P., Bakker, A.M., Breedveld, F.C., Huizinga, T.W., & Verweij, C.L. (2001) Allele-specific quantification of tumor necrosis factor alpha (TNF) transcription and the role of promoter polymorphisms in rheumatoid arthritis patients and healthy individuals. *Genes and Immunity*, 2, 135–144.

Kaluza, W., Reuss, E., Grossmann, S., Hug, R., Schopf, R.E., Galle, P.R., Maerker-Hermann, E., & Hoehler, T. (2000) Different transcriptional activity and in vitro TNF-alpha production in psoriasis patients carrying the TNF-alpha 238A promoter polymorphism. *Journal of Investigative Dermatology*, 114, 1180–1183.

Karplus, T.M., Jeronimo, S.M., Chang, H., Helms, B.K., Burns, T.L., Murray, J.C., Mitchell, A.A., Pugh, E.W., Braz, R.F., Bezerra, F.L., & Wilson, M.E. (2002) Association between the tumor necrosis factor locus and the clinical outcome of *Leishmania chagasi* infection. *Infection and Immunity*, 70, 6919–6925.

Kim, Y.J., Lee, H.S., Yoon, J.H., Kim, C.Y., Park, M.H., Kim, L.H., Park, B.L., & Shin, H.D. (2003) Association of TNF-alpha promoter polymorphisms with the clearance of hepatitis B virus infection. *Human Molecular Genetics*, 12, 2541–2546.

Kindler, V., Sappin, A.P., Grau, G.E., Piguet, P.F., & Vassali, P. (1989) The inducing role of tumor necrosis factor in the development of the bactericidal

granulomas during BCG infection. *Cell*, 56, 731–740.

Knight, J.C., Keating, B.J., Rockett, K.A., & Kwiatkowski, D.P. (2003) In vivo characterization of regulatory polymorphisms by allele-specific quantification of RNA polymerase loading. *Nature Genetics*, 33, 469–475.

Knight, J.C., Udalova, I., Hill, A.V., Greenwood, B.M., Peshu, N., Marsh, K., & Kwiatkowski, D. (1999) A polymorphism that affects OCT-1 binding to the TNF promoter region is associated with severe malaria. *Nature Genetics*, 22, 145–150.

Koss, K., Satsangi, J., Fanning, G.C., Welsh, K.I., & Jewell, D.P. (2000) Cytokine (TNF alpha, LT alpha and IL-10) polymorphisms in inflammatory bowel diseases and normal controls: differential effects on production and allele frequencies. *Genes and Immunity*, 1, 185–190.

Kroeger, K.M., Carville, K.S., & Abraham, L.J. (1997) The −308 tumor necrosis factor-alpha promoter polymorphism effects transcription. *Molecular Immunology*, 34, 391–399.

Kunstmann, E., Epplen, C., Elitok, E., Harder, M., Suerbaum, S., Peitz, U., Schmiegel, W., & Epplen, J.T. (1999) *Helicobacter pylori* infection and polymorphisms in the tumor necrosis factor region. *Electrophoresis*, 20, 1756–1761.

Kusumoto, K., Uto, H., Hayashi, K., Takahama, Y., Nakao, H., Suruki, R., Stuver, S.O., Ido, A., & Tsubouchi, H. (2006) Interleukin-10 or tumor necrosis factor-alpha polymorphisms and the natural course of hepatitis C virus infection in a hyperendemic area of Japan. *Cytokine*, 34, 24–31.

Kwiatowski, D., Hill, A.V.S., Sambou, I., Twumasi, P., Castracane, J., Manogue, K.R., Cerami, A., Brewster, D.R., & Greenwood, B.M. (1990) TNF concentrations in fatal cerebral, non-fatal cerebral, and uncomplicated *Plasmodium falciparum* malaria. *Lancet*, 336, 1201–1204.

Lee, Y.H., Harley, J.B., & Nath, S.K. (2006) Meta-analysis of TNF-alpha promoter −308 A/G polymorphism and SLE susceptibility. *European Journal of Human Genetics*, 14, 364–371.

Li, H.Q., Li, Z., Liu, Y., Li, H.J., Dong, J.Q., Gao, J.R., Gou, C.Y., & Li, H. (2005) Association of polymorphism of tumor necrosis factor-alpha gene promoter region with outcome of hepatitis B virus infection. *World Journal of Gastroenterology*, 11, 5213–5217.

Louis, E., Franchimont, D., Piron, A., Gevaert, Y., Schaaf-Lafontaine, N., Roland, S., Mahieu, P., Malaise, M., De Groote, D., Louis, R., & Belaiche, J. (1998) Tumour necrosis factor (TNF) gene polymorphism influences TNF-alpha production in lipopolysaccharide (LPS)-stimulated whole blood cell culture in healthy humans. *Clinical Experimental Immunology*, **113**, 401–406.

Lu, C.C., Sheu, B.S., Chen, T.W., Yang, H.B., Hung, K.H., Kao, A.W., Chuang, C.H., & Wu, J.J. (2005) Host TNF-alpha-1031 and −863 promoter single nucleotide polymorphisms determine the risk of benign ulceration after *H. pylori* infection. *American Journal of Gastroenterology*, **100**, 1274–1282.

Machado, J.C., Figueiredo, C., Canedo, P., Pharoah, P., Carvalho, R., Nabais, S., Castro Alves, C., Campos, M.L., Van Doorn, L.J., Caldas, C., Seruca, R., Carneiro, F., & Sobrinho-Simoes, M. (2003) A proinflammatory genetic profile increases the risk for chronic atrophic gastritis and gastric carcinoma. *Gastroenterology*, **125**, 364–371.

Maier, L.A., Sawyer, R.T., Bauer, R.A., Kittle, L.A., Lympany, P., McGrath, D., Dubois, R., Daniloff, E., Rose, C.S., & Newman, L.S. (2001) High beryllium-stimulated TNF-alpha is associated with the −308 TNF-alpha promoter polymorphism and with clinical severity in chronic beryllium disease. *American Journal of Respiratory and Critical Care Medicine*, **164**, 1192–1199.

Majetschak, M., Obertacke, U., Schade, F.U., Bardenheuer, M., Voggenreiter, G., Bloemeke, B., & Heesen, M. (2002) Tumor necrosis factor gene polymorphisms, leukocyte function, and sepsis susceptibility in blunt trauma patients. *Clinical and Diagnostic Laboratory Immunology*, **9**, 1205–1211.

Makela, S., Hurme, M., Ala-Houhala, I., Mustonen, J., Koivisto, A.M., Partanen, J., Vapalahti, O., Vaheri, A., & Pasternack A. (2001) Polymorphism of the cytokine genes in hospitalized patients with Puumala hantavirus infection. *Nephrology Dialysis Transplantation*, **16**, 1368–1373.

Mattey, D.L., Hassell, A.B., Dawes, P.T., Ollier, W.E., & Hajeer, A. (1999) Interaction between tumor necrosis factor microsatellite polymorphisms and the HLA-DRB1 shared epitope in rheumatoid arthritis: influence on disease outcome. *Arthritis Rheumatism*, **42**, 2698–2704.

McGuire, W., Hill, A.V., Allsopp, C.E., Greenwood, B.M., & Kwiathowski, D. (1994) Variation in the TNF-alpha promoter region associated with susceptibility to cerebral malaria. *Nature*, **371**(6497), 508–510.

Meddeb-Garnaoui, A., Gritli, S., Garbouj, S., Ben Fadhel, M., El Kares, R., Mansour, L., Kaabi, B., Chouchane, L., Ben Salah, A., & Dellagi, K. (2001) Association analysis of HLA-class II and class III gene polymorphisms in the susceptibility to mediterranean visceral leishmaniasis, *Human Immunology*, **62**, 509.

Mira, J.P., Cariou, A., Grall, F., Delclaux, C., Losser, M.R., Heshmati, F., Cheval, C., Monchi, M., Teboul, J.L., Riche, F., Leleu, G., Arbibe, L., Mignon, A., Delpech, M., & Dhainaut, J.F. (1999) Association of TNF2, a TNF-alpha promoter polymorphism, with septic shock susceptibility and mortality: a multicenter study. *Journal of the American Medical Association*, **282**, 561–568.

Mira, M.T., Alcais, A., Van Thuc, N., Thai, V.H., Huong, N.T., Ba, N.N., Verner, A., Hudson, T.J., Abel, L., & Schurr, E. (2003) Chromosome 6q25 is linked to susceptibility to leprosy in a Vietnamese population. *Nature Genetics*, **33**, 412–415.

Mobley, J.L. (2004) Is rheumatoid arthritis a consequence of natural selection for enhanced tuberculosis resistance? *Medical Hypotheses*, **62**, 839–843.

Molvig, J., Pociot, F., Baek, L., Worsaae, H., Dall Wogensen, L., Christensen, P., Staub-Nielsen, L., Mandrup-Poulsen, T., Manogue, K., & Nerup, J. (1990) Monocyte function in IDDM patients and healthy individuals. *Scandinavian Journal of Immunology*, **32**, 297–311.

Moraes, M.O., Duppre, N.C., Suffys, P.N., Santos, A.R., Almeida, A.S., Nery, J.A., Sampaio, E.P., & Sarno, E.N. (2001) Tumor necrosis factor-alpha promoter polymorphism TNF2 is associated with a stronger delayed-type hypersensitivity reaction in the skin of borderline tuberculoid leprosy patients. *Immunogenetics*, **53**, 45–47.

Nakada, T.A., Hirasawa, H., Oda, S., Shiga, H., Matsuda, K., Nakamura, M., Watanabe, E., Abe, R., Hatano, M., & Tokuhisa, T. (2005) Influence of toll-like receptor 4, CD14, tumor necrosis factor, and interleukin-10 gene polymorphisms on clinical outcome in Japanese critically ill patients. *Journal of Surgery Research*, **129**, 322–328.

Nedospasov, S.A., Udalova, I.A., Kuprash, D.V., & Turetskaya, R.L. (1991) DNA sequence polymorphism at the human tumor necrosis factor (TNF) locus. Numerous TNF/lymphotoxin alleles tagged by two closely linked microsatellites in the upstream region of the lymphotoxin (TNF-beta) gene. *Journal of Immunology*, **147**, 1053–1059.

Ozaki, K., Ohnishi, Y., Iida, A., Sekine, A., Yamada, R., Tsunoda, T., Sato, H., Sato, H., Hori, M., Nakamura, Y., & Tanaka T. (2002) Functional SNPs in the lymphotoxin-alpha gene that are associated with susceptibility to myocardial infarction. *Nature Genetics*, **32**, 650–654.

Petrovsky, N., & Harrison, L.C. (1997) HLA class II-associated polymorphism of interferon-gamma production. Implications for HLA-disease association. *Human Immunology*, **53**, 12–16.

Plevy, S.E., Targan, S.R., Yang, H., Fernandez, D., Rotter, J.I., & Toyoda, H. (1996) Tumor necrosis factor microsatellites define a Crohn's disease-associated haplotype on chromosome 6. *Gastroenterology*, **110**, 1053–1060.

Pociot, F., Briant, L., Jongeneel, C.V., Molvig, J., Worsaae, H., Abbal, M., Thomsen, M., Nerup, J., & Cambon-Thomsen, A. (1993) Association of tumor necrosis factor (TNF) and class II major histocompatibility complex alleles with the secretion of TNF-alpha and TNF-beta by human mononuclear cells: a possible link to insulin-dependent diabetes mellitus. *European Journal of Immunology*, **23**, 224–231.

Rauchschwalbe, S.K., Maseizik, T., Mittelkotter, U., Schluter, B., Patzig, C., Thiede, A., & Reith, H.B. (2004) Effect of the LT-alpha (+250 G/A) polymorphism on markers of inflammation and clinical outcome in critically ill patients. *Journal of Trauma*, **56**, 815–822.

Rodriguez-Perez, J.M. Cruz-Robles, D., Hernandez-Pacheco, G., Perez-Hernandez, N., Murguia, L.E., Granados, J., Reyes, P.A., & Vargas-Alarcon, G. (2005) Tumor necrosis factor-alpha promoter polymorphism in Mexican patients with Chagas' disease. *Immunology Letters*, **98**, 97–102.

Rollinger-Holzinger, I., Eibl, B., Pauly, M., Griesser, U., Hentges, F., Auer, B., Pall, G., Schratzberger, P., Niederwieser, D., Weiss, E.H., & Zwierzina, H. (2000) LST1: a gene with extensive alternative splicing and immunomodulatory function. *Journal of Immunology*, **64**, 3169–3176.

Rood, M.J., van Krugten, M.V., Zanelli, E., van der Linden, M.W., Keijsers, V., Schreuder, G.M.T., Verduyn, W., Westendorp, R.G.J., de Vries, R.R.P., Breedvenl, F.C., Verweij, C.L., & Huizinga, T.W.J. (2000) TNF-308A and HLA-DR3 alleles contribute independently to susceptibility in systemic lupus erythematosus. *Arthritis and Rheumatism*, **43**, 129–134.

Rothschild, B.M., Rothschild, C., & Helbling, M. (2003) Unified theory of the origins of erosive arthritis: conditioning as a protective/directing mechanism? *Journal of Rheumatology*, **30**, 2095–2102.

Roy, S., McGuire, W., Mascie-Taylor, C.G., Saha, B., Hazra, S.K., Hill, A.V., & Kwiatkowski, D. (1997) Tumor necrosis factor promoter polymorphism and susceptibility to lepromatous leprosy. *Journal of Infectious Diseases*, **176**, 530–532.

Santos, A.R., Almeida, A.S., Suffys, P.N., Moraes, M.O., Filho, V.F., Mattos, H.J., Nery, J.A., Cabello, P.H., Sampaio, E.P., & Sarno, E.N. (2000) Tumor necrosis factor promoter polymorphism (TNF2) seems to protect against development of severe forms of leprosy in a pilot study in Brazilian patients. *International Journal Leprosy and Other Mycobacterial Diseases*, **68**, 325–327.

Santos, A.R., Suffys, P.N., Vanderborght, P.R., Moraes, M.O., Vieira, L.M., Cabello, P.H., Bakker, A.M., Matos, H.J., Huizinga, T.W., Ottenhoff, T.H. Sampaio, E.P., & Sarno, E.N. (2002) Role of tumor necrosis factor-alpha and interleukin-10 promoter gene polymorphisms in leprosy. *Journal of Infectious Diseases*, **186**, 1687–1691.

Sarno, E.N., Santos, A.R., Jardim, M.R., Suffys, P.N., Almeida, A.S., Nery, J.A., Vieira, L.M., & Sampaio, E.P. (2000) Pathogenesis of nerve damage in leprosy: genetic polymorphism regulates the production of TNF alpha. *Leprosy Reviews*, **71** (Suppl.), S154–S158.

Selvaraj, P., Sriram Mathan, U., Kurian, S., Reetha, A.M., & Narayanan, P.R. (2001) Tumor necrosis factor alpha (−238 and −308) and gene polymorphisms in pulmonary tuberculosis: haplotype analysis with HLA-A, B and DR genes. *Tuberculosis*, **81**, 335–341.

Shaw, M.A., Donaldson, I.J., Collins, A., Peacock, C.S., Lins-Lainson, Z., Shaw, J.J., Ramos, F., Silveira, F.& Blackwell, J.M. (2001) Association and linkage of leprosy phenotypes with HLA class II and tumour necrosis factor genes. *Genes and Immunity*, **2**, 196–204.

Skoog, T., van't Hooft, F.M., Kallin, B., Jovinge, S., Boquist, S., Nilsson, J., Eriksson, P., & Hamsten, A. (1999) A common functional polymorphism (C → A substitution at position −863) in the promoter region of the tumour necrosis factor-alpha (TNF-alpha) gene associated with reduced circulating levels of TNF-alpha. *Human Molecular Genetics*, **8**, 1443–1449.

Skoog, T., Eriksson, P., Hoffstedt, J., Ryden, M., Hamsten, A., & Armer, P. (2001) Tumour necrosis factor-alpha (TNF-alpha) polymorphisms −857C/A and −863C/A are associated with TNF-alpha secretion from human adipose tissue. *Diabetologia*, **44**, 654–655.

Somoskovi, A., Zissel, G., Seitzer, U., Gerdes, J., Schlaak, M., & Muller-Quernheim, J. (1999) Polymorphisms at position −308 in the promoter region of the TNF-alpha and in the first intron of the TNF-beta genes and spontaneous and lipopolysaccharide-induced TNF-alpha release in sarcoidosis. *Cytokine*, **11**, 882–887.

Stuber, F., Udalova, I.A., Book, M., Drutskaya, L.N., Kuprash, D.V., Turetskaya, R.L., Schade, F.U., Nedospasov, S.A. (1995) −308 tumor necrosis factor (TNF) polymorphism is not associated with survival in severe sepsis and is unrelated to lipopolysaccharide inducibility of the human TNF promoter. *Journal of Inflammation*, **46**, 42–50.

Suryaprasad, A.G., & Prindiville, T. (2003) The biology of TNF blockade. *Autoimmunity Reviews*, **2**, 346–357.

Temple, S.E., Cheong, K.Y., Almeida, C.M., Price, P., & Waterer, G.W. (2003) Polymorphisms in lymphotoxin alpha and CD14 genes influence TNFalpha production induced by Gram-positive and Gram-negative bacteria. *Genes and Immunity*, **4**, 283–288.

Thio, C.L., Goedert, J.J., Mosbruger, T., Vlahow, D., Strathdee, S.A., O'Brien, S.J., Astemborski, J., & Thomas, D.L. (2004) An analysis of tumor necrosis factor alpha gene polymorphisms and haplotypes with natural clearance of hepatitis C virus infection. *Genes and Immunity*, **5**, 294–300.

Udalova, I.A., Nedospasov, S.A., Webb, G.C., Chaplin, D.D., & Turetskaya, R.L. (1993) Highly informative typing of the human TNF locus using six adjacent polymorphic markers. *Genomics*, **16**, 180–186.

Vadlamani, L., & Iyengar, S. (2004) Tumor necrosis factor alpha polymorphism in heart failure-cardiomyopathy. *Congestive and Heart Failure*, **10**, 289–292.

Van Den Biggelaar, A.H., De Craen, A.J., Gussekloo, J., Huizinga, T.W., Heijmans, B.T., Frolich, M., Kirkwood, T.B., & Westendorp, R.G. (2004) Inflammation underlying cardiovascular mortality is a late consequence of evolutionary programming. *FASEB Journal*, **18**, 1022–1024.

Vanderborght, P.R., Matos, H.J., Salles, A.M., Vasconcellos, S,E., Silva-Filho, V.F., Huizinga, T.W.J., Ottenhoff, T.H.M., Sampaio, E.P., Sarno, E.N., Santos A.R., & Moraes, M.O. (2004) Single nucleotide polymorphisms (SNPs) at −238 and −308 positions in TNFα promoter: clinical and bacteriological evaluation in leprosy. *International Journal of Leprosy*, **72**, 143–148.

van Dissel, J.T., van Langevelde, P. Westendorp, R.G., Kwappenberg, K., & Frolich, M. (1998) Anti-Inflammatory cytokine profile and mortality in febrile patients. *Lancet*, **351**, 950–953.

van Krugten, M.V., Huizinga, T.W., Kaijzel, E.L., Zanelli, E., Drossaers-Bakker, K.W., van de Linde, P., Hazes, J.M., Zwinderman, A.H., Breedveld, F.C., & Verweij, C.L. (1999) Association of the TNF +489 polymorphism with susceptibility and radiographic damage in rheumatoid arthritis. *Genes and Immunity*, **1**, 91–96.

Vassalli, P. (1992) The pathophysiology of tumor necrosis factor. *Annual Reviews of Immunology*, **10**, 411–452.

Waldron-Lynch, F., Adams, C., Shanahan, F., Molloy, M.G., & O'Gara, F. (1999) Genetic analysis of the 3' untranslated region of the tumour necrosis factor shows a highly conserved region in rheumatoid arthritis affected and unaffected subjects. *Journal of Medical Genetics*, **36**, 214–226.

Warle, M.C., Farhan, A., Metselaar, H.J., Hop, W.C., Perrey, C., Zondervan, P.E., Kap, M., Kwekkeboom, J., Ijzermans, J.N., Tilanus, H.W., Pravica, V., Hutchinson, I.V., & Bouma, G.J. (2003) Are cytokine gene polymorphisms related to in vitro cytokine production profiles? *Liver Transplantation*, **9**, 170–181.

Wattavidanage, J., Carter, R., Perera, K.L., Munasingha, A., Bandara, S., McGuinness, D., Wickramasinghe, A.R., Alles, H.K., Mendis, K.N., & Premawansa, S. (1999) TNFalpha*2 marks high risk of severe disease during Plasmodium falciparum malaria and other infections in Sri Lankans. *Clinical and Experimental Immunology*, **115**, 350–355.

Weissensteiner, T., & Lanchbury, J.S. (1997) TNFB polymorphisms characterize three lineages of TNF region microsatellite haplotypes. *Immunogenetics*, **47**, 6–16.

Westendorp, RG.J., Langermans, J.A.M., Huizinga, T.W.J., Elouali, A.H., Verweij, C.L., Boomsma, D.I., & van den Brouke, J.P. (1997a) Genetic influence on cytokine production in fatal meningococcal disease. *Lancet*, **349**, 170–173.

Westendorp, R.G., Langermans, J.A., Huizinga, T.W., Verweij, C.L., & Sturk, A. (1997b) Genetic influence on cytokine production in meningococcal disease. *Lancet*, **349**, 1912–1913.

Wilson, A.G., Symons, J.A., McDowell, T.L., McDevitt, H.O., & Duff, G.W. (1997) Effects of a polymorphism in the human tumor necrosis factor alpha promoter on transcriptional activation. *Proceedings of the National Academy Sciences of the United States of America*, **94**, 3195–3199.

Wu, M.S., Chen, L.T., Shun, C.T, Huang, S.P., Chiu, H.M., Wang, H.P., Lin, M.T., Cheng, A.L., & Lin, J.T. (2004) Promoter polymorphisms of tumor necrosis factor-alpha are associated with risk of gastric mucosa-associated lymphoid tissue lymphoma. *International Journal of Cancer*, **110**, 695–700.

Yea, S.S., Yang, Y.I., Jang, W.H., Lee, Y.J., Bae, H.S., & Paik, K.H. (2001) Association between TNF-alpha promoter polymorphism and *Helicobacter pylori* cagA subtype infection. *Journal of Clinical Pathology*, **54**, 703–706.

Zambon, C.F., Basso, D., Navaglia, F., Belluco, C., Falda, A., Fogar, P., Greco, E., Gallo, N., Rugge, M., Di Mario, F., & Plebani, M. (2005) Pro- and anti-inflammatory cytokines gene polymorphisms and Helicobacter pylori infection: interactions influence outcome. *Cytokine*, **29**, 141–152.

15

Cytokine Genes I

IL10, IL6, IL4, and the *IL1* Family

Milton O. Moraes, Janet M. McNicholl,
Tom W. J. Huizinga, & Tom H. M. Ottenhoff

There is growing recognition that cytokine production is under tight genetic control and that variations in cytokine genes play a direct role in regulating cytokine production, disease pathogenesis, and host resistance to infectious diseases, particularly those due to intracellular pathogens. This hypothesis has led to epidemiological and functional studies of variant alleles at different polymorphic sites in many human populations. Promoter polymorphism studies, especially of single nucleotide polymorphisms (SNPs), have been conducted in association studies (mostly case–control) in many diseases, including autoimmune/inflammatory diseases such as rheumatoid arthritis, multiple sclerosis, ankylosing spondylitis, and asthma, and infectious diseases such as malaria, hepatitis B (HBV), hepatitis C (HCV), HIV infection, tuberculosis (TB), leprosy, and sepsis/septic shock. Polymorphisms in *TNF, IL12,* and *IFNG* genes are reviewed in other chapters. Here we focus on *IL10, IL6, IL4,* and the *IL1* gene cluster, including available evidence on the functional role of some promoter polymorphisms. Case–control studies

have produced variable results, with little consensus on whether any polymorphisms are actually associated with disease, although results have been more consistent in the case of certain infectious diseases. Functional studies have also sometimes produced discrepant results. More recently, instead of focusing on single promoter polymorphisms in isolation, investigators have appropriately begun to examine extended haplotypes, which can better capture the true genetic functional variation. This has led to notable success in the identification of new functional loci and set a new standard, replacing smaller case–control studies using single markers with integrative large-scale studies focusing on haplotype analyses.

Cytokine-Mediated Regulation of Host Defense to Intracellular Pathogens

The outcome of infection is influenced by many factors beyond the exposure to the environmental microbes themselves, including such factors as nutritional status, co-infections, and previous vaccinations. Of course, host genetic factors also play an important role, and cytokine genes are prime candidates. As extreme examples, causative mutations in genes that encode major proteins in the type-1 cytokine (IL-12/23–IFN-γ) axis (IL-12/23p40, IL-12/23Rβ1, IFN-γR1, IFN-γR2 or Stat-1) have been identified in patients with severe infections due to weakly virulent (nontuberculous) mycobacteria or *Mycobacterium bovis* Bacille Calmette-Guérin [BCG]) or *Salmonella* species (Ottenhoff et al., 2002; see chapter 16). The IL-12/23–IFN-γ axis is a major immunoregulatory system that bridges innate and adaptive immunity. The mutations found related to those infections emphasize the essential role of this regulatory pathway in host defense against intracellular pathogens. However, these mutations are rare and unlikely to account for genetic susceptibility to major diseases, such as TB and leprosy, at the population level.

In infectious diseases, it is clear that many genes and genetic polymorphisms are involved in controlling signaling pathways critical to the host resistance and disease susceptibility and severity (Segal and Hill, 2003). Besides the type 1 cytokine axis described above, other important cytokines with a role in innate or adaptive immunity are tumor necrosis factor (TNF; see chapter 14), interleukin-10 (IL-10), IL-6, IL-4, and the IL-1 cluster (IL-1α, IL-1β, and receptor antagonist, Ra). The prominent role played by these cytokines in inflammatory, infectious, and autoimmune diseases has heightened interest in the possibility that polymorphism or differential regulation of the cytokine genes may be associated with the pathogenesis of those diseases.

The broad spectrum of cytokine actions suggests that they are key components in protective and pathological immune responses. The synthesis of many cytokines is triggered by a number of stimuli such as gram-negative bacterial lipopolysaccharide (LPS), gram-positive bacteria, viruses, parasites, and other cytokines. However, given the deleterious side effects of excessive production of some cytokines, it is clear that cytokine gene expression must be tightly regulated at different levels (epigenetic, transcription, posttranscription, translation, and secretion) in order to ensure optimal host defense.

SNPs as tools for association studies are mostly biallelic point mutations, present with a frequency of >1% in the population, and typically observed at least every 500–1,000 bp in the human genome. The total number of SNPs is currently estimated to exceed $2–4 \times 10^6$. Most variations are located in noncoding regions, either intergenic or intragenic (Zhao et al.,

2003; Cargill et al., 1999). Fewer SNPs are observed in translated stretches of DNA, and the majority of these encode changes that are synonymous (i.e., do not modify the amino acid). SNPs have major applications in genetics and biology, including use as genetic markers in disease association/linkage studies. A large number of SNPs in cytokine loci have been described and studied in infectious, autoimmune, and neoplastic diseases (Wilson et al., 1995; Hurme et al., 1998; Bayley et al., 2004). Fortunately, a growing number of helpful online databases (see appendix 1) cover human genetic variation and often include tools for customized queries of those databases. One such site focusing on cytokine genes is disease associations of cytokine gene variants (Bidwell et al., 1999, 2001; Haukim et al., 2002; www.nanea.dk/cytokinesnps/).

Functional Implications of SNPs and Studies to Evaluate SNP Activity

Much of what is known about the variation in cytokine genes associated with infectious disease susceptibility points to the importance of noncoding regions. It is therefore worth emphasizing the methodological approaches particularly applicable to the study of variation in these regulatory elements. Depending on the position of a SNP, different types of experiments can be performed to measure the effect of a specific SNP on regulating the expression or function of a given gene. Experiments to analyze promoter SNP functions can evaluate *in vitro* binding capacity of oligonucleotides to transcription factors (in gel-shift assays) or, alternatively, assess the inducibility of a reporter gene in cells transfected with different promoter constructs containing various allelic SNPs. Other approaches employed to study the functional relevance of promoter SNPs rely on the direct detection of the product (either mRNA or protein) *in vivo* using biological samples such as plasma, serum, tissue (immunohistochemistry), or *in vitro* cell culture systems. This approach uses a more physiological environment but could also reflect the effect of different SNPs in linkage disequilibrium with the SNP under study. Regardless, most of these techniques have high variability, and the results are often difficult to interpret. Some of the approaches to examining the physiological role of cytokine SNPs and the emerging results are discussed below.

Models of TB and leprosy are particularly useful since they are chronic infectious diseases in which host

TABLE 15.1. Cytokine gene polymorphisms.

Gene ID (NCBI)	Common Name(s)	Entrez Gene ID (Locus Link)	Map Position[a]	Common Polymorphisms[b]	NM ID (mRNA)
IL10	HGNC:5962, CSIF, IL-10, IL10A, MGC126450, MGC126451, tumor growth-inhibiting factor, cytokine synthesis inhibitory factor;	3586	1q31-q32	−592, −819, −1082, −2763, −2849, −3575[c]	NM00572
IL6	HGNC:6018, BSF2, HGF, HSF, IFNB2	3569	7p21	−174, −634, −1749	NM000600
IL4	HGNC:6014, BSF1, IL-4, MGC79402, B-cell stimulatory factor 1; lymphocyte stimulatory factor 1	3565	5q31.1	−549, −589, +33,	NM000589
IL1A	HGNC: 5991; IL1; IL-1A; IL1F1; IL-1α	3552	2q14	−889, +4845	NM000575
IL1B	HGNC:5992, IL-1, IL1F2, IL-1β	3553	2q14	−31, −511, +3953	NM00576
IL1RN	HGNC:6000, ICIL-1RA, IL1F3, IL-1ra3, IL1RA, IRAP	3557	2q14.2	86 bp VNTR (intron 6)	NM000577

[a]To view a map of any of these genes, use the following Web link, where the gene ID is inserted as the last digits of the string. For example, to see a map of the IL-10 locus use the following link: www.ncbi.nlm.nih.gov/mapview/map_search.cgi?direct = on&idtype = gene&id = 3586

[b]Summary information only is provided here since the number of variants for these genes is long and ever growing. SNP counts are as of January 2006 in dbSNP (which includes short changes of several bases as well as single base changes). Not all reported SNPs have been validated. To access gene dbSNP data, a useful strategy is to go to www.ncbi.nlm.nih.gov/entrez, select the "Gene" database in the search field, and insert the gene name in the "for" field. When the gene information is retrieved, click on links, select "Gene view in dbSNP," and view the polymorphisms using the various "view rs (reference sequence number)" choices. Population frequencies for several of these genes in different racial/ethnic groups are maintained at www.allelefrequencies.net, pga.gs.washington.edu/finished_genes.html, and linked Web sites. For additional information, see also www.ensembl.org.

[c]There are different nomenclatures for many SNPs. The figure 15.2 legend and the NCBI Web site provide additional information.

genetic contributions to disease can be particularly evident. We focus on the most frequent polymorphisms in IL10, IL6, and IL4 and in genes of the IL-1 cluster (table 15.1) and review infectious disease associations (table 15.2). Other chapters review TNF, IL12, and IFNG (see chapters 14 and 16).

IL10

Gene Product in Infection

IL-10 is an 18-kDa immunoregulatory cytokine classified as a type II cytokine since it has some structural similarity to the interferons (IFNs). It binds in dimers to an IL-10 receptor and is generally considered a potent anti-inflammatory cytokine that counterbalances TNF. IL-10 production is under tight regulatory control. Although IL-10 is primarily secreted by cells of the monocyte/macrophage lineage, many cell types express IL-10 mRNA. Not all of these produce detectable amounts of protein, and levels of protein expression vary. Recently, T-regulatory-1 (Tr1) cells that are CD4 positive, secrete IL-10, and suppress T-helper (Th) cells have been defined (Kemper et al., 2003), and these cells are critical in controlling autoimmune and pathogen-driven response. IL-10 has multiple immunoregulatory effects, such as the down-regulation of Th1 cytokines and of MHC class II antigens and co-stimulatory molecules on macrophages. IL-10 also expands IL-4–producing T cells (Volk et al, 2001) and regulates B-cell proliferation and differentiation (Llorente et al., 1995). In this sense, it can be considered pro-inflammatory in that it can enhance B-cell survival and proliferation and promote antibody production. The dominance of one effect over another may be influenced by other signals in the cytokine milieu.

Pathogenesis

Several experimental and clinical observations point to the critical role of IL-10 in infectious disease. IL-10

TABLE 15.2. Cytokine polymorphisms and infectious disease associations.

Allele/Genotype/Haplotype[a]	Pathogen/Disease	Association; Population/Country[b]	Reference
IL10			
−1082 A, −592 C	M. tuberculosis	Variable effects on risk or disease in different populations	Lopez-Maderuelo et al, 2003; Bellamy et al, 1998; Delgado et al, 2002; Scola et al, 2003; Fitness et al, 2004a; Shin et al, 2005; Tso et al, 2005; Henao et al, 2006
−819TT	M. leprae	Variable effects	Santos et al, 2002; Fitness et al, 2004b
−3575A/−2849G/−2763C	M. leprae	Resistance; Brazil	Moraes et al, 2004
−1082G	C. trachomatis	Scarring form; Mandinkas, The Gambia	Mozzato-Chamay et al, 2000
−1082AA	Meningococcemia	Severe outcome/death; Ireland	Balding et al, 2003
−592A	HIV	Increased risk of HIV infection; United States	Shin et al, 2000
−592A and others	HIV	Inconsistent effects on HIV progression; United States, France	Shin et al, 2000; Vasilescu et al, 2003
−592 and others	HTLV	Inconsistent effects on viral load and disease; Japan	Nishimura et al, 2002, 2003
−1082A	EBV	Susceptibility; Finland	Helminen et al, 1999 et al, 2001
−1117 and −3585	RSV	Need for mechanical ventilation	Wilson et al, 2005b
Haplotype/−1082GG/ other SNPs	HCV	Inconsistent effects on clearance/recovery	Liu et al, 2003; Oleksyk et al, 2005; Minto et al, 2005; Barrett et al, 2005
ht2	HBV	Progression to hepatocellular carcinoma; United States	Shin et al, 2003
−1082A	HBV	Reduced disease severity; Japan	Miyazoe et al, 2002
−1082A/−819T/−592A	IFN-γ therapy of HCV	Improved response	Edwards-Smith et al, 1999; Yee et al, 2001
−592-containing haplotype	Severe malaria	Increased risk but not confirmed in transmission disequilibrium test; The Gambia	Wilson et al, 2005a
Microsatellite markers	Chagas' disease	May be due to epistasis with MHC; Colombia	Moreno et al, 2004
IL6			
−174GG	Streptococcus pneumoniae	Reduced extrapulmonary spread	Schaaf et al, 2005
−174GG	Septicemia	Severity	Harding et al, 2003
−174GG	Meningococcemia	Nonsurvival; Ireland	Balding et al, 2003
−174G	Infection in leukemia patients	Increased	Lehrnbecher et al, 2005
−174C	Appendiceal infection /inflammation	Reduced	Rivera-Chavez et al, 2004

(continued)

TABLE 15.2. (continued)

Allele/Genotype/Haplotype[a]	Pathogen/Disease	Association; Population/Country[b]	Reference
Various	Hepatitis C clearance	Inconsistent observations	Barrett et al, 2003; Minton et al, 2005
−634	HTLV	Susceptibility, disease	Nishimura et al, 2003
−1749	KSHV	Kaposi sarcoma	Foster et al, 2000
IL4			
31B1 genotype	Cerebral malaria	Increased risk	Gyan et al, 2004
+33T/−590T	IgE levels in malaria	Increased	Gyan et al, 2004
−589 TT	Vulvovaginal candidiasis	Increased risk	Babula et al, 2005
−589T	RSV	Severe disease	Choi et al, 2002
−549T-containing haplotype	HIV	Rapid disease progression	Vasilescu et al, 2003
-589T	HIV	No effect on severity	Singh et al, 2004
−1089T/−590T/+33C	Hepatitis B vaccine	Responder	Wang et al, 2004
IL4R			
exon 5 position 50 IV variant	HIV	Long-term nonprogression	Soriano et al, 2005
IL1A			
−889TT	Osteomyelitis	Increased risk, weak effect	Asensi et al, 2003
−889TT	Periodontitis	Increased risk, weak effect	Kornman et al, 1997; Diehl et al, 1999
IL-1A +4845G/T	Malaria	Weak association with mild disease	Walley et al, 2004
−899, allele 2	HIV	Good response to antiretroviral therapy	Price et al, 2004
IL1B			
−31T, −511T	H. pylori	Infection and gastric cancer, response to clarithromycin	El-Omar et al, 2000; Uno et al, 2002
−511C	Tuberculosis	Reduced risk of pulmonary TB	Awomoyi et al, 2005
+3953C/T	Malaria	Weak association with mild disease	Walley et al, 2004
+3953C/T	Adult periodontitis	Severity	Galbraith et al, 1999
−511C/T allele	HBV	Viral loads	Zhang et al, 2004
−511C	HBV	Hepatocellular carcinoma	Zhang et al, 2004
IL1RA			
IL1Ra intron 2 86-bp VNTR	Malaria (P. falciparum): severity		Bellamy et al, 1998
*2 homozygosity	Septicemia	High risk for death	Arnalich et al, 2002
Allele 2	HBV	Reduced risk of infection risk	Zhang et al, 2004

[a]The SNP or other genetic designation used in the publication is reported here. Alternate designations, reference sequence (rs) numbers, or other base information can be retrieved from dbSNP via www.ncbi.nlm.nih.gov/entrez, using the search strategy in the table 15.1 note and information in figure 15.2 legend. "−" indicates a promoter site unless otherwise indicated; "/" between SNPs usually indicates haplotypes.

[b]The association listed is with increased risk unless otherwise indicated.

can prevent experimental endotoxemia (Gerard et al., 1993). On the other hand, IL-10 promotes establishment of chronic infection by *Leishmania major* in mice (Belkaid et al., 2001). T-regulatory cells are constitutively presented in anergic TB patients even after long-term TB treatment (Boussiotis et al., 2000). Pathogens may directly influence IL-10–dependent pathways through the production of IL-10 homologs. For example, the Epstein-Barr virus (EBV) protein BCRF-1 is an IL-10 homolog that has many of the same *in vitro* effects on B cells and macrophages as human IL-10, leading to the assumption that its production by EBV promotes infection or latency with this virus. Human cytomegalovirus also has an IL-10 homolog (Gealy et al., 2005). On the other hand, viral proteins such as HIV-1 Tat and Vpr appear to regulate IL-10 production through NF-κB–dependent mechanisms (Bennasser and Bahraoui, 2002; Ayyavoo et al., 1997).

Gene Organization and Sequence

The IL-10 gene is located on chromosome 1q32 (figure 15.1). Table 15.1 provides links to the latest National Center for Biotechnology Information (NCBI) gene map. The gene has five exons. IL-19, -20, and -24 are paralogs located nearby on chromosome 1. IL-10 also has some similarities to IL-22, -26, -28, and -29.

Polymorphism, Populations, and Disease Associations

Variations in the IL-10 promoter were first reported by Turner et al. (1997). The most studied SNPs are G-1082A, C-819T, and C-592A (table 15.1), but recent studies have identified additional SNPs and extended haplotypes (figure 15.2; Kurreeman et al., 2004; Moraes et al., 2004; Vasilescu et al., 2003; Wilson et al., 2005a). Many studies implicating IL-10 promoter variation in infectious diseases have been performed either with isolated SNPs or with haplotypes built on combinations of proximal SNPs in the same chromosomes (table 15.2). Here, we focus on a few well-documented infectious disease associations, some of which illustrate the problems that can occur in case–control studies.

Population genetic studies of TB have led to conflicting results. For example, whereas Lopez-Maderuelo et al. (2003), in a Spanish population with pulmonary TB, and Bellamy et al. (1998), in a Gambian population, found no association between TB and IL-10 promoter SNPs, Delgado et al. (2002) reported that the

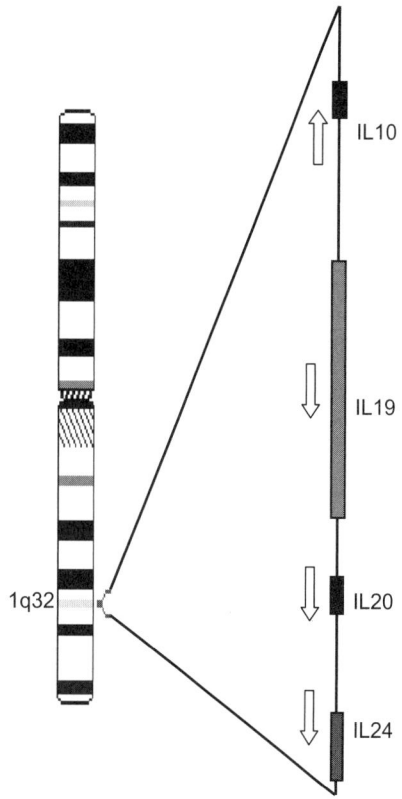

FIGURE 15.1. IL-10 location and structure. The IL-10 gene is located on chromosome 1q32 and clusters with other structurally or functionally related cytokines of IL-10 family (IL-19, IL-20, and IL-24).

−1082A allele was increased among Cambodian pulmonary TB patients, and Scola et al (2003) reported that the same allele was associated with chronic TB in Sicilian patients. Henao et al. (2006) found weak associations of this allele with TB, and similar results were found in Malawian HIV[+] TB patients when compared to HIV[−] controls (Fitness et al., 2004a). In Koreans, the −592C allele is associated with TB protection (Shin et al., 2005), and in a Chinese population, no association with promoter SNPs and TB was found (Tso et al., 2005).

The −819TT genotype was found to be associated with risk of leprosy (Santos et al., 2002). Another case–control study in Malawi did not confirm these data since no association was observed with any polymorphism of the proximal −1082/−819/−592 haplotype and leprosy susceptibility (Fitness et al., 2004b). However, a combination of novel distal SNPs in the

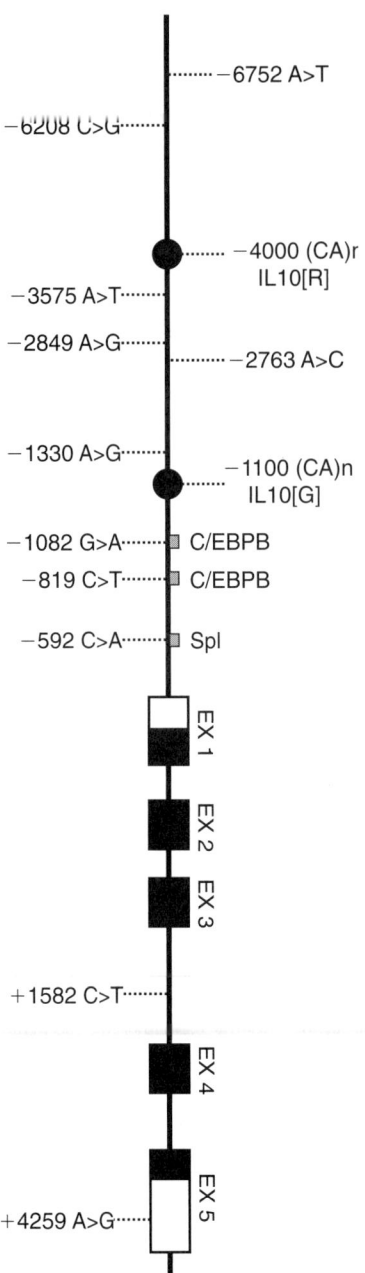

FIGURE 15.2. IL-10 SNPs, microsatellites, and haplotypes. Depiction of the approximately 15-kb promoter/gene region shows that some SNPs (dashed lines) are in transcription factor binding sites (small gray boxes). Microsatellites are represented as black circles. Most known SNPs are in the promoter. Variants include (alternate name or reference sequence [rs] number) −592 (−597,−627, rs1800872);−819 (−824,−854, rs1800871);−1082 (−1087,−1117, rs1800896);−1330 (−1354),−2763 (−2736);−3575 (−3538,−3785).

−3575A/−2849G/−2763C haplotype was associated with resistance to leprosy, while the −3575T/−2849A/−2763C haplotype was associated with susceptibility (Moraes et al., 2001). Extended haplotype analysis showed that the combination −3575T/−2849A/−2763C segregates with −819T. A replication study in Indians also found that the proximal −819T allele was associated with susceptibility, although another distal haplotype (−3575T/−2849G/−2763C) was associated with resistance (Malhotra et al., 2005). From these results, it is not yet clear whether a specific SNP is involved in leprosy susceptibility or disease severity. Overall, the findings indicate a role for the IL-10 locus in influencing both TB and leprosy outcomes (see chapter 22).

Studies of *Chlamydia trachomatis* and *Neisseria meningitidis* have also implicated the −1082 IL-10 SNP. In one West African study, an association between an IL-10 high-producing allele (−1082G) was noted with scarring trachoma in a *C. trachomatis*–endemic population of Mandinkas (Mozzato-Chamay et al., 2000), suggesting that Th2-type immune responses are associated with risk of disease, whereas another West African study found the −1082G allele in both resistance and susceptibility haplotypes. In a study of meningococcemia, the −1082AA genotype was more frequently associated with severe outcome and with lack of survival (Balding et al., 2003).

IL-10 promoter polymorphisms have also been studied in relation to several viral infections. Microsatellite-based studies (of markers linked to known promoter SNPs) showed that individuals with the −592A promoter allele had an increased risk of HIV-1 infection and, once infected, progressed to AIDS more rapidly than homozygotes with the −592CC genotype (Shin et al., 2000). A role for polymorphisms at the IL-10 locus influencing HIV-1 disease progression was also confirmed in another cohort (Vasilescu et al., 2003), although the allelic and haplotypic associations were not identical to those observed in the Shin et al. (2000) study.

Studies of IL-10 SNPs have shown some associations with human T-cell leukemia virus (HTLV) viral load or myelopathy (Nishimura et al., 2002, 2003). Studies of associations with EBV infection and disease severity have suggested that −1082A allele (or a haplotype with 1082A) is associated with increased susceptibility/severity, likely because of lower IL-10 production (Helminen et al., 1999, 2001). A study of respiratory syncytial virus (RSV) infection indicated that IL-10 −1082 and −3575 influenced the need for mechanical ventilation (Wilson et al., 2005b).

Some hepatitis studies have also implicated the *IL10* locus. Clearance of or recovery from HCV infection may be more likely in the presence of high IL-10 (−1082GG) producing genotypes (Oleksyk et al., 2005; Lio et al., 2003). However, the latter association was not replicated in two other HCV studies analyzing multiple cytokine gene types (Minton et al., 2005; Barrett et al., 2003). In chronic HBV infection, progression to hepatocellular carcinoma has been linked to genotypes associated with higher IL-10 production (IL-10 ht2) (Shin et al., 2003) whereas an IL-10 −1082A-containing haplotype was associated with milder disease (Miyazoe et al., 2002).

IL-10 polymorphisms may also influence responses to parasitic infections. In one study of Chagas' disease, associations were found between certain IL-10 microsatellites and infection (Moreno et al., 2004), and analysis in conjunction with polymorphism in the MHC suggested the possibility of epistasis between IL-10 and that region. In a malaria study protection against severe disease was associated with one IL-10 haplotype containing −592C (Wilson et al., 2005a); however, transmission disequilibrium testing did not confirm the association. Additional studies of both Chagas' disease and malaria that address interaction and confounding variables should be performed.

Functional Relationships of IL-10 Variants

Experiments have been inconsistent with regard to promoter variations and quantitative IL-10 secretion. On the one hand, some studies have indicated the IL-10 −1082G SNP (or the IL-10 −1082G/−819C/−592C haplotype) as being associated with high IL-10 production (Turner et al., 1997). These results were confirmed by other studies (Lopez-Maderuelo et al., 2003; Koss et al., 2000; Rieth et al., 2004) showing that IL-10 production was lower among −1082A carriers in patients with TB or inflammatory bowel disease (Lopez-Maderuelo et al., 2003; Koss et al., 2000). Together, these data suggested that the presence of the −1082G allele (or haplotypes containing it) might impair the development of a Th1 response. Another study demonstrated that IL-10 −592A (which generally segregates with −1082A) was associated with low IL-10 release in critically ill patients (Lowe et al., 2003), but Eskdale et al. (1999) demonstrated that IL-10 production was

higher in −1082A individuals. Warle et al. (2003) provided additional opposing evidence for the role of the −1082 SNP in regulating IL-10 production since concanavalin A (con-A)–stimulated peripheral blood mononuclear cells (PBMCs) from healthy individuals carrying the −1082GG genotype released less IL-10 than cells from −1082GA/AA genotypes. Several additional studies using con-A stimulated PBMCs observed no differences in IL-10 production of carriers and noncarriers of −1082G (Rees et al., 2002; Cartwright et al., 2001). The only SNP in the IL-10 promoter for which a clear correlation with LPS-induced IL-10 production was observed is the A-2849G SNP (Westendorp et al., 2001). Interestingly, the nature of the stimulus may also influence IL-10 effects. In two studies (Mormann et al., 2004; Rieth et al., 2004), the −1082G allele was found to influence production only when LPS was used to stimulate PBMCs. In peripheral blood high lymphoproliferative T-cell responses to an antigen from a filarial worm (*Onchocerca volvulus*), but not to phytohemagglutinin, were associated with the −1082A/−819T/−592A haplotype (Timmann et al., 2004).

The level of IL-10 seems to be differentially regulated if haplotypes consisting of the distal or the extended promoter region are considered. The fact that −1082G can be linked to both −2849G and A (the majority of the −1082A alleles are linked to −2849G, and some are linked to −2849A) demonstrates that haplotype composition probably influences the findings of association studies between the IL-10 SNPs and IL-10 production. SNPs at A-6752T, C-6208G, T-3575A, G-2849A, and C-2763A, which are linked to IL-10 microsatellites, form major haplotypes that influence IL-10 expression (Mormann et al., 2004; Eskdale et al., 1999; Gibson et al., 2001). In these studies, the −3575A/−2849A/−2763A haplotype was associated with lower secretion of IL-10 (Eskdale et al., 1999). It is doubtful that all of the SNPs driving differential allelic expression have been identified. Functionally relevant SNPs may well be located in other sequence areas than the regions currently studied, and analysis of associations of polymorphisms with IL-10 production will need to take this extended region into account.

The mechanisms by which the IL-10 promoter −1082/−819/−592 region influences IL-10 production may include gene transcription, since the region contains several putative binding sites for transcription factors (Kube et al., 1995; Ma et al., 2001; Crawley et al., 1999). Promoter analysis has provided evidence that −1082A can either increase (in EBV-transformed B cells; Rees et al., 2002) or decrease (in U937 monocytic cell line; Reuss et al., 2002) IL-10 transcriptional activity, and that this region can bind nuclear proteins (Reuss et al., 2002). It has been reported that IL-10 mRNA synthesis requires p38 MAP kinase and mobilization of the transcription factor Sp1 in human monocytic cells stimulated with LPS (Ma et al., 2001) and also an Sp1-like factor in mouse cells (Brightbill et al., 2000). Moreover, in a B-cell lineage, a region flanking the −120 bp sequence of the human IL-10 promoter has been implicated in IL-10 mRNA induction. This sequence binds STAT3 but not other STAT proteins, and the mutagenesis of the motif inhibits promoter activation (Benkhart et al., 2000).

These data suggest that the stimuli, the cell type, and the length and strength of stimulation all may differentially regulate promoter activity, depending on the signaling pathways activated. The data also suggest that polymorphisms lying in or nearby cis-acting elements in the IL-10 promoter may regulate IL-10 gene activation in ways that are influenced by the microenvironmental conditions to which the cell is exposed.

Animal Studies

The mouse IL-10 gene is located, as in humans, on chromosome 1, but in contrast to human IL-10, it is a monomer, and is not active on human cells. Murine IL-10 has similar immunosuppressive effects on IFN-γ and granulocyte-macrophage colony-stimulating factor production as human IL-10. Mice deficient in IL-10 have excessive inflammatory responses, can get enterocolitis, and become anemic. Databases of murine cytokine gene variants are maintained at the Jackson Laboratories, including the Mouse Genome Informatics database (MGI; www.informatics.jax.org/searches/allele_report.cgi) and the International Mouse Strain Resource (IMSR; www.informatics.jax.org/imsr/index.jsp). Search terms of interest such as a gene, allele, or phenotype can be inserted.

IL6

Gene Product

IL-6 is a long-chain type I immunoregulatory cytokine with pleiotropic actions in adaptive and innate immunity and important effects on bone, liver, and endothelial cells. It is synthesized by many cell types and activates the JAK/STAT signaling pathway via a cell-surface signaling assembly composed of IL-6, IL-6RA, and gp130, the shared signaling receptor. In innate immunity, it contributes to the acute phase response by activating hepatocytes to release C-reactive protein (CRP) and fibrinogen. In adaptive immunity, it is a B-cell growth factor.

Pathogenesis

IL-6 is involved in pathogen-induced host response, as well as host defenses against the pathogen. For example, IL-6 production is a consequence of exposure to LPS from gram-negative bacteria, HIV Tat induces IL-6 expression (Ambrosino et al., 1997), and human cytomegalovirus suppresses posttranscriptional IL-6 production (Gealy et al., 2005). Induction of acute phase reactants by IL-6 could contribute to excessive production of fibrinogen and intravascular thrombosis, particularly in septic patients. On the other hand, IL-6–induced production of antigen-specific antibodies can enhance pathogen clearance and restoration of health. Interestingly, the Kaposi-sarcoma-associated herpes virus (KSHV) encodes a functional homolog of IL-6 (vIL-6; Chow et al., 2001) that can induce some of the effects of IL-6 *in vitro* and may therefore play a role in KSHV pathogenesis *in vivo*. Homozygosity for the IL-6 −174G allele (see below) may be associated with increased risk for Kaposi sarcoma (Foster et al., 2000).

Gene Organization and Sequence

The gene is located on 7p21-p15 and has five exons spanning 5.0 kb in the genome. The mRNA is 1,125 bp long. Unlikely *IL10*, *IL1*, and *IL4*, the *IL6* locus is flanked by several others that are not clearly associated with immune and inflammatory responses. Curiously, some of these genes are associated with spermatogenesis such as a microtubule-dependent motor ATPase, a phosphoribosylpyrophosphate synthetase, and a serine/threonine kinase among other hypothetical genes.

Polymorphism, Populations, and Disease Associations

Updated information on *IL6* gene variation can be found at the NCBI and other Web sites (see table 15.1). Commonly studied variants include G-174C, G-572C, G-597A, and C-634G, or variable tandem repeats linked to these SNPs (table 15.1).

Several studies of *IL6* genotypes and sepsis or bacterial infection have been performed (reviewed in Dahmer et al., 2005). In one study, the IL-6 −174GG genotype was associated with reduced extrapulmonary spread of *Streptococcus pneumoniae* (Schaaf et al., 2005), while the same genotype was associated with increased risk of septicemia in preterm infants (Harding et al., 2003) and with lack of survival from menigococcemia (Balding et al., 2003). In acute appendicitis, a strong protective effect against severe local infection-inflammation was associated with the IL-6 −174C allele, and individuals with this allele had lower levels of plasma and peritoneal fluid IL-6 *in vivo*. (Rivera-Chavez et al., 2004). In children undergoing therapy for acute myeloid leukemia, −174G allele carriers had an increased risk of infection that affected morbidity and mortality (Lehrnbecher et al., 2005).

Inconsistent associations between *IL6* genotypes and clearance of HCV infection have been observed (Barrett et al., 2003; Minton et al., 2005), and so far, no associations of IL-6 genotypes with HBV progression have been noted (Park et al., 2003). The *IL6* −634 genotype appears to influence susceptibility to infection with HTLV-1 and risk of HTLV-1–associated myelopathy (Nishimura et al., 2002) but not HTLV-1 viral load levels (Nishimura et al., 2003; see chapters 20 and 21).

In vitro studies examining the regulation or production of IL-6 have generally linked the haplotype −597G/−174G or the −174G allele to high IL-6 production (Rivera-Chavez et al., 2003). Electrophoretic mobility shift assays demonstrated a higher binding capacity of oligonucleotides for −174G-containing sequences, and in a reporter gene assay, lower expression was observed with −174C than −174G, supporting the G allele being associated with higher IL-6 synthesis (Rivera-Chavez et al., 2003). Nevertheless, as observed for IL-10, some contrasting results have been reported. In an *in vivo* study where subjects were exposed to intravascular LPS, no differences in IL-6 responses were noted in persons with or without the −174G allele (Endler et al., 2004), and no influence of this polymorphism on IL-6 production was found in septic patients (Schluter et al., 2002). In contrast, Heesen et al. (2002) demonstrated that IL-6 production was higher in −174CC healthy blood donors. In babies, the −174 genotype was not associated with IL-6 concentrations in one study of preterm delivered infants (Jamie et al., 2005), while in another group of vaginally delivered neonates, higher levels of IL-6 were found in −174CC individuals than in −174G carriers, either in plasma or in LPS-stimulated PBMCs. Curiously, no influence of this SNP was observed in adults (Kilpinen et al., 2001). Finally, a study of the IL-6–induced protein CRP in women found that among IL-6 −572 genotypes, CRP was 37% higher in the presence of the C allele (Ferrari et al., 2003).

Animal Studies

Animal studies have confirmed the importance of IL-6 in influencing outcomes. IL-6 knockout mice poorly control several infections such as vaccinia virus, *Listeria monocytogenes*, and other bacteria. Mechanisms such as impaired T-cell recruitment, reduced expression of chemokines may be involved as evidenced by studies of IL-6$^{-/-}$ mice with *Staphylococcus epidermidis*–induced peritoneal inflammation (McLoughlin et al., 2005).

IL4 and *IL4R*

Gene Product in Infection

IL-4 is considered the classic Th2 cytokine, whereas the Th1 pathway is defined by IFN-γ. IL-4 was identified as a B-cell stimulatory factor, but it has pleiotropic actions, including T-cell and mast cell growth factor activities and an ability to down-regulate CCR5 expression. It is produced by activated T cells, and IL-10 promotes the expansion of IL-4–producing T cells. IL-4 binds the IL-4 receptor, as does IL-13, explaining some of the IL-4-like activities of this cytokine.

Pathogenesis

Studies of helminthic infections in mice and man have generally led to the finding that these infections are characterized by a Th2 response, with production of IL-4, -5, -9, -10, and -13, and of antibodies such as IgG4 and IgE. Similar types of responses are observed in allergy and atopy. Recently, this infectious disease paradigm has been questioned, with data from gene-deficient mice showing that Th2 responses can be induced by helminthic infection in the absence of IL-4. Whether this can be explained by redundancy in the Th2-triggered responses or of upstream events at the pathogen-antigen–presenting cell level remains to be determined.

Gene Organization and Sequence

The IL-4 gene (*IL4*) maps to chromosome 5q31.1, is approximately 10 kb in size, has four exons, and has two alternately spliced transcript variants. Together with four nearby genes (*IL3, IL5, IL13,* and *CSF2*), *IL4* forms a cluster of cytokine genes on chromosome 5. The first three appear to be co-coordinately regulated by several regulatory elements spread over 120 kb on the chromosome, known as the Th2 locus control region. The IL-4 receptor has two chains. The a-chain gene is located on chromosome 16p12. The second subunit (the β-chain) is a common subunit of several cytokine receptors, including the IL-2 receptor.

Polymorphism, Populations, and Disease Associations

The most commonly studied variant of *IL4* is the promoter variant, C-589T (also referred to as C-590T; table 15.1). The T allele has been previously shown to influence transcriptional activity and enhance IL-4 production. Additional promoter variants (including C+33T) and intronic variants (based on a repeat sequence) have been identified. In the *IL4* receptor, several variants in exons 5 and 12 have been identified. Updated information on these variants and allele frequencies can be found at the Web sites listed in table 15.1. Because IL-4 is such a classic marker of the Th2 response, studies of genetic polymorphisms have focused on infections where dysregulation of Th1/2 balance appears to influence disease susceptibility or outcome.

Since IL-4 influences IgE levels and high IgE levels are associated with severe malaria, one group studied associations between *IL4* intron 3 and promoter polymorphisms in children with severe malaria. Associations were observed between the intron 3 B1B1 genotype and cerebral malaria (Gyan et al., 2004). In a small study of vulvovaginal candidiasis, a very strong association of the *IL4* promoter genotype −589TT was noted with recurrent infection (Babula et al., 2005).

Dysregulation of the Th1/2 axis has been implicated in HIV/AIDS and RSV infection. One study of *IL4* genotypes and HIV disease progression showed associations of an *IL4* haplotypes (containing the −589T allele, also referred to as IL-4 −549T) with rapid disease progression (Vasilescu et al., 2003). In a pediatric study, no association with the IL-4 −589T allele with HIV disease progression or with central

nervous system impairment was found (Singh et al., 2004). In a study of *IL4R* polymorphisms in exon 5, the I50V polymorphism was found most frequently in HIV-1–infected persons who were long-term nonprogressors (Soriano et al., 2005). Interestingly, in RSV infection, an *IL4* promoter haplotype, including the −589T allele, was associated with severe disease (Choi et al., 2002), providing a potential mechanistic explanation for the association between RSV infection and subsequent wheezing.

Some studies have examined the influence of *IL4* polymorphisms on IL-4 production. The IL-4 −590T allele has been associated with higher IL-4 production in PBMCs from healthy volunteers or in vaginal fluid from recurrent candidiasis patients (Pawlik et al., 2006; Babula et al., 2005). The same variation was associated with higher IgE levels in patients with cerebral malaria (Gyan et al., 2004; Verra et al., 2004). On the other hand, some reports do not confirm the association of the −590T allele with either IL-4 production (Cartwright et al., 2001) or IgE secretion (Dizier et al., 1999). An SNP located in the second intron (G+3017T) has also been analyzed in relation to serum IgE. Lower levels were associated with the T allele and higher levels with the G allele.

Animal Studies

Knockout studies have confirmed the important role of IL-4 in regulating antibody levels and in T-cell responses. In a mouse model with a phenotype resembling human X-linked severe combined immunodeficiency where the genes for IL-4 and IL-2 receptor were knocked out, mice had normal IgM but low IgG and IgA levels and did not up-regulate IgE production on antigen exposure (Ozaki et al., 2002). Interestingly, IL-4 also appears to be required for antigen-specific CD8 T-cell responses, as evidenced by murine IL-4 knockout or blocking studies, where lack of IL-4 diminished CD8 responses to a malaria antigen (Carvalho et al., 2002).

The IL-1 Cluster: *IL1A, IL1B,* and *IL1RN*

Gene Products in Infection

The genes of the IL-1 cluster participate in the innate immune response. IL-1α and β are endogenous pyrogens and potent inflammatory mediators of the acute phase response. They are produced by multiple cell types, including B lymphocytes, macrophages, keratinocytes, and fibroblasts. Both cytokines also stimulate osteoclast activity and are involved in hematopoiesis. They are both 17-kDa proteins, but they are structurally different and coded for by different genes. The IL-1 receptor antagonist (IL-1Ra or IL-1RN) is also a 17-kDa protein that binds to IL-1 receptors and thus inhibits the binding and activity of IL-1α and β. IL-1 receptor antagonist levels are elevated in the blood of patients with a variety of infectious, immune, and traumatic conditions. There is a second 18-kDa IL-1RN isoform that remains in the cytoplasm. The IL-1 receptor belongs to the immunoglobulin gene superfamily.

Pathogenesis

LPS and other pathogen-derived products can increase production of IL1-α or IL1-β through transcription or other mechanism. Some studies suggest that HIV-1 Tat influences IL-1α expression, although the findings have not been consistent (Biswas et al., 1995; Sharma et al., 1995; Philippon et al., 1994).

Gene Organization and Sequence

The genes are located on chromosome 2q14. The *IL1A* and *IL1B* genes have seven exons while *IL1RA* has four. They have sequence and organizational similarities that suggests that the three genes have evolved from a duplication event.

Polymorphism, Populations, and Disease Associations

In *IL1A*, variable numbers (ranging from 5 to 18) of repeats of a 46-bp sequence within intron 6 have been noted (Bailly et al., 1993). The repeats contain potential transcription binding sites, which may explain functional associations. The most frequent allele (62%) in that study contained nine repeats. The IL-1A −889T allele is in linkage disequilibrium with the IL-1B +3953TT genotype (Asensi et al., 2003). In the *IL1B* gene, three biallelic C→T base transition polymorphisms at positions −511, −31, and +3954 (or 3953) have been reported. The C→T transition at position −31 creates a TATA box. *IL1RN* has a variable number of tandem repeat (VNTR) polymorphism of an 86-bp sequence in intron 2, generating five

known alleles of between two and six repeats (Tarlow et al., 1993). The most common alleles are the four-repeat (IL-1RN*1) and two-repeat (IL-1RN*2). The other alleles had a combined frequency of <5% in one study (Blakemore et al., 1996).

Because of the importance of the proteins produced by the IL-1 gene cluster in innate immunity, many infectious disease association studies have been conducted (table 15.2). The IL-1A −889TT genotype influences risk for osteomyelitis (Asensi et al., 2003) and periodontitis (Kornman et al., 1997). However, in a sib-pair analysis, the periodontitis associations were weak. Diehl et al (1999). The IL-1B −31T has been implicated in increasing risk for *Helicobacter pylori* infection and gastric cancer, both in Caucasian and in Japanese Brazilian patients (El-Omar et al., 2000; Uno, 2004). This may be due to a specific host–pathogen interaction in that in healthy normal people IL-1β may regulate gastric antral acid levels since low acid levels have been linked to the IL-1B −31T (El-Omar, 2000). The low acid levels may predispose to chronic *H. pylori* infection, gastric atrophy, and eventual development of cancer. The IL-1B −511C allele, but not the +3953 allele or the 86-bp IL-1RN repeat, was associated with reduced risk of pulmonary TB in The Gambia (Awomoyi et al., 2005), although the high frequency of the −31C allele in TB cases suggested that this locus is not the major genetic determinant. Associations of *IL1RN* genotypes with severe septicemia have been sought (Arnalich et al., 2002). In one study, patients homozygous for IL-1RN*2 had the highest risk of death and produced lower IL-1Ra levels.

A study of malaria severity in The Gambia showed weak associations of the IL-1A +4845G/T and the IL-1B +3953C/T markers with mild malaria. The associations were not present when *IL1A* or *IL1B* haplotypes were analyzed, suggesting a minor role for these loci (Walley et al., 2004). Moreover, in a previous study of the IL-1RN intron 2 86-bp VNTR, no association with malaria severity was noted (Bellamy et al., 1998), and another study in Ghana (Gyan et al., 2002) did not find any association with *IL1B* exon 5 or *IL1RN* markers and severe malaria, although a possible association with parasitemia was observed.

Fewer studies have investigated the role of the IL-1 gene cluster in viral infections. In chronic HBV-infected subjects, one study suggested that the IL-1RN allele 2 provides protection against HBV infection and that the IL-1B −511C/T alleles influence viral loads (Zhang et al., 2004).

To determine mechanisms for allelic associations, evaluations of IL-1 levels have been performed *in vivo* and *in vitro*. Asensi et al (2003) noted that IL-1A serum levels were not significantly higher in patients with the IL-1A −889TT genotype than in those without it. In an *ex vivo* whole-blood assay, healthy Gambians homozygous for the IL-1B −511T allele (associated with extrapulmonary TB) did not significantly respond to LPS stimulation after priming with IFN-γ (Awomoyi et al., 2005). However, previous studies using electrophoretic mobility shift analysis showed that DNA binding to the IL-1B −31T allele increased 5-fold after LPS stimulation (El-Omar et al., 2000). Arnalich et al. (2002) noted that PBMCs from IL-1RN*2 homozygotes produced low IL-1RA levels in PBMCs, and in studies of epithelial cell growth, Dewberry et al. (2003) showed that the same allele was associated with increased numbers of senescent epithelial cells. On the other hand, stimulation of PBMCs with purified protein derivative led to higher levels of IL-1RN in individuals carrying IL-1RN*2 allele (Wilkinson et al., 1999).

Animal Studies

Multiple knockout or allelic variants of genes in the IL-1 cluster have been constructed in mice to examine the role of this locus in animal models. As expected, immune system effects are observed, but effects also include abnormalities of growth and development and of cardiovascular and reproductive systems.

Pharmacogenetics and Cytokine Genes

Cytokine-based treatments for infectious diseases are increasingly being used, and it is logical that cytokine genotypes would influence these responses. In chronic HCV infection, patients with the IL-10 −1082A/ −819T/−592A haplotype have been found to have improved or sustained responses to treatment with IFN-α (Edwards-Smith et al, 1999; Yee, 2001; table 15.2). Interestingly, cytokines genotypes may also influence responses to traditional antimicrobial agents. For example, in one study, presence of the IL-1A −889 allele 2 in HIV-infected subjects treated with highly active antiretroviral therapy predicted control of viral loads to less than 400 copies/ml after initiation of treatment (Price et al., 2004). In another study, IL-1B polymorphisms influenced responses of *H. pylori*–infected patients to clarithromycin in that the IL-1B −511T allele (and the *CYP2C19* metabolizing geno-

type) was associated with successful *H. pylori* eradication (Furuta et al., 2004).

Responses to vaccines are also likely to be influenced by cytokine genotypes, although few studies have been carried out in this area. In one study, the IL-4 TTC haplotype (based on positions −1089, −590, and +33) was strongly associated with HBV responsiveness, even after adjustment for nongenetic factors (Wang et al., 2004). These findings expand on previously documented effects of human leukocyte antigen class II alleles on HBV responsiveness (chapter 5).

Conclusions, Prospects, and Needs

These studies confirm the diverse effects of cytokine gene polymorphism on infectious disease outcomes. Given the complex interactions between the cytokines and the often disparate or inconclusive findings of some associations, it is clear that future work is needed. This will include replication, often in larger populations, of initial associations, consideration of gene–gene interactions along known biological pathways and careful design of studies to account for differences in race or ethnicity. Use of family studies to confirm associations is desirable, although not always possible given the nature of some infectious diseases. Continued evaluation of functional relationships of the polymorphisms is essential to provide biological explanations for the disease associations. Until all relevant functional SNPs have been identified (in known and newly identified cytokine genes), high-throughput techniques will be required to determine the precise haplotypes that are functional and associated with disease. It is now feasible to type up to one million SNPs per person (chapter 2). Thus, future studies will be far more complex, generating a need for more sophisticated statistical tools and biological confirmation of the epidemiological findings. New areas of focus include evaluation of the role of cytokine gene polymorphisms in responses to vaccines and antimicrobials. These studies may open new approaches to the prevention and treatment of infectious disease.

Acknowledgments

The assistance of Elizabeth Sampaio, Euzenir Sarno, Wanna Leelawiwat, Theerawit Tasaneeyapan, and Baranee Balmongkol in preparing the manuscript is gratefully acknowledged.

References

Ambrosino C, Ruocco MR, Chen X, Mallardo M, Baudi F, Trematerra S, Quinto I, Venuta S, Scala G. 1997. HIV-1 Tat induces the expression of the interleukin-6 (IL6) gene by binding to the IL6 leader RNA and by interacting with CAAT enhancer-binding protein beta (NF-IL6) transcription factors. *J Biol Chem* 272: 14883–92.

Arnalich F, Lopez-Maderuelo D, Codoceo R, Lopez J, Solis-Garrido LM, Capiscol C, Fernandez-Capitan C, Madero R, Montiel C. 2002. Interleukin-1 receptor antagonist gene polymorphism and mortality in patients with severe sepsis. *Clin Exp Immunol* 127(2):331–36.

Asensi V, Alvarez V, Valle E, Meana A, Fierer J, Coto E, Carton JA, Maradona JA, Paz J, Dieguez MA, de la Fuente B, Moreno A, Rubio S, Tuya MJ, Sarasua J, Llames S, Arribas JM. 2003. IL-1 alpha (–889) promoter polymorphism is a risk factor for osteomyelitis. *Am J Med Genet* A 119:132–36.

Awomoyi AA, Charurat M, Marchant A, Miller EN, Blackwell JM, McAdam KP, Newport MJ. 2005. Polymorphism in IL1B: IL1B-511 association with tuberculosis and decreased lipopolysaccharide-induced IL-1beta in IFN-gamma primed ex-vivo whole blood assay. *J Endotoxin Res* 11:281–86.

Ayyavoo V, Mahboubi A, Mahalingam S, Ramalingam R, Kudchodkar S, Williams WV, Green DR, Weiner DB. 1997. HIV-1 Vpr suppresses immune activation and apoptosis through regulation of nuclear factor kappa B. *Nat Med* 3(10):1117–23.

Babula O, Lazdane G, Kroica J, Linhares IM, Ledger WJ, Witkin SS. 2005. Frequency of interleukin-4 (IL-4) −589 gene polymorphism and vaginal concentrations of IL-4, nitric oxide, and mannose-binding lectin in women with recurrent vulvovaginal candidiasis. *Clin Infect Dis* 40(9):1258–62.

Bailly S, di Giovine FS, Blakemore AI, Duff GW. 1993. Genetic polymorphism of human interleukin-1 alpha. *Eur J Immunol* 1993 23(6):1240–45.

Balding J, Healy CM, Livingstone WJ, White B, Mynett-Johnson L, Cafferkey M, Smith OP. 2003. Genomic polymorphic profiles in an Irish population with meningococcaemia: is it possible to predict severity. *Genes Immun* 4(8):533–40.

Barrett S, Collins M, Kenny C, Ryan E, Keane CO, Crowe J. 2003. Polymorphisms in tumour necrosis factor-alpha, transforming growth factor-beta, interleukin-10, interleukin-6, interferon-gamma, and outcome of hepatitis C virus infection. *J Med Virol* 71(2):212–18.

Bayley J-P, Ottenhoff THM, Verweij CL. 2004. Is there a future for TNF promoter polymorphisms? *Genes Immun* 5(5):315–29.

Belkaid Y, Hoffmann KF, Mendez S, Kamhawi S, Udey MC, Wynn TA, Sacks DL. 2001. The role of interleukin (IL)10 in the persistence of the Leishmania major in the skin after healing and the therapeutic potential of anti-IL-10 receptor antibody for sterile cure. *J Exp Med* 194:1497–1506.

Bellamy R, Ruwende C, Corrah T, McAdam KP, Whittle HC, Hill AV. 1998. Assessment of the interleukin 1 gene cluster and other candidate gene polymorphisms in host susceptibility to tuberculosis. *Tuber Lung Dis* 79:83–89.

Benkhart EM, Siedlar M, Wedel A, Werner T, Ziegler-Heitbrock HW. 2000. Role of Stat3 in lipopolysaccharide-induced IL-10 gene expression. *J Immunol* 165:1612–17.

Bennasser Y, Bahraoui E. 2002. HIV-1 Tat protein induces interleukin-10 in human peripheral blood monocytes: involvement of protein kinase C-betaII and -delta. *FASEB J* 16(6):546–54.

Bidwell J, Keen L, Gallagher G, Kimberly R, Huizinga T, McDermott MF, Oksenberg J, McNicholl J, Pociot F, Hardt C, D'Alfonso S. 1999. Cytokine gene polymorphism in human disease: on-line databases. *Genes Immun* 1:3–19.

Bidwell J, Keen L, Gallagher G, Kimberly R, Huizinga T, McDermott MF, Oksenberg J, McNicholl J, Pociot F, Hardt C, D'Alfonso S. 2001. Cytokine gene polymorphism in human disease: on-line databases, supplement 1. *Genes Immun* 2:61–70.

Biswas DK, Salas TR, Wang F, Ahlers CM, Dezube BJ, Pardee AB. 1995. A Tat-induced auto-up-regulatory loop for superactivation of the human immunodeficiency virus type 1 promoter. *J Virol* 69(12):7437–44.

Blakemore AI, Cox A, Gonzalez AM, Maskil JK, Hughes ME, Wilson RM, Ward JD, Duff GW. 1996. Interleukin-1 receptor antagonist allele (IL1RN*2) associated with nephropathy in diabetes mellitus. *Hum Genet* 97(3):369–74.

Boussiotis VA, Tsai EY, Yunis EJ, Thim S, Delgado JC, Dascher CC, Berezovskaya A, Rousset D, Reynes JM, Goldfeld AE. 2000. IL-10-producing T cells suppress immune responses in anergic tuberculosis patients. *J Clin Invest* 105:1317–25.

Brightbill HD, Plevy SE, Modlin RL, Smale ST. 2000. A prominent role for Sp1 during lipopolysaccharide-mediated induction of the IL-10 promoter in macrophages. *J Immunol* 164:1940–51.

Cargill M, Altshuler D, Ireland J, Sklar P, Ardlie K, Patil N, Shaw N, Lane CR, Lim EP, Kalyanaraman N, Nemesh J, Ziaugra L, Friedland L, Rolfe A, Warrington J, Lipshutz R, Daley GQ, Lander ES. 1999. Characterization of single-nucleotide polymorphisms in coding regions of human genes. *Nat Genet* 22:231–38.

Cartwright NH, Keen LJ, Demaine AG, Hurlock NJ, McGonigle RJ, Rowe PA, Shaw JF, Szydlo RM, Kaminski ER. 2001. A study of cytokine gene polymorphisms and protein secretion in renal transplantation. *Transpl Immunol* 8:237–44.

Carvalho LH, Sano G, Hafalla JC, Morrot A, Curotto de Lafaille MA, Zavala F. 2002. IL-4-secreting CD4+ T cells are crucial to the development of CD8+ T-cell responses against malaria liver stages. *Nat Med* 2: 166–70.

Choi EH, Lee HJ, Yoo T, Chanock SJ. 2002. A common haplotype of interleukin-4 gene IL4 is associated with severe respiratory syncytial virus disease in Korean children. *J Infect Dis* 186(9):1207–11.

Chow D, He X, Snow AL, Rose-John S, Garcia KC. 2001. Structure of an extracellular gp130 cytokine receptor signaling complex. *Science* 291:2150–55.

Crawley E, Kay R, Sillibourne J, Patel P, Hutchinson I, Woo P. 1999. Polymorphic haplotypes of the interleukin-10 5' flanking region determine variable interleukin-10 transcription and are associated with particular phenotypes of juvenile rheumatoid arthritis. *Arthritis Rheum* 42:1101–08.

Dahmer MK, Randolph A, Vitali S, Quasney MW. 2005. Genetic polymorphisms in sepsis. *Pediatr Crit Care Med* 6(3 suppl):S61–73.

Delgado JC, Baena A, Thim S, Goldfeld AE. 2002. Ethnic-specific genetic associations with pulmonary tuberculosis. *J Infect Dis* 186:1463–68.

Dewberry RM, Crossman DC, Francis SE. 2003. Interleukin-1 receptor antagonist (IL-1RN) genotype modulates the replicative capacity of human endothelial cells. *Circ Res* 92(12):1285–87.

Diehl SR, Wang Y, Brooks CN, Burmeister JA, Califano JV, Wang S, Schenkein HA. 1999. Linkage disequilibrium of interleukin-1 genetic polymorphisms with early-onset periodontitis. *J Periodontol* 70(4):418–30.

Dizier MH, Sandford A, Walley A, Philippi A, Cookson W, Demenais F. 1999. Indication of linkage of serum IgE levels to the interleukin-4 gene and exclusion of the contribution of the (–590 C to T) interleukin-4 promoter polymorphism to IgE variation. *Genet Epidemiol* 16(1):84–94.

Edwards-Smith CJ, Jonsson JR, Purdie DM, Bansal A, Shorthouse C, Powell EE. 1999. Interleukin-10 promoter polymorphism predicts initial response of chronic hepatitis C to interferon alfa. *Hepatology* 30(2): 526–30.

El-Omar EM, Carrington M, Chow W-H, McColl KEL, Bream JH, Young HA, Herrera J, Lissowska J, Yuan C-C, Rothman N, Lanyon G, Martin M, Fraumeni JF Jr, Rabkin CS. 2000. Interleukin-1 polymorphisms associated with increased risk of gastric cancer. *Nature* 404:398–402.

Endler G, Marsik C, Joukhadar C, Marculescu R, Mayr F, Mannhalter C, Wagner OF, Jilma B. 2004. The interleukin-6 G(–174)C promoter polymorphism does not determine plasma interleukin-6 concentrations in experimental endotoxemia in humans. *Clin Chem* 50(1):195–200.

Eskdale J, Keijsers V, Huizinga T, Gallagher G. 1999. Microsatellite alleles and single nucleotide polymorphisms (SNP) combine to form four major haplotype families at the human interleukin-10 (IL-10) locus. *Genes Immun* 1:151–55.

Ferrari SL, Ahn-Luong L, Garnero P, Humphries SE, Greenspan SL. 2003. Two promoter polymorphisms regulating interleukin-6 gene expression are associated with circulating levels of C-reactive protein and markers of bone resorption in postmenopausal women. *J Clin Endocrinol Metab* 88(1):255–59.

Fitness J, Floyd S, Warndorff DK, Sichali L, Malema S, Crampin AC, Fine PE, Hill AV. 2004a. Large-scale candidate gene study of tuberculosis susceptibility in the Karonga district of northern Malawi. *Am J Trop Med Hyg* 71(3):341–49.

Fitness J, Floyd S, Warndorff DK, Sichali L, Mwaungulu L, Crampin AC, Fine PE, Hill AV. 2004b. Large-scale candidate gene study of leprosy susceptibility in the Karonga district of northern Malawi. *Am J Trop Med Hyg* 71(3):330–40.

Foster CB, Lehrnbecher T, Samuels S, Stein S, Mol F, Metcalf JA, Wyvill K, Steinberg SM, Kovacs J, Blauvelt A, Yarchoan R, Chanock SJ. 2000. An IL6 promoter polymorphism is associated with a lifetime risk of development of Kaposi sarcoma in men infected with human immunodeficiency virus. *Blood* 96(7):2562–67.

Furuta T, Shirai N, Xiao F, El-Omar EM, Rabkin CS, Sugimura H, Ishizaki T, Ohashi K. 2004. Polymorphism of interleukin-1beta affects the eradication rates of Helicobacter pylori by triple therapy. *Clin Gastroenterol Hepatol* 2(1):22–30.

Gealy C, Denson M, Humphreys C, McSharry B, Wilkinson G, Caswell R. 2005. Posttranscriptional suppression of interleukin-6 production by human cytomegalovirus. *J Virol* 79(1):472–85.

Gerard C, Bruyns C, Marchant A, Abramowicz D, Vandenbeele P, Delvaux A, Fiers W, Goldman M, Velu T. 1993. Interleukin 10 reduces the release of tumor necrosis factor and prevents lethality in experimental endotoxemia. *J Exp Med* 177:547–50.

Gibson AW, Edberg JC, Wu J, Westendorp RG, Huizinga TW, Kimberly RP. 2001. Novel single nucleotide polymorphisms in the distal IL-10 promoter affect IL-10 production and enhance the risk of systemic lupus erythematosus. *J Immunol* 166:3915–22.

Gyan B, Goka B, Cvetkovic JT, Perlmann H, Lefvert AK, Akanmori B, Troye-Blomberg M. 2002. Polymorphisms in interleukin-1beta and interleukin-1 receptor antagonist genes and malaria in Ghanaian children. *Scand J Immunol* 56(6):619–22.

Gyan BA, Goka B, Cvetkovic JT, Kurtzhals JL, Adabayeri V, Perlmann H, Lefvert AK, Akanmori BD, Troye-Blomberg M. 2004. Allelic polymorphisms in the repeat and promoter regions of the interleukin-4 gene and malaria severity in Ghanaian children. *Clin Exp Immunol* 138(1):145–50.

Harding D, Dhamrait S, Millar A, Humphries S, Marlow N, Whitelaw A, Montgomery H. 2003. Is interleukin-6 −174 genotype associated with the development of septicemia in preterm infants? *Pediatrics* 112(4): 800–03.

Haukim N, Bidwell JL, Smith AJ, Keen LJ, Gallagher G, Kimberly R, Huizinga T, McDermott MF, Oksenberg J, McNicholl J, Pociot F, Hardt C, D'Alfonso S. 2002. Cytokine gene polymorphism in human disease: on-line databases, supplement 2. *Genes Immun* 3:313–30.

Heesen M, Bloemeke B, Heussen N, Kunz D. 2002. Can the interleukin-6 response to endotoxin be predicted? Studies of the influence of a promoter polymorphism of the interleukin-6 gene, gender, the density of the endotoxin receptor CD14, and inflammatory cytokines. *Crit Care Med* 30(3):664–69.

Helminen M, Lahdenpohja N, Hurme M. 1999. Polymorphism of the interleukin-10 gene is associated with susceptibility to Epstein-Barr virus infection. *J Infect Dis* 180(2):496–9.

Helminen ME, Kilpinen S, Virta M, Hurme M. 2001. Susceptibility to primary Epstein-Barr virus infection is associated with interleukin-10 gene promoter polymorphism. *J Infect Dis* 184(6):777–80.

Henao MI, Montes C, Paris SC, Garcia LF. 2006. Cytokine gene polymorphisms in Colombian patients with different clinical presentations of tuberculosis. *Tuberculosis (Edinb)* 86(1):11–19.

Hurme M, Lahdenpohja N, Santtila S. 1998. Gene polymorphisms of interleukins 1 and 10 in infectious and autoimmune diseases. *Ann Med* 30:469–73.

Jamie WE, Edwards RK, Ferguson RJ, Duff P. 2005. The interleukin-6–174 single nucleotide polymorphism: cervical protein production and the risk of preterm delivery. *Am J Obstet Gynecol* 192(4):1023–27.

Kemper C, Chan A. C, Green JM, Brett KA, Murphy KM, Atkinson JP. 2003. Activation of human CD4+ cells with CD3 and CD46 induces a T-regulatory cell 1 phenotype. *Nature* 421:388–92.

Kilpinen S, Hulkkonen J, Wang XY, Hurme M. 2001. The promoter polymorphism of the interleukin-6 gene regulates interleukin-6 production in neonates but not in adults. *Eur Cytokine Netw* 12(1): 62–68.

Kornman KS, Crane A, Wang HY, di Giovine FS, Newman MG, Pirk FW, Wilson TG Jr, Higginbottom FL, Duff GW. 1997. The interleukin-1 genotype as a severity factor in adult periodontal disease. *J Clin Periodontol* 24(1):72–77.

Koss K, Satsangi J, Fanning GC, Welsh KI, Jewell DP. 2000. Cytokine (TNF alpha, LT alpha and IL-10) polymorphisms in inflammatory bowel diseases and normal controls: differential effects on production and allele frequencies. *Genes Immun* 1:185–90.

Kube D, Platzer C, von Knethen A, et al. 1995. Isolation of the human interleukin 10 promoter. Characterization of the promoter activity in Burkitt's lymphoma cell lines. *Cytokine* 7:1–7.

Kurreeman FA, Schonkeren JJ, Heijmans BT, Toes RE, Huizinga TW. 2004. Transcription of the IL10 gene reveals allele-specific regulation at the mRNA level. *Hum Mol Genet* 13(16):1755–62.

Lehrnbecher T, Bernig T, Hanisch M, Koehl U, Behl M, Reinhardt D, Creutzig U, Klingebiel T, Chanock SJ, Schwabe D. 2005. Common genetic variants in the interleukin-6 and chitotriosidase genes are associated with the risk for serious infection in children undergoing therapy for acute myeloid leukemia. *Leukemia* 19(10):1745–50.

Lio D, Caruso C, Di Stefano R, Colonna Romano G, Ferraro D, Scola L, Crivello A, Licata A, Valenza LM, Candore G, Craxi A, Almasio PL. 2003. IL-10 and TNF-alpha polymorphisms and the recovery from HCV infection. *Hum Immunol* 64(7): 674–80.

Llorente L, Zou W, Levy Y, Richaud-Patin Y, Wijdenes J, Alcocer-Varela J, Morel-Fourrier B, Brouet JC, Alarcon-Segovia D, Galanaud P. 1995. Role of interleukin-10 in the lymphocyte hyperactivity and autoantibody production in human systemic lupus erythematosus. *J Exp Med* 1:839–44

Lopez-Maderuelo D, Arnalich F, Serantes R, Gonzalez A, Codoceo R, Madero R, Vazquez JJ, Montiel C. 2003. Interferon-gamma and interleukin-10 gene polymorphisms in pulmonary tuberculosis. *Am J Respir Crit Care Med* 167:970–75.

Lowe PR, Galley HF, Abdel-Fattah A, Webster NR. 2003. Influence of interleukin-10 polymorphisms on interleukin-10 expression and survival in critically ill patients. *Crit Care Med* 31:34–38.

Ma W, Lim W, Gee K, et al. 2001. The p38 mitogen-activated kinase pathway regulates the human interleukin-10 promoter via the activation of Sp1 transcription factor in lipopolysaccharide-stimulated human macrophages. *J Biol Chem* 276:13664–74.

Malhotra D, Darvishi K, Sood S, Sharma S, Grover C, Relhan V, Reddy BS, Bamezai RN. 2005. IL-10 promoter single nucleotide polymorphisms are significantly associated with resistance to leprosy. *Hum Genet* 118(2):295–300.

McLoughlin RM, Jenkins BJ, Grail D, Williams AS, Fielding CA, Parker CR, Ernst M, Topley N, Jones SA. 2005. IL-6 trans-signaling via STAT3 directs T cell infiltration in acute inflammation. *Proc Natl Acad Sci USA* 102(27):9589–94.

Minton EJ, Smillie D, Smith P, Shipley S, McKendrick MW, Gleeson DC, Underwood JC, Cannings C, Wilson AG, Trent Hepatitis C Study Group 2005. Clearance of hepatitis C virus is not associated with single nucleotide polymorphisms in the IL-1, -6, or -10 genes. *Hum Immunol* 66(2):127–32.

Miyazoe S, Hamasaki K, Nakata K, Kajiya Y, Kitajima K, Nakao K, Daikoku M, Yatsuhashi H, Koga M, Yano M, Eguchi K. 2002. Influence of interleukin-10 gene promoter polymorphisms on disease progression in patients chronically infected with hepatitis B virus. *Am J Gastroenterol* 97:2086–92.

Moraes MO, Pacheco AG, Schonkeren JJ, Vanderborght PR, Nery JA, Santos AR, Moraes ME, Moraes JR, Ottenhoff TH, Sampaio EP, Huizinga TW, Sarno EN. 2004. Interleukin-10 promoter single-nucleotide polymorphisms as markers for disease susceptibility and disease severity in leprosy. *Genes Immun* 5(7):592–95.

Moreno M, Silva EL, Ramirez LE, Palacio LG, Rivera D, Arcos-Burgos M. 2004. Chagas' disease susceptibility/resistance: linkage disequilibrium analysis suggests epistasis between major histocompatibility complex and interleukin-10. *Tissue Antigens* 64(1):18–24.

Mormann M, Rieth H, Hua TD, Assohou C, Roupelieva M, Hu SL, Kremsner PG, Luty AJ, Kube D. 2004. Mosaics of gene variations in the Interleukin-10 gene promoter affect interleukin-10 production depending on the stimulation used. *Genes Immun* 5(4):246–55

Mozzato-Chamay N, Mahdi OS, Jallow O, Mabey DC, Bailey RL, Conway DJ. 2000. Polymorphisms in candidate genes and risk of scarring trachoma in a *Chlamydia trachomatis*–endemic population. *J Infect Dis* 182(5):1545–48

Nishimura M, Maeda M, Yasunaga J, Kawakami H, Kaji R, Adachi A, Uchiyama T, Matsuoka M. 2003. Influence of cytokine and mannose binding protein gene polymorphisms on human T-cell leukemia virus type I (hTLV-I) provirus load in HTLV-I asymptomatic carriers. *Hum Immunol* 64(4):453–57.

Nishimura M, Matsuoka M, Maeda M, Mizuta I, Mita S, Uchino M, Matsui M, Kuroda Y, Kawakami H, Kaji R, Adachi A, Uchiyama T. 2002. Association between interleukin-6 gene polymorphism and human T-cell leukemia virus type I associated myelopathy. *Hum Immunol* 63(8):696–700.

Oleksyk TK, Thio CL, Truelove AL, Goedert JJ, Donfield SM, Kirk GD, Thomas DL, O'Brien SJ, Smith MW.

2005. Single nucleotide polymorphisms and haplotypes in the IL10 region associated with HCV clearance. *Genes Immun* 6(4):347–57.

Ottenhoff THM, Verreck FAW, Lichtenauer-Kaligis EGR, Hoeve MA, Sanal O, van Dissel JT. 2002. Genetics, cytokines and human infectious disease: lessons from weakly pathogenic mycobacteria and salmonellae. *Nat Genet* 32:97–105.

Ozaki K, Ohnishi Y, Iida A, Sekine A, Yamada R, Tsunoda T, Sato H, Sato H, Hori M, Nakamura Y, Tanaka T. 2002. Functional SNPs in the lymphotoxin-alpha gene that are associated with susceptibility to myocardial infarction. *Nat Genet* 32:650–54.

Park BL, Lee HS, Kim YJ, Kim JY, Jung JH, Kim LH, Shin HD. 2003. Association between interleukin 6 promoter variants and chronic hepatitis B progression. *Exp Mol Med* 35(2):76–82.

Pawlik A, Baskiewicz-Masiuk M, Machalinski B, Gawronska-Szklarz B. 2006. Association of cytokine gene polymorphisms and the release of cytokines from peripheral blood mononuclear cells treated with methotrexate and dexamethasone. *Int Immunopharmacol* 6(3):351–57.

Philippon V, Vellutini C, Gambarelli D, Harkiss G, Arbuthnott G, Metzger D, Roubin R, Filippi P. 1994. The basic domain of the lentiviral Tat protein is responsible for damages in mouse brain: involvement of cytokines. *Virology* 205(2):519–29.

Price P, James I, Fernandez S, French MA. 2004. Alleles of the gene encoding IL-1alpha may predict control of plasma viraemia in HIV-1 patients on highly active antiretroviral therapy. *AIDS* 18(11):1495–501.

Rees LE, Wood NA, Gillespie KM, Lai KN, Gaston K, Mathieson PW. 2002. The interleukin-10–1082 G/A polymorphism: allele frequency in different populations and functional significance. *Cell Mol Life Sci* 59:560–69.

Reuss E, Fimmers R, Kruger A, Becker C, Rittner C, Hohler T. 2002. Differential regulation of interleukin-10 production by genetic and environmental factors—a twin study. *Genes Immun* 3:407–13.

Rieth H, Mormann M, Luty AJ, Assohou-Luty CA, Roupelieva M, Kremsner PG, Kube D. 2004. A three base pair gene variation within the distal 5'-flanking region of the interleukin-10 (IL-10) gene is related to the *in vitro* IL-10 production capacity of lipopolysaccharide-stimulated peripheral blood mononuclear cells. *Eur Cytokine Netw* 15:153–8.

Rivera-Chavez FA, Peters-Hybki DL, Barber RC, Lindberg GM, Jialal I, Munford RS, O'Keefe GE. 2004. Innate immunity genes influence the severity of acute appendicitis. *Ann Surg* 240(2):269–77.

Rivera-Chavez FA, Peters-Hybki DL, Barber RC, O'Keefe GE. 2003. Interleukin-6 promoter haplotypes and interleukin-6 cytokine responses. *Shock* 20(3): 218–23.

Santos AR, Suffys PN, Vanderborght PR, Moraes MO, Vieira LM, Cabello PH, Bakker AM, Matos HJ, Huizinga TW, Ottenhoff TH, Sampaio EP, Sarno EN. 2002. Role of tumor necrosis factor-alpha and interleukin-10 promoter gene polymorphisms in leprosy. *J Infect Dis* 186:1687–91.

Schaaf B, Rupp J, Muller-Steinhardt M, Kruse J, Boehmke F, Maass M, Zabel P, Dalhoff K. 2005. The interleukin-6 −174 promoter polymorphism is associated with extrapulmonary bacterial dissemination in *Streptococcus pneumoniae* infection. *Cytokine* 31(4):324–28.

Scola L, Crivello A, Marino V, Gioia V, Serauto A, Candore G, Colonna-Romano G, Caruso C, Lio D. 2003 IL-10 and TNF-a polymorphisms in a sample of Sicilian patients affected by tuberculosis: implication for ageing and life span expectancy. *Mech Ageing Dev* 124(4):569–72.

Schluter B, Raufhake C, Erren M, Schotte H, Kipp F, Rust S, Van Aken H, Assmann G, Berendes E. 2002. Effect of the interleukin-6 promoter polymorphism (−174 G/C) on the incidence and outcome of sepsis. *Crit Care Med* 30(1):32–37.

Segal S, Hill AVS. 2003. Genetic susceptibility to infectious disease. *Trends Microbiol* 11:445–48.

Sharma V, Knobloch TJ, Benjamin D. 1995. Differential expression of cytokine genes in HIV-1 tat transfected T and B cell lines. *Biochem Biophys Res Commun* 208(2):704–13.

Shin HD, Park BL, Kim YH, Cheong HS, Lee IH, Park SK. 2005. Common interleukin 10 polymorphism associated with decreased risk of tuberculosis. *Exp Mol Med* 37(2):128–32.

Shin HD, Park BL, Kim LH, Jung JH, Kim JY, Yoon JH, Kim YJ, Lee HS. 2003. Interleukin 10 haplotype associated with increased risk of hepatocellular carcinoma. *Hum Mol Genet* 12:901–06.

Shin HD, Winkler C, Stephens JC, Bream J, Young H, Goedert JJ, O'Brien TR, Vlahov, D, Buchbinder S, Giorgi J, Rinaldo C, Donfield S, Willoughby A, O'Brien SJ, Smith MW. 2000 Genetic restriction of HIV-1 pathogenesis to AIDS by promoter alleles of IL10. *Proc Nat Acad Sci USA* 97:14467–72.

Singh KK, Hughes MD, Chen J, Spector SA. 2004. Lack of protective effects of interleukin-4 −589-C/T polymorphism against HIV-1-related disease progression and central nervous system impairment, in children. *J Infect Dis* 189(4):587–92.

Soriano A, Lozano F, Oliva H, Garcia F, Nomdedeu M, De Lazzari E, Rodriguez C, Barrasa A, Lorenzo JI, Del Romero J, Plana M, Miro JM, Gatell JM, Vives J, Gallart T. 2005. Polymorphisms in the interleukin-

4 receptor alpha chain gene influence susceptibility to HIV-1 infection and its progression to AIDS. *Immunogenetics* 57(9):644–54.

Tarlow JK, Blakemore AI, Lennard A, Solari R, Hughes HN, Steinkasserer A, Duff GW. 1993. Polymorphism in human IL-1 receptor antagonist gene intron 2 is caused by variable numbers of an 86-bp tandem repeat. *Hum Genet* 91(4):403–04.

Timmann C, Fuchs S, Thoma C, Lepping B, Brattig NW, Sievertsen J, Thye T, Muller-Myhsok B, Horstmann RD. 2004. Promoter haplotypes of the interleukin-10 gene influence proliferation of peripheral blood cells in response to helminth antigen. *Genes Immun* 5(4): 256–60.

Tso HW, Ip WK, Chong WP, Tam CM, Chiang AK, Lau YL. 2005 Association of interferon gamma and interleukin 10 genes with tuberculosis in Hong Kong Chinese. *Genes Immun* 6(4):358–63.

Turner DM, Williams DM, Sankaran D, Lazarus M, Sinnott PJ, Hutchinson IV. 1997. An investigation of polymorphism in the interleukin-10 gene promoter. *Eur J Immunogenet* 24:1–8.

Uno M, Ito LS, Oba-Shinjo SM, Marie SK, Shinjo SK, Hamajima N. 2004. Possible association of interleukin 1B C-31T polymorphism among Helicobacter pylori seropositive Japanese Brazilians with susceptibility to atrophic gastritis. *Int J Mol Med* 14(3):421–26.

Vasilescu A, Heath SC, Ivanova R, Hendel H, Do H, Mazoyer A, Khadivpour E, Goutalier FX, Khalili K, Rappaport J, Lathrop GM, Matsuda F, Zagury JF. 2003. Genomic analysis of Th1-Th2 cytokine genes in an AIDS cohort: identification of IL4 and IL10 haplotypes associated with the disease progression. *Genes Immun* 4(6):441–49.

Verra F, Luoni G, Calissano C, Troye-Blomberg M, Perlmann P, Perlmann H, Arca B, Sirima BS, Konate A, Coluzzi M, Kwiatkowski D, Modiano D. 2004. IL4–589C/T polymorphism and IgE levels in severe malaria. *Acta Trop* 90(2):205–09.

Volk H, Asadullah K, Gallagher G, Sabat R, Grutz G. 2001. IL-10 and its homologs: important immune mediators and emerging immunotherapeutic targets. *Trends Immunol* 22:414–17

Walley AJ, Aucan C, Kwiatkowski D, Hill AV. 2004. Interleukin-1 gene cluster polymorphisms and susceptibility to clinical malaria in a Gambian case-control study. *Eur J Hum Genet* 12(2):132–38.

Wang C, Tang J, Song W, Lobashevsky E, Wilson CM, Kaslow RA. 2004. HLA and cytokine gene polymorphisms are independently associated with responses to hepatitis B vaccination. *Hepatology* 39(4):978–88.

Warle MC, Farhan A, Metselaar HJ, Hop WC, Perrey C, Zondervan PE, Kap M, Kwekkeboom J, Ijzermans JN, Tilanus HW, Pravica V, Hutchinson IV, Bouma

GJ. 2003. Are cytokine gene polymorphisms related to *in vitro* cytokine production profiles? *Liver Transpl* 9:170–81.

Westendorp, RG, van Dunne FM, Kirkwood TB, Helmerhorst FM, Huizinga TW. 2001. Optimizing human fertility and survival. *Nat Med* 7:873.

Wilkinson RJ, Patel P, Llewelyn M, Hirsch CS, Pasvol G, Snounou G, Davidson RN, Toossi Z. 1999. Influence of polymorphism in the genes for the interleukin (IL)-1 receptor antagonist and IL-1beta on tuberculosis. *J Exp Med* 189(12):1863–74.

Wilson AG, di Giovine FS, Duff GW. 1995. Genetics of tumour necrosis factor-alpha in autoimmune, infectious, and neoplastic diseases. *J Inflamm* 45:1–12

Wilson JN Rockett K, Jallow M, Pinder M, Sisay-Joof F, Newport M, Newton J, Kiatkowski D. 2005a. Analysis of IL-10 haplotypic associations with severe malaria *Genes Immun* 6(6):462–66.

Wilson J, Rowlands K, Rockett K, Moore C, Lockhart E, Sharland M, Kwiatkowski D, Hull J. 2005b. Genetic variation at the IL10 gene locus is associated with severity of respiratory syncytial virus bronchiolitis. *J Infect Dis* 191(10):1705–09.

Yee LJ, Tang J, Gibson AW, Kimberly R, Van Leeuwen DJ, Kaslow RA. 2001. Interleukin 10 polymorphisms as predictors of sustained response in antiviral therapy for chronic hepatitis C infection. *Hepatology* 33:708–12.

Zhang PA, Li Y, Xu P, Wu JM. 2004. Polymorphisms of interleukin-1B and interleukin-1 receptor antagonist genes in patients with chronic hepatitis B. *World J Gastroenterol* 10(12):1826–29

Zhao Z, Fu YX, Hewett-Emmett D, Boerwinkle E. 2003. Investigating single nucleotide polymorphism (SNP) density in the human genome and its implications for molecular evolution. *Gene* 312:207–13.

16

Cytokine Genes II

IL12, IFNG, and Their Receptor Genes

Margje H. Haverkamp & Stephen M. Holland

The host immune response is divided into early innate (nonspecific) and adaptive (later) phases. The latter aims at sustained control of infection (Janeway 1992). The interleukin-12/interferon-γ (IL-12/IFN-γ) signaling axis encourages T-helper-1 (Th1) and discourages T-helper-2 (Th2) development. Genetic deficiencies in IL-12, its receptor (IL-12R), the IFN-γ receptor (IFN-γR), and in STAT-1 all cause susceptibility to weakly pathogenic mycobacteria, *Mycobacterium tuberculosis* and *Salmonella* (Ottenhoff et al. 2002). About 140 patients suffering from Mendelian defects in IL-12p40, IL-12Rβ1, IFN-γR1, IFN-γR2, or STAT-1 have been reported (Mendelian susceptibility to mycobacterial disease; Casanova and Abel 2002, Dorman and Holland 2000, Ottenhoff et al. 2002).

The beginning of this century saw the origin of extensive single nucleotide polymorphism (SNP) databases (e.g., the SNP Consortium), detected by an expanding variety of molecular techniques (see chapter 2) (Miller and Kwok 2001). To analyze these and other genetic data, many statistical and data analytic methods are used, including linkage disequilibrium (LD), odds ratios (ORs), goodness of fit (χ^2-tests), and *t*-tests (see chapter 1). Large data sets are necessary to have adequate statistical power. Biological plausibility, clear-cut phenotype definitions, independent replication studies, and consistent functional data are even more essential.

IL-12 Pathway

Gene Product and Role in Infection

IL-12 Structure

IL-12 is a heterodimeric cytokine, evolutionarily linked to IL-6 and its receptor (Trinchieri 2003), consisting of two disulfide-linked polypeptide chains: p35 and p40. Together, they form IL-12p70 (Kobayashi et al. 1989). IL-12p40, together with p19, is part of IL-23, another heterodimeric cytokine. IL-23 and IL-12 have

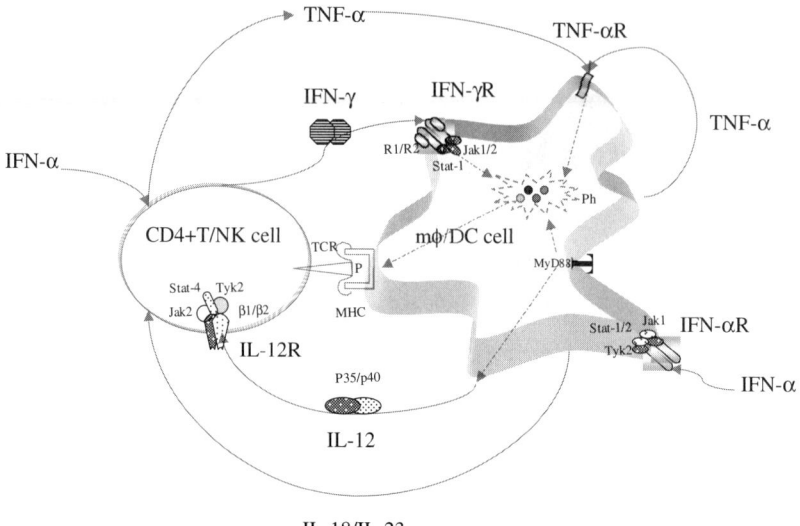

FIGURE 16.1. Macrophage/T-cell interactions. DC, dendritic cell; MHC, MHCII Ag presentation; Mφ, macrophage; P, foreign protein; Ph, Phagosome containing mycobacteria; TCR, T-cell receptor; T, TLR signaling inducing costimulatory factors.

comparable functions (Trinchieri 2003) and share use of IL-12Rβ1. IL-12p35 is thought to be the rate-limiting protein in IL-12p70 heterodimer formation (Snijders et al. 1996). Overproduction of IL-12p40 leads to free IL-12p40 chains or IL-12p40 homodimers, the function of which is unclear (Trinchieri 2003). IL-12p40 is expressed only in activated phagocytes, whereas IL-12p35 is expressed in many cell types, including lymphocytes that do not produce IL-12p70. Expression of both IL-12p35 and IL-12p40 is required for biologically active IL-12p70 (Gubler et al. 1991). IFN-γ production by activated T cells and natural killer (NK) cells up-regulates transcription and expression of IL-12p40 and IL-12p35 by remodeling nucleosome 1 of the promoter of IL-12p40, making it more accessible for the transcription factor C/EBP (Trinchieri 2003). Moreover, in a complex with the nuclear factor-κB (NF-κB) subunit cRel, C/EBP binds to the transcription factor site of NF-κB on IL-12p40, also leading to enhanced production. The IL-12p35 promoter binds the transcription factor SP1, γIRE (IFN-γ response element), and PU.1 (Trinchieri 2003). After executing its stimulatory function, IL-12p70 is translocated to the endoplasmic reticulum, where p35 is cleaved twice and glycosylated.

IL-12 Role in Infection

IL-12 links the innate and adaptive phases of the immune response (figure 16.1). In the innate phase, phagocytes (CD40+ macrophages, monocytes, neutrophils, and other antigen-presenting cells [APCs]) migrate to the place of infection due to a change in vascular permeability. They recognize conserved microbial patterns via surface receptors (e.g., Toll-like receptors [TLRs]) and bind to CD40L on activated T cells (Trinchieri 2003). IL-12, granulocyte-macrophage colony-stimulating factor and tumor necrosis factor-α (TNF-α) are released. IL-12 binds to its cognate receptor on the surface of the T and NK cells. NK cells proliferate and produce IFN-γ. In the adaptive phase, antigen-specific T- and B-cell populations expand clonally. In lymph nodes, naive antigen-specific CD4+ T cells encounter APCs presenting antigens bound to MHC class II molecules and become committed to Th1 or Th2 phenotypes (Mosmann et al. 1989). IL-12, in synergy with IL-18, IL-23, and IL-27, plays a significant role in differentiation of CD4+ T cells toward Th1. However, both the quality of T cell receptor (TCR) antigen binding and the up-regulation of T-bet (a transcription factor controlled by IFN-γ that up-regulates IL-12Rβ2 expression; Afkarian et al. 2002) are triggers for Th1 development. IFN-γ production by a variety of cells (CD4$^+$ Th1 lymphocytes, CD8$^+$ cytotoxic lymphocytes, NK cells, APCs) forms a critical defense against intracellular microorganisms.

IL-12 exerts its influence in several ways: induction of adhesion factors on endothelium and matrix proteins to facilitate cell migration; enhancement of Th1 cytokine secretion (e.g., IFN-γ) by activated T and NK cells and of lipopolysaccharide (LPS)-induced transcription of IL-12p35 and IL-12p40; promotion of proliferation and differentiation of T and B cells and of T- and NK-cell cytotoxicity via increased perforin and granzymes (Ottenhoff et al. 2002, Trinchieri 2003).

The effects of IL-12 are balanced by several Th2 cytokines: IL-4, IL-10, and transforming growth factor-β (TGF-β). Although defects in the IFN-y/IL-12 axis might be expected to skew toward Th2 profiles, this is not supported by observations in human disease (Doffinger et al. 1999). Mycobacterium-specific T cells from IL-12Rβ1–deficient patients display clear Th1 phenotypes (Verhagen et al. 2000).

IL-12R Structure

The IL-12R is composed of two type I transmembrane glycoproteins: IL-12Rβ1 (100 kDa, with 54% homology to mouse IL-12Rβ1, and also part of the IL-23R) and IL-12Rβ2 (130 kDa, 68% homology to the mouse counterpart; Presky et al. 1996). The IL-12R is present not only on NK and activated T cells, but also on dendritic and B cells. Low constitutive levels of functional IL-12R on resting NK cells accounts for their quick activation (Trinchieri 2003). IL-12Rβ2 is only present in Th1 T cells. Co-expression of both IL-12Rβ1 and IL-12Rβ2 is required for biological activity and high-affinity binding of IL-12 (50 pM) (Presky et al. 1996). IL-12p40 binds IL-12Rβ1, whereas p35 mainly interacts with IL-12Rβ2. Both IL-12R and IL-23R are STAT-4 dependent receptors and have overlapping functions.

IL-12R Role in Infection

Both IL-12R and IL-23R activate the Jak/Stat pathway. The IL-12R chains bind and phosphorylate Tyk2 and Jak2 (figure 16.1). These in turn phosphorylate STAT-4, but also activate STAT-1, -3, and -5. STAT-4 translocates to the nucleus, where it activates transcription of IL-12–induced genes such as IFN-γ and IL-18R. The expression of IL-12Rβ2 is regulated by cytokines (IFN-γ), steroids, and accessory signals. Activated mo-

nocytes only possess IL-12Rβ1, which is up-regulated by IL-2 and CD28, and these cells therefore do not bind IL-12 well. IL-12/CD28 synergy stimulates IFN-γ production (Trinchieri 2003). Dexamethasone, and also Th2 cytokines such as IL-4 and TGF-β, down-regulate IL-12R.

Pathogenesis

IL-12

IL-12p40 deficiency leads to a lack of IL-12 and therefore of IL-23; these are the only cytokine ligands known to be genetically deficient in humans thus far (Ottenhoff et al. 2002).

By 2003, 73 patients were known to have defects in the IL-12 axis; 19 patients from various kindreds were reported with complete deficiency in IL-12p40 (Fieschi and Casanova, 2003). Defects in IL-12p35 have not been recognized. Most IL-12p40 deficient patients survive. Residual IL-12–independent IFN-γ activity may explain their relatively good outcomes (Ottenhoff et al. 2002). Patients deficient in IL-12 or IL-12R are most vulnerable to Bacille Calmette-Guérin (BCG), nontuberculous mycobacteria (NTM), and *Salmonella* (Fieschi et al., 2003). Stimulated cellular secretion of IL-12, and subsequently of IFN-γ, is reduced (Casanova and Abel 2002). Clinical infections with pathogens other than mycobacteria and *Salmonella* (e.g., herpes, Epstein-Barr virus, cytomegalovirus, but also chlamydia, *Toxoplasma gondii*) in humans deficient for IL-12 or IL-12R have not been seen (Ottenhoff et al. 2002, Fieschi and Casanova 2003). The incidence of *M. tuberculosis* is low, but this may reflect exposure.

Penetrance and expressivity are variable in these defects. Infections with BCG occurred in all 16 inoculated IL-12p40 deficient patients, but BCG infection did not recur after treatment, nor were those patients subsequently infected with NTM. Therefore, BCG infection appears to protect against NTM infection in patients with defects in IL-12. Seven out of 19 (37%) IL-12p40–deficient patients died, all because of NTM infections. One patient suffered from *M. tuberculosis* (Casanova and Abel, 2002), and five patients (26%) had multiple episodes of *Salmonella* (Fieschi and Casanova 2003). The frequency of *Salmonella* infections in IL-12/IL-12R–deficient patients is much higher than in patients with IFN-γR deficiency, suggesting that there are IFN-γ–independent roles for IL-

12 and IL-12–independent roles for IFN-γ where *Salmonella* is concerned.

IL-12R

To date, all mutations in the IL-12R are in IL-12Rβ1 (Ottenhoff et al. 2002). Mutations are recessive and mostly due to the formation of premature stop codons in the extracellular domain, eliminating surface expression of IL-12Rβ1 in the 54 patients identified so far (Ottenhoff et al. 2002, Fieschi et al. 2003). IL-12Rβ1– deficient NK and T cells still produce low amounts of IFN-γ (1–10%) under the influence of IL-18, IFN-α, and IL-27 (Ottenhoff et al. 2002). Therefore, granuloma formation is normal (Casanova and Abel 2002). Both penetrance and expressivity are incomplete. Most patients can be effectively treated with antibiotics, often in combination with IFN-γ (Dorman and Holland 2000). Seventy percent of the 35 BCG-vaccinated IL-12Rβ1 patients suffered from BCG infection. The protection conferred by a first BCG or NTM infection in combination with response to antibiotics in IL-12Rβ1–deficient patients paralleled IL-12p40 deficiency, suggesting that IL-12 is somewhat redundant for adaptive immunity to mycobacteria (Fieschi and Casanova 2003, Fieschi et al. 2003). Twenty-two percent of patients, all BCG naive, developed clinically apparent NTM infection (Fieschi and Casanova 2003), while some IL-12Rβ1–deficient patients did not develop BCG-itis, despite vaccination. Three IL-12Rβ1- deficient patients developed *M. tuberculosis*, all of whom were cured with appropriate antibiotic therapy (Fieschi and Casanova 2003). Deaths (15%) were from NTM. Almost half of IL-12Rβ1 patients developed *Salmonella*, usually before 12 years of age, and susceptibility remained after clearance of first infection. Therefore, there are different roles for IL-12 in secondary immunity to *Salmonella* and mycobacteria.

Gene Organization and Sequence

IL12A is 7.18 kb and has seven exons (mRNA 1,436 bp), with flanking noncoding mRNAs. *IL12B* is 15.69 kb; the first and the last of eight exons are noncoding, leaving a 987-base mRNA encoding 328 amino acids. All disease-causing mutations to date have been found in *IL12B*, including p40del4.4, a 373-bp deletion involving two exons (Dorman and Holland 2000).

IL12RB1 encodes 17 exons in 27.33 kb; the mRNA is 2,100 bases. More than 20 mutations lead to pre-

mature stop codons or deletions in the extracellular domain. R213W (C701T) precludes expression of IL-12Rβ1, probably due to mRNAs mechanisms (Sakai et al. 2001). C198R (T656C) precludes surface expression but allows high intracellular levels of IL-12Rβ1 and is capable of an IL-12 response (Verhagen et al. 2000).

IL12RB2 has 16 exons, the first of which is not translated (Trinchieri et al. 2003). The gene is 89.54 kb, and the mRNA 4,040 bases. Three cytoplasmic tyrosine residues in IL-12Rβ2 suggest an important role in IL-12 signal transduction (Chua et al. 1995). To date, no mutations have been found in IL-12Rβ2.

Animal Studies

Animal studies parallel observations in humans. IL-12p40–deficient mice are more susceptible to BCG, *M. tuberculosis*, *Salmonella*, and, to a lesser extent, *M. avium*. Mice have poor granuloma formation and defective IFN-γ production (Dorman and Holland 2000, Fieschi 2003). Neutralization of IL-12 impairs production of IFN-γ, permitting overwhelming infection and mortality due to *Histoplasmosis capsulatum* and *T. gondii* (Khan et al. 1994, Zhou et al. 1995). Leishmaniasis and viral infections are also increased by IL-12 signaling defects (Trinchieri 1997). Mice deficient in either IL-12p40 or STAT-4 display defective induction of IFN-γ, defective NK cytotoxicity, and abrogated Th1 differentiation (Kaplan et al. 1996, Thierfelder et al. 1996). This holds true for IL-12p35–deficient mice, as well, but to a lesser extent (Ottenhoff et al. 2002). *T. gondii*–infected mice deficient in both IL-10 and IL-12 survive, suggesting a role for Th1/Th2 balance. When both TLR (MyD88) and IL-12 signaling is absent, no IFN-γ is detected and a full-blown Th2 response develops (Jankovic et al. 2002).

Polymorphisms and Populations

IL12

Although regulatory regions of cytokine genes are generally polymorphic, *IL12A* and *IL12B* have highly conserved promoter regions. C-916T is a rare polymorphism in the *IL12A* promoter (Pravica et al. 1999); only two others are identified in the *IL12B* promoter (Huang et al. 2000, Zwiers et al. 2004) (table 16.1). In two studies, IL12B-pro (allele 1 = CTCTAA; allele 2 = GC, slightly more frequent) has been associated with se-

TABLE 16.1. Polymorphisms found in IFN-γ, IL-12, and their receptors.

NCBI Gene ID	Common Name	Entrez Gene ID	Map Position	Polymorphisms	References (See Also Tables 16.2–16.4)
IL12A	IL-12p35, CLMF, NKSF1	3592	3p12-q13.2	Promoter: C-916T Intronic: 4 SNPs Exon 6: A/G(L189L) Exon 7: T/C(D244D), T/C (M247T) 3′ UTR: three SNPs, one insertion (–/A)	Ensemble, Pravica et al. 2000a
IL12B	IL-12p40, CLMF2, NKSF2	3593	5q31–33	Promoter: IL-12Bpro, G-1287T 5′ UTR: G-806T Exon 3: G/A(V33I), deletion (A/–, frame shift) Exon 5: C/T(G182R), (S226N) Exon 7: G/T (V298F) Intronic: nine SNPs, (ATT)$_n$ in intron 2, TA repeat in intron 4 3′ UTR (exon 8): C1188A, eight other SNPs, one insertion (–/T)	Ensemble, Huang et al. 2000, Pravica et al. 2000a, Randolph et al. 2004, Zwiers et al. 2004
IL12RB1	IL12Rβ1	3594	19p13.1	Promoter: A-111T, 5′ UTR: C-2T, one other SNP Exon 1: C/A (P3Q) Exon 3: C/T (P47S), C/G (S74R) Exon 4: G387C (V129V) Exon 5: G467A (R156H) Exon 7: C684T, A705G (Q214R),[a] C/T (P228P) Exon 8: G/A (V245V) Exon 9: C/G (H339Q) Exon 10: T1158C (M365T), G1196C (G378R) Exon 11: G/A (Y414Y) Exon 13: G/A (A525T), 1664T (P534S) Exon 15: C/T (A673A) intronic: 41 SNPS, among others C409 + 21A, T1791 + 46C, C1983 + 24T, G1983 + 47T, 3′ UTR: 11 SNPs, among others C1989 + 34T frequency < 5%: C-430T, C240 + 20T, G700 + 22A, C1021 + 24T, G1098A, G1327 + 84A, C1376T, G1637A, G1845A	Ensemble, Sakai et al. 2001, Bassuny et al. 2003, Remus et al. 2004
IL12RB2	IL-12Rβ2	3595	1p31.2	5′ flanking region: C-237T, A-465G, A-1023G, C-1033T, A-1035G Exon 2: A/G (M13V) Exon 3: T/C (D26D), C/G S(38) Exon 4: G/A (R149Q) Exon 5: A/G (I185V), C/T (T201I)	

(continued)

TABLE 16.1. (continued)

NCBI Gene ID	Common Name	Entrez Gene ID	Map Position	Polymorphisms	References (See Also Tables 16.2–16.4)
				Exon 6: A/G (P238L)	Ensemble
				Exon 9: G/A (G420R)	
				Exon 10: G/C (Q426H), G/A (G465D)	
				Exon 12: C/A (G524G), G/A (G535G)	
				Exon 14: C/T (A625V), G2569A (A643T)	
				Exon 16: C2977A (P779P), T3283G (L808R), G/A (T787T)	
				Intronic: seven SNPs	
				3′UTR: three SNPs	
IFNG	IFN-γ	3458	12q14	Promoter: C-793T, C-778T, C-756G, C-333T, G-183T, G-179T, A-155G	Ensemble, Giedraitis et al. 1999, Henri et al. 2002, Iwasaki et al. 2001
				intron 1: (CA)$_n$, A874T, C455T, 1480 + T	
				intron 3: A2109G, G3810A, A2118G, T2326C, A2459G, T3177G, G3273A, G3812A, C4766T	
				exon 4: A5199T, A5272G	
				3′ UTR: seven SNPs, oa A5644T, G5134A	
IFNGR1	IFN-γR1	3459	6q23-q24	Promoter: A-611G, G-527A, -470delTT, T-270C, T-255C, C-169A, C-72T, T-56C, T + 95C, TE7 + 189G	Ensemble
				5′ UTR: 1 SNP	
				Exon 1: G83A (V14M), G91A (R16R), 12-allele polymorphism	
				Exon 3: C/A (S116*)	
				Exon 7: H318P, T1443C (L450P), (S350S)	
				Intronic: (CA)$_n$ in intron 6, two other SNPs 3′ UTR: six SNPs, one deletion	
IFNGR2	IFN-γR2	3460	21q22.1-q22.2	5′ UTR: four SNPs	Ensemble
				Exon 2: C/G (T58R), TA839G (R64Q)	
				Exon 4: G/A (E147K), A/G (K182E), C/G (S191C)	
				Exon 6: T/G (V260G)	
				Exon 7: C/A (D322E), C/T (I330I), G/A (P333P)	
				Intronic: seven SNPs	
				3′ UTR: seven SNPs	

Tables in this chapter include only polymorphisms (variants occurring at >1%) in the IFN-γ and IL-12 pathways. Mutations such as those associated with Mendelian susceptibility to mycobacterial disease (MSMD) produce defects in IL-12p40, IL-12Rβ1, IFN-γR1, IFN-γR2, or STAT-1. In those diseases, penetrance due to mutations in a single gene is very high. For more information, see the Ensemble Genome Browser, to search for genes within human species, at www.ensembl.org/. Search the NCBI Map Viewer (www.ncbi.nlm.nih.gov/mapview/) for IL-12p40 (ID 3593), IL-12p35 (ID 3592), IL-12Rβ1 (ID 3594), IL-12Rβ2 (ID 3595), IFN-γ (ID 3458), IFN-γR1 (ID 3459), and IFN-γR2 (ID 3460).

[a]Q214R was initially identified as a mutation (Altare et al. 1998), but Q214R homo- and heterozygosity are high (n = 33 whites; AA/AG/GG: 13/13/6). Moreover, two healthy 214R-homozygous subjects expressed normal IL-12Rβ1 and produced normal levels of IFN-γ (Sakai et al. 2001).

verity but not with susceptibility to disease itself (e.g., cerebral malaria, asthma) (table 16.2). CD40L-stimulated dendritic cells from IL12B-pro-1–homozygous subjects secrete 10-fold less heterodimeric IL-12 than do those from IL12B-pro-2 homozygotes, possibly due to IL-12–inhibiting homodimer formation (Trinchieri 2003, Bergholdt et al. 2004, Muller-Berghaus et al. 2004). The interaction between allele 1 and allele 2 isoforms may play a role, but promoter polymorphisms do not change protein sequence (table 16.2).

The 1188A polymorphism in the 3′ UTR of *IL12B* is more common in Caucasians (80%); 1188C prevails among African Americans (Hall et al. 2000, Ma et al. 2003). The 1188A polymorphism affects IL-12p40 mRNA stability and transcriptional activity and creates a Taq-1 restriction site (Hall et al. 2000, Seegers et al. 2002, Houldsworth et al. 2005). Results of studies linking C1188A to IL12B mRNA expression and IL-12 production in different cell types have been contradictory and inconclusive (Dahlman et al. 2001, Davoodi-Semiromi et al. 2002, Morahan et al. 2002b, Seegers et al. 2002, Bergholdt et al. 2004). SNPs in intron 4 and exon 5 are in LD with the 3′ UTR polymorphism

C1188A. Recently, six new IL12B polymorphisms have been added (Randolph et al. 2004).

IL12R

Almost 30 polymorphisms have been found in *IL12RB1* (table 16.1). The *IL12RB1* polymorphisms −111T and −2T are in strong LD and linked to pulmonary tuberculosis, as found in a Moroccan study ($p = 0.013$/OR = 2.69 and $p = 0.019$/OR = 2.03, respectively) (Remus et al. 2004). The SNPs R214/T365/R378 are in almost complete LD, and homozygosity for this combination is also associated with tuberculosis ($p = 0.013$, OR = 2.45), most likely following from observed functionally reduced IL-12 signaling (reduced IFN-γ production and CD2$^+$ T-cell proliferation). STAT-4 phosphorylation is normal (Akahoshi et al. 2003). The association between R214/T365/R378 and tuberculosis was not found in the Moroccan study (in both studies also a silent replacement C684T links to RTR/QMG; Remus et al. 2004) or in a smaller Japanese study (Sakai et al. 2001). Also, a Korean study did not find associations between

TABLE 16.2. Associations between infectious diseases and IL-12–related polymorphisms in IL12B.

Polymorphism	Disease	Number of Subjects[a]	Population	Outcome	References
IL12B-pro1	Cerebral malaria	82 cases	Tanzanian	Increased mortality ($p = 0.013$), reduced nitric oxide excretion	Morahan et al. 2002a
	HCV	142 cases	European Caucasian	No association	Houldsworth et al. 2005
(ATT)8 (83.5%)	TB	516 cases	Hong Kong Chinese	2-fold increased risk for TB in homozygous individuals ($p < 0.001$) (homozygosity for the TB-susceptible (ATT)8 genotype in combination with heterozygosity for IL12B-pro/intron 4 SNP/3′UTR is also strongly TB associated)	Tso et al. 2004
3′ UTR-A	HCV	72 resolved, 123 chronic cases	Caucasian	Frequency of homozygosity ↓ in resolved cases ($p = 0.04$)	Houldsworth et al. 2005
		133 cases	Chinese	Frequency ↑ in chronic infection	Yin et al. 2004
		186 resolved, 501 chronic cases	German	No association with incidence or liver histology.	Mueller et al. 2004

HCV, hepatitis C virus; TB, tuberculosis. For details, see table 16.1 note.

[a]Only diseased subjects are represented. Cases = case–control study; families = informative families.

leprosy, another mycobacterial disease, and Q214R, G3789R, A525T (a SNP with low frequency), or P534S (a novel SNP; Lee et al., 2003).

IL12RB2 polymorphisms C-1033T and A-1035G together create a GATA (T-cell transcription factor) site, while the −465G allele disrupts the integrity of a GATA consensus site, increasing IL-12Rβ2 promoter activity (van Rietschoten et al. 2004).

Pharmacogenetics

The Th1-promoting character of IL-12 makes this interleukin a therapeutic candidate in infectious diseases (e.g., mycobacteria and *Salmonella*) and cancer. However, IL-12 has hardly been used in humans and has not been tested in patients with mutations or genetic variations in the IFN-γ/IL-12 pathway. Use of IL-12 in human HIV, cancer, and infections has been disappointing (Trinchieri 2003). IL-12 may induce autoimmunity and can be toxic. Low-dose IL-12 (60 ng/kg subcutaneous, 2/week) in a patient with pulmonary *M. abscessus*, refractory to IFN-γ therapy, helped clear the patient's sputum (Holland 2000). It is not clear to what extent these effects of IL-12 therapy were IFN-γ dependent.

Summary and Conclusions

The IL-12/IL-23 pathway appears crucial to prevention of infection with mycobacteria and *Salmonella* but redundant for prevention of other infections. IL-12 has a role in Th1 development but is not the initial trigger. Penetrance of IL-12/IL-12R defects is not 100%, and phenotypes vary, possibly due to other immune mechanisms and variable levels of residual IFN-γ production. The importance of polymorphisms in IL-12/IL-12R remains unresolved in tuberculosis, disseminated mycobacterial infection, malaria, asthma, dermatologic diseases, multiple sclerosis, and viral hepatitis. Larger studies using different patient populations are necessary.

IFN-γ pathway

Gene Product and Role in Infection

IFN-γ Structure

IFN-γ is 143 amino acids long, forming six α-helices and functioning as a noncovalently linked homo-dimeric cytokine. The final basic 21 residues loosely hang outside the core structure (Pestka et al. 2004). IFN-γ transcription in NK and T cells is enhanced by IL-12 and IL-18, among others, in response to infection. IFN-γ is also produced by B cells and other APCs (Schroder et al. 2004).

IFN-γ Role in Infection

IFN-γ, like IL-12, is pivotal in host defense because it activates both the innate and adaptive immune responses. Numerous genes are up-regulated, including its own inducers. Binding of IFN-γ to IFN-γR, has important consequences (Schroder et al. 2004): (1) Innate immunity is boosted by up-regulation of complement-factors and nonspecific macrophage activation. TNF-α and IL-12 production by the macrophage are up-regulated, while the production of IL-4 is decreased. (2) Adaptive immunity is augmented by increased antigen processing and presentation. IFN-γ up-regulates the expression of both MHC class I and II on APCs. In addition, IFN-γ activates the proteosome in a way that increases quantity, diversity, and quality of the peptides for MHC loading. Further, IFN-γ stimulates Ig production and class switching by B cells, maturing the adaptive response. (3) Apoptosis is favored. IFN-γ slows cell growth by increasing *mad1* levels and by diminishing levels of c-myc and essential cell-cycle transcription factors. However, it induces apoptosis in cells that carry high numbers of functional IFN-γR2. Th2 cells carry a surplus of IFN-γR2, making them susceptible to apoptosis, while Th1-differentiated CD4$^+$ T cells are unresponsive to IFN-γ. (4) Leukocyte–endothelial interaction and attraction are orchestrated via up-regulation of adhesion molecules (e.g., ICAMs) and chemokines (e.g., RANTES, IP-10). (5) IFN-γ synergizes with LPS signaling. In cross-talk with the LPS signaling pathway, IFN-γ primes quick degradation of IκBα and NF-κB activation in response to low doses of endotoxin and other TLR agonists. IFN-γ induces NF-κB p65 mRNA (Held et al. 1999, de Wit et al. 1996) and promotes TLR transcription and expression (Mita et al. 2001). Synergy and priming by IFN-γ and LPS may occur through STAT-1- and NF-κB response elements present in the promoters of responsive genes (e.g., IRF-1, ICAM, IP-10, iNOS). (6) Mycobacterial killing is facilitated. Mycobacteria reside within macrophage phagosomes. IFN-γ enhances pinocytosis, receptor-mediated phagocytosis, NADPH-oxidase component expression and activity, and iNOS expression. However, nitric oxide and O_2^- are not critical for control of tuberculosis or NTM infection (Holland 2000, Schroder et al. 2004). IFN-γ can inhibit the growth of *M. bovis* BCG in human macrophages but may require the assistance of other factors such as vitamin D_3, TNF-α, or human lymphocytes to prevent growth of *M. tuberculosis* (Fortune et al. 2004, van de Vosse et al. 2004).

IFN-γR Structure

The IFN-γR complex is a member of the class II cytokine receptor family. Two IFN-γR1s bind to one IFN-γ dimer. Each IFN-γR1 has two fibronectin-like modules, consisting of two antiparallel β-sheets, made up of seven β-strands. IFN-γR1 (90 kDa) has 489 amino acids and harbors several seronine/threonine-rich regions, but no intrinsic kinase/phosphatase activity. Association with signaling machinery and IFN-γR2 is essential for signal transduction. IFN-γR2 (62 kDa) exhibits the same general structure as IFN-γR1 but is angled such that extra- and transmembrane parts are closer to each other (Pestka et al. 2004). IFN-γR2 is thought to be the limiting moiety for signal transduction. IFN-γ signaling causes IFN-γR2 gene downregulation (Schroder et al. 2004).

IFN-γR Role in Infection

Binding of IFN-γ causes the intracellular domains of the receptor chains to open and allow closer associa-tion of IFN-γR1 and IFN-γR2 with their respective Janus kinases, Jak1 and Jak2 (figure 16.2). The Jak-binding sites are in the intracellular domains encoded by exon 7 of both receptor genes (Rosenzweig et al. 2004a). The precise molecular mechanism of Jak activation upon cytokine stimulation is not understood, but Jak1 subsequently phosphorylates Y440 of the intracellular domain of IFN-γR1. P-Y440 serves as a docking site for SH2 domains of STAT-1. Within 1 minute of IFN-γ binding, STAT-1 is phosphorylated at Y701 and S727, probably by Jak2. Phosphorylated STAT-1 molecules homodimerize to form the transcription factor γ-activated factor (GAF). In addition, IFN-stimulated γ-factor 3 (ISGF3, composed of STAT-1, STAT-2, and IRF-9/p48) may form. GAF rapidly dissociates from the receptor complex and moves to the nucleus, without identified transport proteins. GAF induces IFN-γ target genes containing γ-activating sequence elements within 15–30 minutes of IFN-γ binding (Schroder et al. 2004). Inhibition of the signaling pathway within 1 hour of IFN-γ binding can be accomplished by protein tyrosine phosphatases, suppressors of cytokine signaling proteins, anti-inflammatory cytokines (e.g., IL-4, IL-10, TGF-β), and glucocorticoids.

Receptor–ligand endocytosis for IFN-γR1 and subsequent dissociation of the complex is thought to be mediated by specific isoleucine–leucine sequences in the intracellular IFN-γR1 chain; IFN-γR2 has its

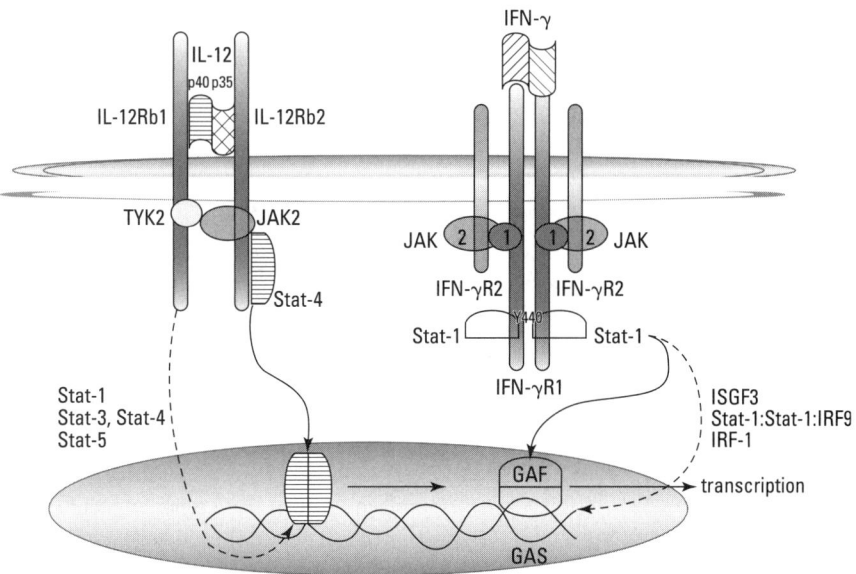

FIGURE 16.2. The IL-12 and IFN-γ signaling pathways.

own similar recycling domain. How coordinated the recycling of the two IFN-γR components is remains unclear. Dephosphorylated IFN-γR1 recycles to the cell surface (Schroder et al. 2004), while IFN-γ is degraded (Dorman and Holland 2000).

Pathogenesis

IFN-γ

Although disease-causing mutations in the IFN-γ gene have not been found, patients with acquired IFN-γ deficiency due to autoantibody formation have been reported (Patel et al. 2004, Hoflich et al. 2004).

IFN-γR

More than 60 individuals are known to be affected by defects in the IFN-γ pathway from mutations in *IFNGR* (reviewed in van de Vosse et al. 2004). Most have been identified through infection by NTM (mostly *Mycobacterium avium*) or through disseminated infection after BCG vaccination. There is a tight correlation between genotype (partial vs. complete), cellular and pathological phenotype, and clinical phenotype. The largest group consists of patients with a dominant-partial (DP) IFN-γR1 deficiency (IFN-γR1-DP). IFN-γ responsiveness is affected but not abolished (Jouanguy et al. 1997). In almost every sphere, patients with recessive complete mutations have done worse than patients with partial defects (Jouanguy et al. 2000, Dorman et al. 2004). Some IFN-γR1-DP patients have remained healthy until adulthood, while complete penetrance and a typically fatal outcome at early age occurs in recessive complete (RC) IFN-γR1 deficiency (IFN-γR1-RC). In IFN-γR1-DP, infection limited to bone was common, often in the form of a multifocal osteomyelitis (Sasaki et al. 2002). Histologically, mature, tuberculoid granulomata with few acid-fast bacilli are typical features of partial IFN-γR–deficient patients (Jouanguy et al. 1997, Fremond et al. 2004).

In contrast to those with partial defects that preserve some signaling, patients with complete IFN-γR deficiencies tend to have granulomata that are less well circumscribed, necrotic, and poorly differentiated (Jouanguy et al. 1997, van de Vosse et al. 2004). Partial and complete IFN-γR deficiencies are mirrored by partially or completely absent cellular responses to IFN-γ. In IFN-γR-RC patients, no significant response to IFN-γ (e.g., phosphorylation of STAT-1, STAT-1 translo-cation to the nucleus, MHC expression, TNF-α production) occurs *in vitro* (Newport et al. 1996, Dorman and Holland 1998, Jouanguy et al. 2000, Fieschi et al. 2001, Dorman et al. 2004, Rosenzweig et al. 2004a, van de Vosse et al. 2004). Paradoxically, since IFN-γ is not cleared by receptor binding and internalization, high circulating IFN-γ levels are found (Newport et al. 1996, Fieschi et al. 2001). On the other hand, responses to IFN-γ of IFN-γR-DP and recessive-partial (RP) IFN-γR deficient (IFN-γR-RP) patients are intermediate (Dorman et al. 2004, Fremond et al. 2004).

In IFN-γR–deficient patients, BCG infection after vaccination delays the onset of first NTM disease. The rates of *Salmonella* infection in IFN-γR1 deficiency are much lower than those in IL-12R deficiency, suggesting that there are IFN-γ–independent roles for IL-12 and IL-12–independent roles for IFN-γ where *Salmonella* is concerned. There is no apparent *in vitro* or *in vivo* phenotype for haplo-insufficiency of IFN-γR1 (Dorman and Holland 1998, Holland et al. 1998, Dorman et al. 2004, Rosenzweig et al. 2004a).

In IFN-γR2, a dominant partial mutation has been identified in one family (IFN-γR2-DP). Two homozygous siblings lacked all IFN-γR activity, while their heterozygous parents showed intermediate levels of IFN-γ–induced STAT-1 phosphorylation, similar to those found in heterozygous IFN-γR1-DP patients. The clinical history of both parents was unremarkable, and bone marrow transplantation from a heterozygous parent cured one patient's disseminated mycobacterial infection (Rosenzweig et al. 2004a). Recessive complete IFN-γR2 deficiency (IFN-γR2-RC) was identified in a boy without IFN-γ responses *in vitro*, whereas his heterozygous parents were normal (Dorman and Holland 1998). IFN-γR2-RP patients exhibited partial IFN-γ signaling. These few IFN-γR2 patients display genotype–phenotype characteristics (partial vs. complete) similar to those of IFN-γR1–defective patients. Infections reported have been limited to mycobacteria, cytomegalovirus, and herpes simplex (Dorman et al. 1999, Rosenzweig et al. 2004a), despite serologic evidence of exposure to *Chlamydia pneumoniae*, varicella zoster virus, and Epstein-Barr virus. Strikingly, three IFN-γR2-RC patients required splenectomy (Dorman and Holland 1998, Rosenzweig et al. 2004a). In IFN-γR1– and IFN-γR2–deficient patients, clinical viral infections have been reported, confirming some role for type II IFN in host defense against viruses, in addition to the protection provided by type I interferons (α/β) (Dorman et al. 1999, Schroder et al. 2004).

Gene Organization and Sequence

The *IFNA* and *IFNB* genes do not have introns, whereas *IFNG* contains three. The four exons encode 166 amino acids. There are repetitive DNA elements just upstream from the 5′ end of the mRNA: TATAAATA, a Goldberg-Hogness box, and GTCACCATCT, both important for transcription activity of RNA polymerase II (Gray and Goeddel 1982).

IFNGR1 encodes 489 amino acids (seven exons). A deletion hotspot around nucleotide 818 is due to two direct repeats that facilitate deletions during DNA replication, commonly denoted 818del4 (Jouanguy et al. 1999). This leads to truncation after the transmembrane domain but eliminates the intracellular domain. While IFN-γ and IFN-γR2 binding sites are preserved, the Jak1 and STAT-1 binding sites in exon 7 are eliminated, as well as the receptor-recycling domain. Overaccumulation of IFN-γR1 on the cell surface occurs in 818del4 and other mutations (811del4, 818delT, 817insA, T832G). Mutations in the extracellular domain of IFN-γR1 (both RC and RP) may lack or retain the transmembrane region, destabilize the IFN-γ binding site (C77Y), and/or alter contact points between IFN-γR1 and IFN-γ (295del12) (Holland and Gallin 2003). I87T modifies a critical residue for IFN-γ signaling, affecting IFN-γ binding to IFN-γR1, IFN-γR1 dimerization, IFN-γR1 association with IFN-γR2, and subsequent activation of Jak–STAT-1. Homozygous I87T leads to impaired but not absent IFN-γ signal transduction (Jouanguy et al. 1997).

The gene *IFNGR2* spans 33 kb and has also seven exons. The 5′ UTR and signal peptide are encoded by exons 1 and 2; exons 2–6 form the extracellular domain. The transmembrane domain includes parts of exons 6 and 7, while the remainder of exon 7 encodes the intracellular domain. There are multiple transcription initiation sites (GC boxes) but no TATA/CAAT (Rhee et al. 1996). The few mutations in IFN-γR2 reside in the extracellular domain (IFN-γR2-RC, 287delAG; IFN-γR2-RP, C340T) or the transmembrane region (IFN-γR2-DP, 719delG). The mutation 287delAG truncates the receptor. C340T encodes a full-length receptor with diminished affinity for IFN-γ–bound, dimerized IFN-γR1 (Dorman and Holland 1998, Fremond et al. 2004). The 719delG mutation lacks the intracellular domain (Rosenzweig et al. 2004a). IFN-γRs are expressed on almost all nucleated cells (Younes and Amsden 2001).

Animal Studies

Mice deficient for IFN-γ, IFN-γR1, and IFN-γR2 have similar phenotypes (e.g., increased susceptibility to *M. bovis*, NTM, other bacteria, viruses, and parasites) but have normal growth and are resistant to normal flora (Dorman et al. 1999, Holland and Gallin 2003). Their laboratory susceptibility patterns are broader than those in humans. In mice, *Toxoplasma* resistance depends on IFN-γ; in humans with defects in the IFN-γ/IL-12 pathway, *T. gondii* infection has not been reported, despite serological evidence of previous infection. Killing of *T. gondii* by monocytes of partially deficient IFN-γR1 individuals can partly be compensated by TNF-α (Janssen et al. 2002), whereas compensation by TNF-α does not occur in the context of *Salmonella*. Deficient mice were highly susceptible to *M. tuberculosis* (van de Vosse et al. 2004) but resistant to LPS-induced toxicity, suggesting cross-talk between LPS- and IFN-γ signaling pathways (Schroder et al. 2004). In mouse models, IFN-γ is mainly produced later in the course of the immune response and is necessary for tumor rejection (Holland and Gallin 2003).

Polymorphisms and Populations

IFNG

A plethora of studies have been performed trying to link IFN-γ polymorphisms to disease (table 16.3). Several SNPs have been identified in the *IFNG* promoter (table 16.1), which contains important binding sites for nuclear factor of activated T cells (NFAT) and NF-κB and has been conserved through evolution (Ackerman et al. 2002). G183T may create an activator protein-1 (AP-1) binding domain and influence the regulation of transcription. A-155G may affect the stability of the NFAT site (Chevillard et al. 2002). The −179T polymorphism also creates a potential AP-1 binding element, although it was incapable of competing for AP-1 binding to a consensus site. Only −179T (4% of African Americans) is TNF-α inducible (Bream et al. 2002, An et al. 2003).

A repeated dinucleotide in intron 1, $(CA)_n$, shows population variations (table 16.3): 10 alleles have been reported, but >90% of Europeans carry either $(CA)_{12}$ (mainly southern Europe) or $(CA)_{13}$ (northern Europe) (Goris et al. 1999, Reynard et al. 2000, Tso et al. 2005). $(CA)_{12}$ is in strong LD with +874T (Pravica et al. 1999,

TABLE 16.3. Associations between infectious diseases and IFN-γ–related polymorphisms.

Polymorphism	Disease	Number of Subjects[a]	Population	Functionality/Outcome	References
Promoter −179T	CD4[+] depletion in HIV	298 seroconverted cases	African Americans	Accelerated HIV progression	An et al. 2003, Bream et al. 2002
Intron 1 (CA)$_n$[b]	Tuberculoid leprosy	96 cases	Brazilian	$n = 15$–17	Reynard et al. 2003
874A[b]	Longevity	174 cases >99 y/o	Italian	↑ frequency in high age in women ($p = 0.02$)	Lio et al. 2002b
	Tuberculosis	112 cases	Sardinian	No association	Pes et al. 2003
		313 cases, 131 families	South African, Colored	Frequency ↑ ($p = 0.0062$)	Rossouw et al. 2003
		113 cases	Spain	Frequency ↑ ($p = 0.0017$)	Lopez-Maderuelo et al. 2003
		385 cases	Hong Kong	Frequency ↑ (p < 0.001)	Tso et al. 2005
		45 cases	Sicilian	A/A frequency ↑ ($p = 0.0243$)	Lio et al. 2002a
		190 cases	Colombian	Frequency ↑ in pulmonary TB[+] controls in relation to pleural/miliary	Henao et al. 2005
		451 cases (HIV[+]/HIV[−])	Malawi	TB, no association	Fitness et al. 2004
	Brucellosis	83 cases	Spanish	A/A freq ↑ ($p = 0.0023$) A/A frequency ↑ ($p = 0.0015$)	Bravo et al. 2003
	Recurrent HCV-posttransplant	31 cases	Israeli	A/A frequency ↑ (otitis media, $p = 0.04$)	Ben-Ari et al. 2004
	RSV	77 cases	VS infant	Frequency ↓ if anti-B19 NS1 antibody ($p = 0.04$)	Gentile et al. 2003
	Parvovirus	36 cases	English	(Disease severity)	Kerr et al. 2003
Intron 3 2109G	PPF[c]	93 cases	Sudan	Susceptibility ↑ ($p = 0.035$)	Chevillard et al. 2003
3810A	PFF	93 cases	Sudan	Protection ↑ ($p = 0.035$)	Chevillard et al. 2003
Exon 4 A5299G	Viliusk encephalo-myelitis	83 families, 69 cases	Siberian	No association	Oleksyk et al. 2004

Abbreviations: HCV, hepatitis C virus; PPF, severe periportal fibrosis, a marker for severe infection with schistosomes and associated with diminished IFN-γ production; RSV, respiratory syncytial virus; VS, vesicular stomatitis virus, . For details, see table 16.1 note.

[a]Only diseased subjects are represented. Cases = case control study; Families = informative families (TDT, transmission disequilbrium test).

[b] +874T is in complete LD with (CA)$_{12}$, therefore, results are inversely overlapping and associations cannot be attributed to an individual marker.

Fitness et al. 2004, Tso et al. 2005) and associated with increased production of IFN-γ *in vitro* (Pravica et al. 1999, Lee et al. 2001). Surprisingly, (CA)$_{12}$ may be a risk factor for some neoplasms (Lai et al. 2005, Saha et al. 2005) but not for human papillomavirus infection (Lai et al. 2005). IFN-γ knockout mice suffer from accelerated acute graft-versus-host disease. (CA)$_n$ polymorphism studies suggest posttransplantation problems in association with low–IFN-γ–producing alleles (Cavet et al. 2001, Mlynarczewska et al. 2004).

The SNP A874T has been extensively studied; 874T creates a putative NF-κB binding site, leading to an increased transcriptional effect of 874T/T and a diminishing effect of 874A/A on IFN-γ production (Pravica et al. 2000b, Rossouw et al. 2003; reviewed in Vandenbroeck and Goris 2003). Europeans carry T and A alleles equally (Poli et al. 2001, Costeas et al. 2003); A/A is more frequent in some Africans and Hong Kong Chinese (Hassan et al. 2003, Rossouw et al. 2003, Delaney et al. 2004, Tso et al. 2005). The 874A polymorphism is associated with longevity, but mostly with disease (table 16.3).

STAT-1 binding site, while T56C may lead to additional methylation close to a transcriptional initiation and AP-4 binding site (Koch et al. 2002, Thye et al. 2003, Rosenzweig et al. 2004b). The −56T ($p < 0.016$) and −611G ($p < 0.001$) alleles are more frequent in Caucasians than in African Americans or Koreans (Rosenzweig et al. 2004b); −611G, and possibly −56T, enhances promoter activity *in vitro* (Juliger et al. 2003, Rosenzweig et al. 2004b). There are no polymorphisms in exons 2 and 3 of IFN-γR1, emphasizing the evolutionary importance of this cytokine-binding region (Tang et al. 2000, Juliger et al. 2003) (table 16.4).

IFNGR

Out of the 10 detected *IFNGR* promoter polymorphisms (table 16.1), −470delTT partly abolishes a

Pharmacogenetics

Human recombinant IFN-γ (hIFN-γ) is produced via recombinant techniques in both *Escherichia coli* and

TABLE 16.4. Associations between infectious diseases and IFN-γR–related polymorphisms.

Disease	Polymorphism	Number of Subjects	Population	Outcome	References
	Promoter R1				
Severe malaria	−470delTT	238 cases, 62 families	Gambian, Mandinka	Protection ($p = 0.017$)	Koch et al. 2002
	T-56C	238 cases, 52 families	Gambian, Mandinka	Heterozygosity protects from development ($p = 0.016$) and death ($p = 0.006$) from cerebral malaria	Koch et al. 2002
Helicobacter pylori	T-56 +	184 cases	Gabonese	No association	Juliger et al. 2003
	H318P + L450P	111 cases	Senegalese	Susceptibility ↑ ($p = 0.03$)	Thye et al. 2003
Mycobacterial disease	−470delTT, T255C, C169A, G611A, C72T, T56C	156 pulmonary TB, 25 disseminated NTM, 53 pulmonary NTM cases	Caucasian	No association	Rosenzweig et al. 2004b
	−470delTT, G611A, C270T, T56C, T95C, TE7 + 189G	320 pulmonary TB cases	Gambian	No association	Awomoyi et al. 2004
	Gene R1-R2				
Leprosy	V14M, L450P	93 cases	Korean	No association	Lee et al. 2003
Periodontitis	(CA)$_n$, 192 bp	46 smokers	Norwegian	Frequency ↑ ($p = 0.014$)	Fraser et al. 2003a
Tuberculosis	(CA)$_n$, 192 bp	120 cases	Croatian	Frequency ↓ ($p = 0.02$)	Fraser et al. 2003b
Dermal leishmaniasis	alleles 10 + 11	351 cases	Gambian	No association	Newport et al. 2003
	allele 12 (from 12-allele polymorphisms)	138 families	Sudanese	Frequency ↑ ($p = 0.03$)	Mohamed et al. 2003

TB, tuberculosis. For details, see table 16.1 note.

cultured animal cells (Younes and Amsden 2001) and is less toxic than IL-12 (Holland 2000). Side effects include fever, nausea, neurotoxicity, and leukopenia (Younes and Amsden 2001), but hIFN-γ is mostly well tolerated. Partial IFN-γR–deficient patients generally show a favorable response to a combination of antimycobacterial chemotherapy and exogenous IFN-γ (Dorman et al. 2004). In contrast, IFN-γR-RC patients respond poorly to IFN-γ and antimycobacterial chemotherapy; bone marrow transplantation for IFN-γR1-RC and IFN-γR2-RC has theoretical advantages, but it has been difficult to achieve cure (Dorman et al. 2004, Roesler et al. 2004). Patients with diminished IFN-γ signaling due to IL-12 pathway deficiencies are responsive to IFN-γ, as this bypasses IL-12 (Holland and Gallin 2003). Some patients with severe mycobacterial infection due to deficiency in NEMO, a protein involved in NF-κB signaling causing abnormally low levels of IL-12 and IFN-γ, have had mycobacterial infections that improved dramatically on IFN-γ. (Holland et al. 1994).

Summary and Conclusions

Genetically controlled STAT-1–dependent, IFN-γ–mediated signaling critically influences the outcome of infection with NTM. The genotype and phenotype relationships in patients with these deficiencies are clear and guide genetic counseling and clinical management. In contrast, the IFN-γ–dependent pathway appears less critical for *Salmonella* susceptibility than for NTM and is not critical for *Toxoplasma* in humans. In addition, all the host factors that influence responses to NTM and to *M. tuberculosis* have not been determined. Patients with defects in IFN-γ signaling are not markedly affected by atopy, asthma, eczema, or other forms of allergy.

There are far fewer patients identified with mutations in IFN-γR2 than in IFN-γR1. IFN-γR2 mutations may be incompletely penetrant or have early lethal effects, such that only few survivors are seen with NTM infection. Mutations in the gene for IFN-γ have not been found, but polymorphisms in the gene and gene promoter leading to altered IFN-γ production appear to be linked to tuberculosis susceptibility.

The same polymorphism may have opposite effects (antagonistic pleiotrophy). For instance, the A allele of the SNP A874T may help in reaching old age by its anti-inflammatory effect (Lio et al. 2002b; table 16.3) but may therefore diminish host defense to mycobacteria. There is a protective effect on tuberculosis susceptibility of a combination of the T allele of A874T with the CA-repeat polymorphism $(CA)_{12}$. This link is repeatedly shown, highly significant, and biologically relevant. A874T is often cited in the context of gender differences, reinforcing the regulation of IFN-γ promoter activity by estrogen (Fox et al. 1991).

Concluding Remarks

Patients with single gene defects in IFN-γ signaling are few, but the profound genetic, immunological, and clinical information derived from these defects has illuminated human control of intracellular pathogens, including mycobacteria. The growing number of studies of the IFN-γ/IL-12 pathway and its SNPs requires the development of better methods to analyze complex data across populations.

Acknowledgments

M.H. has been supported by the intramural Research Program of the National Institute of Allergy and Infectious Diseases, NIH, and by grants from the Dutch scientific organization (NWO), the Fulbright/Netherlands-America Foundation, the Stichting Doctor Catharine van Tussenbroek, the Prins Bernhard Cultuurfonds, the Leids Universiteits Fonds, the Stichting Dr Hendrik Muller's Vaderlandsch Fonds, the Stichting Fundatie Vrijvrouwe van Renswoude, and the Stichting Algemeen Studiefonds.

References

Ackerman, H., Udalova, I., Hull, J., Kwiatkowski, D. (2002) Evolution of a polymorphic regulatory element in interferon-γ through transposition and mutation. *Molecular Biology and Evolution*, 19, 884–890.

Afkarian, M., Sedy, J.R., Yang, J., Jacobson, N.G., Cereb, N., Yang, S.Y., Murphy, T.L., Murphy, K.M. (2002) T-bet is a STAT1-induced regulator of IL-12R expression in naïve CD4+ T cells. *Nature Immunology*, 3, 549–557.

Akahoshi, M., Nakashima, H., Miyake, K., Inoue, Y., Shimizu, S., Tanaka, Y., Okada, K., Otsuka, T., Harada, M. (2003) Influence of interleukin-12 receptor beta1 polymorphisms on tuberculosis. *Human Genetics*, 112, 237–243.

Altare F., Durandy, A., Lammas, D., Emile J.F., Lamhamedi, S., Le Deist, F., Drysdale, P., Jouanguy, E.,

Doffinger, R., Bernaudin, F., Jeppsson, O., Gollob, J.A., Meinl, E., Segal, A.W., Fischer, A., Kumararatne, D., Casanova, J.L. (1998) Impairment of mycobacterial immunity in human interleukin-12 receptor deficiency. *Science,* 280, 1432–4135.

An, P., Vlahov, D., Margolick, J.B., Phair, J., O'Brien, T.R., Lautenberger, J., O'Brien, S.J., Winkler, C.A. (2003) A tumor necrosis factor-α-inducible promoter variant of interferon-γ accelerates CD4+ T cell depletion in human immunodeficiency virus-1-infected individuals. *Journal of Infectious Diseases,* 188, 228–231.

Awomoyi, A.A., Nejentsev, S., Richardson, A., Hull, J., Koch, O., Podinovskaia, M., Todd, J.A., McAdam, K.P.W.J., Blackwell, J.M., Kwiatkowski, D., Newport, M.J. (2004) No association between interferon-γ receptor-1 gene polymorphism and pulmonary tuberculosis in a Gambian population sample. *Thorax,* 59, 291–294.

Bassuny, W.M., Ihara, K., Kimura, J., Ichikawa, S., Kuromaru, R., Miyako, K., Kusahara, K., Sasaki, Y., Kohno, H., Mutsuura, N., Nishima, S., Hara, T. (2003) Association study between interleukin-12 receptor beta1/beta2 genes and type 1 diabetes or asthma in the Japanese population. *Immunogenetics,* 55, 189–192.

Ben-Ari, Z., Pappo, O., Druzd, t., Sulkes, J., Klein, T., Samra, Z., Gadba, R., Tambur, A.R., Tur-Kaspa, R., Mor, E. (2004) Role of cytokine gene polymorphism and hepatic transforming growth factor β1 expression in recurrent hepatitis C after liver transplantation. *Cytokine,* 27, 7–14.

Bergholdt, R., Johannesen, J., Kristiansen, O.P., Kockum, I., Luthman, H., Ronningen, K.S., Nerup, J., Julier, C., Pociot, F. (2004) Genetic and functional evaluation of an Interleukin-12 polymorphism (IDDM18) in families with type 1 diabetes. *Journal of Medical Genetics,* 41, e39.

Bravo, M.J., de Dios Colmenero, J., Alonso, A., Cabellero, A. (2003) Polymorphisms of the interferon gamma and interleukin 10 genes in human brucellosis. *European Journal of Immunogenetics,* 30, 433–435.

Bream, J.H., Ping, A., Zhang, X., Winkler, C., Young, H.A. (2002) A single nucleotide polymorphism in the proximal IFN-gamma promoter alters control of gene transcription. *Genes and Immunity,* 3, 165–169.

Casanova, J.L., Abel, L. (2002) Genetic dissection of immunity to mycobacteria: The human model. *Annual Review of Immunology,* 20, 581–620.

Cavet, J., Dickinson, A.M., Norden, J., Taylor, P.R.A., Jackson, G.H., Middleton, P.G. (2001) Interferon-γ and interleukin-6 gene polymorphisms associate with graft-versus-host disease in HLA-matched sibling bone marrow transplantation. *Blood,* 98, 1594–1600.

Chevillard, C., Henri, S., Stefani, F., Parzy, D., Dessein, A. (2002) Two new polymorphisms in the human interferon gamma promoter. *European Journal of Immunogenetics,* 29, 53–56.

Chevillard, C., Moukoko, C.E., Elwali, N.-E.M.A., Bream, J.H., Kouriba, B., Argiro, L., Rahoud, S., Mergani, A., Henri, S., Gaudart, J., Mohamed-Ali, Q., Young, H.A., Dessein, A.J. (2003) IFN-γ polymorphisms (IFN-γ +2109 and IFN-γ +3810) are associated with severe hepatic fibrosis in human hepatic schistosomiasis (*Schistosoma mansoni*). *Journal of Immunology,* 171, 5596–5601.

Chua, A.O., Wilkinson, V.L., Presky, D.H., Gubler, U. (1995) Cloning and characterization of a mouse IL-12 receptor-β component. *Journal of Immunology,* 155, 4286–4294.

Costeas, P.A., Koumas, L., Koumouli, A., Kyriakou-Giantsiou, A., Papaloizou, A. (2003) Cytokine polymorphism frequencies in the Greek Cypriot population. *European Journal of Immunogenetics,* 30, 341–343.

Dahlman, E., Eaves, I.A., Kosoy, R., Morrison, A.V., Heward, J., Gough, S.C.L., Allahabadia, A., Franklyn, J.A., Tuomilehto, J., Tuomilehto-Wolf, E., Cucca, F., Guja, C., Ionescu-Tirgoviste, C., Stevens, H., Carr, P., Nutland, S., McKinney, P., Shield, J.P., Wang, W., Cordell, H.J., Walker, N., Todd, J.A., Concannon, P. (2001) Parameters for reliable results in genetic association studies in common disease. *Nature Genetics,* 30, 149–150.

Davoodi-Semiromi, A., Yang, J.J., Jin-Xiong, S. (2002) IL-12p40 is associated with type 1 diabetes in Caucasian-American families. *Diabetes,* 51, 2334–2336.

Delaney, N.L., Esquenazi, V., Lucas, D.P., Zachary, A.A., Leffell, M.S. (2004) TNF-α, TGF-β, IL-10, IL-6, and IFN-γ alleles among African Americans and Cuban Americans. Report of the ASHI minority workshops: Part IV. *Human Immunology,* 65, 1413–1419.

de Wit, H., Hoogstraten, D., Halie, R.M., Vellenga, E. (1996) Interferon gamma modulates the lipopolysaccharide-induced expression of AP-1 and NF-kappa B at the mRNA and protein level in human monocytes. *Experimental Hematology,* 24, 228–235.

Doffinger, R., Jouanguy, E., Altere, F., Wood, P., Shirakawa, T., Novelli, F., Lammas, D., Kumararatne, D., Casanova, J.L. (1999) Inheritable defects in interleukin-12-and interferon-gamma-mediated immunity and the Th1/Th2 paradigm in man. *Allergy,* 54, 409–412.

Dorman, S.E., Holland, S.M. (1998) Mutation in the signal-transducing chain to the interferon γ receptor and susceptibility to mycobacterial infection. *Journal of Clinical Investigation,* 101, 2364–2369.

Dorman, S.E., Holland, S.M. (2000) Interferon-γ and interleukin-12 pathway defects and human disease. *Cytokine and Growth Factor Reviews*, 11, 321–333.

Dorman, S.E., Uzel, G., Roesler, J., Bradley, J.S., Bastian, J., Billman, G., King, S., Filie, A., Schermerhorn, J., Holland, S.M. (1999) Viral infections in interferon-γ receptor deficiency. *Journal of Pediatrics*, 135, 640–643.

Dorman, S.E., Picard, C., Lammas, D., Heyne, K., Dissel, J.T.van, Baretto, R., Rosenzweig, S.D., Newport, M., Levin, M., Roesler, J., Kumararatne, D., Casanova, J.L., Holland, S.M. (2004) Clinical features of dominant and recessive interferon γ receptor 1 deficiencies. *Lancet*, 364, 2113–1221.

Fieschi, C., Casanova, JL. (2003) The role of interleukin-12 in human infectious diseases: Only a faint signature. *European Journal of Immunology*, 33, 1461–1464.

Fieschi, C., Dupuis, S., Catherinot, E., Feinber, J., Bustamante, J., Breiman, A., Altare, F., Baretto, R., Le Deist, F., Kayal, S., Koch, H., Richter, D., Brezina, M., Aksu, G., Wood, P., Al-Jumaah, S., Raspall, M., da Silva Duarte, A.J., Tuerlinckx, D., Virelizier, JL., Fischer, A., Enright, A., Bernoft, J., Cleary, A.M., Vermylen, C., Rodriquez-Gallego, C., Davies, G., Blutters-Sawatzki, R., Siegrist, CA., Ehlayel, M.S., Novvelli, V., Haas, W.H., Levy, J., Freihorst, J., AL-Hajjar, S., Nadal, D., deMoraes Vasconcelos, D., Jeppsson, O., Kutukculer, N., Frecerova, K., Caragol, I., Lammas, D., Kumararatne, D.S., Abel, L., Casanova, JL. (2003) Low penetrance, broad resistance and favorable outcome of interleukin 12 receptor β1 deficiency: Medical and immunological implications. *Journal of Experimental Medicine*, 197, 527–535.

Ficschi, C., Dupuis, S., Picard, C., Smith, C.I., Holland, S.M., Casanova, J.L. (2001) High levels of Interferon gamma in the plasma of children with complete interferon gamma receptor deficiency. *Pediatrics*, 107, E48.

Fitness, J., Floyd, S., Warndorff, D.K., Sichali, L., Maleema, S., Crampin, A.C., Fine, P.E.M., Hill, A.V.S. (2004) Large-scale candidate gene study of tuberculosis susceptibility in the Karonga district of northern Malawi. *American Journal of Tropical Medicine*, 71, 341–349.

Fortune, S.M., Solache, A., Jaeger, A., Hill, P.J., Belisle, J.T., Bloom, B.R., Rubin, E.J., Ernst, J.D. (2004) *Mycobacterium tuberculosis* inhibits macrophage responses to IFNγ through myeloid differentiation factor 88-dependent and -independent mechanisms. *Journal of Immunology*, 172, 6272–6280.

Fox, H.S., Bond, B.L., Parslow, T.G. (1991) Estrogen regulates the IFN-gamma promoter. *Journal of Immunology*, 146, 4362–4367.

Fraser, D.A., Bulat-Kardum, L., Knezevic, J., Babarovic, P., Matakovic-Mileusnic, N., Dellavasagrande, J., Matanic, D., Pavelic, J., Beg-Zec, Z., Dembic, Z. (2003b) Interferon-γ receptor-1 gene polymorphism in tuberculosis patients from Croatia. *Scandinavian Journal of Immunology*, 57, 480–484.

Fraser, D.A., Loos, B.G., Boman, U., van Winkelhoff, A.J., van der Velden, U., Schenck, K., Dembic, Z. (2003a) Polymorphisms in an interferon-γ receptor-1 gene marker and susceptibility to periodontitis. *Acta Odontologica Scandinavica*, 61, 297–302.

Fremond, C., Yeremeev, V., Nicolle, D.M., Jacobs, M., Quesniaux, V.F., Ryffel, B. (2004) Fatal *Mycobacterium tuberculosis* infection despite adaptive immune response in the absence of Myd88. *Journal of Clinical Investigation*, 114, 1790–1799.

Gentile, D.A., Doyle, W.J., Zeevi, A., Howe-Adams, J., Kapadia, S., Trecki, J., Skoner, D.P. (2003) Cytokine gene polymorphisms moderate illness severity in infants with respiratory syncytial virus infection. *Human Immunology*, 64, 338–344.

Giedraitis, V., He, B., Hillert, J. (1999) Mutation screening of the interferon-gamma gene as a candidate gene for multiple sclerosis. *European Journal of Immunogenetics*, 26, 257–259.

Goris, A., Epplen, C., Fiten, P., Andersson, M., Murru, R., Sciacca, F.L., Ronsse, I., Jackel, S., epplen, J.T., Marrosu, M.G., Olsson, T., Grimaldi, L.M.E., Opdenakker, G., Billiau, A., Vandenbroeck, K. (1999) Analysis of an IFN-γ gene (IFNG) polymorphism in multiple sclerosis in Europe: Effect of population structure on association with disease. *Journal of Interferon and Cytokine Research*, 19, 1037–1046.

Gray, P.W., Goeddel, D.V. (1982) Structure of the human immune interferon gene. *Nature*, 298, 859–863.

Gubler, U., Chua, A.O., Schoenhaut, D.S., Dwyer, C.M., McComas, W., Motyka, R., Nabavi, N., Wolitzky, A.G., Quinn, P.M., Familetti, P.C., Gately, M.K. (1991) Coexpression of two distinct genes is required to generate secreted bioactive cytotoxic lymphocyte maturation factor. *Proceedings of the National Academy of Sciences of the United States of America*, 88, 4143–4147.

Hall, M.A., McGlinn, E., Coakley, G., Fisher, S.A., Boki, K., Middleton, D., Kaklamani, E., Moutsopoulos, H., Loughran, T.P., Jr., Ollier, W.E.R., Panayi, G.S., Lanchbury, J.S. (2000) Genetic polymorphism of IL-12 p40 gene in immunemediated disease. *Genes and Immunity*, 1, 219–224.

Hassan, M.I., Aschner, Y., Manning, C.H., Xu, J., Aschner, J.L. (2003) Racial differences in selected cytokine allelic and genotypic frequencies among healthy, pregnant women in North Carolina. *Cytokine*, 21, 10–16.

Held, T.K., Weihua, X., Yuan, L., Kalvakolanu, D.V., Cross, A.S. (1999) Gamma interferon augments macrophage activation by lipopolysaccharide by two distinct mechanisms, at the signal transduction level and via an autocrine mechanism involving tumor necrosis factor alpha and interleukin-1. *Infection and Immunity,* **67,** 206–212.

Henao, M.I., Montes, C., Paris, S.C., Garcia, L.F. (2005) Cytokine gene polymorphisms in Colombian patients with different clinical presentations of tuberculosis. *Tuberculosis.* **86,** 11–19.

Henri, S., Stefani, F., Parzy, D., Eboumbou, C., Dessein, A., Chevillard, D. (2002) Description of three new polymorphisms in the intronic and 3/UTR regions of the human interferon gamma gene. *Genes and Immunity,* **3,** 1–4.

Hoflich, C., Sabat, R., Rosseau, S., Temmesfeld, B., Slevogt, H., Docke, W.D., Grutz, G., Meisel, C., Halle, E., Gobel, U.B., Vold, H.D., Suttorp, N. (2004) Naturally occurring anti-IFN-gamma autoantibody and severe infections with *Mycobacterium cheloneae* and *Burkholderia cocovenenans. Blood,* **103,** 673–675.

Holland, S.M. (2000) Treatment of infections in the patient with Mendelian susceptibility to mycobacterial infection. *Microbes and Infection,* **2,** 1579–1590.

Holland, S.M., Dorman, S.E., Kwon, A., Pitha-Rowe, I.F., Frucht, D.M., Gerstberger, S.M., Noel, G.J., Vesterhus, P., Brown, M.R., Fleisher, T.A. (1998) Abnormal regulation of IFN-γ, IL-12, and TNFα in human IFN-γreceptor 1 deficiency. *Journal of Infectious Diseases,* **178,** 1095–1104.

Holland, S.M., Eisenstein, E.M., Kuhns, D.B., Turner, M.L., Fleisher, T.A., Strober, W., Gallin, J.I. (1994) Treatment of refractory disseminated nontuberculous mycobacterial infection with interferon gamma. A preliminary report. *New England Journal of Medicine,* **330,** 1348–1355.

Holland, S.M., Gallin, J.I. (2003) Interferon-γ in the treatment of infectious diseases. In: *Cytokines and chemokines in infectious diseases handbook.* M. Kotb and T. Calandra, eds. Humana Press, Totowa, NJ.

Houldsworth, A., Metzner, M., Rossol, S., Shaw, S., Kaminski, E., Demaine, A.G., Cramp, M.E. (2005) Polymorphisms in the IL-12B gene and outcome of HCV infection. *Journal of Interferon and Cytokine Research,* **25,** 271–276.

Huang, D., Cancilla, M.R., Morahan, G. (2000) Complete primary structure, chromosomal localization and definition of polymorphisms of the gene encoding the human interleukin-12 p40 subunit. *Genes and Immunity,* **1,** 515–520.

Iwasaki, H., Ota, N., Nakajima, T., Shinohara, Y., Kodaira, M., Kajita, M., Emi, M. (2001) Five novel single-nucleotide polymorphisms of human interferon gamma identified by sequencing the entire gene. *Journal of Human Genetics,* **46,** 32–34.

Janeway, C.A., Jr. (1992) The immune system evolved to discriminate infectious nonself from noninfectious self. *Immunology Today,* **13,** 11–16.

Jankovic, D., Kulberg, M.C., Hieny, S., Caspar, P., Collazo, C.M., Sher, A. (2002) In the absence of IL-12, CD4(+)T cell responses to intracellular pathogens fail to default to a Th2 pattern and are host protective in an IL-10(-/-) setting. *Immunity,* **16,** 429–439.

Janssen, R., van Wengen, A., Verhard, E., de Boer, T., Zomerdijk, T., Ottenhoff, T.H.M., van Dissel, J.T. (2002) Divergent role for TNFα in IFN-γ induced killing of *Toxoplasma gondii* and *Salmonella typhimurium* contributes to selective susceptibility of patients with partial IFN-γ Receptor 1 deficiency. *Journal of Immunology,* **169,** 3900–3907.

Jouanguy, E., Lamhamedi-Cherrade, S., Altare, F., Fondaneche, M.-C., Tuerlinckx, D., Blanche, S., Emile, J.F., Gaillard, J.L., Schreiber, R., Levin, M., Fischer, A., Hivroz, C., Casanova, J.L. (1997) Partial IFN-γR1 deficiency in a child with tuberculoid Bacillus Calmette-Guerin infection and a sibling with clinical tuberculosis. *Journal of Clinical Investigation,* **100,** 2658–2664.

Jouanguy, E., Lamhamedi-Cherradi, S., Lammas, D., Dorman, S.E., Fondaneche, M.-C., Dupuis, S., Doffinger, R., Altare, F., Girdlesstone, J., Emile, J.F., Ducoulombier, H., Edgar, D., Clarke, J., Oxelius, V.A., Brai, M., Novelli, V., Heyne, K., Fischer, A., Holland, S.M., Kumararatne, D.S., Schreiber, R.D., Casanova, J.L. (1999) A human IFNGR1 small deletion hotspot associated with dominant susceptibility to mycobacterial infection. *Nature Genetics,* **21,** 370–178.

Jouanguy, E., Dupuis, S., Pallier, A., Doffinger, R., Fondanech, M.-C., Fieschi, C., Lamhamedi-Cherradi, S., Altare, F., Emile, J.F., Lutz, P., Bordigoni, P., Cokugras, H., Akcakaya, N., Landman-Parker, J., Donnadieu, J., Camcioglu, Y., Casanova, J.L. (2000) In a novel form of IFN-γ receptor 1 deficiency, cell surface receptors fail to bind IFN-γ. *Journal of Clinical Investigation,* **105,** 1429–1436.

Juliger, S., Bongartz, M., Luty, A.J.F., Kremsner, P.G., Kun, J.F.J. (2003) Functional analysis of a promoter variant of the gene encoding the interferon-gamma receptor chain 1. *Immunogenetics,* **54,** 675–680.

Kaplan, M.H., Sun, Y.L., Hoey, Y., Grusby, M.J. (1996) Impaired IL-12 responses and enhanced development of Th2 cells in Stat4-deficient mice. *Nature,* **382,** 174–177.

Kerr, J.R., McCoy, M., Burke, B., Mattey, D.L., Pravica, V., Hutchinson, I.V. (2003) Cytokine gene polymorphisms associated with symptomatic parvovirus B19 infection. *Journal of Clinical Pathology,* **56,** 725–727.

Khan, I.A., Matsuura, F., Kasper, K.H. (1994) Interleukin −12 enhances murine survival against acute toxoplasmosis. *Infection and Immunity*, 62, 1639–1642.

Kobayashi, M., Fitz, L., Ryan, M., Hewick, R.M., Clark, S.C., Chan, S., Loudon, R., Sherman, F., Perussia, B., Trinchieri, G. (1989) *Journal of Experimental Medicine*, 170, 827–845.

Koch, O., Awomoyi, A., Usen, S., Jallow, M., Richardson, A., Hull, J., Pinder, M., Newport, M., Kwiatkowski, D. (2002) IFNGR1 gene promoter polymorphisms and susceptibility to cerebral malaria. *Journal of Infectious Diseases*, 185, 1684–1687.

Lai, H.-C., Chang, C-C, Lin, Y-W, Chen, S-F, Yu, M-H, Nieh, S., Chu, T.-W., Chu, T.-Y. (2005) Genetic polymorphism of the interferon-γ gene in cervical carcinogenesis. *International Journal of Cancer*, 113, 712–718.

Lee, J.Y., Goldman, D., Piliero, L.M., Petri, M., Sullivan, K.E. (2001) Interferon-γ polymorphisms in systemic lupus erythematosus. *Genes and Immunity*, 2, 254–257.

Lee, S.B., Kim, B.C., Jin, S.H., Park, Y.G., Kim, S.K., Kang, T.J., Chae, G.T. (2003) Missense mutations of the interleukin-12 receptor beta 1 (IL12RB1) and interferon-gamma receptor 1 (IFNGR1) genes are not associated with susceptibility to lepromatous leprosy in Korea. *Immunogenetics*, 55, 177–181.

Lio, D., Marino, V., Serauto, A., Gioia, V., Scola, L., Crivello, A., forte, G.I., Colonna-Romano, G., Candore, G., Caruso, C. (2002a) Genotype frequencies of the +874T → A single nucleotide polymorphism in the first intron of the interferon-γ gene in a sample of Sicilian patients affected by tuberculosis. *European Journal of Immunogenetics*, 29, 371–374.

Lio, D., Scola, L., Crivello, A., Bonafe, M., Franceschi, C., Olivieri, F., Colonna-Romano, G., Candore, G., Caruso, C. (2002b) Allele frequencies of +874T → A single nucleotide polymorphism at the first intron of interferon-γ gene in a group of Italian centenarians. *Experimental Gerontology*, 37, 315–319.

Lopez-Maderuelo, D., Arnalich, F., Serantes, R., Gonzalez, A., Codoceo, R., Madero, R., Vazquez, J.J., Montiel, C. (2003) Interferon-γ and interleukin-10 gene polymorphisms in pulmonary tuberculosis. *American Journal of Respiratory Critical Care Medicine*, 167, 970–975.

Ma, X., Reich, R.A., Gonzalez, O., Pan, X., Fothergill, A.K., Starke, J.R., Teeter, L.D., Musser, J.M., Graviss, A.E. (2003) No evidence for association between the polymorphism in the 3' untranslated region of interleukin-12B and human susceptibility to tuberculosis. *Journal of Infectious Diseases*, 188, 1116–1118.

Miller, R.D., Kwok, P.-Y. (2001) The birth and death of human single-nucleotide polymorphisms: New experimental evidence and implications for human history and medicine. *Human Molecular Genetics*, 10, 2195–2198.

Mita, Y., Dohashi, K., Shimizu, Y., Nakazawa, T., Mori, M. (2001) Toll-like receptor 2 and 4 surface expressions on human monocytes are modulated by interferon-γ and macrophage colony-stimulating factor. *Immunology Letters*, 78, 97–101.

Mlynarczewska, A., Wysoczanska, B., Karabon, L., Bogunia-Kubik, K., Lange, A. (2004) Lack of IFN-gamma 2/2 homozygous genotype independently of recipient age and intensity of conditioning regimen influences the risk of a GVHD manifestation after HLA-matched sibling haematopoietic stem cell transplantation. *Bone Marrow Transplantation*, 34, 339–334.

Mohamed, H.S., Ibrahim, M.E., Miller, E.N., Peacock, C.S., Khalil, E.A.G., Cordell, H.J., Howson, J.M.M., El Hassan, A.M., Bereir, R.E.H., Blackwell, J.M. (2003) Genetic susceptibility to visceral leishmaniasis in The Sudan: Linkage and association with IL4 and IFNGR1. *Genes and Immunity*, 4, 351–355.

Morahan, G., Boutlis, C.S., Huang, D., Pain, A., Saunders, J.R., Hobbs, M.R., Granger, D.L., Weinberg, J.B., Peshu, N., Mwaikambo, E.D., Marsh, K., Roberts, D.j., Anstey, N.M. (2002a) A promoter polymorphism in the gene encoding interleukin-12 p40 (IL12B) is associated with mortality from cerebral malaria and with reduced nitric oxide production. *Genes and Immunity*, 3, 414–418.

Morahan, G., Huang, D., Wu, M., Holt, B., White, G.P., Kendall, G., Sly, P.D., Holt, P.G. (2002b) Asssociation of IL12B promoter polymorphism with severity of atopic and non-atopic asthma in children. *Lancet*, 360, 455–459.

Mosmann, T.R., Coffman, R.L. (1989) Th1 and Th2 cells: Different patterns of lymphokine secretion lead to different functional properties. *Annual Review of Immunology*, 7, 145–173.

Mueller, T., Mas-Marques, A., Sarrazin, C., Wiese, M., Halangk, J., Witt, H., Ahlenstiel, G., Spengler, U., Goebel, U., Wiedenmann, B., Schreier, E Berg, T. (2004) Influence of interleukin 12B (IL12B) polymorphisms on spontaneous and treatment-induced recovery from hepatitis C virus infection. *Journal of Hepatology*, 41, 652–658.

Muller-Berghaus, J., Kern, K., Paschen A., Nguyen, X.D., Kluter, H., Morahan, G., Schadendorf, D. (2004) Deficient IL-12p70 secretion by dendritic cells based on IL12B promoter genotype. *Genes and Immunity*, 5, 431–434.

Newport, M.J., Awomoyi, A.A., Blackwell, J.M. (2003) Polymorphism in the interferon-γ receptor-1 gene and susceptibility to pulmonary tuberculosis in The

Gambia. *Scandinavian Journal of Immunology,* **58,** 383–385.

Newport, M.J., Huxley, C.M., Huston, S., Hawrylowicz, C.M., Oostra, B.A., Williamson, R., Levin, M. (1996) A mutation in the interferon-receptor gene and susceptibility to mycobacterial infection. *New England Journal of Medicine,* **335,** 1941–1949.

Oleksyk, T.K., Goldfarb, L.G., Sivtseva, T., Danilova, A.P., Osakovsky, V.L., Shrestha, S., O'Brien, S.J., Smith, M.W. (2004) Evaluating association and transmission of eight inflammatory genes with Viliuisk encephalomyelitis susceptibility. *European Journal of Immunogenetics,* **31,** 121–128.

Ottenhoff, T.H.M., Verreck, F.A.W., Lichtenauer-Kaligis, E.G.R., Hoeve, M.A., Sanal, O.S., van Dissel, J.T. (2002) Genetics, cytokines and human infectious disease: Lessons from weakly pathogenic mycobacteria and salmonellae. *Nature Genetics,* **32,** 97–105.

Patel, S.Y., Ding, L., Holland, S.M. (2004) Anti-interferon gamma autoantibodies in extrapulmonary tuberculosis and nontuberculous mycobacterial infections. *Abstract no 4472 Focis Montreal*

Pes, G.M., Lio, D., Carru, C., Deiana, L., Baggio, G., Franceschi, C., Ferrucci, L., Oliveri, F., Scola, L., Crivello, A., Candore, G., Colonna-Romano, G., Caruso, C. (2003) Association between longevity and cytokine gene polymorphisms. A study in Sardinian centenarians. *Aging Clinical and Experimental Research,* **16,** 244–248.

Pestka, S., Krause, C.D., Walter, M.R. (2004) Interferons, interferon-like cytokines, and their receptors. *Immunological Reviews,* **202,** 8–32.

Poli, F., Nocco, A., Berra, S., Scalamogna, M., Taioli, E., Longhi, E., Sirchia, G. (2001) Allele frequencies of polymorphisms of TNFA, IL-6, IL-10 and IFNG in an Italian Caucasian population. *European Journal of immunogenetics,* **29,** 237–240.

Pravica, V., Asderakis, A., Perrey, C., Hajeer, A., Sinnott, P.J., Hutchinson, I.V. (1999) In vitro production of IFN-γ correlates with CA repeat polymorphism in the human IFN-γ gene. *European Journal of Immunogenetics,* **26,** 1–3.

Pravica, V., Brogan, I.J., Hutchinson, I.V. (2000a) Rare polymorphisms in the promoter regions of the human interleukin-12 p35 and interleukin-12 p40 subunit genes. *European Journal of Immunogenetics,* **27,** 35–36.

Pravica, V., Perrey, C., Stevens, A., Lee, J.-H., Hutchinson, I.V. (2000b) A single nucleotide polymorphism in the first intron of the human IFN-γ gene: Absolute correlation with a polymorphic CA microsatellite marker of high IFN-γ production. *Human Immunology,* **61,** 863–866.

Presky, D.H., Yang, H., Minetti, L.J., Chua, A.O., Nabavi, N., Wu, C.Y., Gately, M.K., Gubler, U. (1996) A functional interleukin 12 receptor complex is composed of two beta-type cytokine receptor subunits. *Proceeding of the National Academy of Sciences of the United States of America,* **93,** 14002–14007.

Randolph, A.G., Lange, C., Silverman, E.K., Lazarus, R., Silverman, E.S., Raby, B., Brown, A., Ozonoff, A., Richter, B., Weiss, S.T. (2004) The IL12B gene is associated with asthma. *American Journal of Human Genetics,* **75,** 709–715.

Remus, N., Baghdadi, J.E., Fieschi, C., Feinberg, J., Quintin, T., Chentoufi, M., Schurr, E., Benslimane, A., Casanova, J.L., Abel, L. (2004) Association of IL12RB1 polymorphisms with pulmonary tuberculosis in adults in Morocco. *Journal of Infectious Diseases,* **190,** 580–587.

Reynard, M.P., Turner, D., Junqueira-Kipnis, A.P., Ramos de Souza, M., Moreno, C., Navarrete, C.V. (2003) Allele frequencies for an interferon-γ microsatellite in a population of Brazilian leprosy patients. *European Journal of Immunogenetics,* **30,** 149–151.

Reynard, M.P., Turner, D., Navarrete, C.V. (2000) Allele frequencies of polymorphisms of the tumor necrosis factor-α, interleukin-10, interferon-γ and interleukin-2 genes in a North European Caucasoid group from the UK. *European Journal of Immunogenetics,* **27,** 241–249.

Rhee, S., Ebensperger, C., Dembic, Z., Pestka. (1996) The structure of the gene for the second chain of the human interferon-γ receptor. *Journal of Biological Chemistry,* **271,** 28947–28952.

Roesler, J., Horwitz, M.E., Picard, C., Bordigoni, P., Davies, G., Koscielniak, E., Levin, M., Veys, P., Reuter, U., Schulz A., Thiede, C., Klingebiel, T., Fischer, A., Holland, S.M., Casanova, J.L., Friedrich, W. (2004) Hematopoietic stem cell transplantation for complete IFN-γ receptor 1 deficiency: A multi-institutional survey. *Journal of Pediatrics,* **145,** 806–812.

Rosenzweig, S.D., Dorman, S.E., Uzel, G., Shaw, S., Scurlock, A., Brown, M.R., Buckley, R.H., Holland, S.M. (2004a) A Novel mutation in IFN-γ receptor 2 with dominant negative activity: Biological consequences of homozygous and heterozygous states. *Journal of Immunology,* **173,** 4000–4008.

Rosenzweig, S.D., Schaffer, A.A., Ding, L., Sullivan, R., Enyedi, B., Yim, J.-J., Cook, J.L., Musser, J.M., Holland, S.M. (2004b) Interferon-γ receptor 1 promoter polymorphisms: Population distribution and functional implications. *Clinical Immunology,* **112,** 113–119.

Rossouw, M., Nel, H.J., Cooke, G.S., van Helden, P.D., Hoal, E.G. (2003) Association between tuberculosis and a polymorphic NFκB binding site in the interferon-γ gene. *The Lancet*, **361**, 1871–1872.

Saha, A., Dhir, A., Ranjan, A., Gupta, V., Bairwa, N., Bamezai, R. (2005) Functional IFNG polymorphism in intron 1 in association with an increased risk to promote sporadic breast cancer. *Immunogenetics*, **57**, 165–171.

Sakai, T., Matsuoka, M., Aoki, M., Nosaka, K., Mitsuya, H. (2001) Missense muation of the interleukin-12 receptor beta 1 chain-encoding gene is associated with impaired immunity against *Mycobacterium avium* complex infection. *Blood*, **97**, 2688–2694.

Sasaki, Y., Nomura, A., Kusuhara, K., Takada, H., Ahmed, S., Obinata, K., Hamada, K., Okimoto, Y., Hara, T. (2002) Genetic basis of patients with BCG osteomyelitis in Japan: Identification of dominant partial interferon-γ receptor 1 deficiency as a predominant type. *Journal of Infectious Diseases*, **185**, 706–709.

Schroder, K., Hertzog, P.J., Ravasi, T., Hume, D.A. (2004) Interferon-gamma: An overview of signals, mechanisms and functions. *Journal of Leukocyte Biology*, **75**, 163–189.

Seegers, D., Zwiers, A., Strober, W., Pena, A.S., Bouma, G. (2002) A TaqI polymorphism in the 3'UTR of the IL-12 p40 gene correlates with increased IL-12 secretion. *Genes and Immunity*, **3**, 419–423.

Snijders, A., Hilkens, C.M., van der Pouw Kraan, T.C., Engel, M., Aarden, L.A., Kapsenberg, M.L. (1996) Regulation of bioactive IL-12 production in lipopolysaccharide-stimulated human monocytes is determined by the expression of the p35 subunit. *Journal of Immunology*, **156**, 1207–1212.

Tang, Y.-W., Cleavinger, P.J., Li, H., Mitchell, P.S., Smith, T.F., Persing, D.H. (2000) Analysis of candidate-host immunogenetic determinants in herpes simplex virus-associated Mollaret's meningitis. *Clinical Infectious Diseases*, **30**, 176–178.

Thierfelder, W.E., van Deursen, J.M., Yamamoto, Y., Tripp, R.A., Sarawar, S.R., Carson, R.T., Sangster, M.Y., Vignali, D.A., Doherty, P.C., Grosveld, G.C., Ihle, J.N. (1996) Requirement for Stat4 in interleukin-12-mediated responses of natural killer and T cells. *Nature*, **382**, 171–174.

Thye, T., Burchard, G.D., Nilius, M., Muller-Myhsok, B., Horstmann, R.D. (2003) Genomewide linkage analysis identifies polymorphism in the human interferon-γ receptor affecting *Helicobacter pylori* infection. *American Journal of Human Genetics*, **72**, 448–453.

Trinchieri, G. (1997) Cytokines acting on or secreted by macrophages during intracellular infection (IL-10, IL-12, IFN-γ). *Current Opinion in Immunology*, **9**, 17–23.

Trinchieri, G. (2003) Interleukin-12 and the regulation of innate resistance and adaptive immunity. *Nature Reviews Immunology*, **3**, 133–146.

Tso, H.W., Ip, W.K., Chong, W.P., Tam, C.M., Chiang, A.K.S., Lau, Y.L. (2005) Association of interferon gamma and interleukin 10 genes with tuberculosis in Hong Kong Chinese. *Genes and Immunity*, **6**, 358–363.

Tso, H.W., Lau, Y.L., Tam, C.M., Wong, H.S., Chiang, A.K. (2004) Associations between IL12B polymorphisms and tuberculosis in the Hong Kong Chinese population. *Journal of Infectious Diseases*, **190**, 913–919.

Vandenbroeck, K., Goris, A. (2003) Cytokine gene polymorphisms in multifactorial diseases: Gateways to novel targets for immunotherapy? *Trends in Pharmacological Sciences*, **24**, 284–289.

van de Vosse, E., Hoeve, M.A., Ottenhoff, T.H.M. (2004) Human genetics of intracellular infectious diseases: Molecular and cellular immunity against mycobacteria and salmonellae. *Lancet Infectious Diseases*, **4**, 139–149.

van Rietschoten, J.G.I., Westland, R., van den Bogaard, R., Nieste-Otter, M.A., van Veen, A., Jonkers, R.E., van der Pouw Kraan, T.C.T.M., den Hartog, M.T., Wierenga, E.A. (2004) A novel polymorphic GATA site in the human IL-12Rβ2 promoter region affects transcriptional activity. *Tissue Antigens*, **63**, 538–546.

Verhagen, C.E., de Boer, T., Smits, H.H., Verreck, F.A.W., Wierenga, E.A., Kurimoto, M., Lammas, A.D., Kumararatne, D.S., Sanal, O., Kroon, F.P., van Dissel, J.T., Sinigaglia, F., Ottenhoff, T.H.M. (2000) Residual type 1 immunity in patients genetically deficient for interleukin 12 receptor β1 (IL-12Rβ1): Evidence for an IL-12β1-independent pathway of IL-12 responsiveness in human T cells. *Journal of Experimental Medicine*, **192**, 517–528.

Yin, L.M., Zhu, W.F., Wei, L., Xu, Z.Y., Sun, D.C., Wang, Y-B, Fan, W-M, Yu, M., Tian, X-L, Wang, Q-X, Gao, Y., Zhuang, H. (2004) Association of interleukin-12 p40 gene 3'untranslated region polymorphism and outcome of HCV infection. *World Journal of Gastroenterology*, **10**, 3330–3333.

Younes, H.M., Amsden, B.G. (2001) Interferon-γ therapy: Evaluation of routes of administration and delivery systems. *Journal of Pharmaceutical Sciences*, **91**, 2–17.

Zhou, P., Sieve, M.C., Bennet, J., Kwon-Chung, K.J., Tewari, R.P., Gazzinelli, R.T., Sher, A., Seder, R.A. (1995) IL-12 prevents mortality in mice infected with Histoplasma capsulatum through induction of IFN-γ. *Journal of Immunology*, **155**, 785–795.

Zwiers, A., Seegers, D., Heijmans, R., Koch, A., hampe, J., Nikolaus, S., Pena, A.S., Schreiber, S., Bouma, G. (2004) Definition of polymorphisms and haplotypes in the interleukin-12B gene: Association with IL-12 production but not with Crohn's disease. *Genes and Immunity*, **5**, 675–677.

17

Chemokine Receptor and Ligand Genes

Jianming "James" Tang

As members of the cytokine superfamily, small and inducible chemokine ligands (CLs) and their G-protein–coupled, transmembrane receptors (CRs) form a complex entity in their own right. Some 44 structurally and functionally related CL genes and 20 CR genes have been identified in the human genome. Their protein products interact either on a strict one-to-one basis or with varying degrees of promiscuity and redundancy (Devalaraja and Richmond 1999; Luster 1998; Rossi and Zlotnik 2000). Signal transduction following CL–CR binding and receptor dimerization is responsible for a wide range of biological phenomena, including angiogenesis, inflammation, graft-versus-host disease, and immune defense against microbial infections.

Within the context of infection and immunity, the CL/CR system is important at least in three ways. First, receptor–ligand interactions regulate the development, trafficking, and function of B- and T-lymphocytes (Baggiolini 1998; DeVries et al. 1999; Luther and Cyster 2001; Thelen 2001). Second, chemokines can directly block the entry of pathogens that rely on CRs for invasion into host cells. Third, production of CL-like and CR-like products by human pathogens (e.g., herpesviruses) is a common mechanism that facilitates latent infections (Arvanitakis et al. 1997; Endres et al. 1999; Gompels et al. 1995; Liston and McColl 2003; Shan et al. 2000; Zhou et al. 2000). More thorough understanding of these interactive pathways will have multiple implications, both basic and translational. Due to the complex and rapidly evolving discoveries about the CR/CL system, this chapter focuses on illustrative work rather than providing gene-by-gene coverage.

Nomenclatures by Structure and Function

Based on the positioning of structurally conserved cysteine residue(s) in the various ligands, CLs and CRs are now systematically divided into C-X-C (α), C-C (β), C (γ), and C-XXX-C (C-X$_3$-C or δ) subfamilies, with X denoting any amino acid that separates the cysteines in CL molecules (table 17.1). In humans, the C-X-C subfamily consists of 15 CL genes and 6 CR genes, while the C-C subfamily has 26 CLs and 11 CRs. The remaining three CL and three CR genes fall into the minor C and C-X₃-C subfamilies. Phylogenetic analyses suggest that C-X-C and C-C chemokine subfamilies and their respective receptors diverged from each other before the emergence of placental mammals (Hughes and Yeager 1999). In addition, most of the C-X-C chemokines in mammals are not seen in other vertebrate species.

Alternative classification by function can group CLs as inflammatory, homeostatic, or dually functional to reflect the major biological consequences. Likewise, CRs can be categorized as specific (e.g., CXCR4), shared (e.g., CCR5), or promiscuous according to the specificity of receptor–ligand interactions. Sequence similarities in the extracellular (EC) domains EC3 and EC4 may account for activities of the shared C-C-motif CRs (CCRs), such as CCR2 and CCR3 (Alkhatib et al. 1997). Additional separation of agonist from antagonist receptors emphasizes differences in signal transduction following the receptor–ligand binding process. Other nomenclatures based on cell types and/or observed function seem less reliable. For example, division of the C-C-motif chemokine subfamily into the macrophage inflammatory proteins (MIPs) and monocyte chemoattractant proteins (MCPs) appears to contradict their evolutionary relationships (Hughes and Yeager 1999).

The nomenclatures used here are those recommended by the International Union of Immunological Societies (IUIS)/WHO Nomenclature Committee (Bacon et al. 2002) and the International Union of Pharmacology (Murphy 2002). Widely recognized common names (table 17.1) are also used throughout this chapter to assist with gradual transition in terminology.

Chemokine Gene Expression and Posttranslational Modification

CLs are primarily produced by mononuclear cells. Unlike prototype T-helper type 1 (T$_H$1) and T$_H$2 cytokines such as the interferons, interleukin-4 (IL-4), and tumor necrosis factor alpha (TNF-α), many of the CLs are found in stable, high concentrations in human peripheral blood (figure 17.1). The specific expression pattern does not correlate with sequence similarity or chromosomal location. Members of the C-C-motif CL (CCL) gene cluster at chromosome 17q11.2-q21.2 demonstrate a wide range of circulating levels. CCL5 (RANTES) is abundant in serum/plasma, but CCL2 (MCP-1) is often detected at low concentrations. There is some evidence that a few CCL-like genes (e.g., CCL3L1) with copy number variation (from 0 to 11 copies per individual) may have an additional advantage in gene expression and function, especially when the copy number exceeds the population average (Gonzalez et al. 2005; Townson et al. 2002).

The expression of CRs is highly variable and often cell specific (Locati et al. 2002); this degree of specificity dictates the cellular responses to chemokine gradients (table 17.1). For instance, memory T-cells respond to CCL27 and CCL28 due to their expression of CCR3 and CCR10. Among those well-studied CRs, in vitro CCR5 and CCR3 production has been shown to follow the two major T$_H$ lineages (with CCR5 on T$_H$1 and CCR3 on T$_H$2 cells) (Bonecchi et al. 1998a, 1998b; Loetscher et al. 1998; Sallusto et al. 1997, 1998), while CXCR4 is expressed in T$_H$1 as well as T$_H$2 cell types (Romagnani et al. 2000). Selective in vivo receptor (e.g., CCR2, CCR3, and CCR5) expression by polarized effector T-cells has been more difficult to prove; this difficulty probably implies tissue-specific regulation. Quantitatively, many T$_H$1 cells express CXCR3 in vivo, whereas most T$_H$2 cells express CCR4. Dual expression of CCR4 and CXCR3 is also seen in a small proportion of polarized T-cells (Campbell et al. 2003).

The newly recognized T$_H$17 lineage, which defines distinct effector (pro-inflammatory) T-cell subset with regulatory function (Bettelli et al. 2007; Steinman 2007; Weaver et al. 2006), has been shown to bear the CCR2+CCR5- phenotype (Sato et al. 2007). More recent studies suggest that co-expression of CCR6 and CCR4 specifies human memory CD4$^+$ T-cells that produce IL-17, while CCR6 and CXCR3 jointly define T$_H$-1 cells that produce interferon-gamma (IFN-γ) (Acosta-Rodriguez et al. 2007). T-helper cells producing both IFN-γ and IL-17 can also have the CCR6 and CXCR3 markers (Acosta-Rodriguez et al. 2007).

Alternative splicing is a common feature in CL and CR gene expression. For example, dozens of CCR5 mRNA transcripts have been described, many of which carry novel 5′ UTRs (Liu et al. 1998; Mummidi et al. 2000). The variety of mRNA transcripts often results from the use of alternative promoters (e.g., proximal

TABLE 17.1. Chemokine ligands (CLs, $n = 44$) and their respective chemokine receptors (CRs, $n = 20$) identified in humans.

Subfamily	Ligand (Acronym), Mapping	Agonist Receptor(s) [Cell Type(s)]	Antagonist Receptor
C-X-C (α):	CXCL1 (GROα), 4q21	CXCR2 [N]	DARC
15 CLs	CXCL2 (GROβ), 4q21	CXCR2 [N]	
6 CRs	CXCL3 (GROγ), 4q21	CXCR2 [N]	
	CXCL4 (PF4), 4q12-q21	Heparin [F, N], CXCR3 [AT, NK]	
	CXCL5 (ENA78), 4q12-q13	CXCR2 [N]	DARC
	CXCL6 (GCP2), 4q21	CXCR1 [N], CXCR2 [N]	
	CXCL7 (NAP-2), 4q12-q13	CXCR2 [N]	DARC
	CXCL8 (IL-8), 4q13-q21	CXCR1 [N], CXCR2 [N]	DARC
	CXCL9 (Mig), 4q21	CXCR3 [AT, NK]	CCR3
	CXCL10 (IP10), 4q21	CXCR3 [AT, NK]	CCR3
	CXCL11 (IP9), 4q21.2	CXCR3 [AT, NK]	CCR3
	CXCL12 (SDF-1), 10q11.1	CXCR4 (fusin) [DC, M, RT]	
	CXCL13 (BLC, BCA1), 4q21	CXCR5 [B]	
	CXCL14 (BRAK), 5q31	Unknown [M]	
	CXCL16, 17p13	CXCR6 [DC, ET, NKT]	
C-C (β):	CCL1 (I-309), 17q12	CCR8 [M]	
25 CLs	CCL2 (MCP-1), 17q11.2-q21.2	CCR2 [AT, B, DC, M, NK], CCR10 [MT]	DARC
11 CRs	CCL3 (MIP-1α, LD78α), 17q11-q21	CCR5 [AT, DC, M, NK]	
	CCL3L1 (LD78β), 17q21.1	CCR5 [AT, DC, M, NK]	
	CCL4 (MIP-1β), 17q12	CCR5 [AT, DC, M, NK]	
	CCL4L1 (MIP-1β), 17q12	CCR5 [AT, DC, M, NK]?	
	CCL5 (RANTES), 17q11.2-q12.1	CCR5 [AT, DC, NK]	DARC
	CCL7 (MCP-3), 17q11.2-q12	CCR1, CCR2, CCR3 [AT, B, DC, E, M]	CCR5, DARC
	CCL8 (MCP-2), 3p22	CCR1, CCR2, CCR3 [AT, B, DC, E, M]	
	CCL11 (Eotaxin-1), 17q21.1-q21.2	CCR3 [B, DC, E]	CCR2
	CCL13 (MCP-4), 17q11.2	CCR2 [AT, B, DC, M, NK]	
	CCL14 (HCC-1), 17q11.2	CCR1 [AT, DC, E]	
	CCL15 (MIP-1δ, HCC-2), 17q11.2	CCR1 [AT, DC, E]	
	CCL16 (LEC), 17q11.2	CCR1 [AT, DC, E]	
	CCL17 (TACK), 16q13	CCR4 [AT, DC]	
	CCL18 (PARC), 17q11.2	Unknown [NT]	
	CCL19 (ELC, MIP-3β), 9p13	CCR7 [AT], CCR1L1 [DC]	
	CCL20 (LARC, MIP-3α), 2q33-q37	CCR6 [DC]	
	CCL21 (SLC), 9p13	CCR7 [AT], CCR1L1 [DC]	
	CCL22 (MDC), 16q13	CCR4 [AT, DC]	
	CCL23 (CKb8), 17q21.1	CCR1 [AT, DC, E]	CCR2
	CCL24 (Eotaxin-2), 7q11.23	CCR3 [B, DC, E]	
	CCL25 (TECK), 19p13.2	CCR9 [M], CCR1L1 [DC]	CCR2
	CCL26 (eotaxin-3), 7q11.23	CCR3 [B, DC, E]	
	CCL27 (CTACK), 9p13	CCR10 [MT]	
	CCL28 (MEC), 5p12	CCR3 [B, DC, E], CCR10 [MT]	
X-C (γ):	XCL1 (lymphotactin), 1q23	XCR1 [RT]	
2 CLs, 2 CRs	XCL2 (SCYC2), 1q23-q25	XCR2 [AT, RT]	
C-X-X-X-C (d):	CX3L1 (fractalkine), 16q13	C-X$_3$-CR1 [AT, M, NK]	

Abbreviations, in alphabetical order: AT, activated T-cells; B, B-lymphocytes; BLC, B-cell-homing chemokine; BRAK, breast and kidney cell chemokine; CKb8, C6 β-chemokine; CTACK, cutaneous T-cell–attracting chemokine; DARC, Duffy antigen receptor of chemokine; DC, dendritic cells; E, eosinophils; ELC, EBI1-ligand chemokine; ENA, epithelial cell–derived neutrophil attractant; ET, effector T-cells; F, fibroblasts; GCP2, granulocyte chemotactic protein 2; GRO, growth-related oncogene; HCC, hemofiltrate CC chemokine; I-309, inflammatory cytokine I-309; IL-8, IL-8; IP, IFN-γ–inducible protein; LARC, liver and activation-regulated chemokine; LEC, liver-expressed chemokine; M, monocytes; MCP, monocyte chemoattractant protein; MDC, monocyte-derived chemokine; MEC, mucosae-associated epithelial chemokine; Mig, monokine induced by interferon; MIP, macrophage inflammatory protein; MT, memory T-cells; N, neutrophils; NAP, neutrophil-activated peptide; NK, natural killer cells; NKT, natural killer T-cells; PARC, pulmonary and activation-regulated chemokine; PF4, platelet factor 4; RANTES, regulated upon regulation, normal T-cell expressed and secreted; RT, resting T-cells; SCYC2, small inducible cytokine subfamily C, member 2; SDF-1 stromal cell–derived factor 1; SLC, secondary lymphoid tissue chemokine; TACK, thymus and activation-regulated chemokine; TECK, thymus-expressed chemokine. Additional acronyms can be found at NCBI Entrez Gene (www.ncbi.nlm.nih.gov/entrez/query.fcgi?db=gene). Last accessed on June 5, 2007.

a

Pos.	Pos.	Neg.	Neg.	ENA-78	GCSF	GM-CSF	GRO	GRO-α	I-309	IL-1α	IL-1β
Pos.	Pos.	Neg.	Neg.	ENA-78	GCSF	GM-CSF	GRO	GRO-α	I-309	IL-1α	IL-1β
IL-2	IL-3	IL-4	IL-5	IL-6	IL-7	IL-8	IL-10	IL-12	IL-13	IL-15	IFN-γ
IL-2	IL-3	IL-4	IL-5	IL-6	IL-7	IL-8	IL-10	IL-12	IL-13	IL-15	IFN-γ
MCP-1	MCP-2	MCP-3	MCSF	MDC	MIG	MIP-1δ	RANTES	SCF	SDF-1	TARC	TGF-β
MCP-1	MCP-2	MCP-3	MCSF	MDC	MIG	MIP-1δ	RANTES	SCF	SDF-1	TARC	TGF-β
TNF-α	TNF-β	EGF	IGF-1	ANG	OSM	Tpo	VEGF	PDGF BB	Leptin	Neg.	Pos.
TNF-α	TNF-β	EGF	IGF-1	ANG	OSM	Tpo	VEGF	PDGF BB	Leptin	Neg.	Pos.

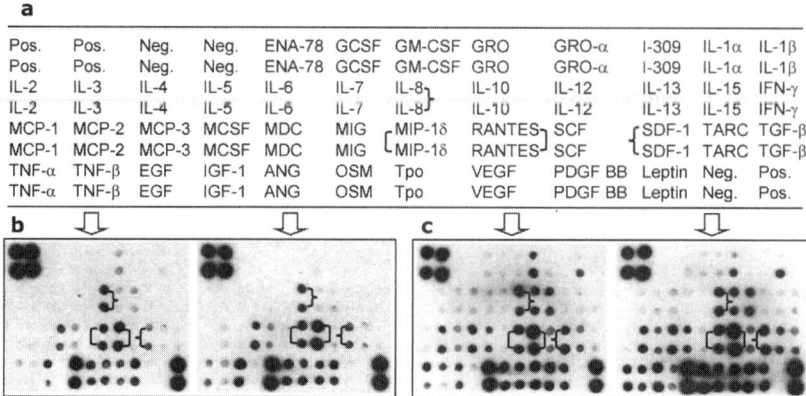

FIGURE 17.1. Detection of cytokines, chemokines, growth factors, and related products with monoclonal antibodies and enhanced chemiluminescence (Huang 2001a,b; Lin et al. 2002). Based on an 8 (rows) by 12 (columns) format (a), each antibody array tests 42 serum products, along with positive (Pos.) and negative (Neg.) controls that gauge the quality of reagents for enhanced chemiluminescence detection. Results as shown are based on serum samples from two individuals (b and c) before and after HIV-1 infection (left to right, drawn at <9-month intervals). Chemokines like IL-8 (CXCL8), MIP-1δ (CCL15), RANTES (CCL5), and SDF-1 (CXCL12) are detected at high concentrations: duplicates of these products are grouped by }, [,], and {, respectively. In contrast, classical cytokines (e.g., INF-γ, IL-2, IL-4, and IL-5) are present at much lower levels.

and distal) and multiple splicing sites (Mummidi et al. 2000); they may also account for cell-specific regulation of transcription. However, the protein products predicted from multiple mRNA species for each locus can be identical (e.g., CCR5), when the entire open reading frame is within a single exon. Different protein isoforms can also function in similar ways (e.g., SDF-1α and SDF-1β from the CXCL12 locus) when the critical domains are retained in different transcripts. However, CXCR3 appears to be one exception, since two splicing variants, CXCR3-A and CXCR3-B, differ enough (in the first two exons) to be functionally distinct (Romagnani et al. 2004), with CXCR3-B having high affinity for CXCL4 in addition to its usual high affinity for CXCL10 and low affinity for CXCL9 and CXCL11. Coincidentally, all four CXC chemokines that bind to CXCR3-B are angiostatic; their ability to reduce angiogenesis is being explored for antitumor therapy.

For CLs, their potency can be significantly altered by posttranslational modification mediated by cell-surface dipeptidyl peptidase (DPP) IV (CD26) and its homologues (DPP8 and FAP), which hydrolyze amino (N)-terminal Ala-Pro, Arg-Pro, and Gly-Pro residues seen in one-third of mature (secreted) chemokine

polypeptides. Notably, compared with the full-length CCL3L1 (LD78β or MIP-1α), CCL3L1 without the N-terminal Ala-Pro dipeptide has a 10-fold higher efficiency in binding CCR5 (Struyf et al. 2001). In contrast, removal of the N-terminal dipeptide from RANTES reduces its chemotactic potency for monocytes and eosinophils (Proost et al. 2000; Struyf et al. 1998). Introduction of N-terminal pyroglutamic acid (pGlu) protects against degradation by DPP IV, as shown for pGlu-modified CCL8 (MCP-2), which retains its chemotactic activity (Van Coillie et al. 1998). This feature applies to all MCPs and CCL4 (MIP-1β) (Moser et al. 2004).

Mature chemokines can also be modified by other proteases, including matrix metalloproteases (MMP), cathepsin D, cathepsin G, cathepsin L, elastase, and urokinase plasminogen activator (Moser et al. 2004). In particular, cleavage of CCL7 (NAP-2) by MMP-1, MMP-2, MMP-3, MMP-13, and MMP-14 turns this chemokine into an antagonist ligand, whereas CXCL12 (SDF-1) modified by MMP-1, MMP-2, MMP-3, MMP-9, MMP-13, MMP-14, cathepsin G, and elatase completely loses its bioactivity. Loss of function also extends to modified CCL3, CCL4, CCL5, CCL21, CCL22, CXCL1, and CXCL4, with multiple enzymes being involved in this process (Moser et al. 2004).

Signal Transduction, Decoy Receptors, and Virally Encoded Homologs

Depending on the gradient of CL concentration, receptor–ligand complex formation may lead to hetero- and homodimerization (Mellado et al. 2001a, 2001b; Rodriguez-Frade et al. 2001), followed by internal signal transduction mediated by G-proteins, Janus kinases (JAKs), phospholipase isoforms, and tyrosine kinases. Cell adhesion and migration into sites of inflammation are the major actions after signal transduction, while involvement of adaptin and phosphatases contributes to receptor sequestration, recycling, and degradation. Subsequent downstream gene expression is often accompanied by polarization of T-helper cells into the T_H1 and T_H2 effector lineages. However, these pathways are blocked by antagonist ligands (Blanpain et al. 1999; Loetscher and Clark-Lewis 2001; Ogilvie et al. 2001) or decoy receptors (Mantovani et al. 2001).

The erythrocyte decoy receptor DARC (Duffy antigen and receptor for chemokines) has been studied extensively in the context of transfusion medicine (Mantovani et al. 2001). Promiscuous binding of DARC with various ligands like CCL2, CCL5, CXCL1, CXCL5, CXCL7, and CXCL8 (IL-8) triggers endocytosis without signal transduction. This kind of decoy action may promote lymphocyte homeostasis by clearing excess chemokines from the peripheral blood and inflammatory tissues.

Generation of CL-like and CR-like products by human and animal viruses is considered one of the common strategies used by microbial pathogens to subvert the host immune system (Alcami 2003; Liston and McColl 2003). CR-like proteins (e.g., vCXCR, vCCR-1, vCCR-2, and vCCR-3) encoded by human herpesviruses (Liston and McColl 2003) demonstrate promiscuous specificity for human chemokines (Arvanitakis et al. 1997; Beisser et al. 2002; Endres et al. 1999; Gompels et al. 1995; Zhou et al. 2000), and that property presumably facilitates persistent viral survival. Kaposi's sarcoma–associated herpesvirus (KSHV or HHV-8) also encodes three products (vMIP-I, vMIP-II, and vMIP-III) similar (~40% sequence identity) to human MIPs. In experimental studies, vMIP-II has been shown to be a chemokine antagonist with a broader spectrum of receptor binding affinity than any known mammalian chemokines (Kledal et al. 1997). Delayed onset of AIDS in patients concurrently infected with HIV-1 and KSHV may be attributable to vMIP-II because binding of vMIP-II for several HIV-1 co-receptors (CCR5, CXCR4, and CCR3) would be expected to retard HIV-1 dissemination (Boshoff et al. 1997; Kledal et al. 1997).

Findings in Animal Models

Studies based on transgenic and knockout mice have provided some of the most convincing evidence that elimination of single CLs only partially affects T-cell recruitment and function, as exemplified by normal development of mice with MIP-1α (CCL3) or eotaxin deficiency. Defective B-cell lymphopoiesis in mice with mutated *CXCL12* (SDF-1) is mostly restricted to the bone marrow, and this model supports the suspected role of SDF-1 in mediating progenitor cell homing or development.

Disruption of individual CRs tends to have more severe outcomes. Mice lacking CXCR4 show a wide range of defects in vascular development, hematopoiesis, and cardiogenesis. CXCR2 deficiency leads to abnormal lymphoid and myeloid tissues, while null CXCR5 is accompanied by the lack of inguinal lymph nodes and Peyer's patches, along with impaired B-cell trafficking. Likewise, depletion of CCR1, CCR2, CCR4, or CCR5 leads to defective monocyte chemotaxis, reduced response to lipopolysaccharides, and imbalanced T_H1 and T_H2 cytokine responses. Overall, CR deficiency affects both T-cell migration and T-cell differentiation.

Transgenic and knockout models have been tested for at least eight C-C-motif and C-X-C-motif CRs (CCR1, CCR2, CCR4, CCR5, CCR7, CXCR2, CXCR4, and CXCR5) and six related CLs (CCL2, CCL3, CCL11, CCL21, CXCL12, and CXCL13). The findings do not always support the expected effect; again, the complexity of receptor–ligand function precludes straightforward interpretations.

In murine models that test modified chemokines as promising candidates for targeted therapy, recombinant Met-RANTES, which retains the full-length sequence starting from the first methionine residue, potently inhibits chemotaxis induced by naturally processed RANTES and MIP-1α. This effect is apparently mediated through CCR1 and not CCR3 or

CCR5. In addition, Met-RANTES blocks monocyte chemotaxis in mice by competing with MIP-1β for CCR5 binding. In rats, use of Met-RANTES can prevent rejection of kidney transplants.

Overall, studies based on animals (mostly rodents and primates) should improve the understanding of immune-mediated inflammatory reaction (Ransohoff 1997) and help identify novel strategies for effective intervention (Rosenberg et al. 2005; Veasey et al., 2005), especially for diseases (e.g., HIV and malaria) known to have originated from animals.

Chromosomal Location (Physical Mapping) of CR and CL Loci

With few exceptions, the CXCL and CCL genes and several pseudogenes are tandemly arranged on chromosomes 4q12-q21 and 17q11, respectively (table 17.1), quite likely as a result of multiple gene duplication (Maho et al. 1999b; Naruse et al. 1996; Nomiyama et al. 1999; Rollins et al. 1991) and gene fusion (Tasaki et al. 1999). Indeed, multiple copies of CCL3- and CCL4-like genes are readily detected as functional units (Colobran et al. 2005; Gonzalez et al. 2005; Townson et al. 2002). As for the CR genes, many reside on chromosomes 2q34-q35 and 3p21 (Ahuja et al. 1992; Daugherty and Springer 1997; Maho et al. 1999a; Raport et al. 1996; Samson et al. 1996). As with other paired receptor–ligand gene clusters such as the human leukocyte antigen complex and the killer cell immunoglobulin receptor loci, complexity of CL and CR gene content is augmented by allelic and haplotypic diversity (Clark and Dean 2004a, 2004b).

Structurally, CL and CR genes typically consist of three exons and two introns. Their cis- and trans-regulatory elements can be found in both upstream (promoter) and downstream (intron 1) of exon 1 sequences. The smallest genes (CCL21, CCR2, CXCL4, and XCR1) in this system are around 2 kb; the largest ones (CCL28, CCR1, and CXCL13) range from 32 kb to 123 kb in size. Not surprisingly, information about the simpler (i.e., smaller) genes has accumulated more rapidly because they are much easier to characterize and manipulate.

Genetic Variations

Among the three forms of genetic variations reported for genes in the CL and CR family, gene duplication

and nucleotide insertion/deletion variants are not as well documented as are single nucleotide polymorphisms (SNPs). The profusion of SNP data in the CL and CR genes cannot be easily summarized. Following are a few of the informative Web sites where these data are being catalogued and updated regularly (see also appendix 1). The dbSNP database (www.ncbi.nih.gov/SNP/) at the National Center for Biotechnology Information (NCBI) hosts a large number of SNPs, with each having an annotated reference sequence (rs) number within the context of neighboring nucleotides. The SNP Consortium (snp.cshl.org/) is another useful resource, with more than 1.8 million SNPs to date. These databases can be searched simultaneously via the Web-based SNPper program (snpper.chip.org/bio/snpper-explain). For example, SNPper catalogues more than 200 SNPs for the CCR3-CCR2-CCR5 gene cluster (figure 17.2). However, few of these are considered informative in terms of their relevance to gene function or their ability to tag local haplotypes, and even fewer have been studied for disease associations. It is also noteworthy that more recently assembled genotyping arrays for genome-wide association studies, such as the Affymetrix 500K chip and Illumina 550K array, target relatively few SNPs at these CCR loci.

The SNPs retrievable through SNPper or PupasView (Conde et al. 2005) require adequate validation at the population level. For a more focused approach, SNP data from the International HapMap Project (www.hapmap.org/) and the Perlegen Genotype Browser (genome.perlegen.com/browser/index.html) are especially valuable for sorting genotypes by individuals or ethnic groups and for analyzing linkage disequilibrium (LD) (figure 17.2). Of note, populations that deviate from the typical European, African, and Asian ancestries (as targeted by the HapMap and Perlegen databases) have not been well characterized for genetic variations.

Several ongoing projects funded by the National Institutes of Health have mapped functionally relevant SNPs in certain CL and CR genes. The products derived from these projects are freely available at SeattleSNPs (pga.gs.washington.edu/finished_genes.html) and its linked pages, including GeneSNPs (www.genome.utah.edu/genesnps/). Each SNP map (e.g., the CCR2 SNP map at pga.gs.washington.edu/data/ccr2/) covers all known exons and intron–exon boundaries, plus 10-kb upstream and 10-kb downstream at each locus. These maps and associated data (e.g.,

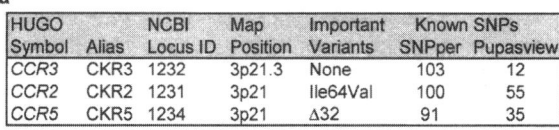

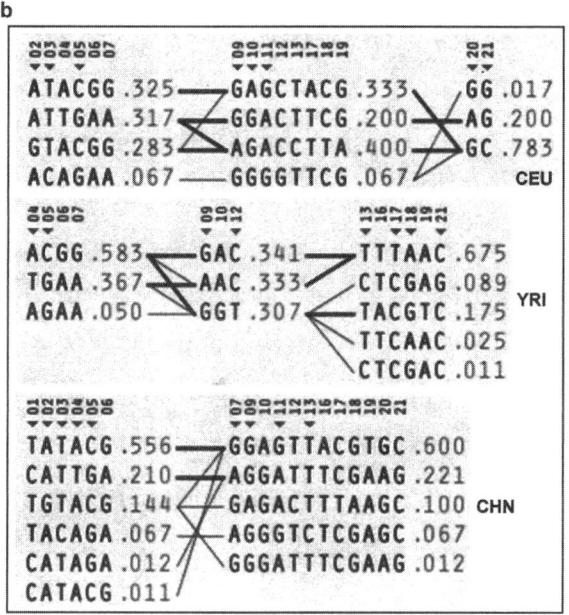

FIGURE 17.2. Examples of genetic variations in the chemokine ligand and receptor system. For the gene cluster of *CCR3*, *CCR2*, and *CCR5* on chromosme 3, a search through SNPpper (snpper.chip.org/bio/snpper-explain) yield hundreds of SNPs in public databases (a), including some that are predicted by Pupas-View (Conde et al., 2005) as potentially relevant to gene function. To date, immuonogenetic studies in human populations have dealt with rather limited numbers of variants (SNPs and a deletion mutant). A survey of the International HapMap Project database (www.hapmap.org/) reveals just 21 SNPs (listed as 01 to 21) for the *CCR3* locus (b), with very little information for the *CCR2* and *CCR5* loci. Importantly, the structure of haplotype blocks (Gabriel et al. 2002) differs between populations represented by Centre d'Etude du Polymorphisme Humain Europeans (CEU), Africans (Yoruba from Nigeria, YRI), and Han Chinese (CHN). The haplotype-tagging SNPs (htSNPs, indicated by arrow heads) within each block are often considered informative (adequate) for the purpose of genotyping.

genotypes and haplotypes) for individuals can immediately guide studies involving European Americans and African Americans, where the production of CRs and CLs is known to vary greatly (Paxton et al. 1996, 2001).

Disease Associations and Their Implications

Associations of *DARC* and *CCR5* mutations with resistance to malaria and HIV-1 infection, respectively, are the best known and most frequently cited examples of genotype–phenotype relationships in infectious diseases (table 17.2). Findings in these two diseases are detailed elsewhere in this volume (chapters 19 and 24). Novel genetic effects, which are mostly preliminary, have also been reported but not uniformly verified in several other disease models (table 17.2), including hepatitis C virus (HCV) infection (Hellier et al. 2003; Woitas et al. 2002, Mascheretti et al. 2004), response to therapy in HCV and HIV-1 patients (Dorak et al. 2002; Guerin et al. 2000; O'Brien et al. 2000; Valdez et al. 1999, Wasmuth et al. 2004), bronchiolitis

after respiratory syncytial virus (RSV) infection (Hacking et al. 2004; Hull et al. 2000), and *Helicobacter pylori*–induced diseases (Gyulai et al. 2004; Lu et al. 2005).

For *DARC*, both promoter and coding sequence variants have been shown to reduce the amount of cell surface expression, leading to protection from *Plasmodium vivax* malaria as the parasite relies on DARC for invasion into human erythrocytes. Resistance to HIV-1 infection conferred by a 32-bp deletion ($\triangle$32) and a nonsynonymous nucleotide substitution (m303) in the *CCR5* open reading frame works in a similar way: Both mutations introduce a premature stop codon, so individuals with homozygous $\triangle$32 mutation or $\triangle$32 plus m303 only produce truncated CCR5 that fails to reach cell surface (Liu et al. 1996; Quillent et al. 1998). These observations corroborate the notion that primary HIV-1 infection mostly involves CCR5-using viruses (Meng et al. 2002). Such viral co-receptor specificity has led to the design of synthetic CCR5 antagonist as therapeutic agents for HIV patients (Barbaro et al. 2005; Schols 2004) (see chapter 19).

The *CCR5-*$\triangle$32 mutation may have been introduced into the Caucasian populations about 1,000 years ago (Stephens et al. 1998). Its rapid spread from northern Europe to the South and to certain Jewish populations is more likely a result of strong selection than random genetic drift or migration (Libert et al. 1998; Maayan et al. 2000). The possibility of positive selection pressure from widespread infection with smallpox virus or the plague bacillus has apparently been refuted recently in studies of transgenic animal models (Elvin et al. 2004; Mecsas et al. 2004); additional hypotheses await formal testing.

In contrast to the more prominent effects of null alleles and gene duplication variants (Gonzalez et al. 2005; Liu et al. 1996; Quillent et al. 1998), common SNPs in CL and CR genes have demonstrated modest associations with disease outcomes. The majority of these findings still require independent confirmation, but they do begin to convey some consensus messages.

First, frequent differences in the distribution of many SNPs and their haplotypes between racial/ethnic groups (Bamshad et al. 2002; Gonzalez et al. 1999; Mummidi et al. 1998; Tang et al. 1999) may lead to population-specific effects (table 17.2), as clearly exemplified by the CCR5-△32 mutation and the Duffy null allele. Thus, the importance of genetic contribution depends on the frequency of specific mutation/variant as well as the prevalence of associated infections. More important, genetic advantage in one setting may become disadvantageous in others, as exemplified by a study of CCR5-△32 mutation in relation to West Nile virus infection in the United States (Glass et al. 2006).

Second, traditional analyses of recessive and dominant effects may no longer be sufficient since there is some empirical support (e.g., figure 17.3) for disease associations with both individual haplotypes and haplotype pairs (diplotypes) (Tang and Kaslow 2004). For example, nine major human haplotypes (HHA through HHG*2; figure 17.3) (see also chapter 19) defined by CCR2 and CCR5 variants on chromosome 3 can yield up to 45 genotypes (diplotypes) (Mummidi et al. 1998); two of these, HHC/HHE and HHE/HHE, have demonstrated very different associations with HIV-1 infection and disease progression than the HHE haplotype alone or other genotypic combinations involving HHE (e.g., HHA/HHE and HHE/HHF*2). Studies of CCL2 and CCL5 variants on chromosome 17 have come to similar conclusions for the HIV/AIDS model (An et al. 2002; Liu et al. 1999; Modi et al. 2003), suggesting that more generalizable

findings should be based on complete resolution of informative SNPs and haplotypes (figure 17.2), followed by comprehensive statistical analyses. Independent replication of findings in other well-defined cohorts is also of great importance (Kaslow et al. 2004).

Third, mechanisms underlying the immunogenetic findings can be both direct and indirect (Mackay 2005). For instance, codon 64 polymorphism (GTC → ATC) in CCR2 leads to a conservative amino acid change from valine (V) to isoleucine (I); association of CCR2-64I with various outcomes during HIV-1 infection may be due to interaction between CCR5 and CXCR4 (Lee et al. 1998; Mellado et al. 1999) rather than to the loss of CCR2 function per se. Partial resistance to HIV-1 infection conferred by heterozygous CCR5-△32 mutation may result from the interference of the truncated product with the function of the wild-type (full-length) CCR5 through the formation of defective heterodimers (Benkirane et al. 1997).

Targets for Interventions

Strategies to enhance or block CR and CL interactions may become feasible, as demonstrated by the use of CR antagonist to inhibit HIV-1 dissemination (Proudfoot 2002) and chimeric simian-human immunodeficiency virus infection (Lederman et al. 2004; Veasey et al., 2005). At least two small-molecule antagonists (TAK779 and SCH-C, Schering Plough) have been tested with some success in animal models, but their practical values seem quite limited because HIV-1 mutates rapidly to acquire either enhanced binding affinity for CCR5 or expand usage of alternative coreceptors (e.g., CXCR4 and CCR2) (Cilliers et al. 2005; Trkola et al. 2001, 2002). Additional co-receptor inhibitors (e.g., AMD3100) that target CXCR4 are confronted by problems ranging from insufficient delivery to adverse effects (Hatse et al. 2005). While new products continue to emerge, randomized human trials to test their clinical usefulness are still lagging behind. Two recent human trials actually yielded unexpectedly discouraging results (Honey 2007).

Close examination of the level of constitutively expressed and induced CR and CL profile is also critical to the assessment of therapeutic success, especially when individuals can be primed either sequentially or concurrently by multiple pathogens. For example, a reduction in HIV-related mortality rate in patients coinfected with HIV-1 and GB virus C (GBV-C) has

TABLE 17.2. Well-known CR and CL gene variants associated with human infectious diseases and/or related outcomes.

Locus: Variants/Mutations[a]	Population Distribution	Associations[a]	Apparent or Possible Mechanisms
CCR2: homozygous or heterozygous CCR2-64I (CCR2-190A)	Common (>10%) in all ethnic groups	(1) Delayed onset of AIDS in HIV-1–infected subjects	May influence CCR2–CCR5 dimerization or CCR5/CXCR4 signaling
		(2) Inability to clear HCV infection	Unknown
CCR5: homozygous CCR5-Δ32 mutation	~1% of Caucasians	Resistance to HIV-1 infection	Truncated CCR5 (primary co-receptor for HIV-1) not present on cell surface
CCR5: heterozygous CCR5-Δ32 mutation	<20% of Caucasians	Partial resistance to HIV-1 infection, along with reduced viral load or delayed onset of AIDS	Reduced CCR5 on cell surface, especially in subjects with certain CCR5 promoter variants
CCR5: promoter variants (e.g., haplotypes)	Highly variable	Differences in viral load and rates of disease progression in HIV-1–infected subjects	Variability in CCR5 expression on surface of cells targeted by HIV-1
CCL3L1: copy number	Highly variable (0–11)	Reduced viral load and delayed onset of AIDS in HIV-1–infected subjects with copy numbers greater than the population average	CCL3L1 (MIP-1β) potently inhibits HIV-1 binding to the CCR5 co-receptor
CCL5: promoter and intron 1 SNPs and haplotypes	Highly variable	Contrasting viral load and rates of disease progression in HIV-1–infected subjects	Differential expression of CCL5 influences the CCR5 function as HIV-1 co-receptor
CXCL8 (IL8): −251A/A or A/T	Frequencies range from 10% to 50%	(1) Helicobacter pylori–related disease manifestations	Elevated, persistent inflammation mediated by IL-8 (CXCL8)
		(2) Bronchiolitis caused by RSV	
CXCL12: homozygous SDF-1 3'A (CXCL12 801A)	<10% in any population	Delayed onset of AIDS in HIV-1–infected subjects	3' UTR polymorphism may increase SDF-1 (CXCL12) expression?
DARC: homozygous FY*O (Duffy null)	Near fixation in most Africans but rare elsewhere	Resistance to Plasmodium vivax malaria	No or reduced Duffy antigen (P. vivax receptor) on red blood cells

Abbreviations (in alphabetical order): HCV, hepatitis C virus; HIV-1, human immunodeficiency virus, type 1; RSV, respiratory syncytial virus; UTR, untranslated region. Additional abbreviations are listed in table 17.1.

[a]Restricted to those reported for large cohorts ($n \geq 800$) or showing some consistency in different studies and supported by experimental evidence. Key references are cited in the text.

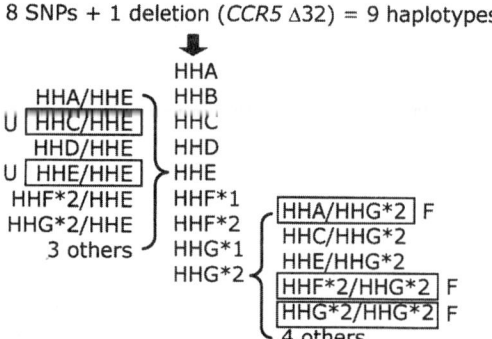

FIGURE 17.3. Genetic association analyses of human haplogroups (HH) defined at the neighboring CCR2 and CCR5 loci on chromosome 3. Several studies have revealed favorable (F) and unfavorable (U) haplotypes and haplotype pairs (boxed) in relation to human immunodeficiency virus (HIV-1) infection and/or disease progression (see table 17.2). The effects of diplotypes (i.e., pairs of haplotypes from opposite chromosomes) can be considered novel because their influence can not be identified through conventional dominant and recessive models.

been attributed to up-regulation of CCL3 (MIP-1α), CCL4 (MIP-1β), CCL5 (RANTES), and CXCL12 (SDF-1), apparently induced by GBV-C rather than HIV-1 (Xiang et al. 2004). Local and systemic inflammation not related to infection can lead to similar complications.

Conclusions and Prospects

The CL/CR system resembles the classic cytokine and cytokine receptor systems in terms of complexity and role in regulating lymphocyte trafficking, activation, and differentiation. In the peripheral blood, persistent presence of high-level CLs contrasts with the often transient presence of low-level cytokines. Circulating CLs will likely serve as useful diagnostic biomarkers for occurrence, severity and course of infectious as well as other diseases.

The importance of genes and gene products in the CL/CR system can vary from one infectious disease to another. Documented success in relating alleles, haplotypes, and diplotypes to variable disease outcomes is encouraging. Concerted efforts to confirm and refine genetic factors within the CL/CR system will benefit from the newly established SNP databases, readily accessible bioinformatics software, and advanced tech-niques designed for high-throughput genotyping. Assays that can unambiguously assign individual haplotypes in heterozygous ndividuals should further expedite the analyses of genotype–phenotype relationships.

Acknowledgments

I thank members of the Program in Epidemiology of Infection and Immunity, University of Alabama at Birmingham Schools of Medicine and Public Health, for frequent discussions and reviews of current literature. The manuscript was written during a period of support by grants AI51173, AI41951, AI40591, AI41530, HD32842, CA73475, and CA097247 from National Institute of Allergy and Infectious Diseases and the National Cancer Institute.

References

Acosta-Rodriguez, E. V., Rivino, L., Geginat, J., Jarrossay, D., Gattorno, M., Lanzavecchia, A., Sallusto, F., and Napolitani, G.: Surface phenotype and antigenic specificity of human interleukin 17-producing T helper memory cells. *Nat Immunol* 8: 639–646, 2007.

Ahuja, S. K., Ozcelik, T., Milatovitch, A., Francke, U., and Murphy, P. M.: Molecular evolution of the human interleukin-8 receptor gene cluster. *Nat Genet* 2: 31–36, 1992.

Alcami, A.: Viral mimicry of cytokines, chemokines and their receptors. *Nat Rev Immunol* 3: 36–50, 2003.

Alkhatlb, G., Ahuja, S. S., Light, D., Mummidi, S., Berger, E. A., and Ahuja, S. K.: CC chemokine receptor 5-mediated signaling and HIV-1 co-receptor activity share common structural determinants. Critical residues in the third extracellular loop support HIV-1 fusion. *J Biol Chem* 272: 19771–19776, 1997.

An, P., Nelson, G. W., Wang, L., Donfield, S., Goedert, J. J., Phair, J., Vlahov, D., Buchbinder, S., Farrar, W. L., Modi, W., O'Brien, S. J., and Winkler, C. A.: Modulating influence on HIV/AIDS by interacting RANTES gene variants. *Proc Natl Acad Sci USA* 99: 10002–10007, 2002.

Arvanitakis, L., Geras-Raaka, E., Varma, A., Gershengorn, M. C., and Cesarman, E.: Human herpesvirus KSHV encodes a constitutively active G-protein-coupled receptor linked to cell proliferation. *Nature* 385: 347–350, 1997.

Bacon, K., Baggiolini, M., Broxmeyer, H., Horuk, R., Lindley, I., Mantovani, A., Maysushima, K., Murphy, P., Nomiyama, H., Oppenheim, J., Rot, A.,

Schall, T., Tsang, M., Thorpe, R., Van Damme, J., Wadhwa, M., Yoshie, O., Zlotnik, A., and Zoon, K.: Chemokine/chemokine receptor nomenclature. *J Interferon Cytokine Res* 22: 1067–1068, 2002.

Baggiolini, M.: Chemokines and leukocyte traffic. *Nature* 392: 565–568, 1998.

Bamshad, M. J., Mummidi, S., Gonzalez, E., Ahuja, S. S., Dunn, D. M., Watkins, W. S., Wooding, S., Stone, A. C., Jorde, L. B., Weiss, R. B., and Ahuja, S. K.: A strong signature of balancing selection in the 5′ cis-regulatory region of CCR5. *Proc Natl Acad Sci USA* 99: 10539–10544, 2002.

Barbaro, G., Scozzafava, A., Mastrolorenzo, A., and Supuran, C. T.: Highly active antiretroviral therapy: current state of the art, new agents and their pharmacological interactions useful for improving therapeutic outcome. *Curr Pharm Des* 11: 1805–1843, 2005.

Beisser, P. S., Goh, C. S., Cohen, F. E., and Michelson, S.: Viral chemokine receptors and chemokines in human cytomegalovirus trafficking and interaction with the immune system: CMV chemokine receptors. *Curr Top Microbiol Immunol* 269: 203–234, 2002.

Benkirane, M., Jin, D. Y., Chun, R. F., Koup, R. A., and Jeang, K. T.: Mechanism of transdominant inhibition of CCR5-mediated HIV-1 infection by CCR5 delta32. *J Biol Chem* 272: 30603–30606, 1997.

Bettelli, E., Oukka, M., and Kuchroo, V. K.: T(H)-17 cells in the circle of immunity and autoimmunity. *Nat Immunol* 8: 345–350, 2007.

Blanpain, C., Migeotte, I., Lee, B., Vakili, J., Doranz, B. J., Govaerts, C., Vassart, G., Doms, R. W., and Parmentier, M.: CCR5 binds multiple CC-chemokines: MCP-3 acts as a natural antagonist. *Blood* 94: 1899–1905, 1999.

Bonecchi, R., Bianchi, G., Bordignon, P. P., D'Ambrosio, D., Lang, R., Borsatti, A., Sozzani, S., Allavena, P., Gray, P. A., Mantovani, A., and Sinigaglia, F.: Differential expression of chemokine receptors and chemotactic responsiveness of type 1 T helper cells (Th1s) and Th2s. *J Exp Med* 187: 129–134, 1998a.

Bonecchi, R., Sozzani, S., Stine, J. T., Luini, W., D'Amico, G., Allavena, P., Chantry, D., and Mantovani, A.: Divergent effects of interleukin-4 and interferon-gamma on macrophage-derived chemokine production: an amplification circuit of polarized T helper 2 responses. *Blood* 92: 2668–2671, 1998b.

Boshoff, C., Endo, Y., Collins, P. D., Takeuchi, Y., Reeves, J. D., Schweickart, V. L., Siani, M. A., Sasaki, T., Williams, T. J., Gray, P. W., Moore, P. S., Chang, Y., and Weiss, R. A.: Angiogenic and HIV-inhibitory functions of KSHV-encoded chemokines. *Science* 278: 290–294, 1997.

Campbell, D. J., Kim, C. H., and Butcher, E. C.: Chemokines in the systemic organization of immunity. *Immunol Rev* 195: 58–71, 2003.

Cilliers, T., Willey, S., Sullivan, W. M., Patience, T., Pugach, P., Coetzer, M., Papathanasopoulos, M., Moore, J. P., Trkola, A., Clapham, P., and Morris, L.: Use of alternate coreceptors on primary cells by two HIV-1 isolates. *Virology* 339: 136–144, 2005.

Clark, V. J., and Dean, M.: Characterisation of SNP haplotype structure in chemokine and chemokine receptor genes using CEPH pedigrees and statistical estimation. *Hum Genomics* 1: 195–207, 2004a.

Clark, V. J., and Dean, M.: Haplotype structure and linkage disequilibrium in chemokine and chemokine receptor genes. *Hum Genomics* 1: 255–273, 2004b.

Colobran, R., Adreani, P., Ashhab, Y., Llano, A., Este, J. A., Dominguez, O., Pujol-Borrell, R., and Juan, M.: Multiple products derived from two *CCL4* loci: high incidence of a new polymorphism in HIV+ patients. *J Immunol* 174: 5655–5664, 2005.

Conde, L., Vaquerizas, J. M., Ferrer-Costa, C., de la Cruz, X., Orozco, M., and Dopazo, J.: PupasView: a visual tool for selecting suitable SNPs, with putative pathological effect in genes, for genotyping purposes. *Nucleic Acids Res* 33: W501–505, 2005.

Daugherty, B. L., and Springer, M. S.: The beta-chemokine receptor genes CCR1 (CMKBR1), CCR2 (CMKBR2), and CCR3 (CMKBR3) cluster within 285 kb on human chromosome 3p21. *Genomics* 41: 294–295, 1997.

Devalaraja, M. N., and Richmond, A.: Multiple chemotactic factors: fine control or redundancy? *Trends Pharmacol Sci* 20: 151–156, 1999.

DeVries, M. E., Ran, L., and Kelvin, D. J.: On the edge: the physiological and pathophysiological role of chemokines during inflammatory and immunological responses. *Semin Immunol* 11: 95–104, 1999.

Dorak, M. T., Folayan, G. O., Niwas, S., Yee, L. J., Tang, J., van Leevan, D. J., and Kaslow, R. A.: C-C chemokine receptor 2 (*CCR2*) and *CCR5* genotypes in patients treated for hepatitis C virus infection. *Immunol Res* 26: 167–175, 2002.

Elvin, S. J., Williamson, E. D., Scott, J. C., Smith, J. N., Perez De Lema, G., Chilla, S., Clapham, P., Pfeffer, K., Schlondorff, D., and Luckow, B.: Evolutionary genetics: ambiguous role of CCR5 in Y. pestis infection. *Nature* 430: 1 p following 417, 2004.

Endres, M. J., Garlisi, C. G., Xiao, H., Shan, L., and Hedrick, J. A.: The Kaposi's sarcoma-related herpesvirus (KSHV)-encoded chemokine vMIP-I is a specific agonist for the CC chemokine receptor (CCR)8. *J Exp Med* 189: 1993–1998, 1999.

Gabriel, S. B., Schaffner, S. F., Nguyen, H., Moore, J. M., Roy, J., Blumenstiel, B., Higgins, J., DeFelice, M.,

Lochner, A., Faggart, M., Liu-Cordero, S. N., Rotimi, C., Adeyemo, A., Cooper, R., Ward, R., Lander, E. S., Daly, M. J., and Altshuler, D.: The structure of haplotype blocks in the human genome. *Science* 296: 2225–2229, 2002.

Glass, W. G., McDermott, D. H., Lim, J. K., Lekhong, S., Yu, S. F., Frank, W. A., Pape, J., Cheshier, R. C., and Murphy, P. M.: CCR5 deficiency increases risk of symptomatic West Nile virus infection. *J Exp Med* 203: 35–40, 2006.

Gompels, U. A., Nicholas, J., Lawrence, G., Jones, M., Thomson, B. J., Martin, M. E., Efstathiou, S., Craxton, M., and Macaulay, H. A.: The DNA sequence of human herpesvirus-6: structure, coding content, and genome evolution. *Virology* 209: 29–51, 1995.

Gonzalez, E., Bamshad, M., Sato, N., Mummidi, S., Dhanda, G., Catano, G., Cabrera, S., McBride, M., Cao, X.-H., Merrill, G., O'Connell, P., Bowden, D. W., Frredman, B. I., Anderson, S. A., Walters, E. A., Evans, J. S., Stephan, K. T., Clark, R. A., Tyagi, S., Ahuja, S. S., Dolan, M. J., and Ahuja, S. K.: Race-specific HIV-1 disease modifying effects associated with CCR5 haplotypes. *Proc Natl Acad Sci USA* 96: 12004–12009, 1999.

Gonzalez, E., Kulkarni, H., Bolivar, H., Mangano, A., Sanchez, R., Catano, G., Nibbs, R. J., Freedman, B. I., Quinones, M. P., Bamshad, M. J., Murthy, K. K., Rovin, B. H., Bradley, W., Clark, R. A., Anderson, S. A., O'Connell R, J., Agan, B. K., Ahuja, S. S., Bologna, R., Sen, L., Dolan, M. J., and Ahuja, S. K.: The influence of *CCL3L1* gene-containing segmental duplications on HIV-1/AIDS susceptibility. *Science* 307: 1434–1440, 2005.

Guerin, S., Meyer, L., Theodorou, I., Boufassa, F., Magierowska, M., Goujard, C., Rouzioux, C., Debre, P., and Delfraissy, J. F.: CCR5 Δ32 deletion and response to highly active antiretroviral therapy in HIV-1-infected patients. *AIDS* 14: 2788–2790, 2000.

Gyulai, Z., Klausz, G., Tiszai, A., Lenart, Z., Kasa, I. T., Lonovics, J., and Mandi, Y.: Genetic polymorphism of interleukin-8 (IL-8) is associated with Helicobacter pylori-induced duodenal ulcer. *Eur Cytokine Netw* 15: 353–358, 2004.

Hacking, D., Knight, J. C., Rockett, K., Brown, H., Frampton, J., Kwiatkowski, D. P., Hull, J., and Udalova, I. A.: Increased *in vivo* transcription of an IL-8 haplotype associated with respiratory syncytial virus disease-susceptibility. *Genes Immun* 5: 274–282, 2004.

Hatse, S., Princen, K., Clercq, E. D., Rosenkilde, M. M., Schwartz, T. W., Hernandez-Abad, P. E., Skerlj, R. T., Bridger, G. J., and Schols, D.: AMD3465, a monomacrocyclic CXCR4 antagonist and potent HIV entry inhibitor. *Biochem Pharmacol* 70: 752–761, 2005.

Hellier, S., Frodsham, A. J., Hennig, B. J., Klenerman, P., Knapp, S., Ramaley, P., Satsangi, J., Wright, M., Zhang, L., Thomas, H. C., Thursz, M., and Hill, A. V.: Association of genetic variants of the chemokine receptor CCR5 and its ligands, RANTES and MCP-2, with outcome of HCV infection. *Hepatology* 38: 1468–1476, 2003.

Honey, K.: Microbicide trial screeches to a halt. *J Clin Invest* 117: 1116, 2007.

Huang, R. P.: Detection of multiple proteins in an antibody-based protein microarray system. *J Immunol Methods* 255: 1–13, 2001a.

Huang, R. P.: Simultaneous detection of multiple proteins with an array-based enzyme-linked immunosorbent assay (ELISA) and enhanced chemiluminescence (ECL). *Clin Chem Lab Med* 39: 209–214, 2001b.

Hughes, A. L., and Yeager, M.: Coevolution of the mammalian chemokines and their receptors. *Immunogenetics* 49: 115–124, 1999.

Hull, J., Thomson, A., and Kwiatkowski, D.: Association of respiratory syncytial virus bronchiolitis with the interleukin 8 gene region in UK families. *Thorax* 55: 1023–1027, 2000.

Kaslow, R. A., Tang, J., and Dorak, M. T.: Chapter 12: The role of host genetic variation in HIV infection and its manifestations. *In* G. P. Wormser (ed.): *AIDS and Other Manifestations of HIV Infection*, pp. 285–302, Elsevier Science, New York, 2004.

Kledal, T. N., Rosenkilde, M. M., Coulin, F., Simmons, G., Johnsen, A. H., Alouani, S., Power, C. A., Luttichau, H. R., Gerstoft, J., Clapham, P. R., Clark-Lewis, I., Wells, T. N., and Schwartz, T. W.: A broad-spectrum chemokine antagonist encoded by Kaposi's sarcoma-associated herpesvirus. *Science* 277: 1656–1659, 1997.

Lederman, M. M., Veazey, R. S., Offord, R., Mosier, D. E., Dufour, J., Mefford, M., Piatak, M., Jr., Lifson, J. D., Salkowitz, J. R., Rodriguez, B., Blauvelt, A., and Hartley, O.: Prevention of vaginal SHIV transmission in rhesus macaques through inhibition of CCR5. *Science* 306: 485–487, 2004.

Lee, B., Doranz, B. J., Rana, S., Yi, Y., Mellado, M., Frade, J. M., Martinez, A. C., O'Brien, S. J., Dean, M., Collman, R. G., and Doms, R. W.: Influence of the CCR2-V64I polymorphism on human immunodeficiency virus type 1 coreceptor activity and on chemokine receptor function of CCR2b, CCR3, CCR5, and CXCR4. *J Virol* 72: 7450–7458, 1998.

Libert, F., Cochaux, P., Beckman, G., Samson, M., Aksenova, M., Cao, A., Czeizel, A., Claustres, M., de la

Rua, C., Ferrari, M., Ferrec, C., Glover, G., Grinde, B., Guran, S., Kucinskas, V., Lavinha, J., Mercier, B., Ogur, G., Peltonen, L., Rosatelli, C., Schwartz, M., Spitsyn, V., Timar, L., Beckman, L., and Vassart, G.: The Dccr5 mutation conferring protection against HIV-1 in Caucasian populations has a single and recent origin in Northeastern Europe. *Hum Mol Genet* 7: 399–406, 1998.

Lin, Y., Huang, R., Santanam, N., Liu, Y. G., Parthasarathy, S., and Huang, R. P.: Profiling of human cytokines in healthy individuals with vitamin E supplementation by antibody array. *Cancer Lett* 187: 17–24, 2002.

Liston, A., and McColl, S.: Subversion of the chemokine world by microbial pathogens. *Bioessays* 25: 478–488, 2003.

Liu, H. L., Chao, D., Nakayama, E. E., Taguchi, H., Goto, M., Xin, X. M., Takamatsu, J., Saito, H., Ishikawa, Y., Akaza, T., Juji, T., Takebe, Y., Ohishi, T., Fukutake, K., Maruyama, Y., Yashiki, S. J., Sonoda, S., Nakamura, T., Nagai, Y., Iwamoto, A., and Shioda, T.: Polymorphism in RANTES chemokine promoter affects HIV-1 disease progression. *Proc Natl Acad Sci USA* 96: 4581–4585, 1999.

Liu, R., Paxton, W. A., Choe, S., Ceradini, D., Martin, S. R., Horuk, R., MacDonald, M. E., Stuhlmann, H., Koup, R. A., and Landau, N. R.: Homozygous defect in HIV-1 coreceptor accounts for resistance of some multiply-exposed individuals to HIV-1 infection. *Cell* 86: 367–377, 1996.

Liu, R., Zhao, X. Q., Gurney, T. A., and Landau, N. R.: Functional analysis of the proximal CCR5 promoter. *AIDS Res Hum Retroviruses* 14: 1509–1519, 1998.

Locati, M., Otero, K., Schioppa, T., Signorelli, P., Perrier, P., Baviera, S., Sozzani, S., and Mantovani, A.: The chemokine system: tuning and shaping by regulation of receptor expression and coupling in polarized responses. *Allergy* 57: 972–982, 2002.

Loetscher, P., and Clark-Lewis, I.: Agonistic and antagonistic activities of chemokines. *J Leukoc Biol* 69: 881–884, 2001.

Loetscher, P., Uguccioni, M., Bordoli, L., Baggiolini, M., Moser, B., Chizzolini, C., and Dayer, J. M.: CCR5 is characteristic of Th1 lymphocytes. *Nature* 391: 344–345, 1998.

Lu, W., Pan, K., Zhang, L., Lin, D., Miao, X., and You, W.: Genetic polymorphisms of interleukin (IL)-1B, IL-1RN, IL-8, IL-10 and tumor necrosis factor {alpha} and risk of gastric cancer in a Chinese population. *Carcinogenesis* 26: 631–636, 2005.

Luster, A. D.: Chemokines: chemotactic cytokines that mediate inflammation. *N Engl J Med* 338: 436–445, 1998.

Luther, S. A., and Cyster, J. G.: Chemokines as regulators of T cell differentiation. *Nat Immunol* 2: 102–107, 2001.

Maayan, S., Zhang, L., Shinar, E., Ho, J., He, T., Manni, N., Kostrikis, L. G., and Neumann, A. U.: Evidence for recent selection of the CCR5-delta 32 deletion from differences in its frequency between Ashkenazi and Sephardi Jews. *Genes Immun* 1: 358–361, 2000.

Mackay, C. R.: CCL3L1 dose and HIV-1 susceptibility. *Trends Mol Med* 11: 203–206, 2005.

Maho, A., Bensimon, A., Vassart, G., and Parmentier, M.: Mapping of the CXCR1, CX3CR1, CCBP2 and CCR9 genes to the CCR cluster within the 3p21.3 region of the human genome. *Cytogenet Cell Genet* 87: 265–268, 1999a.

Maho, A., Carter, A., Bensimon, A., Vassart, G., and Parmentier, M.: Physical mapping of the CC-chemokine gene cluster on the human 17q11. 2 region. *Genomics* 59: 213–223, 1999b.

Mantovani, A., Locati, M., Vecchi, A., Sozzani, S., and Allavena, P.: Decoy receptors: a strategy to regulate inflammatory cytokines and chemokines. *Trends Immunol* 22: 328–336, 2001.

Mascheretti, S., Hinrichsen, H., Ross, S., Buggisch, P., Hampe, J., Foelsch, U. R., and Schreiber, S.: Genetic variants in the CCR gene cluster and spontaneous viral elimination in hepatitis C-infected patients. *Clin Exp Immunol* 136: 328–333, 2004.

Mecsas, J., Franklin, G., Kuziel, W. A., Brubaker, R. R., Falkow, S., and Mosier, D. E.: Evolutionary genetics: CCR5 mutation and plague protection. *Nature* 427: 606, 2004.

Mellado, M., Rodriguez-Frade, J. M., Manes, S., and Martinez, A. C.: Chemokine signaling and functional responses: the role of receptor dimerization and TK pathway activation. *Annu Rev Immunol* 19: 397–421, 2001a.

Mellado, M., Rodriguez-Frade, J. M., Vila-Coro, A. J., de Ana, A. M., and Martinez, A. C.: Chemokine control of HIV-1 infection. *Nature* 400: 723–724., 1999.

Mellado, M., Rodriguez-Frade, J. M., Vila-Coro, A. J., Fernandez, S., Martin de Ana, A., Jones, D. R., Toran, J. L., and Martinez, A. C.: Chemokine receptor homo- or heterodimerization activates distinct signaling pathways. *EMBO J* 20: 2497–2507, 2001b.

Meng, G., Wei, X.-P., Wu, X.-Y., Sellers, M. T., Deckers, J. M., Moldoveanu, Z., Orenstein, J. M., Graham, M. F., Kappes, J. C., Mestecky, J., Shaw, G. M., and Smith, P. D.: Primary intestinal epithelial cells selectively transfer R5 HIV-1 to CCR5[+] cells. *Nat Med* 8: 150–156, 2002.

Modi, W. S., Goedert, J. J., Strathdee, S., Buchbinder, S., Detels, R., Donfield, S., O'Brien, S. J., and Winkler,

C.: MCP-1-MCP-3-eotaxin gene cluster influences HIV-1 transmission. *AIDS* 17: 2357–2365, 2003.

Moser, B., Wolf, M., Walz, A., and Loetscher, P.: Chemokines: multiple levels of leukocyte migration control. *Trends Immunol* 25: 75–84, 2004.

Mummidi, S., Ahuja, S. S., Gonzalez, E., Anderson, S. A., Santiago, E. N., Stephan, K. T., Craig, F. E., O'Connell, P., Tryon, V., Clark, R. A., Dolan, M. J., and Ahuja, S. K.: Genealogy of the CCR5 locus and chemokine system gene variants associated with altered rates of HIV-1 disease progression. *Nat Med* 4: 786–793, 1998.

Mummidi, S., Bamshad, M., Ahuja, S. S., Gonzalez, E., Feuillet, P. M., Begum, K., Galvis, M. C., Kostecki, V., Valente, A. J., Murthy, K. K., Haro, L., Dolan, M. J., Allan, J. S., and Ahuja, S. K.: Evolution of human and non-human primate CC chemokine receptor 5 gene and mRNA. Potential roles for haplotype and mRNA diversity, differential haplotype-specific transcriptional activity, and altered transcription factor binding to polymorphic nucleotides in the pathogenesis of HIV-1 and simian immunodeficiency virus. *J Biol Chem* 275: 18946–18961, 2000.

Murphy, P. M.: International Union of Pharmacology. XXX. Update on chemokine receptor nomenclature. *Pharmacol Rev* 54: 227–229, 2002.

Naruse, K., Ueno, M., Satoh, T., Nomiyama, H., Tei, H., Takeda, M., Ledbetter, D. H., Coillie, E. V., Opdenakker, G., Gunge, N., Sakaki, Y., Iio, M., and Miura, R.: A YAC contig of the human CC chemokine genes clustered on chromosome 17q11.2. *Genomics* 34: 236–240, 1996.

Nomiyama, H., Fukuda, S., Iio, M., Tanase, S., Miura, R., and Yoshie, O.: Organization of the chemokine gene cluster on human chromosome 17q11.2 containing the genes for CC chemokine MPIF-1, HCC-2, HCC-1, LEC, and RANTES. *J Interferon Cytokine Res* 19: 227–234, 1999.

O'Brien, T. R., McDermott, D. H., Ioannidis, J. P., Carrington, M., Murphy, P. M., Havlir, D. V., and Richman, D. D.: Effect of chemokine receptor gene polymorphisms on the response to potent antiretroviral therapy. *AIDS* 14: 821–826, 2000.

Ogilvie, P., Bardi, G., Clark-Lewis, I., Baggiolini, M., and Uguccioni, M.: Eotaxin is a natural antagonist for CCR2 and an agonist for CCR5. *Blood* 97: 1920–1924, 2001.

Paxton, W. A., Martin, S. R., Tse, D., O'Brien, T. R., and al., e.: Relative resistance to HIV-1 infection of CD4 lymphocytes from persons who remain uninfected despite multiple high-risk sexual exposures. *Nature Med* 2: 412–417, 1996.

Paxton, W. A., Neumann, A. U., Kang, S., Deutch, L., Brown, R. C., Koup, R. A., and Wolinsky, S. M.:

RANTES production from CD4+ lymphocytes correlates with host genotype and rates of human immunodeficiency virus type 1 disease progression. *J Infect Dis* 183: 1678–1681, 2001.

Proost, P., Menten, P., Struyf, S., Schutyser, E., De Meester, I., and Van Damme, J.: Cleavage by CD26/dipeptidyl peptidase IV converts the chemokine LD78beta into a most efficient monocyte attractant and CCR1 agonist. *Blood* 96: 1674–1680, 2000.

Proudfoot, A. E.: Chemokine receptors: multifaceted therapeutic targets. *Nat Rev Immunol* 2: 106–115, 2002.

Quillent, C., Oberlin, E., Braun, J., Rousset, D., Gonzalez-Canali, G., Metais, P., Montagnier, L., Virelizier, J.-L., Arenzana-Seisdedos, F., and Beretta, A.: HIV-1 resistance phenotype conferred by combination of two separate inherited mutations of CCR5 gene. *Lancet* 351: 14–18, 1998.

Ransohoff, R. M.: Chemokines in neurological disease models: correlation between chemokine expression patterns and inflammatory pathology. *J Leukoc Biol* 62: 645–652, 1997.

Raport, C. J., Gosling, J., Schweickart, V. L., Gray, P. W., and Charo, I. F.: Molecular cloning and functional characterization of a novel human CC chemokine receptor (CCR5) for RANTES, MIP-1beta, and MIP-1alpha. *J Biol Chem* 271: 17161–17166, 1996.

Rodriguez-Frade, J. M., Mellado, M., and Martinez, A. C.: Chemokine receptor dimerization: two are better than one. *Trends Immunol* 22: 612–617, 2001.

Rollins, B. J., Morton, C. C., Ledbetter, D. H., Eddy, R. L., Jr., and Shows, T. B.: Assignment of the human small inducible cytokine A2 gene, SCYA2 (encoding JE or MCP-1), to 17q11.2–12: evolutionary relatedness of cytokines clustered at the same locus. *Genomics* 10: 489–492, 1991.

Romagnani, P., Annunziato, F., Piccinni, M. P., Maggi, E., and Romagnani, S.: Cytokines and chemokines in T lymphopoiesis and T-cell effector function. *Immunol Today* 21: 416–418, 2000.

Romagnani, P., Lasagni, L., Annunziato, F., Serio, M., and Romagnani, S.: CXC chemokines: the regulatory link between inflammation and angiogenesis. *Trends Immunol* 25: 201–209, 2004.

Rosenberg, H. F., Bonville, C. A., Easton, A. J., and Domachowske, J. B.: The pneumonia virus of mice infection model for severe respiratory syncytial virus infection: identifying novel targets for therapeutic intervention. *Pharmacol Ther* 105: 1–6, 2005.

Rossi, D., and Zlotnik, A.: The biology of chemokines and their receptors. *Annu Rev Immunol* 18: 217–242, 2000.

Sallusto, F., Lenig, D., Mackay, C. R., and Lanzavecchia, A.: Flexible programs of chemokine receptor expression on human polarized T helper 1 and 2 lymphocytes. *J Exp Med* 187: 875–883, 1998.

Sallusto, F., Mackay, C. R., and Lanzavecchia, A.: Selective expression of the eotaxin receptor CCR3 by human T helper 2 cells. *Science* 277: 2005–2007, 1997.

Samson, M., Soularue, P., Vassart, G., and Parmentier, M.: The genes encoding the human CC-chemokine receptors CC-CKR1 to CC-CKR5 (CMKBR1-CMKBR5) are clustered in the p21.3-p24 region of chromosome 3. *Genomics* 36: 522–526, 1996.

Sato, W., Aranami, T., and Yamamura, T.: Cutting Edge: Human Th17 cells are identified as bearing CCR2+CCR5- phenotype. *J Immunol* 178: 7525–7529, 2007.

Schols, D.: HIV co-receptors as targets for antiviral therapy. *Curr Top Med Chem* 4: 883–893, 2004.

Shan, L., Qiao, X., Oldham, E., Catron, D., Kaminski, H., Lundell, D., Zlotnik, A., Gustafson, E., and Hedrick, J. A.: Identification of viral macrophage inflammatory protein (vMIP)-II as a ligand for GPR5/XCR1. *Biochem Biophys Res Commun* 268: 938–941, 2000.

Steinman, L.: A brief history of T(H)17, the first major revision in the T(H)1/T(H)2 hypothesis of T cell-mediated tissue damage. *Nat Med* 13: 139–145, 2007.

Stephens, J. C., Reich, D. E., Goldstein, D. B., Shin, H. D., Smith, M. W., Carrington, M., Winkler, C., Huttley, G. A., Allikmets, R., Schriml, L., Gerrard, B., Malasky, M., Ramos, M. D., Morlot, S., Tzetis, M., Oddoux, C., di Giovine, F. S., Nasioulas, G., Chandler, D., Aseev, M., Hanson, M., Kalaydjieva, L., Glavac, D., Gasparini, P., Dean, M., et al.: Dating the origin of the CCR5-Δ32 AIDS-resistance allele by the coalescence of haplotypes. *Am J Hum Genet* 62: 1507–1515, 1998.

Struyf, S., De Meester, I., Scharpe, S., Lenaerts, J. P., Menten, P., Wang, J. M., Proost, P., and Van Damme, J.: Natural truncation of RANTES abolishes signaling through the CC chemokine receptors CCR1 and CCR3, impairs its chemotactic potency and generates a CC chemokine inhibitor. *Eur J Immunol* 28: 1262–1271, 1998.

Struyf, S., Menten, P., Lenaerts, J. P., Put, W., D'Haese, A., De Clercq, E., Schols, D., Proost, P., and Van Damme, J.: Diverging binding capacities of natural LD78beta isoforms of macrophage inflammatory protein-1alpha to the CC chemokine receptors 1, 3 and 5 affect their anti-HIV-1 activity and chemotactic potencies for neutrophils and eosinophils. *Eur J Immunol* 31: 2170–2178, 2001.

Tang, J., and Kaslow, R. A.: Polymorphic chemokine receptor and ligand genes in HIV infection. *In* R. Bellamy (ed.): *Susceptibility to Infectious Diseases: The Importance of Host Genetics*, pp. 185–220, Cambridge University Press, Cambridge, 2004.

Tang, J., Rivers, C., Karita, E., Costello, C., Allen, S., Fultz, P. N., Schoenbaum, E. E., and Kaslow, R. A.: Allelic variants of human beta-chemokine receptor 5 (CCR5) promoter: evolutionary relationships and predictable association with HIV-1 disease progression. *Genes Immun* 1: 20–27, 1999.

Tasaki, Y., Fukuda, S., Lio, M., Miura, R., Imai, T., Sugano, S., Yoshie, O., Hughes, A. L., and Nomiyama, H.: Chemokine PARC gene (SCYA18) generated by fusion of two MIP-1alpha/LD78alpha-like genes. *Genomics* 55: 353–357, 1999.

Thelen, M.: Dancing to the tune of chemokines. *Nat Immunol* 2: 129–134, 2001.

Townson, J. R., Barcellos, L. F., and Nibbs, R. J.: Gene copy number regulates the production of the human chemokine CCL3-L1. *Eur J Immunol* 32: 3016–3026, 2002.

Trkola, A., Ketas, T. J., Nagashima, K. A., Zhao, L., Cilliers, T., Morris, L., Moore, J. P., Maddon, P. J., and Olson, W. C.: Potent, broad-spectrum inhibition of human immunodeficiency virus type 1 by the CCR5 monoclonal antibody PRO 140. *J Virol* 75: 579–88, 2001.

Trkola, A., Kuhmann, S. E., Strizki, J. M., Maxwell, E., Ketas, T., Morgan, T., Pugach, P., Xu, S., Wojcik, L., Tagat, J., Palani, A., Shapiro, S., Clader, J. W., McCombie, S., Reyes, G. R., Baroudy, B. M., and Moore, J. P.: HIV-1 escape from a small molecule, CCR5-specific entry inhibitor does not involve CXCR4 use. *Proc Natl Acad Sci USA* 99: 395–400, 2002.

Valdez, H., Purvis, S. F., Lederman, M. M., Fillingame, M., and Zimmerman, P. A.: Association of the CCR5Δ32 mutation with improved response to antiretroviral therapy. *JAMA* 282: 734, 1999.

Van Coillie, E., Proost, P., Van Aelst, I., Struyf, S., Polfliet, M., De Meester, I., Harvey, D. J., Van Damme, J., and Opdenakker, G.: Functional comparison of two human monocyte chemotactic protein-2 isoforms, role of the amino-terminal pyroglutamic acid and processing by CD26/dipeptidyl peptidase IV. *Biochemistry* 37: 12672–12680, 1998.

Veasey, R. S., Springer, M. S., Marx, P. A., Dufour, J., Klasse, P. J., and Moore, J. P.: Protection of macaques from vaginal SHIV challenge by an orally delivered CCR5 inhibitor. *Na Med* 11: 1293–1294, 2005.

Wasmuth, H. E., Werth, A., Mueller, T., Berg, T., Dietrich, C. G., Geier, A., Gartung, C., Lorenzen, J., Matern, S., and Lammert, F.: Haplotype-tagging

RANTES gene variants influence response to anti-viral therapy in chronic hepatitis C. *Hepatology 40*: 327–334, 2004.

Weaver, C. T., Harrington, L. E., Mangan, P. R., Gavrieli, M., and Murphy, K. M.: Th17: an effector CD4 T cell lineage with regulatory T cell ties. *Immunity 24*: 677–688, 2006.

Woitas, R. P., Ahlenstiel, G., Iwan, A., Rockstroh, J. K., Brackmann, H. H., Kupfer, B., Matz, B., Offergeld, R., Sauerbruch, T., and Spengler, U.: Frequency of the HIV-protective CC chemokine receptor 5-Δ32/Δ32 genotype is increased in hepatitis C. *Gastroenterology 122*: 1721–1728, 2002.

Xiang, J., George, S. L., Wunschmann, S., Chang, Q., Klinzman, D., and Stapleton, J. T.: Inhibition of HIV-1 replication by GB virus C infection through increases in RANTES, MIP-1a, MIP-1b, and SDF-1. *Lancet 363*: 2040–2046, 2004.

Zhou, N., Luo, Z., Luo, J., Hall, J. W., and Huang, Z.: A novel peptide antagonist of CXCR4 derived from the N-terminus of viral chemokine vMIP-II. *Biochemistry 39*: 3782–3787, 2000.

PART III

GENETIC DETERMINANTS OF INFECTIOUS DISEASES AND RESPONSE TO VACCINES

18

Immune Deficiency Disorders

Harry W. Schroeder & Janet M. McNicholl

More than 100 primary immunodeficiency syndromes are currently recognized (Rosen, 2001; Glanzmann & Riniker, 1950; Bruton, 1952; Ochs et al, 1999; Buckley, 2002; Conley, 1999). The majority of these disorders result from single gene defects that affect the function of one or more components of the immune system, which includes B cells, T cells, natural killer (NK) cells, phagocytes, complement, and other elements of innate immune system. The presenting complaint is typically a history of recurrent infection, often early in life. Useful Web sites with information on genetic aspects of immunodeficiencies include the Human Gene Mutation Database (www.hgmd.cf.ac.uk) and the Online Mendelian Inheritance of Man database (www.ncbi.nlm.nih.gov/entrez). Other links can be found at these Web sites and at other sites listed in appendix 1.

The primary role of the B cell is to produce antigen-specific immunoglobulin, and the signature of B-cell dysfunction is abnormal, diminished, or absent production of serum or mucosal immunoglobulin. In those

cases marked by a congenital inability to produce immunoglobulin, infections begin soon after maternal immunoglobulin is catabolized to level below that which will afford protection. The infant will then begin to experience otitis media, bronchitis, folliculitis, or, rarely, pneumonia at four to six months of age. For those more common disorders characterized by diminished or abnormal immunoglobulin production, infections and serum immunoglobulin defects may not be observed until puberty, young adulthood, or even old age. Most frequently, the presenting complaint is a history of recurrent pyogenic bacterial infections, infection with certain parasites (e.g., *Giardia lamblia*), and with increased susceptibility to reinfection with viruses. In the absence of IgA, patients suffer an increased incidence of otitis media, sinusitis, bronchitis, and recurrent gastrointestinal discomfort that often manifests as gastrointestinal reflux. In the absence of IgG and IgM, recurrent pneumonia is common. Repeated respiratory infection can lead to bronchiecstasis, pulmonary compromise, and early death. Untreated agammaglobulinemic patients are also at risk for inflammatory arthritis of the large joints. This arthritis may reflect mycoplasma infection. Moderate B-cell disorders can often be clinically controlled with prophylactic antibiotics. Disorders that create severe immunoglobulin deficits are best treated with intravenous infusions of gamma globulin.

T-cell disorders are marked by dysfunction of cell-mediated immunity. Affected patients are at risk for susceptibility to life-threatening opportunistic infections from the time of birth. Severe T-cell disorders tend to require intensive or even heroic therapy, which may range from bone marrow transplantation to thymic transplantation to direct genetic manipulation. Disorders that affect both T cells and B cells are termed severe combined immunodeficiencies (SCID). SCID disorders are uniformly fatal without some form of intensive therapy.

In this overview, primary B-cell deficiencies and the molecular and developmental biology of immunoglobulins are covered in the greatest depth because the most prevalent immunodeficiencies, such as IgA deficiency (IgAD), are of immunoglobulin. Other deficiencies are also discussed, and table 18.1 provides a more extensive list.

Immunoglobulin and Primarily Antibody Deficiencies

Immunoglobulins (Igs) serve as both the receptors and the effectors of the adaptive humoral immune response. As receptors, Igs are able to recognize and distinguish between self and foreign antigens, such as toxins, viruses, and molecules expressed on the surface of pathogenic organisms. As effectors, they can be used to inactivate or eliminate foreign antigens or the cells that bear them (Schroeder, Jr., 2001).

All Igs are heterodimeric proteins composed of two heavy (H) and two light (L) chains (figure 18.1). Each chain consists of a series of globular subunits, or domains, of 110–120 residues. Humans express two types, or classes, of L chains, κ and λ, and five major classes of H chains, μ, γ, α, ε, and δ. Differences in the structure of the region known as the "hinge," which lies between the CH1 and CH2 domains of the γ, δ, and α chains, and the presence of an additional domain in μ and ε chains in place of the "hinge" creates differences in the size, structure, and flexibility of the H chain.

Each H or L chain contains one variable (V) domain followed by one or more constant (C) domains.

V_H and V_L domains pair to form the receptor component of the immunoglobulin. Together, the V_H and V_L domains define the antigen specificity of the antibody. The H chain C domains trigger the effector functions of the antibody. Alternative splicing allows each H chain gene to form either a secretory or a membrane-bound Ig molecule. Soluble antibody effector functions are generally inflammatory reactions that include fixation of complement, activation of complement, and binding of antibody to fragment crystallizable (Fc) receptors on the surface of phagocytes, platelets, mast cells, and other cells of the immune system. The membrane form of the H chain C domain can associate with Igα and Igβ to form the B-cell receptor. Antigen bound to membrane Ig can initiate the various signal transduction events that regulate the development and activity of the B cell.

Each class and subclass of immunoglobulin H chain has a special effector function that allows it to play a specific and sometimes unique role in immunologic defense. IgM is the first antibody to be made during B-cell development. It is the predominant component of the primary humoral immune response. With the aid of the J chain, IgM forms pentamers that avidly fix complement. IgG is the predominant serum antibody in the secondary response to systemic antigens. The four IgG subclasses are numbered in relation to their serum levels relative to each other in healthy individuals, with IgG_1 the most common and IgG_4 the least. Viral antigens tend to elicit IgG_1 and IgG_3 (Skvaril & Schilt, 1984), carbohydrates tend to elicit IgG_2 (Barrett & Ayoub, 1986), and helminthic parasites elicit IgG_4 and IgE (Otteson et al, 1985). Individuals that lack specific subclasses appear more susceptible to specific types of infectious organisms (Preudhomme & Hanson, 1990). For example, deficiency of IgG_2 is associated with susceptibility to infections with encapsulated bacteria such as *Streptococcus pneumoniae* and *Haemophilus influenzae*. IgA is the predominant antibody found on mucosal surfaces and external secretions, including breast milk (Goldblum, 1990). It helps protect the respiratory and gastrointestinal tracts from exogenous organisms and substances. High IgE levels are frequent in parasitic infections. In the presence of antigen, IgE can induce the release of histamine and various other vasoactive substances from mast cells and basophils. In affluent societies, IgE is primarily associated with allergy (Preudhomme & Hanson, 1990). The appearance of IgD on the cell surface is a marker of B-cell maturation.

TABLE 18.1. Primary immunodeficiencies: laboratory and clinical features.

| | | Lymphocytes[a] | | | Cellular Immunity | Humoral Immunity | | | | | |
| | | | | | | Serum Immunoglobulins | | | | Antibody Responses | Common Infections |
	Chromosome/Locus	B*	T*	NK*		M	G	A	E		
Predominantly antibody deficiency											
Autosomal recessive agammaglobulinemia											
Recessive (λ5, Igβ, or BLNK deficiency)	10q23.2, other	−	+	+	+	↓	↓	↓	↓	−	Bacteria, *Giardia lamblia*
Dominant (LRRC8)	9q34	−	+	+	+	↓	↓	↓	↓	−	Bacteria, *Giardia lamblia*
Common variable immune deficiency (CVID)	6p21.3, other	+	+	+	+	↓	↓	↓	↓	+/−	Bacteria, *Giardia lamblia*
Recessive (ICOS, CD19)	2q33, 16p11	+	+	+	+	N/↓	↓	↓	↓?	+/−	–
Dominant (TACI)	17p11	+	+	+	+	↓	↓	↓	↓	+/−	Bacteria, *Giardia lamblia*
Hyper-IgM syndrome											
Activation-induced cytidine deaminase (AID) deficiency	12p13	+	+	+	+	N/↑	↓	↓	↓	+/−	Bacteria
X-linked CD40 ligand deficiency	Xq26	+	+	+	+	N/↑	↓	N/↓	↓	+/−	Bacteria, viruses, fungi, cryptosporidia
X-linked IKK-γ (NEMO) deficiency	Xq28	+	+	+	+	N/↑	↓		↓	+/−	Bacteria, viruses, fungi, cryptosporidia
CD40 deficiency	20q12	+	+	+	+	N/↑	↓	N/↓	↓	+/−	Bacteria, viruses, fungi, cryptosporidia
Uracil-DNA glycolase deficiency	12q23–24.1	+	+	+	+	N/↑	↓	↓	↓	+/−	Bacteria
IgG subclass deficiency	6p21.3, other	+	+	+	+	N	N/↓	N/↓	N	+/−	Bacteria
Selective IgA deficiency (IgAD)	6p21.3	+	+	+	+	N	N	↓	N	+/−	Bacteria, *Giardia lamblia*
X-linked agammaglobulinemia (XLA)	Xq22	−	+	+	+	↓	↓	↓	↓	−	Bacteria, *Giardia lamblia*
Severe combined immunodeficiency (SCID)											
Adenosine deaminase (ADA) deficiency	20q13.11; 21q22	−	−	+		↓	↓	↓	↓	−	Bacteria, viruses, fungi
Artemis deficiency (SCIDA)	10p13	−	−	+		↓	↓	↓	↓	−	Bacteria, viruses, fungi

(continued)

267

TABLE 18.1. (continued)

Chromosome/Locus	Lymphocytes[a]			Cellular Immunity	Humoral Immunity						Common Infections
					Serum Immunoglobulins				Antibody Responses		
	B*	T*	NK*		M	G	A	E			
CD45 deficiency 1q31	+	–	–	–	↓	↓	↓	↓	+/–		Bacteria, viruses, fungi
Interleukin-2 receptor γ-chain deficiency (X-linked SCID) Xq13.1	+	–	–	–	N	↓	↓	↓	+/–		Bacteria, viruses, fungi
Interleukin-7 receptor α-chain deficiency 5p13	+	–	+	–	N	↓	↓	↓	+/–		Bacteria, viruses, fungi
Janus-associated kinase 3 (JAK3) deficiency 19p13.1	+	–	–	–	N	↓	↓	↓	+/–		Bacteria, viruses, fungi
Recombinase-activating gene (RAG) deficiency 11p13	–	–	+	–	–	–	–	–	–		Bacteria, viruses, fungi
Reticular dysgenesis	–	–	–	–	–	–	–	–	–		Bacteria, viruses, fungi
TAP1 or –2 deficiency (MHC class I deficiency) 6p21.3	+	+/–	+	–	N	N	N	N	+		Bacteria, viruses, fungi
Primary T-cell deficiency DiGeorge syndrome (congenital thymic aplasia) 22q11.2	+	–	+	–	N	N	N	N	+/–		Bacteria, viruses, fungi
MHC class II deficiency 1q21, 13q14, 16p13, 19p12	+	+/–	+	+	N	↓	↓	↓	+/–		Bacteria, viruses, fungi
Nude syndrome (wing helix nude deficiency) 17	+	–	+	–	N	N/↓	N/↓	N/↓	+/–		Bacteria, viruses, fungi
Purine nucleotide phosphorylase (PNP) deficiency 14q13.1	+	–	+	–	N	↓	↓	↓	+/–		Bacteria, viruses, fungi

Disorder	Chromosomal location										Associated infections
T-cell receptor deficiency (CD3γ or CD3ε deficiency)	11q23	+	+	+	−	N	N	N	N	+/−	Bacteria, viruses, fungi
Zap70 tyrosine kinase deficiency	2q12	+	+/−	+/−	−	N	N/↓	N/↓	N/↓	+/−	Bacteria, viruses, fungi
CD8 deficiency	2q21	+	+/−	+/−	+/−	N	N	N	N	+	Bacteria
Other well-defined immunodeficiency syndromes											
Ataxia telangiectasia (AT)	11q22	+	+	+	+	N/↑	N/↓	↓	↓	+/−	Bacteria
Chediak Higashi syndrome	1q24	+	+	+	−	N	N	N	N	+	Epstein-Barr virus
Complement and component deficiencies	6p21, Xp11.3, other	+	+	+	+	N	N	N	N	+	Bacteria—*Neisseria* species
Hyper-IgE syndrome	4q21	+	+	+	+	N	N	N	↑↑↑	+	Bacteria—*Neisseria* species
Immunodeficiency with thymoma	?	−	+	+	+/−	↓	↓	↓	↓	+/−	Bacteria—*Neisseria* species
Wiskott-Aldrich syndrome (WAS)	Xp11.2	+	+	+	+/−	↓	N	↑	↑	+/−	Bacteria—*Neisseria* species
Interferon-γ receptor deficiency	6q22	+	+	+	+	N	N	N	N	+	Mycobacteria, viruses
Interleukin-12 and interleukin-12 receptor deficiency	5q31, 19p13	+	+	+	+	N	N	N	N	+	Mycobacteria, *Salmonella*
Mannose-binding lectin (MBL) deficiency	10q11	+	+	+	+	N	N	N	N	+	Bacteria—primarily in childhood
Phagocytic defects (CGD, LAD)											
CGD	1q25, 7q11, 16q24, Xp21	+	+	+	+	N	N	N	N	+	Bacteria
LAD1, LAD2	21q22, 11	+	+	+	+	N	N	N	N	+	Bacteria
X-linked lymphoproliferative syndrome	Xq24–25	+	+	+	+	N	N/↓	N/↓	N/↓	+/−	Epstein-Barr virus

[a]B, B cells; NK, natural killer lymphocytes; T, T cells. N indicates normal levels.

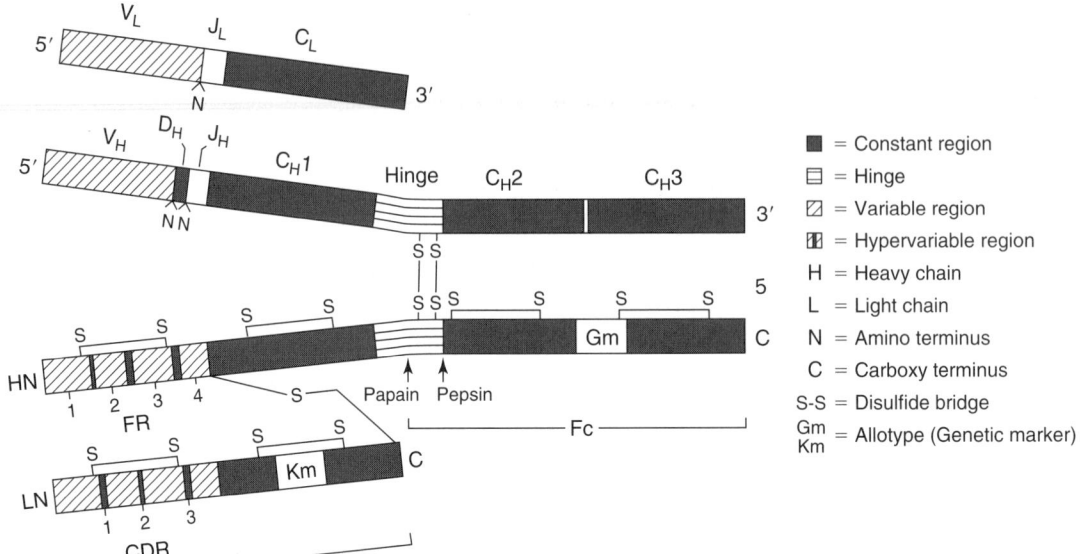

FIGURE 18.1. Two-dimensional model of the immunoglobulin molecule. Immunoglobulins are heterodimeric molecules consisting of two heavy (H) and two light (L) chains. Functionally, each chain can be divided into a variable (V) domain, which engages in antigen binding, and one or more constant (C) domains, which specify effector function. These chains are held together by both intra- and inter-domain cysteine bonds. Digestion with papain or pepsin yields an Fc fragment and either two Fab or one Fab_2 fragment. Some H chains also include a hinge region between the Fc and Fab. (Top) V domains are the product of a complex series of gene rearrangement events. L chain V domains are created by the joining of a V_L to a J_L. H chain V domains include a D_H between the $V_H J_H$. Diversity is enhanced by the insertion of non-germline encoded N nucleotides between these rearranging gene segments. (Bottom) Each V domain includes three complementarity determining regions (CDRs) of highly variable sequence and four framework regions (FRs) of relatively conserved sequence. The three CDRs from the H chain V domain are juxtaposed with the three CDRs from the L chain V domain to form the antigen binding site. The FRs create the scaffold upon which the antigen binding site rests. Polymorphisms in the sequence of the constant domain can be recognized serologically. For κ-light chains, these are identified as Km variants and for IgG these are identified as Gm variants.

Immunoglobulins Genes Are Manufactured

Immunoglobulin variable domains are created by a unique genetic mechanism involving site-directed recombination and rearrangement of individual variable (V), diversity (D), and joining (J) gene segments. Each of these gene segments is flanked by one or two recombination signal sequences. Early in B-cell development in $CD19^+$ pro-B cells, the recombination-activating genes (*RAG1* and *RAG2*) catalyze rearrangement of one of 27 D_H gene segments to one of six JH gene segments. Subsequent rearrangement of one of approximately 50 V_H gene segments to the intermediate DJ join creates a complete H chain V domain. The number of V gene segments can vary among individual IgH

alleles. In-frame VDJ rearrangements that do not include termination codons allow translation of μ H chains, whose appearance in the cytoplasm marks the pre–B-cell stage of development. The μ H chain associates with a noncovalently linked pair of Vλ (VpreB) and Cλ (λ5, λ14.1) homologues, and two adapter proteins termed Igα and Igβ. Together, these five chains form the pre–B-cell receptor. Signals sent through the receptor terminate further H chain rearrangement and allow the cell to initiate L chain rearrangement. The κ locus contains approximately 40 Vκ gene segments, five Jκ gene segments, and one Cκ domain. The λ locus contains approximately 32 Vκ and four functional Jλ-Cλ units. Should Vκ → Jκ rearrangement fail to yield a functional product, successful rearrangement at the λ locus gives the developing cell an additional opportunity to create a functional membrane-bound IgM molecule, which also associates with Igα and Igβ.

The diversity of the initial antibody repertoire in part reflects the apparently stochastic nature of the rearrangement process whereby fewer than 200 V(D)J gene segments can yield more than 10^8 VDJ–VJ combinations. Additional diversity is introduced at the junctions of the rearranging gene segments. There is considerable imprecision in the site of joining, with terminal loss of nucleotides as well as palindromic gain of terminal sequence (P junctions). The enzyme terminal deoxynucleotidyl transferase (TdT) can also act to introduce nucleotides at random (N addition) between the rearranging gene segments. Together, these junctional processes increase the potential diversity by more than 10^8, yielding a potential initial IgM repertoire in excess of 10^{16} sequences.

B-Cell Development and Exposure to Antigen

The appearance of surface IgM marks the immature B cell, which by means of alternative splicing begins to express IgD as well as IgM. These transitional B cells enter the circulation and travel to the spleen and other peripheral lymphoid organs. Mature IgM^+IgD^+ cells circulate between the spleen, the lymphoid organs, and the bone marrow. These naive B cells have only a limited time to encounter a cognate antigen. Failure to do so leads to programmed death.

Cells that encounter antigens containing repeated subunits, such as the polysaccharides that coat the surface capsule of some bacteria, can differentiate into short-lived Ig-secreting cells producing low-affinity IgM. Cells that encounter a T-dependent antigen, such as a protein or peptide, and receive T-cell help can also proliferate to create germinal centers in the follicles of the peripheral lymphoid organs. B-cell–T-cell interactions involve cell contact through surface proteins such as CD40 and CD40 ligand (CD154) and exposure to cytokines such as interleukin-4 (IL-4) or interferon-λ (IFN-λ). Together these signals can induce transcription of downstream C domain genes and expression of activation-induced cytidine deaminase (AID) (Revy et al, 2000). AID (Revy et al, 2000) and uracil-DNA glycosylase (UNG) (Imai et al, 2003) catalyze nonhomologous recombination between upstream and downstream C domains, allowing the cells to switch production from one class of H chain to another. AID and UNG also

catalyze somatic hypermutation of the V domains, the process underlying affinity maturation of the antibody repertoire. B cells that successfully transit these mutational processes and are competitively selected by their inciting antigen may either develop into long-lived plasma cells or memory B cells. Plasma cells lose the expression of CD19 and Ig on their cell surface.

Human memory B cells gain the ability to express CD27 on their cell surface. On average, 40% of the cells in the blood are $CD27^+$ and are thus presumed to be memory cells. The CD27 molecule belongs to the tumor necrosis factor (TNF) receptor family. The interaction between the CD27 and its ligand (CD70) plays a crucial role in plasma cell differentiation. Another key player in late B-cell differentiation is CD278, the product of *ICOS*. This gene is associated with T-cell reactivation.

Agammaglobulinemia

Agammaglobulinemia in the absence of B cells is the hallmark of loss-of-function mutations in the B-cell receptor or components of its signal transduction pathways. Deletions of Cμ, λ5 (λ14.1), and VpreB, which are components of the pre–B-cell receptor, and deletions of Igα and Igβ have all been associated with failure of B-cell development past the early pro–or pre–B-cell stage. X-linked agammaglobulinemia (XLA) is the best-known example of a loss-of-function mutation of a B-cell receptor signal transduction component, in this case Bruton tyrosine kinase (BTK). All of these mutations abort early B-cell development and are thus marked by the absence of $CD19^+$ cells in the blood. T-cell function in these conditions appears to be normal in that delayed-type hypersensitivity, contact hypersensitivity, and homograft rejection is intact.

X-Linked Agammaglobulinemia

In 1952, Bruton identified a young boy with recurrent bacterial infections and pan-hypogammaglobulinemia. Bruton was the first to show that human gammaglobulin replacement therapy could prevent recurrence of infection in a patient with a B-lymphocyte deficiency.

Diagnosis and Clinical Features

XLA, also known as Bruton agammaglobulinemia, is the prototype for selective B-lymphocyte deficiencies (Smith et al, 1998). Among patients with an early onset of recurrent infections, profound hypogammaglobulinemia, and markedly reduced or absent B cells, greater than 90% have loss-of-function mutations in the src family gene for Bruton tyrosine kinase (BTK) (Conley, 2003). Since BTK is located on the X chromosome at position Xq22, XLA is inherited as a Mendelian X-linked recessive trait. Mutations in BTK prevent pre-B cells from progressing from the pre–B-cell stage to the immature B-cell stage. This severe blockage results in an almost complete absence of B cells in the periphery. With their consequent paucity of plasma cells, these patients usually produce very little immunoglobulin. As noted above, T-cell function appears to be unaffected.

Neonates are protected by placental transfer of maternal IgG immunoglobulins (Zinkernagel, 2001). In addition, breast-fed offspring receive IgA in breast milk. However, the half-life of IgG is about 25 days, and after six months of age, when most of the maternal antibodies have been lost to catabolism, the deficiency manifests clinically.

Laboratory Features

The hallmark of XLA is a profound deficit of both B cells and immunoglobulin, usually extending to all of the immunoglobulin isotypes, IgM, IgG, IgA, IgD, and IgE. BTK is expressed in neutrophils, whose function is usually normal. However, in the face of recurrent infections, XLA patients, like other hypogammaglobulinemic individuals, may suffer from severe neutropenia. Other constituents involved in resistance to infection, including serum complement, T cells and NK cells, are normal. Early detection in neonates at risk for XLA is typically focused on the enumeration of CD19+ B cells and the measurement of the levels of non-IgG immunoglobulin isotypes, particularly IgM and IgA. Reduced expression of neutrophil BTK can be evaluated by flow cytometry (Futatani et al, 1998). In those cases where protein is present but the phenotype suggests XLA, sequence analysis of BTK remains the definitive diagnostic procedure. Many different mutations have been found and these have been collected in a disease-specific database known as BTKbase (Vihinen et al, 1998). As with other X-linked lethal diseases, approximately one-third of sporadic cases are due to de novo mutations. Therefore, definitive diagnosis may require individual mutation analysis.

Pathogens

Boys affected with XLA have infections with pyogenic organisms, including staphylococci, pneumococci, streptococci, and *Haemophilus influenzae*. Purulent otitis media, sinusitis, pneumonia, bacteremia, meningitis, and furunculosis may occur. These infections usually can be controlled with antibiotics, but they tend to recur repeatedly until immunoglobulin replacement is undertaken.

Because of their T-cell integrity, agammaglobulinemic children usually overcome varicella in an ordinary fashion and have no difficulty with mycotic infections. In the absence of immunoglobulin replacement therapy, however, they remain susceptible to measles, mumps, and rubella after vaccination. Recurrent infection with latent viruses, such as herpes zoster, is common. Bronchiectasis may result from incomplete treatment of recurrent pulmonary infections. Chronic mucosal inflammation and scarring in patients with severe bronchiectasis can expand the spectrum of pathogens to include enterococci and gram-negative bacilli, even after gammaglobulin replacement is initiated.

Untreated XLA patients may experience inflammation of the large joints. This arthritis may reflect mycoplasma infection and typically resolves with appropriate antibiotics and gammaglobulin replacement. Other clinical manifestations may include a syndrome resembling dermatomyositis, central nervous system involvement occasionally with a potentially fatal neurologic disease, possibly due to echovirus infection (Wilfert et al, 1977). Gammaglobulin and antiviral therapy can be effective in controlling this latter syndrome.

Other Rare Immunodeficiency Syndromes

Mutations of genes involved in the initial VDJ recombination process, such as the RAG proteins, prevent formation of T cells as well as of B cells and are thus grouped under the rubric of severe combined immune deficiency (see below).

Agammaglobulinemia as well as isolated deficiencies of immunoglobulin classes are also seen in the presence of B cells. Abnormalities in CD40–CD40 ligand (CD154) B-cell–T-cell interaction pathway may disrupt class switching and affinity maturation. IgM can accumulate to 1,000 mg/dl, a level that reflects exaggerated polyclonal responses to antigens and accounts for the designation of hyper-IgM syndrome or hyper-IgM immunodeficiency.

The TNFSF5 gene (encoding CD40L) on the X chromosome explains why loss-of-function mutations here show Mendelian X-linked recessive inheritance

(Kroczek et al, 1994). *CD40* on chromosome 12 accounts for similar mutations with Mendelian autosomal recessive inheritance (Ferrari et al, 2001). The signal transduction cascade triggered by CD40–CD40 ligand interactions proceeds in part through a nuclear factor-κB essential modulator (NEMO). This molecule is encoded by *IKBKG*, also located on the X chromosome and subject to X-linked recessive loss-of-function mutations. Loss of function of any one of these three genes yields a hyper-IgM syndrome that raises susceptibility to opportunistic infections, including *Pneumocystis carinii* pneumonia. Loss of function of these genes in other hematopoietic cells may also lead to thrombocytopenia, neutropenia, and aplastic or hemolytic anemia, in which prognosis may be less favorable than for AID or UNG deficiency, and may require bone marrow transplantation (Duplantier et al, 2001).

AICDA (encoding AID) and *UNG* are located in separate regions of chromosome 12 (table 18.1), leading to autosomal recessive loss of function mutations. Immune deficits in patients with AID are strictly limited to the humoral immune system, but the spectrum of functional loss due to changes in *UNG* is still unclear.

Homozygous deletions of IgG constant domain genes have been observed. Interestingly, most patients with selective IgG subclass deficiencies due to deletion have not reported unusual difficulty with infections.

IgA Deficiency and Common Variable Immune Deficiency

The most common primary humoral immunodeficiencies, selective IgAD and common variable immune deficiency (CVID), are the most poorly understood. Most IgA-deficient individuals have normal serum levels of IgM, normal or elevated levels of IgG, normal cell-mediated immunity, and no undue illness early in life. A minority have other evidence of immune dysfunction, including the inability to generate IgG_2 anticarbohydrate antibodies or frank IgG subclass deficiencies. Among IgAD patients referred to immunology clinics, more than 85% present with recurrent pyogenic infections (Morell et al, 1986). IgA-deficient individuals also have a high incidence of celiac disease, systemic lupus erythematosus, rheumatoid arthritis, and allergies (Burrows & Cooper, 1997). Chronic intermittent diarrhea due to *Giardia lamblia* is a com-

mon problem. Some IgAD patients experience recurrent bronchitis, pneumonia, and even bronchiectasis. These patients may also have deficits in IgG_2 and IgG_4. The Cα gene is typically intact in IgAD, and B cells bearing IgA can be found in the blood.

CVID is the most frequent primary immune deficiency requiring clinical care. This immunodeficiency may appear during childhood, but most patients are diagnosed as adults. It often manifests in the third decade of life (Schroeder, Jr., et al, 2004), typically following some years of recurrent sinusitis and bronchitis. Subsequently, recurrent pneumonia may precipitate presentation to the clinical immunologist. Family studies have documented that susceptibility for CVID is inherited and that the degree of immunoglobulin deficiency may change over time (Schroeder, Jr., et al, 2004; Grimbacher et al, 2003). Normal serum immunoglobulin concentrations may evolve into isolated IgAD and then combined with IgG subclass deficits; these may ultimately progress to frank CVID, either sporadic or familial (Johnson et al, 1997). B-cell numbers are typically in the normal range and B cells bearing IgA and IgG can be observed.

Patients with CVID tend to exhibit a distinctive phenotype characterized by a broad deficiency of immunoglobulin isotypes despite the presence of normal numbers of surface immunoglobulin bearing B cells. Most are IgA deficient and, by definition, have serum IgG levels of less than 500 mg/dl. Some IgG subclasses may be more affected than others, with the sequential order of involvement being $IgG_4 > IgG_2 > IgG_1 > IgG_3$. Most CVID patients are also deficient in IgM and IgE. Cell-mediated immunity is usually normal, although dysfunction of T cells (Sneller et al, 1993) and other hematopoietic cell types (Belickova et al, 1994) has been described.

Many CVID patients show failure of affinity maturation and a paucity of circulating memory B cells. These observations suggest that CVID and IgAD are likely disorders of late B-cell regulation. Recently, a series of apparently monogenic disorders has been identified as causing the CVID phenotype. These include a homozygous or heterozygous loss-of-function mutation in TACI, an important growth factor for late B-cell development (Castigli et al, 2005; Salzer et al, 2005), a homozygous loss-of-function mutation in CD19, a pan–B-cell marker that is associated with lowering the threshold for B-cell activation (van Zelm et al, 2006), and a homozygous loss-of-function mutation in *ICOS*, a gene associated with T-cell reactivation. These disorders have been shown to be an infrequent cause of adult-onset CVID (Grimbacher et al, 2003).

Polymorphisms and Populations

Selective IgAD is the most frequently recognized primary immunodeficiency in the Americas, Australia, and Europe. The prevalence is approximately 1 in 600 individuals of European ancestry (Burrows & Cooper, 1997). In these same populations, the estimated prevalence of CVID is 1 in 50,000 (Fasth, 1982). The two disorders occur at about 1/20th the frequency in African Americans (Johnson et al, 1997) and even less commonly among Japanese and other Asian populations. IgAD and CVID are often observed in members of the same family. Susceptibility to IgAD and CVID appears to reside in the MHC in most patients of northern European descent. At least two loci have been identified, one near the class II region (Kralovicova et al, 2003) and one near the class I region (de la Concha et al, 2002; Schroeder et al, 1998). Inheritance of all or a portion of two extended MHC haplotypes, HLA–DQ2–DR7–B44 or HLA–DQ2–DR3(17)–B8, is common. Susceptibility appears to be additive.

Therapy

Patients who suffer from the absence of serum immunoglobulin are targeted for prevention and aggressive treatment of infection. Monthly or more frequent intravenous administration of human IgG (IVIG) is usually effective in preventing severe recurrent pyogenic infections, arthritis, and latent viral infections. Additional one-time infusions may improve recovery from a severe breakthrough infection. Excessive fatigue and depression are frequent symptoms when serum immunoglobulin levels become very low.

Therapeutic replacement of mucosal IgA is not currently possible in patients with selective IgAD or agammaglobulinemia. Prophylactic therapy with antibiotics can diminish the frequency and severity of infections, although complete resolution is rarely achieved.

With aggressive prophylactic IVIG, appropriate antibiotic therapy, and annual assessment of pulmonary function, the prognosis for agammaglobulinemic patients is excellent. Severe complications, such as central nervous system infection with echovirus and the dermatomyositis-like syndrome may also be controlled with aggressive treatment (see above).

Severe Combined Immunodeficiency (SCID)

In 1950, Glanzmann and Riniker described two unrelated infants who succumbed to overwhelming infection during the second year of life after a succession of serious infections, including intractable diarrhea, thrush, and a persistent morbilliform rash. Infants with this clinical presentation have a profound lymphopenia and hypo- or agammaglobulinemia. Untreated, this SCID is uniformly fatal.

Family studies soon demonstrated the heterogeneity of SCID, with two common patterns of inheritance, X-linked and autosomal recessive. Increasingly sophisticated definition of the syndromes has disclosed that in some cases only the T cells are absent (termed $T^-B^+NK^+$ SCID), while in others both T and B cells are affected ($T^-B^-NK^+$ SCID). In those with the most severe lymphopenia, NK cells are also absent ($T^-B^-NK^-$ SCID). Due to the need for T-cell help in generating an efficient antibody response against protein antigens, T-cell deficiency impairs immunoglobulin production even when B cells are present.

Common Clinical Features

The complete absence of T-cell function impairs both cell-mediated immunity and humoral immunity. Infections begin early, between three and six months of age. Diarrhea, bronchitis, and pneumonia with failure to thrive are almost universal. They follow opportunistic infection with *Candida albicans*, *Pneumocystis carinii*, adenovirus, respiratory syncytial virus, parainfluenza 3, Epstein-Barr virus, cytomegalovirus, and other agents (Buckley et al, 1997). Extensive moniliasis of the mouth or diaper area that persists beyond the neonatal period is often the first sign of the disease. Stool cultures frequently reveal strains of *Salmonella* or of enteropathic *Escherichia coli*. Lung abscesses may contain *Pseudomonas aeruginosa*.

Affected infants are also at risk from several routine medical interventions. Immunization with attenuated viral or mycobacterial agents can lead to death because the SCID patients are incapable of limiting or overcoming the relatively benign infections. Inoculation with vaccinia virus or bacille Calmette-Guerin can result in a progressive, ultimately fatal infection. Lymphocytes from transfused blood can induce graft-versus-host disease (GVHD), as can maternal lymphoid cells that have traversed the placental barrier. The characteristic maculopapular rash of GVHD may first appear on the face and then spread rapidly, ultimately involving all skin surfaces including the palms and soles. Thrombocytopenia, leukopenia, jaundice, anasarca, and death from hemorrhage may follow.

Laboratory Features

Progressive lymphopenia and virtual absence of $CD3^+$ cells are characteristic. The rare mature T cells are usually of maternal origin (Reinherz et al, 1981). In affected neonates, lymphocyte counts may begin at normal neonatal levels but decline dramatically. Generation of B cells and NK cells may also lead to variation of lymphocyte counts in SCID patients. Accordingly, a single normal lymphocyte count in newborn peripheral blood cannot exclude the diagnosis of SCID. Platelet and neutrophil counts are typically in the normal range, but eosinophilia is common.

Abnormalities in lymphoid organs include (1) deficiency of bone marrow plasma cells, lymphocytes, and lymphoblasts; (2) a complete lack of germinal center elements, plasma cells, and lymphocytes in secondary lymphoid organs; (3) rudimentary or absent tonsils and missing lymphoid populations in spleen, appendix, and intestinal tract; and (4) occasional mast cells and eosinophils along with rare, unorganized collections of lymphoid cells in lymph node stromata. Diagnostic lymph node biopsies can introduce infection and should be avoided. The minuscule thymus fails to generate T cells and casts no visible shadow on chest X-ray. Nevertheless, the thymus is capable of generating T cells when bone marrow transplantation or specific gene therapy provides lymphoid progenitors

Patients missing T lymphocytes do not display tuberculin or chemically induced delayed type hypersensitivity, their mononuclear cells are unresponsive to phytohemagglutinin or allogenic stimulation, and they do not reject skin allografts. Those patients with B cells are unable to generate a humoral response to protein antigens, including toxins and viral proteins.

SCID Syndromes and Genetics

Classic X-linked SCID comprises approximately 45% of all cases of SCID (Buckley, 2004). This $T^-B^+NK^+$ SCID is caused by a loss-of-function mutation in *IL2RG*, the gene for the γ chain of the IL-2 receptor (Noguchi et al, 1993) on the X chromosome (table 18.1). This γ chain is also an essential component of

the IL-4, IL-7, IL-9, and IL-15 cytokine receptors. This shared usage led to its designation as the common gamma ($γ_c$) chain. Engagement of the IL-7 receptor is required for T-cell development; hence, absence of the common gamma chain leads to a profound T-cell deficiency. When T cells are activated by IL-7, the $γ_c$ chain is phosphorylated by a tyrosine kinase, JAK3. Non-X-linked deficiency of JAK3, a $T^-B^+NK^+$ SCID (Russell et al, 1994), accounts for approximately 6% of all cases of SCID. A similar proportion (9%) of all cases of SCID are due to autosomally inherited deficiency of the *IL7R*-encoded IL-7 receptor α-chain, also a $T^-B^+NK^+$ SCID (Puel et al, 1998). A ζ-associated protein kinase (ZAP70) associates with the CD3ζ chain of the T-cell receptor/CD3 complex and undergoes tyrosine phosphorylation following TCR stimulation. Loss-of-function mutations in the gene for ZAP70 also lead to a $T^-B^+NK^+$ SCID (Colucci et al, 2002).

About 15% of infants with SCID have a deficiency of the *ADA*-encoded adenosine deaminase (ADA), an aminohydrolase that converts adenosine to inosine and thus plays a major role in DNA synthesis (Giblett et al, 1972) (table 18.1). About 2% of SCID infants have a deficiency of purine nucleoside phosphorylase (PNP) encoded by *NP*. In both ADA and PNP deficiency the accumulation of toxic DNA metabolites, dATP or dGTP, inhibits normal T- and B-lymphocyte development, resulting in a $T^-B^-NK^+$ SCID.

$T^-B^-NK^+$ SCID can also result from mutations in enzymes that are involved in the non-homologous end-joining reactions required for the VDJ joining that creates the variable domains of the T-cell receptors and immunoglobulins. Loss-of-function mutations have been reported in *RAG1* and *RAG2* (~3% of SCID cases), which catalyze VDJ recombination and in *DCLRE1C* (~1% of SCID cases), which encodes ARTEMIS, a DNA repair factor (table 18.1). Missense mutations in *RAG1* and *RAG2* can result in a variant of SCID called Omenn's syndrome, which is characterized by marked erythroderma, hyper-IgE, eosinophilia, and oligoclonal expansion of T cells.

Reticular dysgenesis is one of the rarest and most severe forms of SCID. It is a $T^-B^-NK^-$ SCID characterized by congenital agranulocytosis, lymphopenia, lymphoid hypoplasia, and thymic hypoplasia (Bertrand et al, 2002). There is a complete absence of cellular and humoral immune function in affected newborns. This is a rapidly fatal disorder, unless repaired by bone marrow transplantation. A primary genetic etiology remains uncertain.

Therapy

Untreated infection and malnutrition are lethal for SCID patients. Therapy of SCID has been revolutionized by bone marrow transplantation with MHC-matched and, more recently, haplo-identical donors, coupled with the development of techniques for T-cell depletion (Reisner et al, 1983; Buckley et al, 1999). Because infants with SCID cannot reject allografts, bone marrow transplantation usually does not require pretransplant chemotherapeutic conditioning. Because of the high risk of hospital-acquired infection, patients may be transplanted as outpatients.

The accessibility of lymphoid progenitors has made SCID a model for gene therapy. Success has been achieved in X-linked SCID caused by deficiency of the common γ-chain (Fischer et al, 2002) and ADA deficiency (Muul et al, 2003b), although many pitfalls remain (Muul et al, 2003a).

Primary T-Cell Deficiency Syndromes

Congenital Thymic Aplasia (DiGeorge Syndrome)

During early embryonic development, neural crest cell migration into the third and fourth pharyngeal arches leads to the normal development of the thymus, the parathyroid glands, the outflow vessels of the heart, and facial features including the philtrum of the lip and the tubercles of the ear. Chromosomal deletions (table 18.1) are associated with variable disruption of this process, giving rise to a spectrum of phenotypes that include thymic hypoplasia, parathyroid hypoplasia, cardiac defects (including tetralogy of Fallot, truncus arteriosus, and interrupted aortic arch), cleft palate, and facial anomalies (Perez & Sullivan, 2002). Within this spectrum, DiGeorge syndrome is characterized by hypocalcemia due to parathyroid dysfunction, T-cell lymphopenia due to thymic hypoplasia, and cardiac outflow tract defects. DiGeorge syndrome patients thus often present with neonatal tetany, cardiac defects requiring surgical intervention, and a history of increased susceptibility to viral, fungal, and bacterial infections. Speech delay is also a common finding. The variability of this syndrome is emphasized by the observation that up to one-quarter of the patients with DiGeorge syndrome have an asymptomatic parent with a similar chromosomal deletion (Levy et al, 1997).

A variable amount of parathyroid tissue and thymic tissue may be found in ectopic positions in the neck of DiGeorge syndrome patients. The extent of functioning thymic and parathyroid tissue exercises a strong influence on outcome. For patients with sufficient parathyroid tissue, the hypocalcemia tends to ameliorate with development during the first year of life. Patients have variable numbers of $CD3^+$ T cells in the blood, and the severity of susceptibility to infection correlates with the T-cell level. T-cell numbers in the blood vary from normal in approximately one-fifth of patients to total absence in fewer than 1 in 200 affected individuals. Hypersensitivity to common antigens, such as *Candida* or *Trichophyton*, is often delayed or impaired. Skin allograft rejection is abnormally delayed or absent and lymphocyte responses to stimulation with mitogens or allogenic cells are impaired.

Management of the immunodeficiency in DiGeorge syndrome is heavily influenced by the clinical spectrum of symptoms. No therapy is necessary in these patients with only moderately impaired thymic function. In DiGeorge syndrome patients who have T cells, the bone marrow and secondary lymphoid organs may contain normal numbers of germinal centers and plasma cells. Antibody responses to many antigens may be preserved, and serum immunoglobulins levels are usually normal. At the other end of the spectrum, patients with severely impaired thymic function may require transplantation of thymic epithelial tissue that has been depleted of donor thymocytes (Markert et al, 1999).

MHC Class II Deficiency

Patients with MHC class II deficiency, or bare lymphocyte syndrome type II, may appear to have normal numbers of T cells and B cells. Closer examination, however, reveals a deficiency of $CD4^+$ T cells. The T-cell deficiency in these patients is typically more obvious in lymphoid tissues than in the circulation. The interaction of CD4 with MHC class II is required for the development and survival of $CD4^+$ T cells. Loss of these molecules can result from deficiency of any one of four promoter binding proteins that are essential for MHC class II gene regulation and expression. They are encoded by *RFXANK* (19p12), *RFX5* (1q21), *RFXAP* (13q14), and *CIITA* (16p13) (Reith & Mach, 2001) (see chapter 5). All four transcription factor disorders are inherited as Mendelian autosomal recessive traits.

These patients have severe and repeated opportunistic infections that are frequently life threatening.

Without adequate numbers of helper CD4$^+$ T cells, their B cells cannot respond appropriately to protein antigens, including toxins and viral peptides. The *in vitro* response of their T cells to mitogens and to allogeneic lymphocytes in mixed lymphocyte cultures is poor, although they may respond normally to anti-CD3 and anti-CD2. Bone marrow transplantation has proven successful in treating patients with this condition.

Deficiency of Transporter ATP-Binding Cassette (TAP) and MHC Class I Function

Transporter ATP-binding cassette (TAP) is a heterodimeric protein composed of TAP1 and TAP2. These subunits are encoded by the closely linked *TAP1* and *TAP2* genes just upstream of the MHC class II locus on chromosome 6. TAP translocates peptides derived from the cytosolic proteosomes into the endoplasmic reticulum to load the MHC class I molecules (see chapter 4). This peptide loading of the MHC class I β-microglobulin complex is required for stabilization of the MHC class I complex and its transport to the cell surface. Loss-of-function mutations in *TAP1* or *TAP2* are therefore associated with a severe deficit in cell surface expression of MHC class I molecules, which has been termed the bare lymphocyte syndrome, type 1. Since the presentation of peptides by MHC class I molecules is required for normal development and function of cytotoxic CD8$^+$ T cells, patients with certain *TAP1* or *TAP2* mutations are deficient in these cells. Affected patients often appear healthy in the first years of life (de la Salle et al, 1999; Moins-Teisserenc et al, 1999) but in late childhood begin to have recurrent respiratory infections that may lead to bronchiectasis. There is currently no satisfactory therapy for these patients beyond appropriate treatment of their infections and the attendant respiratory complications.

Functional Deficiency of Th1 Cells

The production of IFN-γ by effector Th1 cells within the CD4$^+$ T-cell subpopulation is required for effective elimination of intracellular pathogens. IL-12, a heterodimeric cytokine, interacts with its receptor to play a dominant role in directing the development of Th1 cells. IFN-γ is also produced by NK cells and CD8$^+$ T cells. Patients who demonstrate abnormal induction of IFN-γ because of loss-of-function mutations of the *IFNG* gene (12q14) or the genes for the two IFN-γ receptor chains (6q23 and 21q22) exhibit an increased susceptibility to tuberculosis, atypical mycobacteria, and *Salmonella* (Jouanguy et al, 1999; Rossouw et al, 2003). Patients with loss-of-function mutations in either the genes for IL-12 (3p12 and 5q31) or the gene for the IL-12 receptor β-1 chain (19p13) have similar types of infections. Patients suffering from these infections usually respond well to the appropriate antimicrobial therapy. A detailed overview of the pathogenesis and molecular genetics of these syndromes can be found in chapter 16.

Other Well-Defined Immunodeficiency Syndromes

Ataxia Telangiectasia (AT)

Ataxia telangiectasia (AT) is an autosomal recessive disease that results from mutations in the AT mutated gene (*ATM*) on chromosome 11 (table 18.1) (Gatti et al, 1991; Xu, 1999). *ATM* is involved in the repair of double-stranded DNA breaks. AT patients begin to have progressive cerebellar ataxia early in childhood. Affected individuals later develop conjunctival telangiectasias and eventually fatal sinopulmonary infections or lymphoreticular malignancy by the third decade of life. Heterozygous carriers, estimated at 1.4% of the population, also appear to be at increased risk for malignancy.

AT patients may have both humoral and cell-mediated immunodeficiency. Serum IgG$_2$ or IgA levels are reduced or absent in up to 80% of patients. The thymus is uniformly hypoplastic, and the numbers of αβ T cells are low, especially in the secondary lymphoid tissues. Delayed hypersensitivity reactions and skin allograft rejection are compromised as a reflection of their T-cell deficiency. Immunoglobulin replacement and symptomatic measures may offer limited therapeutic benefit.

Wiscott-Aldrich Syndrome (WAS)

Wiskott-Aldrich syndrome (WAS) is characterized by eczema, thrombocytopenia, and recurrent infections (Kirchhausen & Rosen, 1996). The recessive mutation of the gene for WAS protein (*WASP*) on chromosome X is inherited in a Mendelian pattern. WAS patients have a specific inability to respond normally to polysaccharide antigens. Serum IgM levels are usually low, whereas IgG and IgA levels can be normal or elevated.

With increasing age, affected boys become lymphopenic, develop severely impaired cell-mediated immunity, and rarely survive beyond the first decade of life because of overwhelming infections with gram-positive and gram-negative bacteria, viruses, and fungi. WAS patients may also suffer from hemorrhage and lymphoreticular malignancies.

Deficiencies of Complement Components and Mannose-Binding Lectin (MBL)

The role of these soluble plasma proteins and the consequences of their genetically mediated alteration are extensively reviewed in chapters 10 and 11. Deficiency of complement components in both the early (e.g., C2) and later (C5–C9) pathways are associated primarily with bacterial infections, often due to gram-negative pathogens such as *Neisseria meningitidis* and *N. gonorrheae* that cause meningitis. The autosomal recessive C2 deficiency is the most common. Mannose-binding lectin (MBL) deficiency is also associated with bacterial and possibly other infections. The responsible genes appear to be involved more generally in regulating inflammatory responses.

Deficiencies Related to Phagocyte Function

The most widely known defect of neutrophil (phagocyte) function is chronic granulomatous disease (CGD). It is characterized by recurrent granulomatous lesions of skin, lymph nodes, and lungs, but there is also hypergammaglobulinemia and anemia. This X-linked recessive disorder is caused by *CYBB*. There is also an autosomal recessive form of CGD and several other syndromes associated with abnormalities of neutrophil function with varying inheritance. For some of these, the associated gene has been identified; for example, *ITGB2* on chromosome 21 encodes the β-integrin CD18, a deficiency of which is associated with reduced neutrophil adhesion and necrotic infections.

Conclusion and Prospects

Although the exact MHC-linked genetic lesions in the most common forms of primary humoral immune deficiency, IgAD, and CVID have not been determined, their location is known, and they will likely be identified in the near future. These genes may play a greater role in susceptibility to common infections than currently appreciated (Johnston et al, 2006). If so, the extended syndrome of IgAD/CVID could become the most common cause of susceptibility to infection in individuals of northern European descent. Uncovering the key genes, proteins, and their actions has also provided, and will continue to provide, insight into which genes and responses are critical in controlling pathogens of different types. Progress in defining the molecular basis of many of the rare immunodeficiencies has led to new approaches to therapy for patients with these disorders, ranging from gene therapy and transplantation to replacement therapy with the deficient protein or cells. This understanding may also lead to new immune-based therapies for infections of the general population.

References

Barrett, D.J., & Ayoub, E.M. (1986) IgG2 subclass restriction of antibody to pneumococcal polysaccharides. *Clin. Exp. Immunol.*, **63**, 127–134.

Belickova, M., Schroeder, H.W., Jr., Guan, Y.L., Brierre, J., Berney, S., Cooper, M.D., & Prchal, J.T. (1994) Clonal hematopoiesis and acquired thalassemia in common variable immunodeficiency. *Mol. Med.*, **1**, 56–61.

Bertrand, Y., Muller, S.M., Casanova, J.L., Morgan, G., Fischer, A., & Friedrich, W. (2002) Reticular dysgenesis: HLA non-identical bone marrow transplants in a series of 10 patients. *Bone Marrow Transpl.*, **29**, 759–762.

Bruton, O.C. (1952) Agammaglobulinemia. *Pediatrics* **9** 722–728.

Buckley, R.H. (2002) Primary cellular immunodeficiencies. *J. Allergy Clin. Immunol.*, **109**, 747–757.

Buckley, R.H. (2004) A historical review of bone marrow transplantation for immunodeficiencies. *J. Allergy Clin. Immunol.*, **113**, 793–800.

Buckley, R.H., Schiff, R.I., Schiff, S.E., Markert, M.L., Williams, L.W., Harville, T.O., Roberts, J.L., & Puck, J.M. (1997) Human severe combined immunodeficiency: genetic, phenotypic, and functional diversity in one hundred eight infants. *J. Pediatr.*, **130**, 378–387.

Buckley, R.H., Schiff, S.E., Schiff, R.I., Markert, L., Williams, L.W., Roberts, J.L., Myers, L.A., & Ward, F.E. (1999) Hematopoietic stem-cell transplantation for the treatment of severe combined immunodeficiency. *N. Engl. J. Med.*, **340**, 508–516.

Burrows, P.D., & Cooper, M.D. (1997) IgA deficiency. *Adv. Immunol.*, **65**, 245–276.

Castigli, E., Wilson, S.A., Garibyan, L., Rachid, R., Bonilla, F., Schneider, L., & Geha, R.S. (2005) TACI is mutant in common variable immunodeficiency and IgA deficiency. *Nat. Genet.*, **37**(8), 829–834.

Colucci, F., Schweighoffer, E., Tomasello, E., Turner, M., Ortaldo, J.R., Vivier, E., Tybulewicz, V.L., & di Santo, J.P. (2002) Natural cytotoxicity uncoupled from the Syk and ZAP-70 intracellular kinases. *Nat. Immunol.*, **3**, 288–294.

Conley, M.E. (1999) Diagnostic guidelines—an international consensus document. *Clin. Immunol.*, **93**, 189.

Conley, M.E. (2003) Genes required for B cell development. *J. Clin. Invest.*, **112**, 1636–1638.

de la Concha, E.G., Fernandez-Arquero, M., Gual, L., Vigil, P., Martinez, A., Urcelay, E., Ferreira, A., Garcia-Rodriguez, M.C., & Fontan, G. (2002) MHC susceptibility genes to IgA deficiency are located in different regions on different HLA haplotypes. *J. Immunol.*, **169**, 4637–4643.

de la Salle, H., Zimmer, J., Fricker, D., Angenieux, C., Cazenave, J.P., Okubo, M., Maeda, H., Plebani, A., Tongio, M.M., Dormoy, A., & Hanau, D. (1999) HLA class I deficiencies due to mutations in subunit 1 of the peptide transporter TAP1. *J. Clin. Invest.*, **103**, R9-R13.

Duplantier, J.E., Seyama, K., Day, N.K., Hitchcock, R., Nelson, R.P., Jr., Ochs, H.D., Haraguchi, S., Klemperer, M.R., & Good, R.A. (2001) Immunologic reconstitution following bone marrow transplantation for X-linked hyper IgM syndrome. *Clin. Immunol.*, **98**, 313–318.

Fasth, A. (1982) Primary immunodeficiency disorders in Sweden: cases among children, 1974–1979. *J. Clin. Immunol.*, **2**, 86–92.

Ferrari, S., Giliani, S., Insalaco, A., Al Ghonaium, A., Soresina, A.R., Loubser, M., Avanzini, M.A., Marconi, M., Badolato, R., Ugazio, A.G., Levy, Y., Catalan, N., Durandy, A., Tbakhi, A., Notarangelo, L.D., & Plebani, A. (2001) Mutations of CD40 gene cause an autosomal recessive form of immunodeficiency with hyper IgM. *Proc. Natl. Acad. Sci. U.S.A.*, **98**, 12614–12619.

Fischer, A., Hacein-Bey, S., & Cavazzana-Calvo, M. (2002) Gene therapy of severe combined immunodeficiencies. *Nat. Rev. Immunol.*, **2**, 615–621.

Futatani, T., Miyawaki, T., Tsukada, S., Hashimoto, S., Kunikata, Arai, S., Kurimoto, M., Niida, Y., Matsuoka, H., Sakiyama, Y., Iwata, T., Tsuchiya, S., Tatsuzawa, O., Yoshizaki, K., & Kishimoto, T. (1998) Deficient expression of Bruton's tyrosine kinase in monocytes from X-linked agammaglobulinemia as evaluated by a flow cytometric analysis and its clinical application to carrier detection. *Blood*, **91**, 595–602.

Gatti, R.A., Boder, E., Vinters, H.V., Sparkes, R.S., Norman, A., & Lange, K. (1991) Ataxia-telangiectasia: an interdisciplinary approach to pathogenesis. *Medicine*, **70**, 99–117.

Giblett, E.R., Anderson, J.E., Cohen, F., Pollara, B., & Meuwissen, H.J. (1972) Adenosine-deaminase deficiency in two patients with severely impaired cellular immunity. *Lancet*, **2**, 1067–1069.

Glanzmann, E., & Riniker, P. (1950) Essentielle Lymphocytophtose: ein neues Krankeitsbild aus der Sauglingspathologie. *Ann. Paediatr.*, **9**, 722–728.

Goldblum, R.M. (1990) The role of IgA in local immune protection. *J. Clin. Immunol.*, **10**, 64S–70S.

Grimbacher, B., Hutloff, A., Schlesier, M., Glocker, E., Warnatz, K., Drager, R., Eibel, H., Fischer, B., Schaffer, A.A., Mages, H.W., Kroczek, R.A., & Peter, H.H. (2003) Homozygous loss of ICOS is associated with adult-onset common variable immunodeficiency. *Nat. Immunol.*, **4**, 261–268.

Imai, K., Slupphaug, G., Lee, W.I., Revy, P., Nonoyama, S., Catalan, N., Yel, L., Forveille, M., Kavli, B., Krokan, H.E., Ochs, H.D., Fischer, A., & Durandy, A. (2003) Human uracil-DNA glycosylase deficiency associated with profoundly impaired immunoglobulin class-switch recombination. *Nat. Immunol.*, **4**, 1023–1028.

Johnson, M.L., Keeton, L.G., Zhu, Z.-B., Volanakis, J.E., Cooper, M.D., & Schroeder, H.W., Jr. (1997) Age-related changes in serum immunoglobulins in patients with familial IgA deficiency and common variable immunodeficiency (CVID). *Clin. Exp. Immunol.*, **108**, 477–483.

Johnston, D.T, Mehaffey, G., Thomas, J., Young, K.R., Jr., Wiener, H., Li, J., Go, R.C.P., Schroeder, H.W., Jr. (2006) Increased frequency of HLA -B44 in recurrent sino-pulmonary infections (RESPI). *Clin. Immunol.* 119, 346–350.

Jouanguy, E., Doffinger, R., Dupuis, S., Pallier, A., Altare, F., & Casanova, J.L. (1999) IL-12 and IFN-gamma in host defense against mycobacteria and salmonella in mice and men. *Curr. Opin. Immunol.*, **11**, 346–351.

Kirchhausen, T., & Rosen, F.S. (1996) Disease mechanism: unravelling Wiskott-Aldrich syndrome. *Curr. Biol.*, **6**, 676–678.

Kralovicova, J., Hammarstrom, L., Plebani, A., Webster, A.D., & Vorechovsky, I. (2003) Fine-scale mapping at IGAD1 and genome-wide genetic linkage analysis implicate HLA-DQ/DR as a major susceptibility locus in selective IgA deficiency and common variable immunodeficiency. *J. Immunol.*, **170**, 2765–2775.

Kroczek, R.A., Graf, D., Brugnoni, D., Giliani, S., Korthuer, U., Ugazio, A., Senger, G., Mages, H.W., Villa, A., & Notarangelo, L.D. (1994) Defective expression of CD40 ligand on T cells causes "X-linked immunodeficiency with hyper-IgM (HIGM1)." *Immunol. Rev.*, **138**, 39–59.

Levy, A., Michel, G., Lemerrer, M., & Philip, N. (1997) Idiopathic thrombocytopenic purpura in two mothers of children with DiGeorge sequence: a new component manifestation of deletion 22q11? *Am. J. Med. Genet.*, **69**, 356–359.

Markert, M.L., Boeck, A., Hale, L.P., Kloster, A.L., McLaughlin, T.M., Batchvarova, M.N., Douek, D.C., Koup, R.A., Kostyu, D.D., Ward, F.E., Rice, H.E., Mahaffey, S.M., Schiff, S.E., Buckley, R.H., & Haynes, B.F. (1999) Transplantation of thymus tissue in complete DiGeorge syndrome. *N. Engl. J. Med.*, **341**, 1180–1189.

Moins-Teisserenc, H.T., Gadola, S.D., Cella, M., Dunbar, P.R., Exley, A., Blake, N., Baykal, C., Lambert, J., Bigliardi, P., Willemsen, M., Jones, M., Buechner, S., Colonna, M., Gross, W.L., & Cerundolo, V. (1999) Association of a syndrome resembling Wegener's granulomatosis with low surface expression of HLA class-I molecules. *Lancet*, **354**, 1598–1603.

Morell, A., Muehlheim, E., Schaad, U., Skvaril, F., & Rossi, E. (1986) Susceptibility to infections in children with selective IgA- and IgA-IgG subclass deficiency. *Eur. J. Pediatr.*, **145**, 199–203.

Muul, L.M., Tuschong, L.M., Soenen, S.L., Jagadeesh, G.J., Ramsey, W.J., Long, Z., Carter, C.S., Garabedian, E.K., Alleyne, M., Brown, M., Bernstein, W., Schurman, S.H., Fleisher, T.A., Leitman, S.F., Dunbar, C.E., Blaese, R.M., & Candotti, F. (2003a) Persistence and expression of the adenosine deaminase gene for 12 years and immune reaction to gene transfer components: long-term results of the first clinical gene therapy trial. *Blood*, **101**, 2563–2569.

Noguchi, M., Yi, H., Rosenblatt, H.M., Filipovich, A.H., Adelstein, S., Modi, W.S., McBride, O.W., & Leonard, W.J. (1993) Interleukin-2 receptor gamma chain mutation results in X-linked severe combined immunodeficiency in humans. *Cell*, **73**, 147–157.

Ochs, H.D., Smith, C.I.E., & Puck, J.M. (1999) *Primary Immunodeficiency Diseases: A Molecular and Genetic Approach*, Oxford University Press, Oxford.

Otteson, E.A., Skvaril, F., Tripathy, S.P., Poindexter, R.W., & Hussain, R. (1985) Prominence of IgG4 in the IgG antibody response to human filariasis. *J. Immunol.*, **134**, 2707–2712.

Perez, E., & Sullivan, K.E. (2002) Chromosome 22q11.2 deletion syndrome (DiGeorge and velocardiofacial syndromes). [Review] [44 refs]. *Curr. Opin. Pediatr.*, **14**, 678–683.

Preudhomme, J.L., & Hanson, L.A. (1990) IgG subclass deficiency. *Immunodef. Rev.*, **2**, 129–149.

Puel, A., Ziegler, S.F., Buckley, R.H., & Leonard, W.J. (1998) Defective IL7R expression in T(-)B(+)NK(+)

severe combined immunodeficiency. *Nat. Genet.*, **20**, 394–397.

Reinherz, E.L., Cooper, M.D., Schlossman, S.F., & Rosen, F.S. (1981) Abnormalities of T cell maturation and regulation in human beings with immunodeficiency disorders. *J. Clin. Invest.*, **68**, 699–705.

Reisner, Y., Kapoor, N., Kirkpatrick, D., Pollack, M.S., Cunningham-Rundles, S., Dupont, B., Hodes, M.Z., Good, R.A., & O'Reilly, R.J. (1983) Transplantation for severe combined immunodeficiency with HLA-A, B, D, DR incompatible parental marrow cells fractionated by soybean agglutinin and sheep red blood cells. *Blood*, **61**, 341–348.

Reith, W., & Mach, B. (2001) The bare lymphocyte syndrome and the regulation of MHC expression. *Annu. Rev. Immunol.*, **19**, 331–373.

Revy, P., Muto, T., Levy, Y., Geissmann, F., Plebani, A., Sanal, O., Catalan, N., Forveille, M., Dufourcq-Labelouse, R., Gennery, A., Tezcan, I., Ersoy, F., Kayserili, H., Ugazio, A.G., Brousse, N., Muramatsu, M., Notarangelo, L.D., Kinoshita, K., Honjo, T., Fischer, A., & Durandy, A. (2000) Activation-induced cytidine deaminase (AID) deficiency causes the autosomal recessive form of the Hyper-IgM syndrome (HIGM2). *Cell*, **102**, 565–575.

Rosen, F.S. (2001) Immunodeficiency diseases. In *Textbook of Hematology*, 6th edition (ed. by E Beutler, M.A. Lichtman, B.S. Coller, T.J. Kipps, & U. Seligsohn), pp. 977–983. McGraw-Hill, New York.

Rossouw, M., Nel, H.J., Cooke, G.S., van Helden, P.D., & Hoal, E.G. (2003) Association between tuberculosis and a polymorphic NFkappaB binding site in the interferon gamma gene. *Lancet*, **361**, 1871–1872.

Russell, S.M., Johnston, J.A., Noguchi, M., Kawamura, M., Bacon, C.M., Friedmann, M., Berg, M., McVicar, D.W., Witthuhn, B.A., & Silvennoinen, O. (1994) Interaction of IL-2R beta and gamma c chains with Jak1 and Jak3: implications for XSCID and XCID. *Science*, **266**, 1042–1045.

Salzer, U., Chapel, H.M., Webster, A.D., Pan-Hammarstrom, Q., Schmitt-Graeff, A., Schlesier, M., Peter, H.H., Rockstroh, J.K., Schneider, P., Schaffer, A.A., Hammarstrom, L., Grimbacher, B. (2005) Mutations in TNFRSF13B encoding TACI are associated with common variable immunodeficiency in humans. *Nat. Genet.*, **37**(8), 820–828.

Schroeder, H.W., Jr. (2001) Immunoglobulins and their genes. In *Arthritis and Allied Conditions: A Textbook of Rheumatology* (ed. by W. J. Koopman). Williams & Wilkins, Baltimore.

Schroeder, H.W., Jr., Schroeder, H.W., III, & Sheikh, S.M. (2004) The complex genetics of common variable immunodeficiency. *J. Invest. Med.*, **52**, 90–103.

Schroeder, H.W.J., Zhu, Z.B., March, R.E., Campbell, R.D., Berney, SM, Nedospasov, S.A., Turetskaya, R.L., Atkinson, T.P., Go, R.C., Cooper, M.D., & Volanakis, J.E. (1998) Susceptibility locus for IgA deficiency and common variable immunodeficiency in the HLA-DR3, -B8, -A1 haplotypes. *Mol. Med.*, **4**, 72–86.

Skvaril, F., & Schilt, U. (1984) Characterization of the subclass and light chain types of IgG antibodies to rubella. *Clin. Exp. Immunol.*, **55**, 671–676.

Smith, C.I., Backesjo, C.M., Berglof, A., Branden, L.J., Islam, T., Mattsson, P.T., Mohamed, A.J., Muller, S., Nore, B., & Vihinen, M. (1998) X-linked agammaglobulinemia: lack of mature B lineage cells caused by mutations in the Btk kinase. *Springer Semin. Immunopathol.*, **19**, 369–381.

Sneller, M.C., Strober, W., Eisenstein, E., Jaffe, J.S., & Cunningham Rundles, C. (1993) New insights into common variable immunodeficiency. *Ann. Int. Med.*, **118**, 720–730.

van Zelm, M.C., Reisli, I., van der Burg, M., Castano, D., van Noesel, C.J.M., van Tol, M.J.D., Woellner, C., Grimbacher, B., Patino, P.J., van Dongen, J.J.M., & Franco, J.L. (2006). An antibody-deficiency syndrome due to mutations in the CD19 gene. *N. Engl. J. Med.* 354, 1901–1912.

Vihinen, M., Brandau, O., Branden, L.J., Kwan, S.P., Lappalainen, I., Lester, T., Noordzij, J.G., Ochs, H.D., Ollila, J., Pienaar, S.M., Riikonen, P., Saha, B.K., & Smith, C.I.E. (1998) BTKbase, mutation database for X-linked agammaglobulinemia (XLA) *Nucleic Acids Res.*, **26**, 242–247.

Wilfert, C.M., Buckley, R.H., Mohanakumar, T., Griffith, J.F., Katz, S.L., Whisnant, J.K., Eggleston, P.A., Moore, M., Treadwell, E., Oxman, M.N., & Rosen, F.S. (1977) Persistent and fatal central-nervous-system echovirus infections inpatients with agammaglobulinemia. *N. Engl. J. Med.*, **296**, 1485–1489.

Xu, Y. (1999) ATM in lymphoid development and tumorigenesis. *Adv. Immunol.*, **72**, 179–189.

Zinkernagel, R.M. (2001) Maternal antibodies, childhood infections, and autoimmune diseases. *N. Engl. J. Med.*, **345**, 1331–1335.

19

Human Immunodeficiency Virus Type 1 (HIV-1) and Acquired Immunodeficiency Syndrome (AIDS)

Thomas R. O'Brien, Tania Mara Welzel, & Richard A. Kaslow

HIV-1 Infection and AIDS

Epidemiology

HIV-1 appears to have originated in Central Africa sometime in the first half of the twentieth century (Korber et al., 2000). It was almost surely confined there unrecognized for years before it spread to North America, where its cardinal late complications (*Pneumocystis carinii* pneumonia and Kaposi's sarcoma) appeared among homosexual men in 1981 (CDC, 1981). Once HIV-1 was characterized several years later, the extent of the HIV-1 epidemic was recognized.

HIV-1 is most commonly acquired through sexual intercourse but can also be transmitted parenterally (through needles used for transfusion or drug injection) and perinatally from mother to infant. The epidemic is most severe in sub-Saharan Africa, where about three-fourths of worldwide acquired immunodeficiency syndrome (AIDS) deaths have occurred thus far (Piot et al., 2001). Although HIV-1 reached Asia relatively recently, it has spread rapidly (via sexual transmission and injection drug use) in Southeast Asia and India. The infection is also increasing in China, both among injection drug users and in residents of certain rural areas where the virus was transmitted via contaminated blood collection equipment. In North America, Western Europe, and Australia, the HIV-1 epidemic arose initially among homosexual or bisexual men and then spread to injection drug users and some heterosexuals. HIV-1 infection is also a major problem in parts of the Caribbean and Latin America.

HIV-1 Pathogenesis

HIV-1 infects key components of the immune system, especially macrophages and CD4$^+$ T helper lymphocytes. To enter a cell, HIV-1 requires both the CD4 molecule and one of two chemokine co-receptor molecules encoded by genes named for the backbone motif they display: (chemokine [C-C motif] receptor 5, CCR5) and (chemokine [C-X-C motif] receptor 4,

CXCR4) (Dragic et al., 1996, Feng et al., 1996). CCR5 is the major co-receptor for HIV-1 strains that predominate during early infection (Dragic et al., 1996), and CXCR4 is the major co-receptor for the more pathogenic, syncytium-inducing HIV-1 strains that usually emerge later in infection (Feng et al., 1996). Depletion of CD4$^+$ lymphocytes disrupts various elements of host defense and opens the door to the opportunistic infections, cancers, and other AIDS-defining conditions.

Clinical Course

Acute (primary) HIV-1 infection may be marked by nonspecific symptoms such as fever, sore throat, rash, and aching and swollen lymph nodes, as well as very high levels of circulating HIV-1 and decreased CD4$^+$ lymphocytes. About 6–12 weeks after the initial infection, in the vast majority of cases, the host immune response results in decreased viremia and at least a partial rebound in the CD4$^+$ lymphocyte count. However, in that brief interval of intense viral replication, HIV-1 disseminates widely to lymphoid organs, and chronic infection is established. Thereafter, usually for months or years, persistent viral replication steadily damages the immune system. The rate of HIV-1 replication, as reflected by the HIV-1 RNA level, is the most important determinant of the rate of loss of CD4$^+$ lymphocytes and the clinical prognosis (figure 19.1) (O'Brien et al., 1996). A complex interplay of factors, including genetically determined immune mechanisms, govern the host–virus equilibrium (i.e., HIV-1 RNA level and rate of CD4$^+$ cell loss) relatively early in infection and the subsequent disease course. Without effective treatment, almost all HIV-1–infected patients eventually become severely immunosuppressed and succumb to accompanying clinical manifestations, with an average time from infection to the development of AIDS of 9–10 years (Collaborative Group on AIDS Incubation and HIV Survival, 2000).

Treatment

Combinations of antiretroviral drugs effective at suppressing HIV-1 replication by targeting key viral enzymes became more widely available in 1996. From that point forward in time, the occurrence of AIDS in the United States and elsewhere in the developed countries began to decline markedly (Palella et al., 1998). Mortality among HIV-1–infected patients plummeted. Hopes that treatment might altogether eliminate the virus in infected individuals faded with the finding that the virus remains integrated within resting CD4$^+$ lymphocytes despite years of therapy and that the virus inevitably reactivates after treatment is stopped (Finzi et al., 1999). HIV-1–infected patients will therefore likely require life-long treatment. Furthermore, these regimens do not yield lasting viral suppression for all patients; resistance to the most effective drugs can develop. Because current therapies are imperfect, new control measures that act through novel mechanisms are needed. The discovery of the role of chemokine genes in HIV-1 infection was actu-

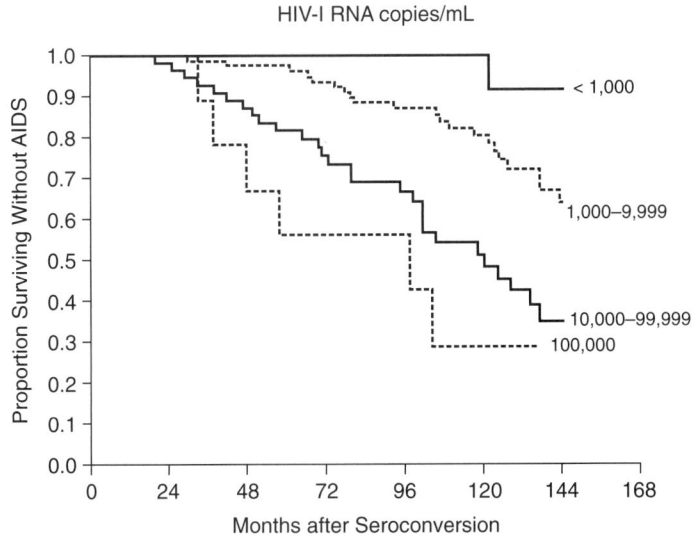

FIGURE 19.1. Proportion of subjects surviving without AIDS, by HIV-1 RNA level, 12–36 months after the estimated date of HIV-1 seroconversion: Multicenter Hemophilia Cohort Study, 1979–1995 (*p*<0.001). (Reprinted from *JAMA*, 1996, 276; 105–110. Copyright © (1996), American Medical Association. All rights reserved.)

ally an impetus for development and implementation of new approaches to therapy. Intense motivation to develop therapeutic as well as preventive vaccines has resulted in meticulous attention to the genetic variation of key human leukocyte antigen (HLA) genes in individuals and in populations (see below).

Molecular Structure and Function of HIV-1

HIV-1 is an RNA virus and a member of the genus *Lentivirus*, family Retroviridae. As a retrovirus, HIV-1 replicates through a double-stranded DNA intermediate by use of a viral reverse transcriptase. The HIV-1 virion contains two copies of the viral genome, and the integrated form of HIV-1 is known as provirus. The four major viral genes (*gag*, *pro*, *pol*, and *env*) encode viral structural proteins. Regulatory proteins and accessory proteins are encoded by other viral genes controlling viral replication and regulating its expression (*tat*, *ref*, *vpr*, *vpu*, *vif*, and *nef*). The viral "negative factor" (nef) can down-regulate CD4 (Garcia and Miller, 1992) and MHC class I expression, particularly human leukocyte antigen-A (HLA-A) and HLA-B molecules (Schwartz et al., 1996); nef can also impair destruction of HIV infected cells by cytotoxic T lymphocytes.

The viral envelope glycoprotein gp160 is translated from a single mRNA and then cleaved into the transmembrane proteins gp41 and gp120, which are located on the virion surface. Gp120 is essential for HIV binding to the CD4 receptor (Landau et al., 1988). The V3 loop sequences of gp120 also interact with CCR5, CXCR4, and, less often, other co-receptors. HIV-1 strains are termed R5, X4, or R5/X4, depending on whether they use one or both of the major co-receptors.

Genetic Determinants

Exploration of the genetic factors driving the occurrence, progression, and clinical manifestations of HIV-1 infection is proceeding rapidly along many paths, and the reports of associations are proliferating. Several classes of host proteins are unequivocally involved in the regulation of viral production, intercellular transmission, and other mechanisms of host–virus interaction (e.g., catalytic mRNA editing enzymes encoded by a family of APOBEC3 genes and a tripartite motif-containing protein called *TRIM5*). However, isolated findings on the impact of polymorphism in these and other candidate human genes require replication or

lack evidence for functional correlation. Genomewide association (GWA) studies of HIV-1 infection are underway.

Chemokine Receptor and Chemokine Genes

Chemokine receptors, including CCR5 and CXCR4 co-receptors mentioned above, are members of the superfamily of seven transmembrane, G-protein-coupled receptors. CCR5 is the natural receptor for three β chemokines, CCL3, -4, and -5 (also known, respectively, as macrophage inflammatory protein [MIP]-1α, MIP-1β, and regulated on activation normal T-cell expressed and secreted [RANTES]) (Shields and Adams, 2002). CXCR4 appears to have a specific relationship with a single chemokine ligand, CXCL12 (also called stromal cell–derived factor-1 [SDF-1]). Other chemokine receptors (e.g., CCR2, CX3CR1) serve as less important HIV-1 co-receptors.

CCR5

The gene that encodes CCR5 is located on the short arm of chromosome 3. The coding region consists of a single open reading frame of 1,055 bp. Soon after the key role of CCR5 in HIV-1 cell entry was reported, several groups found a 32-bp deletion polymorphism (△32) of the *CCR5* gene (Dean et al., 1996, Liu et al., 1996, et al., 1996). A frame shift in this mutant allele results in a protein with a truncated extracellular domain that does not bind chemokines or HIV-1. Homozygotes for the deletion (*CCR5-△32*) express no CCR5; heterozygotes generally express less than people with two functional alleles (Wu et al., 1997). The △32 allele is common in Caucasians of northern European descent (~10–15% allele frequency) but very rare or absent in Asians and Africans. The restricted racial distribution and high frequency of the *CCR5-△32* allele suggest that it arose relatively recently under strong selective pressure, perhaps because it protected against infection by some other lethal agent (Stephens et al., 1998).

Soon after the discovery of the △32 polymorphism, epidemiologic investigations revealed that HIV-1–uninfected persons at high risk of acquiring the virus were considerably more likely to be homozygous for the deletion mutant (Dean et al., 1996, Liu et al., 1996, Samson et al., 1996). Only a handful of HIV-1–infected *CCR5-△32* homozygotes have been reported worldwide (O'Brien et al., 2002). Such high-level resistance to HIV-1 acquisition indicates that CCR5 plays a key role in initiating the infection. Diminished expression of CCR5 on lymphocytes of △32 heterozygotes would predict that those individuals would show a degree of resistance to initial HIV-1 infection, and some studies (Marmor et al., 2001, Philpott et al., 2003, Samson et al., 1996, Tang et al., 2002a), although not all (Dean et al., 1996, O'Brien et al., 1998), have documented such protection. However, heterozygotes for CCR5-△32 who do become infected with HIV-1 are at clear advantage. Compared with wild-type patients, heterozygotes have lower HIV-1 RNA levels and develop AIDS ~25% more slowly (Dean et al., 1996, Ioannidis et al., 2001, Tang et al., 2002a).

Just as the deletion in the CCR5 coding region leads to loss of cell-surface expression of the protein, polymorphism in the promoter region also influences the amount of co-receptor available for attachment of HIV-1, with accompanying clinical consequences. Independent of the CCR5-△32 and the CCR2–64I effects discussed below, a G→A single nucleotide polymorphism (SNP) at position−2459 (previously designated 59029A), most likely in conjunction with other SNPs forming a haplotype from−2733 to−1835

(see below and figure 19.2), is associated with higher viral load and more rapid disease progression when it occurs in the homozygous state among Caucasians (Martin et al., 1998, McDermott et al., 1998).

CCR2

Adjacent to CCR5 on chromosome 3 is CCR2, which encodes a minor HIV-1 co-receptor used by certain HIV-1 strains occasionally appearing late in the course of HIV-1 infection. Although CCR2 is not a key receptor for HIV-1, a common allelic form appears to affect disease prognosis. This polymorphism is a conservative substitution of isoleucine for valine in a transmembrane domain of CCR2 (Smith et al., 1997). Heterozygous Caucasian CCR2–64I carriers have lower levels of HIV-1 viremia and slower progression to AIDS, but the effect has not been quite so uniformly observed in persons of African origin (Ioannidis et al., 2001, Ramaley et al., 2002). The allele frequency of CCR2–64I is about 10% in Caucasians, 15% in African Americans, 17% in Hispanics, and 25% in Asians. In the absence of an important role for CCR2 as a co-

Human Haplotype	CCR2	CCR5							
	46296	58755	58934	59029	59353	59356	59402	59653	62036
A	G	/- A	G	G	T	C	A	C -/	wt
B	-	/- -	T	-	-	-	-	- -/	-
C	-	/- -	T	-	-	-	G	- -/	-
D	-	/- -	T	-	-	T	-	- -/	-
E	-	/- -	-	A	C	-	-	- -/	-
F*1	- (641)	/- -	-	A	C	-	-	T -/	-
F*2	A	/- -	-	A	C	-	-	T -/	-
G*1	-	/- G	-	A	C	-	-	- -/	-
G*2	-	/- G	-	A	C	-	-	- -/	△32
	190	−2733	−2554	−2459	−2135	−2132	−2086	−1835	553-584

FIGURE 19.2. Nine CCR2–CCR5 haplotypes on chromosome 3 (designated human haplotypes A through G*2) after Gonzalez et al. (1999). Nucleotides identical to those in haplotype A are shown as (−). The five-digit numbers (top line) are based on GenBank sequence U95656; three- to four-digit numbers (bottom line) refer to positions relative to the ATCG translation start site in the transcribed CCR2 and CCR5 sequences. Haplotypes are defined by one SNP in CCR2, seven SNPs in the promoter region of CCR5, and a 32-bp deletion in the coding region, designated △32. Haplotypes E, F*1, F*2, G*1, and G*2 include 59029A; haplotype F*2 contains the SNP encoding the CCR2–64V/I polymorphism; and haplotype G*2 contains the 32-bp deletion known as CCR5-△32.

receptor, possible explanations for the CCR2–64I effect include the interaction of the protein product with CCR5 or CXCR4 to decrease expression (Mellado et al., 1999, Sabbe et al., 2001) or linkage disequilibrium with a yet unidentified variant that affects expression of CCR5 (Kostrikis et al., 1998).

Haplotypes in the CCR2–CCR5 Region

The polymorphisms highlighted above lie in close physical proximity on chromosome 3p21 and show strong linkage disequilibrium patterns. The evolution-based classification (figure 19.2) designating nine CCR5-related haplotypes (originally called human haplogroup [HH] A, B, C, D, E, F*1, F*2, G*1, and G*2) are defined by CCR5-△32, CCR5 59029, CCR2–64I, and six additional SNPs (Gonzalez et al., 1999). Investigations in several populations have associated the E haplotype, particularly in the homozygous state, with an unfavorable outcome—both a higher likelihood of infection (Mangano et al., 2001, Tang et al., 2002a) and more rapid progression of disease (Gonzalez et al., 1999, Tang et al., 2002a). Although HIV-1 susceptibility of cells of individuals carrying −2459A, or the E haplotype containing, it has been corroborated experimentally (Kawamura et al., 2003), the precise molecular mechanism by which this combination of variants in CCR5 promoter sequence modulates production of the receptor protein has not been elucidated. Therefore, analysis going beyond the described haplotype relationships to the level of specific genotypic combinations must be interpreted with caution. Genotype effects may be population specific, with persons of European and of African descent showing different associations (Gonzalez et al., 1999), but the likelihood of false-positive results increases with multiple selective analyses of SNP and haplotype combinations in ethnic subgroups. What seems clear is that one or more SNPs in the E promoter haplotype have an effect comparable in magnitude to that of the CCR5 and CCR2 coding-region variants mentioned above, but the relatively high frequencies of E haplotype in all major ethnic groups (28–32% of Caucasians, 13–20% of Africans, and 25–29% of Asians (Gonzalez et al., 2001) imply that it could exert a greater impact at the population level.

CXCR4

The important role of CXCR4 as a co-receptor for more pathogenic X4 HIV-1 strains led to an examination of the gene that codes for this receptor. CXCR4 is highly conserved and the rare variants that have been identified have no apparent functional consequence. Knockout mutations of CXCR4 are lethal in mice (Nagasawa et al., 1996, Zou et al., 1998), which suggests that the gene is essential to normal development.

CX₃CR1

In vitro studies have shown that CX$_3$CR1 (the receptor for the chemokine fractalkine) can act as a co-receptor for certain strains of HIV-1, although its in vivo role appears to be limited. CX$_3$CR1 is located on chromosome 3p21 in the vicinity of the CCR5 and CCR2 genes. Faure et al. (2000) found three haplotypes that involved two altered amino acids (isoleucine-249 and methionine-280) in the coding region of CX$_3$CR1: 249V-280T, 249I-280T, and 249I-280M. Homozygotes for the CX$_3$CR1 249I-280M haplotype had reduced binding for fractalkine in vitro.

Studies attempting to relate these two variants to HIV-1 infection have yielded conflicting data, and their role remains ambiguous. In French patients, homozygosity for the CX$_3$CR1 249I-280M haplotype was associated with increased risk of becoming infected with HIV-1 and with accelerated disease progression after infection occurred (Faure et al., 2000). Furthermore, homozygosity for the 280M variant was rare among HIV-1–seroprevalent subjects in this cohort, which could be consistent with a deleterious selective effect for this genotype (Faure et al., 2003). Another group of investigators failed to find an association between CX$_3$CR1 280M and long term nonprogression, but did find the 249I-280T haplotype in significantly higher frequency among long-term nonprogressors (Vidal et al., 2005b).

On the other hand, several studies have been unable to detect any effects of this haplotype in either direction. McDermott et al. (2000) attempted to confirm these associations in a study of HIV-1–infected men from North America but found no evidence that CX$_3$CR1 genotype was associated with susceptibility to HIV-1 infection or that homozygotes for CX$_3$CR1–280M progressed to AIDS or death faster than subjects who were homozygous for the more common CX$_3$CR1 haplotype. Similarly, Hendel et al. (2001) found no effect of this CX$_3$CR1 polymorphism in a case–control study of AIDS. There was also no evidence for an association between the CX$_3$CR1 polymorphism and the clinical course of HIV infection in the Amsterdam cohort of homosexual men (Kwa et al., 2003).

CCL5

The chemokine RANTES, encoded by *CCL5*, can bind to CCR5 and block infection by R5 HIV-1 strains (Cocchi et al., 1995). Lymphocytes from individuals vary in their secretion of RANTES, and higher levels of RANTES may protect against infection or slow disease progression if infection occurs (Saha et al., 1998). These findings may be mediated through polymorphisms of *CCL5* gene. The−403G/A and−28C/G promoter polymorphisms of this gene did not alter the incidence of HIV-1 infection (Liu et al., 1999; Cocchi et al., 1995), but the−28G allele, which had a frequency of 17% in a Japanese population, was associated with reduced CD4$^+$ lymphocyte depletion rates in HIV-1–infected individuals. Functional analyses indicated that this allele increased transcription of *CCL5*.

McDermott et al. (2000) examined the effect of these promoter polymorphisms among participants in the Multicenter AIDS Cohort Study of American homosexual men. The CCL5−28G variant was much rarer in this cohort, with allele frequencies ranging from 5.7% in Asian Americans to 0.0% in African Americans. The original report could not be confirmed, but these investigators found that those with the−403G/A,−28C/C compound genotype (−403G−28C/−403A−28C diplotype) were more likely to acquire HIV but, paradoxically, less likely to progress to AIDS rapidly (when compared to those with the−403G−28C/−403G−28C diplotype). In a more recent report on disease progression in a Spanish population, no significant effect was observed (Vidal et al., 2006). These studies did not examine regional haplotypes, including an intron SNP that may accelerate the disease process by down-regulating RANTES production (An et al., 2002).

SDF-1 3′A

Stromal cell–derived factor-1 (SDF-1) is the chemokine ligand of CXCR4 (Bjorndal et al., 1997, Lu et al., 1997). Homozygosity for the *SDF-1* 3′A allele, which is found in the 3′ untranslated region of the gene, has been reported to slow disease progression in some studies (Winkler et al., 1998) but not in others (van Rij et al., 1998; Hendel et al., 1998; Mummidi et al., 1998; Vidal et al., 2005a). An international meta-analysis (Ioannidis et al., 2001) found no evidence that *SDF-1* 3′A homozygotes had an altered risk of AIDS, death, or death after AIDS. Reports of relationships have continued to appear, but they have not led to the establishment of any consistent pattern of involvement.

CCL3L1

CCL3 (MIP-1α), a ligand for CCR5, can suppress HIV-1 infection. The *CCL3* gene is subject to segmental duplications and *CCL3L1* represents the duplicated isoforms of the genes encoding CCL3. *CCL3L1* copy number varies both between individuals and between populations. Gonzalez et al. (2005) found that individuals who carry a lower number of *CCL3L1* copies than the population average for their ethnic/racial group had faster progression of HIV-1 infection. This effect was accentuated in individuals who also had an unfavorable *CCR5* genotype. It is unclear why the gene dose relative to the average copy number in each population, rather than the absolute *CCL3L1* copy number, determines the response to HIV-1; however, if this finding is confirmed, it will establish *CCL3L1* copy number as an important consideration in HIV-1 infection and raise the possibility of a wider role for segmental gene duplications in host defense against infectious diseases.

CCL2, CCL7, *and* CCL11

Monocyte chemoattractant protein-1 (MCP-1), MCP-3, and eotaxin all play a role in monocyte recruitment, viral replication, and anti-HIV cytotoxic T-cell responses. Genes for these chemokines (*CCL2*, *CCL7*, and *CCL11*, respectively) are clustered on the long arm of chromosome 17. A haplotype containing two *CCL2*-related SNPs and an SNP in the *CCL11* promoter was found more frequently than expected among uninfected subjects who were repeatedly exposed to HIV-1 through high-risk sexual behavior or contaminated blood products. Because these chemokines are not ligands for CCR5 or CXCR4, any influence they may have on transmission would likely result from activation of the immune system rather than receptor blockage (Modi et al., 2003a).

Chemokine Receptor Gene Polymorphisms as Predictors of Therapeutic Response

Chemokine receptor gene polymorphisms may explain some of the individual differences in response to antiretroviral treatment. Valdez et al. (1999) found that combination therapy reduced the HIV-1 RNA level to low levels in 81% of CCR5-△32 heterozygotes and

57% of wild-type subjects. In a French study, CCR5-△32 heterozygotes had a better virologic and immunologic response to combination therapy at both 6 and 12 months than did wild type patients (Guerin et al., 2000). Another study examined the predictive value of the CCR5-△32, CCR5 59029A, and CCR2–64I polymorphisms among subjects enrolled in a clinical trial of combination therapy (O'Brien et al., 2000). There was a trend toward better response among CCR5-△32 heterozygotes, but stronger evidence was found for the CCR5 promoter allele. Consistent with natural history studies, those who were homozygous for−2459A were less likely to adequately suppress the virus in response to treatment. Polymorphisms in cytokine genes may also predict response to antiviral therapy. In one study, better control of plasma viremia was associated with a variant in the gene IL1A at position−889; this variant is in linkage disequilibrium with a nonsynonymous SNP at IL1A +4845 (Price et al., 2004).

Targeting Chemokine Receptor Expression for Treatment and Prevention

The key roles of CCR5 and CXCR4 in HIV-1 cell entry raise the possibility of treating HIV infection by blocking these chemokine receptors or down-regulating their expression. Several different potential therapeutic approaches have been proposed, including RANTES derivatives (Simmons et al., 1997), low-molecular-weight CCR5 antagonists (Baba et al., 1999), and anti-CCR5 monoclonal antibodies (Trkola et al., 2001). Because blockade of CCR5 might cause selection for more pathogenic X4 HIV-1 strains, a number of potential CXCR4 blockers are also under investigation (Greene, 2004). This approach assumes that CCR5-△32 homozygosity carries no proven deleterious effects and that blockade of CCR5 would be safe. However, a recent report that CCR5 mediates resistance to West Nile virus implies that CCR5-blocking agents could exacerbate the course of those dually infected with this emerging pathogen as well as HIV-1 (Glass et al., 2006).

Other Cytokine Genes

In addition to the chemokines that function as ligands for HIV-1 co-receptors CCR5 or CXCR4, other cytokines may play a role in the response to HIV-1 by stimulating or inhibiting viral replication. A TH2 cytokine profile, determined predominantly by interleukin-4

(IL-4) and IL-10, is associated with a higher rate of HIV-1 replication (Galli et al., 1998) and more advanced HIV-1 infection (Klein et al., 1997, Wasik et al., 1997). Furthermore, IL-4 may also modify viral replication by down-regulating CCR5 and up-regulating CXCR4 (Valentin et al., 1998). The IL-4 gene is located at position 5q31. The IL-4 promoter−589T/T genotype was associated with increased rates of X4 strain acquisition in HIV-1–infected Japanese patients (Nakayama et al., 2000). The−589T allele in either the heterozygous or homozygous state was found to be associated with more favorable clinical course in French and American cohorts (Nakayama et al., 2000, Wang et al., 2004), but that association was not observed in a study based on five HIV-1 cohorts from the United States (Modi et al., 2003b). The IL10 gene lies on the long arm of chromosome 1. Individuals carrying an SNP in the IL10 promoter region (IL10–5′-592A) progressed to AIDS more rapidly than did homozygotes for the alternative (IL10–5′-592C) genotype, particularly in the later stages of HIV-1 infection (Shin et al., 2000). However, this relationship has not been readily reproduced in other HIV-1–infected populations.

HLA

General Considerations

Of the genes so far implicated in HIV/AIDS, the three loci governing the classical class I pathway (HLA-A, -B, and -C) probably have the greatest population impact. Greater detail about the chromosomal organization, physical structure, and functional characteristics of these genes can been found in chapter 4. The enormous polymorphism of the molecules encoded by HLA class I genes are assumed to have developed in response to evolutionary pressure principally from microbial flora that colonize and infect populations and perhaps other local environmental factors (Hughes and Yeager, 1998). In the latest update of the official database, more than 1,400 class I alleles have been catalogued (Marsh et al., 2005), including >700 HLA-B alleles. Only a small fraction of these alleles are present in any specific local population, and each individual in that population has only two at each locus available for the task of recognizing and, when appropriate, attacking cells that display peptides from foreign infectious agents. As elaborated below, the success of this mechanism at controlling HIV-1 infection is transient and rarely complete.

Most studies of class I polymorphisms in HIV/AIDS have concentrated on their ability to control viremia or to determine the rate at which infected individuals deteriorate immunologically or clinically. This review emphasizes those effects. Relatively few investigations have explored the role of these genetic variants in the susceptibility of uninfected hosts, and even less attention has been devoted to the contribution of HLA to late complicating conditions or to the therapeutic response.

Immunopathogenesis: The CD8+ Cytotoxic T-Lymphocyte Response in HIV-1 Evolution and Escape

Among the most thoroughly studied mechanisms available to the host for control of viral replication is the process of stimulation by the antigen-presenting cell (e.g., dendritic cell) and response by a cytotoxic T lymphocyte (CTL). Extensive investigations have now shed considerable light on the dynamic interplay of virus and host class I HLA allele-specific CTL response. Following is a selective summary of the work that has elucidated this process.

The process follows a familiar evolutionary theme: (1) virus encounters a new host immune system, (2) rapid replication and mutation occur under pressure of the individual host class I machinery, (3) host and virus equilibrate on viral replication, (4) escape mutants emerge with replication competence restored (sometimes with the help of nearby compensatory mutations), and (5) newly adapted virus eventually dominates. The evidence for this sequence of events continues to accumulate from studies in primates (Friedrich et al., 2004), as well as humans, particularly from informative cohorts of infected Europeans, Australians, and South Africans infected with HIV-1B, 1B, and 1C, respectively (Allen et al., 2005, Feeney et al., 2005, Leslie et al., 2004, Moore et al., 2002, Pillay et al., 2005). According to this theme, a major proportion of the mutations in nonenvelope sequences from an infected population occur at sites of epitopes for CTLs generated by the HLA alleles prevalent in that population, while another smaller proportion reflect reversion from escape mutations in the absence of HLA pressure (Allen et al., 2005). Escape mutations occur at sites so critical to replication that other specific mutations will compensate; when the CTL pressure is subsequently removed (e.g., by transmission to a new host), the escape mutation may or may not revert to

consensus, but the compensating mutation may remain as a footprint (Leslie et al., 2004).

HLA relationships with absence of a mutation also occur. These "negative" associations are thought to reflect previous HLA-driven mutations that appear to have evolved to consensus and may be detectable only transiently (Leslie et al., 2005). Other variations on the theme continue to be reported; for example, vertically infected infants show patterns of escape that appropriately reflect a joint maternal and paternal HLA contribution (Feeney et al., 2005). These balancing evolutionary forces, in an individual and ultimately in a population, presumably reflect the HLA profile of that population and likely contributed both to the occurrence of the major viral subtypes reflecting founder effects and to the divergence into new strains (circulating recombinant forms) as the pandemic has progressed (Bhattarcharya et al., 2007).

The Role of Individual HLA Class I Alleles

Although dozens of reports describe associations between individual class I alleles and disease control or progression, the findings can be difficult to interpret. Major shortcomings in many of the reports have included (1) assessment of the phenotype (choice of virologic, immunologic, or clinical end point), (2) sample size (low power and unstable effect estimates for many alleles due to the extreme polymorphism), and (3) comparisons across ethnic and HIV-1 subtype boundaries. Nevertheless, the effects of a few alleles have often been consistent enough in larger cohorts to be persuasive, or they have been carefully verified through *ex vivo* immunologic studies. A summary of the alleles whose associations seem more convincing is shown in table 19.1. New additions will undoubtedly occur, particularly for other ethnic groups with distinctive HLA class I profiles and as the prevalent viral quasi species evolves in a given locality.

Two sets of markers have received particular attention and deserve specific comment. Several alleles grouped as the B58 supertype (see below), and most notably B*57, have a protective effect that has been exceptionally strong and uniform in every population studied. Early in the course of infection these protective alleles generate CTL responses to a critical epitope in Gag whose escape mutation seems to be unusually costly to the virus (Leslie et al., 2004).

Another cluster of related alleles, B*35 and B*53, have shown similarly strong deleterious influence on

TABLE 19.1. Replicated associations of HLA class I polymorphism with control and acquisition of HIV-1 infection.

Class I Marker	Disease Control[a]	Acquisition[a]	References
Homozygosity (HLA-A, HLA-B, HLA-C)	Eu−, Af−	Eu0, Af0	(Carrington et al, 1999, Dorak et al, 2004, Keet et al, 1999, Liu et al, 2003, Tang et al, 1999)
A*0205/A*6802	Af+/−	Eu+, Af+/−[b]	(Liu et al, 2003, MacDonald et al, 2001)
A*23	Eu−, Af−	Af−	(Chen et al, 1997, MacDonald et al, 2000, Tang et al, 2002b)
B*13	Af+	Af0	(Honeyborne et al, 2007)
B*18	Af−	Af+, As+	(Beyrer et al, 1999, Farquhar et al, 2004, Kiepiela et al, 2004, MacDonald et al, 2000)
B22 (B*54-*56)	Eu−, As−	—[c]	(Dorak et al, 2003, Hendel et al, 1999, Munkanta et al, 2005)
B*27	Eu+	Eu0	(Hendel et al, 1999, Liu et al, 2003, McNeil et al, 1996)
B*35/*53	Eu+, Af+/−[d]	Eu±, Af0	(Carrington et al, 1999, Hendel et al, 1999, Liu et al, 2003, MacDonald et al, 2000, 2001, Tang et al, 2002c)
B*57	Eu++, Af+	Eu0, Af0	(Hendel et al, 1999, Leslie et al, 2004, MacDonald et al, 2000, 2001, Migueles et al, 2000, Tang et al, 2002b, 2002c)
B*5801	Eu+, Af+	Eu0	(Lazaryan et al, 2006, Leslie et al, 2004, MacDonald et al, 2000, 2001, Trachtenberg et al, 2003)
B*5802	Af−	Af0	(Kiepiela et al, 2004, Lazaryan et al, 2006, MacDonald et al, 2001)
B*8101	Af+	—[c]	(Kiepiela et al, 2004, Lazaryan et al, 2006)
HLA class I allele, HLA-B sharing	Af−	Eu−, Af−[e]	(Dorak et al, 2004, Kiepiela et al, 2004, Lockett et al, 2001, MacDonald et al, 1998)

[a]Disease control is variably assessed among individuals with or without a genetic marker either in survival analysis from early infection to AIDS or a CD4+ cell threshold or in comparisons of differences in plasma HIV-1 RNA concentration or CD4+ cell count. Acquisition is usually assessed either as a comparison of proportions with and without a marker among those at risk or as time from sufficient exposure to infection in those with or without a marker. Eu, Europeans; Af, Africans/African Americans; As, Asians. +, favorable; −, unfavorable; +/−, not uniform for all ethnic groups or viral subtypes; 0, no association reported.

[b]Observations in perinatal and sexual transmission studies have not all yielded consistent results.

[c]Uncertain due to infrequency in Europeans and Africans.

[d]In Caucasian HIV-1B–infected persons, the effect has been attributed to a subset of these closely related alleles that preferentially bind peptides without tyrosine in position 9; in infected persons of African ancestry, the effects of B*53 are not uniform.

[e]Associations with sharing at one or two class I loci have been reported for transmission from mother to infant and for ease of transmission between sex partners; a large study of sex partners showed association with sharing only at the B locus.

Modified and reprinted with permission from Berka, N. and Kaslow, R.A. *Current Opinion in HIV and AIDS*, 2006, Lippincott Williams & Wilkins.

disease control and progression in some but not all European and African cohorts (table 19.1). It has been proposed that the effect is actually confined to certain B*35 as well as B*53 alleles, which prefer motifs with small nonaromatic residues rather than tyrosine at peptide position 9 (Gao et al., 2001). However, for reasons not understood, the disadvantage has not been seen in studies of ample numbers of subtype C–

infected Africans commonly carrying B*53 (Kiepiela et al., 2004, Tang et al., 2002b). An explanation for this discrepancy is eagerly awaited.

Patterns of Class I Allele Involvement

Several broad patterns of involvement are also worth mentioning. First, homozygosity at *HLA-A*, *HLA-B*, or

HLA-C is disadvantageous (Carrington et al., 1999, Keet et al., 1999, Tang et al., 1999), presumably due to the more limited antigen-presenting capacity provided by fewer alleles. Second, the effects of *HLA-B* alleles appear to dominate, elegantly demonstrated through experimental immunologic as well as epidemiologic studies (table 19.1) (Kiepiela et al., 2004). This predominance of B- compared with A- and C-locus effects has been generally recognized in the transplantation setting, and its mechanistic explanation should prove especially instructive for vaccine design. Third, alleles have been categorized in "supertypes" according to similarity in their peptide binding characteristics (Doytchinova et al., 2004, Sette and Sidney, 1999), and a current hypothesis suggests that alleles of uncommon supertypes should be relatively favorable on a population level because the virus has had relatively less opportunity for exposure and adaptation to them. There is evidence for this general pattern of involvement (Scherer et al., 2004, Trachtenberg et al., 2003), but there are exceptions, and how completely the rare supertype advantage holds will depend on the evolving definition of the supertypes.

HLA Class I and Initial Infection

The role of class I molecules in modulating propagation of initial infection has not been extensively studied, and the effects are not as well documented or widely accepted as for disease progression (table 19.1). Perhaps the most striking observation is the discrepancy between the markers of acquisition of the virus and the markers of prognosis. Although class I markers that influence HIV-1 disease progression and viral levels might also affect HIV-1 infectivity, markers common to both have been difficult to demonstrate. In a study of male-to-female HIV-1 transmission, Welzel et al. (2007) found that men who carried *HLA-B* alleles with the Bw4 epitope were less likely to have infected their female sex partners than men who did not carry these alleles. This association of the Bw4 motif with reduced infectivity serves as further evidence that activation of natural killer (NK) cells by interaction between HLA-B ligands and their cognate NK receptors contributes to the control of virus in infected individuals (see below).

Evidence from a few appropriately designed studies suggests that identity of HLA alleles shared between one HIV-1$^+$ and another HIV-1$^-$ partner enhances the risk of infection. Although not observed in every study, the effect has been documented in uninfected sex partners of infected individuals and in infants exposed to infected mothers (Dorak et al., 2004, Kiepiela et al., 2004, Lockett et al., 2001, MacDonald et al., 1998). Allele sharing may even confer a poorer prognosis in the recipient following transmission (Kuhn et al., 2004). A study specifying the disadvantage to sharing of B and not A or C alleles in hastening sexual transmission (Dorak et al., 2004) is consistent with the dominance of the *HLA-B* locus in disease control (see above and figure 19.3). Possible explanations have included

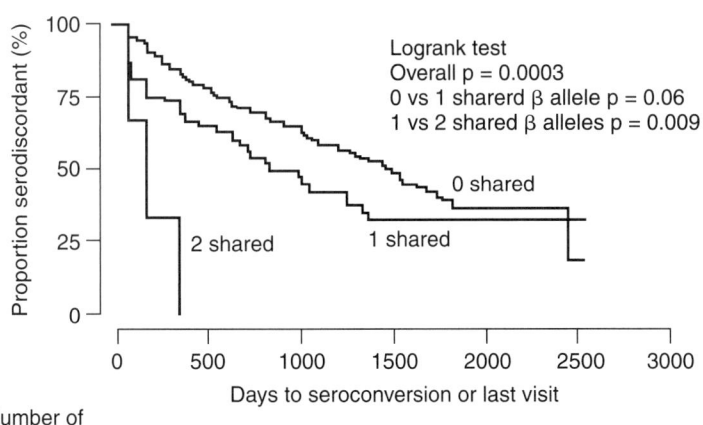

FIGURE 19.3. Kaplan-Meier plot of time to seroconversion of HIV-1–seronegative partners among Zambian couples discordant for HIV-1 infection, according to the number of HLA-B alleles shared between partners. (Reprinted with permission from *Lancet* [Dorak et al., 2004].)

Number of couples at risk

Days	0	300	600	900	1200	1500	1800	2100	2400
2 shared	3	1	0	0	0	0	0	0	0
1 shared	55	40	31	24	17	10	7	4	1
0 shared	171	147	122	96	77	56	36	19	4

both immunologic indifference of the recipient to virus already primed for escape in an HLA-identical donor and less complete alloimmunization of the recipient by donor cells. Beyond corroborating the important role of B-locus polymorphism in controlling HIV-1, this particular investigation re-emphasized that the influence of genetic variation may be less well captured as occurrence or non-occurrence than as a differential effect cumulating over time.

HLA Class I Polymorphism in Natural HIV-1 Infection and Vaccine Response

Many investigators believe that the design and application of efficacious HIV-1 vaccines must take account of the properties of the HLA class I molecular machinery. Distinctive population profiles of class I alleles probably partially account for the different HIV-1 subtypes in populations as a reflection of viral adaptation in each niche where it has propagated. There is minimal evidence that the relationships with individual alleles or the general patterns of involvement described above will modify a vaccine-induced immune response. A study of recombinant HIV-1–canarypox vaccine suggested that B*27 and B*57, the two alleles best known for their protective effects in infected patients (but not highly exposed susceptibles), were also associated with earlier and more exuberant CTL response (Kaslow et al., 2001). However, even vaccines customized for specific class I–mediated response to common viral epitopes may not generate high-level or permanent protection (Altfeld et al., 2005, Betts et al., 2005).

Influence of HLA Class II Genetic Polymorphism on Occurrence and Control of HIV-1 Infection

Antigen presentation and CD4$^+$ T-cell recognition in the class II pathway undoubtedly contributes to HIV-1–specific immune response (Rosenberg et al., 1997). Yet research on the role of class II genetic polymorphism in differential control or progression of HIV-1 infection has yielded rather unconvincing results. Despite similarities across studies (e.g., in apparent advantage of the different alleles of the DR13 gene group), there is little consistency in the population studies and meager support from more direct immunologic investigation (Hendel et al., 1999, Itescu et al., 1995, Keet et al., 1999, Malhotra et al., 2001). Likewise for acquisition of infection, several reports describe differential effects of class II polymorphism, but it is difficult to assess their

significance or draw any general inferences from them (Liu et al., 2004, MacDonald et al., 2000, Tang et al., 2004). The contrast with the unequivocal impact of class I polymorphism on HIV-1 infection and disease is striking. The usual reason given for the failure to detect comparable effects with the two systems is the structural/functional differences between the two types of molecules—the greater plasticity and permissiveness for peptide binding in the class II cleft. However, the fact that class II molecules are capable of binding a larger spectrum of peptides would not explain why their allelic differences would be so difficult to detect for HIV-1 in comparison with their putative effects on other viruses (see chapter 22). This apparent discrepancy may be resolved as ongoing efforts to map epitopes for specific HLA class II molecules mature.

Killer Immunoglobulin-Like Receptor (KIR) Gene Family

Natural killer (NK) cells are components of the innate immune system that respond to viral infections with direct cytotoxic activity and the production of cytokines. NK cell activity is regulated by a variety of receptors (Raulet, 2004), including killer cell immunoglobulin-like receptors (KIRs). The KIR locus on chromosome 19q3 is both highly polygenic and highly polymorphic. As a result, there are many KIR variants, which yield a great variety of receptors (see chapter 9). Different KIRs can stimulate or inhibit NK cell–mediated immune responses.

Some HLA class I molecules are KIR ligands, and KIRs appear to serve a role in the contribution of HLA-B–restricted immune responses in determining the rate of HIV-1 disease progression (Carrington and Martin, 2006). HLA-B alleles can be dichotomized into two serologic groups (Bw4 and Bw6), which are defined by amino acids at positions 79–83 in the heavy chain. HLA-Bw4, but not HLA-Bw6, serves as a KIR ligand. Martin et al. (2002) found that the epistatic interaction between the activating KIR receptor, KIR3DS1, and HLA–B alleles displaying the Bw4 motif with isoleucine at position 80 (HLA-Bw4–80Ile) was associated with delayed progression to AIDS. The presence of HLA-Bw4–80Ile alone did not alter HIV-1 disease progression, but in the absence of Bw4–80Ile, KIR3DS1 was associated with more rapid AIDS progression. These effects have not been replicated elsewhere; however, the same investigative team has made supportive yet seemingly paradoxical observations in a partially independent collection of cohorts of HIV-1-infected individuals (Martin et al., 2007). The alternative form of the *KIR3DS1* gene, *KIR3DL1*, shows further allelic (single nucleotide) variation, and in experimental studies the individual alleles show differential expression upon binding with the Bw4 ligand. In the cohorts excluding carriers of *KIR3DS1*, individuals displaying different combinations of *KIR3DL1* alleles plus the Bw4 motif also showed a range of protection that reflected the allele-specific *in vitro* NK expression and activation. Participants with KIR3DL1*004 and certain other high-expression 3DL1 alleles in combination with HLA-Bw4 showed 1.5 to 2.0-fold lower relative hazards of AIDS as well as correspondingly lower viral loads than did participants with other KIR-HLA combinations. At first pass, this apparent NK "activation" by KIR3DL1 alleles is contrary to what would be expected of a molecule whose structure is thought to confer inhibitory function and presumably diminished NK activity. One explanation offered is that the response is contextual. The level of NK activity under specific stimulatory conditions (i.e., HIV-1 down-regulation of HLA-B expression) is highly dependent on the established underlying balance of inhibitory and activating signals on which the host operates. If the strong inhibitory signal predicted for the *KIR3DL1*-Bw4 under normal conditions is abruptly interrupted, the relatively strong and now unopposed residual activation signals could dominate.

These and other ancillary findings remains to be verified and serve as early milestones on what promises to be a tortuous avenue of inquiry. The elaborate system of KIR and other genes in the chromosome 19 leukocyte receptor complex region coupled with the multifaceted contributions of the HLA region will make HLA–KIR genetic interactions particularly difficult but obviously necessary to disentangle in order to understand fully their contribution to the pathogenesis of HIV/AIDS.

Mannose-Binding Lectin

Mannose-binding lectin (MBL) is a calcium-dependent (C-type) serum lectin that activates complement in response to various infectious agents (Holmskov et al., 2003, Ji et al., 2005). MBL can also directly interact with surface receptors, inducing opsonization and neutralization of pathogens. The *MBL2* gene is located on chromosome 10q (Sastry et al., 1989, Taylor et al., 1989). The products of certain MBL alleles fail to assemble fully functional proteins and, consequently, fail to activate complement. Three *MBL2* variants, located in codons 52, 54, and 57 of exon 1, are associated with MBL deficiencies that impair immunity and increase the risk of various infections (Lipscombe et al., 1992, Madsen et al., 1994, Turner and Hamvas, 2000).

Several epidemiologic studies have addressed the relationship between MBL and HIV transmission or disease progression. Some studies suggest that a person who is homozygous for MBL variants or who has lower MBL levels is more susceptible to HIV-1 infection and more likely to develop AIDS rapidly (Garred et al., 1997, Maas et al., 1998, Pastinen et al., 1998), but other studies failed to confirm these findings (Hundt et al., 2000, Malik et al., 2003, McBride et al., 1998).

Conclusion

The effects of polymorphism in HIV/AIDS have been most convincingly documented for two gene systems: *CCR5* encoding the cell entry co-receptor for HIV-1 and HLA class I genes encoding antigen-presenting molecules. Epidemiologic and experimental evidence for involvement of variants at these two loci is compelling. Caucasians homozygous for a deletion in *CCR5* are at strikingly lower risk of acquiring the infection, while multiple other single markers in that gene and *HLA-B* exert clear but relatively modest influences on occurrence of infection or control of disease. Furthermore, these receptor and antigen-presenting molecules bind ligands (products of CCL and KIR genes) whose polymorphisms also very likely modulate HIV-1 infection. Early epidemiologic indications of interaction between products of polymorphic receptor and ligand genes (e.g., CCR-CCL, HLA-KIR) in HIV/AIDS suggest that epistatic interaction will likely represent a recurrent theme in genetic susceptibility in general. The rapidly replicating retrovirus has already demonstrated successful adaptation to human genetic differences (e.g., in HLA) at both the population level, as reflected in global divergence of HIV-1 subtypes, and at the individual level, as illustrated in CTL escape during propagation from one host to the next. The goal, both for antiretroviral drugs that act more directly on the viral genome and for immunomodulatory agents that exploit human immune response genes, is to raise the cost of successful adaptation beyond what the virus can pay.

References

Allen, T.M., Altfeld, M., Geer, S.C., Kalife, E.T., Moore, C., O'Sullivan K, M., Desouza, I., Feeney, M.E., Eldridge, R.L., Maier, E.L., Kaufmann, D.E., Lahaie, M.P., Reyor, L., Tanzi, G., Johnston, M.N., Brander, C., Draenert, R., Rockstroh, J.K., Jessen, H., Rosenberg, E.S., Mallal, S.A., & Walker, B.D. (2005) Selective escape from CD8$^+$ T-cell responses represents a major driving force of human immunodeficiency virus type 1 (HIV-1) sequence diversity and reveals constraints on HIV-1 evolution. *J Virol*, 79, 13239–13249.

Altfeld, M., Allen, T.M., Kalife, E.T., Frahm, N., Addo, M.M., Mothe, B.R., Rathod, A., Reyor, L.L., Harlow, J., Yu, X.G., Perkins, B., Robinson, L.K., Sidney, J., Alter, G., Lichterfeld, M., Sette, A., Rosenberg, E.S., Goulder, P.J., Brander, C., & Walker, B.D. (2005) The majority of currently circulating human immunodeficiency virus type 1 clade B viruses fail to prime cytotoxic T-lymphocyte responses against an otherwise immunodominant HLA-A2-restricted epitope: Implications for vaccine design. *J Virol*, 79, 5000–5005.

An, P., Nelson, G.W., Wang, L., Donfield, S., Goedert, J.J., Phair, J., Vlahov, D., Buchbinder, S., Farrar, W.L., Modi, W., O'Brien, S.J., & Winkler, C.A. (2002) Modulating influence on HIV/AIDS by interacting RANTES gene variants. *Proc Natl Acad Sci USA*, 99, 10002–10007.

Baba, M., Nishimura, O., Kanzaki, N., Okamoto, M., Sawada, H., Iizawa, Y., Shiraishi, M., Aramaki, Y., Okonogi, K., Ogawa, Y., Meguro, K., & Fujino, M. (1999) A small-molecule, nonpeptide CCR5 antagonist with highly potent and selective anti-HIV-1 activity. *Proc Natl Acad Sci USA*, 96, 5698–5703.

Bhattacharya, T., Daniels, M., Heckerman, D., Foley, B., Frahm, N., Kadie, C., Carlson, J., Yusim, K., McMahon, B., Gaschen, B., Mallal, S., Mullins, J.I., Nickle, D.C., Herbeck, J., Rousseau, C., Learn, G.H., Miura, T., Brander, C., Walker, B., Korber, B. (2007) Founder effects in the assessment of HIV polymorphisms and HLA allele associations. *Science*, 315, 1505–1507.

Betts, M.R., Exley, B., Price, D.A., Bansal, A., Camacho, Z.T., Teaberry, V., West, S.M., Ambrozak, D.R., Tomaras, G., Roederer, M., Kilby, J.M., Tartaglia, J., Belshe, R., Gao, F., Douek, D.C., Weinhold, K.J., Koup, R.A., Goepfert, P., & Ferrari, G. (2005) Characterization of functional and phenotypic changes in anti-Gag vaccine-induced T cell responses and their role in protection after HIV-1 infection. *Proc Natl Acad Sci USA*, 102, 4512–4517.

Beyrer, C., Artenstein, A.W., Rugpao, S., Stephens, H., VanCott, T.C., Robb, M.L., Rinkaew, M., Birx, D.L., Khamboonruang, C., Zimmerman, P.A., Nelson, K.E., Natpratan, C., & Chiang Mai HEPS Working Group (1999) Epidemiologic and biologic characterization of a cohort of human immunodeficiency virus type 1 highly exposed, persistently seronegative female sex workers in northern Thailand. *J Infect Dis*, 179, 59–67.

Bjorndal, A., Deng, H., Jansson, M., Fiore, J.R., Colognesi, C., Karlsson, A., Albert, J., Scarlatti, G., Littman, D.R., & Fenyo, E.M. (1997) Coreceptor usage of primary human immunodeficiency virus type 1 isolates varies according to biological phenotype. *J Virol*, 71, 7478–7487.

Brumme, Z.L., Dong, W.W., Chan, K.J., Hogg, R.S., Montaner, J.S., O'Shaughnessy, M.V., & Harrigan, P.R. (2003) Influence of polymorphisms within the CX3CR1 and MDR-1 genes on initial antiretroviral therapy response. *AIDS*, 17, 201–208.

Carrington, M., & Martin, M.P. (2006) The impact of variation at the KIR gene cluster on human disease. *Curr Top Microbiol*, 298, 225–257.

Carrington, M., Nelson, G.W., Martin, M.P., Kissner, T., Vlahov, D., Goedert, J.J., Kaslow, R., Buchbinder, S., Hoots, K., & O'Brien, S.J. (1999) HLA and HIV-1: Heterozygosity advantage and B*35-Cw*04 disadvantage. *Science*, 283, 1748–1752.

CDC (1981) Kaposi's sarcoma and Pneumocystis pneumonia among homosexual men—New York City and California. *MMWR Morbid Mortal Wkly Rep*, 30, 305–308.

Chen, Y., Winchester, R., Korber, B., Gagliano, J., Bryson, Y., Hutto, C., Martin, N., McSherry, G., Petru, A., Wara, D., & Ammann, A. (1997) Influence of HLA alleles on the rate of progression of vertically transmitted HIV infection in children: Association of several HLA-DR13 alleles with long-term survivorship and the potential association of HLA-A*2301 with rapid progression to AIDS. Long-Term Survivor Study. *Hum Immunol*, 55, 154–162.

Cocchi, F., DeVico, A.L., Garzino-Demo, A., Arya, S.K., Gallo, R.C., & Lusso, P. (1995) Identification of RANTES, MIP-1 alpha, and MIP-1 beta as the major HIV-suppressive factors produced by CD8$^+$ T cells. *Science*, 270, 1811–1815.

Collaborative Group on AIDS Incubation and HIV Survival including the CASCADE EU Concerted Action, Concerted Action on SeroConversion to AIDS and Death in Europe. (2000) Time from HIV-1 seroconversion to AIDS and death before widespread use of highly-active antiretroviral therapy: A collaborative re-analysis. *Lancet*, 355, 1131–1137.

Dean, M., Carrington, M., Winkler, C., Huttley, G.A., Smith, M.W., Allikmets, R., Goedert, J.J., Buchbinder, S.P., Vittinghoff, E., Gomperts, E., Donfield, S., Vlahov, D., Kaslow, R., Saah, A., Rinaldo, C., Detels, R., Hemophilia Growth and Development Study, Multicenter AIDS Cohort Study, Multicenter Hemophilia Cohort Study, San Franscisco Cohort Study, ALIVE Study & O'Brien, S.J. (1996) Genetic restriction of HIV-1 infection and progression to AIDS by a common deletion allele of the chemokine receptor 5 structural gene. *Science*, 273, 1856–1862.

Dorak, M.T., Tang, J., Tang, S., Coutinho, R., Goedert, J., Detels, R., & Kaslow, R.A. (2003) Influence of human leukocyte antigen-B22 alleles on the course of human immunodeficiency virus type 1 infection in 3 cohorts of white men. *J Infect Dis*, 188, 856–863.

Dorak, M.T., Tang, J., Penman-Aguilar, A., Westfall, A.O., Zulu, I., Lobashevsky, E.S., Kancheya, N.G., Schaen, M.M., Allen, S., & Kaslow, R.A. (2004) Transmission of HIV-1 and HLA-B allele-sharing within serodiscordant heterosexual Zambian couples. *Lancet*, 363, 2137–2139.

Doytchinova, I.A., Guan, P., & Flower, D.R. (2004) Identifiying human MHC supertypes using bioinformatic methods. *J Immunol*, 172, 4314–4323.

Dragic, T., Litwin, V., Allaway, G.P., Martin, S.R., Huang, Y., Nagashima, K.A., Cayanan, C., Maddon, P.J., Koup, R.A., Moore, J.P., & Paxton, W.A. (1996) HIV-1 entry into CD4$^+$ cells is mediated by the chemokine receptor CC-CKR-5. *Nature*, 381, 667–673.

Farquhar, C., Rowland-Jones, S., Mbori-Ngacha, D., Redman, M., Lohman, B., Slyker, J., Otieno, P., Obimbo, E., Rostron, T., Ochieng, J., Oyugi, J., Bosire, R., & John-Stewart, G. (2004) Human leukocyte antigen (HLA) B*18 and protection against mother-to-child HIV type 1 transmission. *AIDS Res Hum Retroviruses*, 20, 692–697.

Faure, S., Meyer, L., Costagliola, D., Vaneensberghe, C., Genin, E., Autran, B., Delfraissy, J.F., McDermott, D.H., Murphy, P.M., Debre, P., Theodorou, I., & Combadiere, C. (2000) Rapid progression to AIDS in HIV$^+$ individuals with a structural variant of the chemokine receptor CX3CR1. *Science*, 287, 2274–2277.

Faure, S., Meyer, L., Genin, E., Pellet, P., Debre, P., Theodorou, I., & Combadiere, C. (2003) Deleterious genetic influence of CX3CR1 genotypes on HIV-1 disease progression. *J Acquir Immune Defic Syndr*, 32, 335–337.

Feeney, M.E., Tang, Y., Pfafferott, K., Roosevelt, K.A., Draenert, R., Trocha, A., Yu, X.G., Verrill, C., Allen, T., Moore, C., Mallal, S., Burchett, S., McIntosh, K., Pelton, S.I., St John, M.A., Hazra, R., Klenerman, P., Altfeld, M., Walker, B.D., & Goulder, P.J. (2005) HIV-1 viral escape in infancy followed by emergence of a variant-specific CTL response. *J Immunol*, 174, 7524–7530.

Feng, Y., Broder, C.C., Kennedy, P.E., & Berger, E.A. (1996) HIV-1 entry cofactor: Functional cDNA cloning of a seven-transmembrane, G protein-coupled receptor. *Science*, 272, 872–877.

Finzi, D., Blankson, J., Siliciano, J.D., Margolick, J.B., Chadwick, K., Pierson, T., Smith, K., Lisziewicz, J., Lori, F., Flexner, C., Quinn, T.C., Chaisson, R.E., Rosenberg, E., Walker, B., Gange, S., Gallant, J., & Siliciano, R.F. (1999) Latent infection of CD4$^+$ T cells provides a mechanism for lifelong persistence of HIV-1, even in patients on effective combination therapy. *Nat Med*, 5, 512–517.

Friedrich, T.C., Dodds, E.J., Yant, L.J., Vojnov, L., Rudersdorf, R., Cullen, C., Evans, D.T., Desrosiers, R.C., Mothe, B.R., Sidney, J., Sette, A., Kunstman, K., Wolinsky, S., Piatak, M., Lifson, J., Hughes, A.L., Wilson, N., O'Connor, D.H., & Watkins, D.I. (2004) Reversion of CTL escape-variant immunodeficiency viruses in vivo. *Nat Med*, 10, 275–281.

Galli, G., Annunziato, F., Mavilia, C., Romagnani, P., Cosmi, L., Manetti, R., Pupilli, C., Maggi, E., & Romagnani, S. (1998) Enhanced HIV expression during Th2-oriented responses explained by the opposite regulatory effect of IL-4 and IFN-gamma of fusin/CXCR4. *Eur J Immunol*, 28, 3280–3290.

Gao, X., Nelson, G.W., Karacki, P., Martin, M.P., Phair, J., Kaslow, R., Goedert, J.J., Buchbinder, S., Hoots, K., Vlahov, D., O'Brien, S., & Carrington, M. (2001) Effect of a single amino acid change in MHC class I molecules on the rate of progression to AIDS. *New Engl J Med*, 344, 1668–1675.

Garcia, J.V., & Miller, A.D. (1992) Downregulation of cell surface CD4 by nef. Res Virol, 143, 52–55.

Garred, P., Madsen, H.O., Balslev, U., Hofmann, B., Pedersen, C., Gerstoft, J., & Svejgaard, A. (1997) Susceptibility to HIV infection and progression of AIDS in relation to variant alleles of mannose-binding lectin. *Lancet*, 349, 236–240.

Glass, W.G., McDermott, D.H., Lim, J.K., Lekhong, S., Yu, S.F., Frank, W.A., Pape, J., Cheshier, R.C., Murphy, P.M. (2006) CCR5 deficiency increases risk of symptomatic West Nile virus infection. *J Exp Med*, 203, 35–40.

Gonzalez, E., Bamshad, M., Sato, N., Mummidi, S., Dhanda, G., Catano, G., Cabrera, S., McBride, M., Cao, X.-H., Merrill, G., O'Connell, P., Bowden, D.W., Freedman, B.I., Anderson, S.A., Walters, E.A., Evans, J.S., Stephan, K.T., Clark, R.A., Tyagi, S., Ahuja, S.S., Dolan, M.J., & Ahuja, S.K. (1999) Race-specific HIV-1 disease modifying effects associated with CCR5 haplotypes. *Proc Natl Acad Sci USA*, 96, 12004–12009.

Gonzalez, E., Dhanda, R., Bamshad, M., Mummidi, S., Geevarghese, R., Catano, G., Anderson, S.A., Walter, E.A., Stephan, K.T., Hammer, M.F., Mangano, A., Sen, L., Clark, R.A., Ahuja, S.S., Dolan, M.J., & Ahuja, S.K. (2001) Global survey of genetic variation in CCR5, RANTES, and MIP-1a: Impact on the epidemiology of the HIV-1 pandemic. *Proc Natl Acad Sci USA*, 98, 5199–5204.

Gonzalez, E., Kulkarni, H., Bolivar, H., Mangano, A., Sanchez, R., Catano, G., Nibbs, R.J., Freedman, B.I., Quinones, M.P., Bamshad, M.J., Murthy, K.K., Rovin, B.H., Bradley, W., Clark, R.A., Anderson, S.A., O'Connell R, J., Agan, B.K., Ahuja, S.S., Bologna, R., Sen, L., Dolan, M.J., & Ahuja, S.K. (2005) The influence of CCL3L1 gene-containing segmental duplications on HIV-1/AIDS susceptibility. *Science*, 307, 1434–1440.

Greene, W.C. (2004) The brightening future of HIV therapeutics. *Nat Immunol*, 5, 867–871.

Guerin, S., Meyer, L., Theodorou, I., Boufassa, F., Magierowska, M., Goujard, C., Rouzioux, C., Debre, P., & Delfraissy, J.F. (2000) CCR5 D32 deletion and response to highly active antiretroviral therapy in HIV-1-infected patients. *AIDS*, 14, 2788–2790.

Hendel, H., Caillat-Zucman, S., Lebuanec, H., Carrington, M., O'Brien, S., Andrieu, J.M., Schachter, F., Zagury, D., Rappaport, J., Winkler, C., Nelson, G.W., & Zagury, J.F. (1999) New class I and II HLA alleles strongly associated with opposite patterns of progression to AIDS. *J Immunol*, 162, 6942–6946.

Hendel, H., Henon, N., Lebuanec, H., Lachgar, A., Poncelet, H., Caillat-Zucman, S., Winkler, C.A., Smith, M.W., Kenefic, L., O'Brien, S., Lu, W., Andrieu, J.M., Zagury, D., Schachter, F., Rappaport, J., Zagury, J.F. (1998) Distinctive effects of CCR5, CCR2, and SDF1 genetic polymorphisms in AIDS progression. *J Acquir Immune Defic Syndr Hum Retrovirol*, 19, 381–386.

Hendel, H., Winkler, C., An, P., Roemer-Binns, E., Nelson, G., Haumont, P., O'Brien, S., Khalilli, K., Zagury, D., Rappaport, J., & Zagury, J.F. (2001) Validation of genetic case-control studies in AIDS and application to the CX3CR1 polymorphism. *J Acquir Immune Defic Syndr*, 26, 507–511.

Holmskov, U., Thiel, S., & Jensenius, J.C. (2003) Collections and ficolins: Humoral lectins of the innate immune defense. *Annu Rev Immunol*, 21, 547–578.

Honeyborne, I., Prendergast, A., Pereyra, F., Leslie, A., Crawford, H., Payne, R., Reddy, S., Bishop, K., Moodley, E., Nair, K., van der Stok, M., McCarthy, N., Rousseau, C.M., Addo, M., Mullins, J.I., Brander, C., Kiepiela, P., Walker, B.D., Goulder, P.J.

(2007) Control of human immunodeficiency virus type 1 is associated with HLA-B*13 and targeting of multiple gag-specific CD8+ T-cell epitopes. *J Virol*, 81, 3667–3672.

Hughes, A.L., & Yeager, M. (1998) Natural selection and the evolutionary history of major histocompatibility complex loci. Frontiers in Bioscience, 3, 509–516.

Hundt, M., Heiken, H., & Schmidt, R.E. (2000) Low mannose-binding lectin serum concentrations in HIV long-term nonprogressors? *AIDS Res Hum Retroviruses*, 16, 1927.

Ioannidis, J.P., Rosenberg, P.S., Goedert, J.J., Ashton, L.J., Benfield, T.L., Buchbinder, S.P., Coutinho, R.A., Eugen-Olsen, J., Gallart, T., Katzenstein, T.L., Kostrikis, L.G., Kuipers, H., Louie, L.G., Mallal, S.A., Margolick, J.B., Martinez, O.P., Meyer, L., Michael, N.L., Operskalski, E., Pantaleo, G., Rizzardi, G.P., Schuitemaker, H., Sheppard, H.W., Stewart, G.J., Theodorou, I.D., Ullum, H., Vicenzi, E., Vlahov, D., Wilkinson, D., Workman, C., Zagury, J.F., & O'Brien, T.R. (2001) Effects of CCR5-D32, CCR2-64I and SDF-1 3'A alleles on HIV disease progression: An international meta-analysis of individual-patient data. *Ann Int Med*, 135, 782–795.

Itescu, S., Rose, S., Dwyer, E., & Winchester, R. (1995) Certain HLA-DR5 and -DR6 major histocompatibility complex class II alleles are associated with a CD8 lymphocytic host response to human immunodeficiency virus type 1 characterized by low lymphocyte viral strain heterogeneity and slow disease progression. *Proc Natl Acad Sci USA*, 91, 11472–11476.

Ji, X., Gewurz, H., & Spear, G.T. (2005) Mannose binding lectin (MBL) and HIV. *Mol Immunol*, 42, 145–152.

Kaslow, R.A., Rivers, C.R., Tang J, Bender, T.J., Goepfert, P.A., El Habib, R., Weinhold, K., Mulligan, M.J., & NIAID AIDS Vaccine Evaluation Group (2001) Polymorphisms in HLA class I genes associated with both favorable prognosis of human immunodeficiency virus (HIV) type 1 infection and positive cytotoxic T-lymphocyte responses to ALVAC-HIV recombinant canarypox vaccines. *J Virol*, 75, 8681–8689.

Kawamura, T., Gulden, F.O., Sugaya, M., McNamara, D.T., Borris, D.L., Lederman, M.M., Orenstein, J.M., Zimmerman, P.A., & Blauvelt, A. (2003) R5 HIV productively infects Langerhans cells, and infection levels are regulated by compound CCR5 polymorphisms. *Proc Natl Acad Sci USA*, 100, 8401–8406.

Keet, I.P., Tang, J., Klein, M.R., LeBlanc, S., Enger, C., Rivers, C., Apple, R.J., Mann, D., Goedert, J.J., Miedema, F., & Kaslow, R.A. (1999) Consistent associations of HLA class I and class II and transporter gene products with progression of human immunodeficiency virus-1 infection in homosexual men. *J Infect Dis*, 180, 299–309.

Kiepiela, P., Leslie, A.J., Honeyborne, I., Ramduth, D., Thobakgale, C., Chetty, S., Rathnavalu, P., Moore, C., Pfafferott, K.J., Hilton, L., Zimbwa, P., Moore, S., Allen, T., Brander, C., Addo, M.M., Altfeld, M., James, I., Mallal, S., Bunce, M., Barber, L.D., Szinger, J., Day, C., Klenerman, P., Mullins, J., Korber, B., Coovadia, H.M., Walker, B.D., & Goulder, P.J. (2004) Dominant influence of HLA-B in mediating the potential co-evolution of HIV and HLA. *Nature*, 432, 769–775.

Klein, S.A., Dobmeyer, J.M., Dobmeyer, T.S., Pape, M., Ottmann, O.G., Helm, E.B., Hoelzer, D., & Rossol, R. (1997) Demonstration of the Th1 to Th2 cytokine shift during the course of HIV-1 infection using cytoplasmic cytokine detection on single cell level by flow cytometry. *AIDS*, 11, 1111–1118.

Korber, B., Muldoon, M., Theiler, J., Gao, F., Gupta, R., Lapedes, A., Hahn, B.H., Wolinsky, S., & Bhattacharya, T. (2000) Timing the ancestor of the HIV-1 pandemic strains. *Science*, 288, 1789–1796.

Kostrikis, L.G., Huang, Y., Moore, J.P., Wolinsky, S.M., Zhang, L., Guo, Y., Deutsch, L., Phair, J., Neumann, A.U., & Ho, D.D. (1998) A chemokine receptor CCR2 allele delays HIV-1 disease progression and is associated with a CCR5 promoter mutation. *Nat Med*, 4, 350–353.

Kuhn, L., Abrams, E.J., Palumbo, P., Bulterys, M., Aga, R., Louie, L., & Hodge, T. (2004) Maternal versus paternal inheritance of HLA class I alleles among HIV-infected children: Consequences for clinical disease progression. *AIDS*, 18, 1281–1289.

Kwa, D., Boeser-Nunnink, B., & Schuitemaker, H. (2003) Lack of evidence for an association between a polymorphism in CX3CR1 and the clinical course of HIV infection or virus phenotype evolution. *AIDS*, 17, 759–761.

Landau, N.R., Warton, M., & Littman, D.R. (1988) The envelope glycoprotein of the human immunodeficiency virus binds to the immunoglobulin-like domain of CD4. *Nature*, 334, 159–162.

Lazaryan, A., Lobashevsky, E., Mulenga, J., Karita, E., Allen, S., Tang, J., & Kaslow, R.A. (2006) Human leukocyte antigen B58 supertype and human immunodeficiency virus type 1 infection in native Africans. *J Virol*, 80, 6056–6060.

Leslie, A., Kavanagh, D., Honeyborne, I., Pfafferott, K., Edwards, C., Pillay, T., Hilton, L., Thobakgale, C., Ramduth, D., Draenert, R., Le Gall, S., Luzzi, G., Edwards, A., Brander, C., Sewell, A.K., Moore, S., Mullins, J., Moore, C., Mallal, S., Bhardwaj, N.,

Yusim, K., Phillips, R., Klenerman, P., Korber, B., Kiepiela, P., Walker, B., & Goulder, P. (2005) Transmission and accumulation of CTL escape variants drive negative associations between HIV polymorphisms and HLA. *J Exp Med*, 201, 891–902.

Leslie, A.J., Pfafferott, K.J., Chetty, P., Draenert, R., Addo, M.M., Feeney, M., Tang, Y., Holmes, E.C., Allen, T., Prado, J.G., Altfeld, M., Brander, C., Dixon, C., Ramduth, D., Jeena, P., Thomas, S.A., John, A.S., Roach, T.A., Kupfer, B., Luzzi, G., Edwards, A., Taylor, G., Lyall, H., Tudor-Williams, G., Novelli, V., Martinez-Picado, J., Kiepiela, P., Walker, B.D., & Goulder, P.J. (2004) HIV evolution: CTL escape mutation and reversion after transmission. *Nat Med*, 10, 282–289.

Lipscombe, R.J., Sumiya, M., Hill, A.V., Lau, Y.L., Levinsky, R.J., Summerfield, J.A., & Turner, M.W. (1992) High frequencies in African and non-African populations of independent mutations in the mannose binding protein gene. *Hum Mol Genet*, 1, 709–715.

Liu, C., Carrington, M., Kaslow, R.A., Gao, X., Rinaldo, C.R., Jacobson, L.P., Margolick, J.B., Phair, J., O'Brien, S.J., & Detels, R. (2003) Association of polymorphisms in human leukocyte antigen class I and transporter associated with antigen processing genes with resistance to human immunodeficiency virus type 1 infection. *J Infect Dis*, 187, 1404–1410.

Liu, C., Carrington, M., Kaslow, R.A., Gao, X., Rinaldo, C.R., Jacobson, L.P., Margolick, J.B., Phair, J., O'Brien, S.J., & Detels, R. (2004) Lack of associations between HLA class II alleles and resistance to HIV-1 infection among white, non-Hispanic homosexual men. *J Acquir Immune Defic Syndr*, 37, 1313–1317.

Liu, H., Chao, D., Nakayama, E.E., Taguchi, H., Goto, M., Xin, X., Takamatsu, J., Saito, H., Y Ishikawa, Y., Akaza, T., Juji, T., Takebe, Y., Ohishi, T., Fukutake, K., Maruyama, Y., Yashiki, S., Sonoda, S., Nakamura, T., Nagai, Y., Iwamoto, A., and Shioda, T. (1999) Polymorphism in RANTES chemokine promoter affects HIV-1 disease progression *Proc Natl Acad Sci USA*, 96, 4581–4585

Liu, R., Paxton, W.A., Choe, S., Ceradini, D., Martin, S.R., Horuk, R., MacDonald, M.E., Stuhlmann, H., Koup, R.A., & Landau, N.R. (1996) Homozygous defect in HIV-1 coreceptor accounts for resistance of some multiply-exposed individuals to HIV-1 infection. *Cell*, 86, 367–377.

Lockett, S.F., Robertson, J.R., Brettle, R.P., Yap, P.L., Middleton, D., & Leigh Brown, A.J. (2001) Mismatched human leukocyte antigen alleles protect against heterosexual HIV transmission. *J Acquir Immune Defic Syndr*, 27, 277–280.

Lu, Z., Berson, J.F., Chen, Y., Turner, J.D., Zhang, T., Sharron, M., Jenks, M.H., Wang, Z., Kim, J., Rucker, J., Hoxie, J.A., Peiper, S.C., & Doms, R.W. (1997) Evolution of HIV-1 coreceptor usage through interactions with distinct CCR5 and CXCR4 domains. *Proc Natl Acad Sci USA*, 94, 6426–6431.

Maas, J., de Roda Husman, A.M., Brouwer, M., Krol, A., Coutinho, R., Keet, I., van Leeuwen, R., & Schuitemaker, H. (1998) Presence of the variant mannose-binding lectin alleles associated with slower progression to AIDS. *AIDS*, 12, 2275–2280.

MacDonald, K.S., Embree, J.E., Nagelkerke, N.J., Castillo, J., Ramhadin, S., Njenga, S., Oyug, J., Ndinya-Achola, J., Barber, B.H., Bwayo, J.J., & Plummer, F.A. (2001) The HLA A2/6802 supertype is associated with reduced risk of perinatal human immunodeficiency virus type 1 transmission. *J Infect Dis*, 183, 503–506.

MacDonald, K.S., Embree, J., Njenga, S., Nagelkerke, N.J.D., Ngatia, I., Mohammed, Z., Barber, B.H., Ndinya-Achola, J., Bwayo, J., & Plummer, F.A. (1998) Mother-child class I HLA concordance increases perinatal human immunodeficiency virus type 1 infection. *J Infect Dis*, 177, 551–556.

MacDonald, K.S., Fowke, K.R., Kimani, J., Dunand, V.A., Nagelkerke, N.J.D., Ball, T.B., Oyugi, J., Njagi, E., Gaur, L.K., Brunham, R.C., Wade, J., Luscher, M.A., Hrausa, P., Rowland-Jones, S., Ngugi, E., Bwayo, J.J., & Plummer, F.A. (2000) Influence of HLA supertypes on susceptibility and resistance to human immunodeficiency virus type 1 infection. *J Infect Dis*, 181, 1581–1589.

Madsen, H.O., Garred, P., Kurtzhals, J.A., Lamm, L.U., Ryder, L.P., Thiel, S., & Svejgaard, A. (1994) A new frequent allele is the missing link in the structural polymorphism of the human mannan-binding protein. *Immunogenetics*, 40, 37–44.

Malhotra, U., Holte, S., Dutta, S., Berrey, M.M., Delpit, E., Koelle, D.M., Sette, A., Corey, L., & McElrath, M.J. (2001) Role for HLA class II molecules in HIV-1 suppression and cellular immunity following antiretroviral treatment. *J Clin Invest*, 107, 505–517.

Malik, S., Arias, M., Di Flumeri, C., Garcia, L.F., & Schurr, E. (2003) Absence of association between mannose-binding lectin gene polymorphisms and HIV-1 infection in a Colombian population. *Immunogenetics*, 55, 49–52.

Mangano, A., Gonzalez, E., Dhanda, R., Catano, G., Bamshad, M., Bock, A., Duggirala, R., Williams, K., Mummidi, S., Clark, R.A., Ahuja, S.S., Dolan, M.J., Bologna, R., Sen, L., Ahuja, S.K., & Sen, L. (2001) Concordance between the CC chemokine receptor 5 genetic determinants that alter risks of transmission and disease progression in children exposed perinatally to human immunodeficiency virus. *J Infect Dis*, 183, 1574–1585.

Marmor, M., Sheppard, H.W., Donnell, D., Bozeman, S., Gehm, G., Buchbind, S., Koblin, B.A., Seage, C.R., & HIV Network for Prevention Trials Vaccine Preparedeness Protocol Team. (2001) Homozygous and heterozygous CCR5-D32 genotypes are associated with resistance to HIV infection. *J Acquir Immune Defic Syndr*, 27, 472–481.

Marsh, S.G., Albert, E.D., Bodmer, W.F., Bontrop, R.E., Dupont, B., Erlich, H.A., Geraghty, D.E., Hansen, J.A., Hurley, C.K., Mach, B., Mayr, W.R., Parham, P., Petersdorf, E.W., Sasazuki, T., Schreuder, G.M., Strominger, J.L., Svejgaard, A., Terasaki, P.I., & Trowsdale, J. (2005) Nomenclature for factors of the HLA system, 2004. *Hum Immunol*, 66, 571–636.

Martin, M.P., Dean, M., Smith, M.W., Winkler, C., Gerrard, B., Michael, N.L., Lee, B., Doms, R.W., Margolick, J., Buchbinder, S., Goedert, J.J., O'Rien, T.S., Hilgartner, M.W., Vlahov, D., O'Brien, S., & Carrington, M. (1998) Genetic acceleration of AIDS progression by a promoter variant of CCR5. *Science*, 282, 1907–1911.

Martin, M.P., Gao, X., Lee, J.H., Nelson, G.W., Detels, R., Goedert, J.J., Buchbinder, S., Hoots, K., Vlahov, D., Trowsdale, J., Wilson, M., O'Brien, S.J., & Carrington, M. (2002) Epistatic interaction between KIR3DS1 and HLA-B delays the progression to AIDS. *Nat Genet*, 31, 429–434.

Martin, M.P., Gao, X., Yamada, E., Martin, J.N., Pereyra, F., Colombo, S., Brown, E.E., Shupert, W.L., Phair, J., Goedert, J.J., Buchbinder, S., Kirk, G.D., Telenti, A., Connors, M., O'Brien, S.J., Walker, B.D., Parham, P., Deeks, S.G., McVicar, D.W., Carrington, M. (2007) Innate partnership of HLA-B and KIR3DL1 subtypes against HIV-1. *Nat Genet*, 39, 733–740.

McBride, M.O., Fischer, P.B., Sumiya, M., McClure, M.O., Turner, M.W., Skinner, C.J., Weber, J.N., & Summerfield, J.A. (1998) Mannose-binding protein in HIV-seropositive patients does not contribute to disease progression or bacterial infections. *Int J STD AIDS*, 9, 683–688.

McDermott, D.H., Colla, J.S., Kleeberger, C.A., Plankey, M., Rosenberg, P.S., Smith, E.D., Zimmerman, P.A., Combadiere, C., Leitman, S.F., Kaslow, R.A., Goedert, J.J., Berger, E.A., O'Brien, T.R., & Murphy, P.M. (2000) Genetic polymorphism in CX3CR1 and risk of HIV disease. *Science*, 290, 2031.

McDermott, D.H., Zimmerman, P.A., Guignard, F., Kleeberger, C.A., Leitman, S.F., & Murphy, P.M. (1998) CCR5 promoter polymorphism and HIV-1 disease progression. *Lancet*, 352, 866–870.

McNeil, A.J., Yap, P.L., Gore, S.M., Brettle, R.P., McColl, M., Wyld, R., Davidson, S., Weightman, R., Richardson, A.M., & Robertson, J.R. (1996) Association of HLA types A1-B8-DR3 and B27 with rapid and slow progression of HIV disease. *Q J Med*, 89, 177–185.

Mellado, M., Rodriguez-Frade, J.M., Vila-Coro, A.J., de Ana, A.M., & Martinez, A.C. (1999) Chemokine control of HIV-1 infection. *Nature*, 400, 723–724.

Migueles, S.A., Sabbaghian, M.S., Shupert, W.L., Bettinotti, M.P., Marincola, F.M., Martino, L., Hallahan, C.W., Selig, S.M., Schwartz, D., Sullivan, J., & Connors, M. (2000) HLA B*5701 is highly associated with restriction of virus replication in a subgroup of HIV-infected long term nonprogressors. *Proc Natl Acad Sci USA*, 97, 2709–2714.

Modi, W.S., Goedert, J.J., Strathdee, S., Buchbinder, S., Detels, R., Donfield, S., O'Brien, S.J., & Winkler, C. (2003a) MCP-1-MCP-3-eotaxin gene cluster influences HIV-1 transmission. *AIDS*, 17, 2357–2365.

Modi, W.S., O'Brien, T.R., Vlahov, D., Buchbinder, S., Gomperts, E., Phair, J., O'Brien, S.J., & Winkler, C. (2003b) Haplotype diversity in the interleukin-4 gene is not associated with HIV-1 transmission and AIDS progression. *Immunogenetics*, 55, 157–164.

Moore, C.B., John, M., James, I.R., Christiansen, F.T., Witt, C.S., & Mallal, S.A. (2002) Evidence of HIV-1 adaptation to HLA-restricted immune responses at a population level. *Science*, 296, 1439–1443.

Mummidi, S., Ahuja, S.S., Gonzalez, E., Anderson, S.A., Santiago, E.N., Stephan, K.T., Craig, F.E., O'Connell, P., Tryon, V., Clark, R.A., Dolan, M.J., Ahuja, SK. (1998) Genealogy of the CCR5 locus and chemokine system gene variants associated with altered rates of HIV-1 disease progression. *Nat Med*, 4, 786–793.

Munkanta, M., Terunuma, H., Takahashi, M., Hanabusa, H., Miura, T., Ikeda, S., Sakai, M., Fujii, T., Takahashi, Y., Oka, S., Matsuda, J., Ishikawa, M., Taki, M., Takashima, Y., Mimaya, J., Ito, M., Kimura, A., & Yasunami, M. (2005) HLA-B polymorphism in Japanese HIV-1-infected long-term surviving hemophiliacs. *Viral Immunol*, 18, 500–505.

Nagasawa, T., Hirota, S., Tachibana, K., Takakura, N., Nishikawa, S., Kitamura, Y., Yoshida, N., Kikutani, H., & Kishimoto, T. (1996) Defects of B-cell lymphopoiesis and bone-marrow myelopoiesis in mice lacking the CXC chemokine PBSF/SDF-1. *Nature*, 382, 635–638.

Nakayama, E.E., Hoshino, Y., Xin, X., Liu, H., Goto, M., Watanabe, N., Taguchi, H., Hitani, A., Kawana–Tachikawa, A., Fukushima, M., Yamada, K., Sugiura, W., Oka, S.I., Ajisawa, A., Sato, H., Takebe, Y., Nakamura, T., Nagai, Y., Iwamoto, A., & Shioda, T. (2000) Polymorphism in the interleukin-4 promoter affects acquisition of human immunodeficiency virus type 1 syncytium-inducing phenotype. *J Virol*, 74, 5452–5459.

O'Brien, T.R., Blattner, W.A., Waters, D., Eyster, E., Hilgartner, M.W., Cohen, A.R., Luban, N., Hatzakis, A., Aledort, L.M., Rosenberg, P.S., Miley, W.J., Kroner, B.L., & Goedert, J.J. (1996) Serum HIV-1 RNA levels and time to development of AIDS in the Multicenter Hemophilia Cohort Study. *JAMA*, 276, 105–110.

O'Brien, T.R., McDermott, D.H., Ioannidis, J.P., Carrington, M., Murphy, P.M., Havlir, D.V., & Richman, D.D. (2000) Effect of chemokine receptor gene polymorphisms on the response to potent antiretroviral therapy. *AIDS*, 14, 821–826.

O'Brien, T.R., Michael, N.L., Sheppard, H.W., & Buchbinder, S. (2002) HIV-1 infection in patients with the CCR5-delta32 homozygous genotype. In: Chemokine Receptors and AIDS (ed. by T.R. O'Brien), pp. 215–224. Marcel Dekker, New York.

O'Brien, T.R., Padian, N.S., Hodge, T., Goedert, J.J., O'Brien, S.J., & Carrington, M. (1998) CCR-5 genotype and sexual transmission of HIV-1. *AIDS*, 12, 444–445.

Palella, F.J., Jr., Delaney, K.M., Moorman, A.C., Loveless, M.O., Fuhrer, J., Satten, G.A., Aschman, D.J., & Holmberg, S.D. (1998) Declining morbidity and mortality among patients with advanced human immunodeficiency virus infection. HIV Outpatient Study Investigators. *N Engl J Med*, 338, 853–860.

Pastinen, T., Liitsola, K., Niini, P., Salminen, M., & Syvanen, A.C. (1998) Contribution of the CCR5 and MBL genes to susceptibility to HIV type 1 infection in the Finnish population. *AIDS Res Hum Retroviruses*, 14, 695–698.

Philpott, S., Weiser, B., Tarwater, P., Vermund, S.H., Kleeberger, C.A., Gange, S.J., Anastos, K., Cohen, M., Greenblatt, R.M., Kovacs, A., Minkoff, H., Young, M.A., Miotti, P., Dupuis, M., Chen, C.H., & Burger, H. (2003) CC chemokine receptor 5 genotype and susceptibility to transmission of human immunodeficiency virus type 1 in women. *J Infect Dis*, 187, 569–575.

Pillay, T., Zhang, H.T., Drijfhout, J.W., Robinson, N., Brown, H., Khan, M., Moodley, J., Adhikari, M., Pfafferott, K., Feeney, M.E., St John, A., Holmes, E.C., Coovadia, H.M., Klenerman, P., Goulder, P.J., & Phillips, R.E. (2005) Unique acquisition of cytotoxic T-lymphocyte escape mutants in infant human immunodeficiency virus type 1 infection. *J Virol*, 79, 12100–12105.

Piot, P., Bartos, M., Ghys, P.D., Walker, N., & Schwartlander, B. (2001) The global impact of HIV/AIDS. *Nature*, 410, 968–973.

Price, P., James, I., Fernandez, S., & French, M.A. (2004) Alleles of the gene encoding IL-1alpha may predict control of plasma viraemia in HIV-1 patients on highly active antiretroviral therapy. *AIDS*, 18, 1495–1501.

Ramaley, P.A., French, N., Kaleebu, P., Gilks, C., Whitworth, J., & Hill, A.V. (2002) HIV in Africa (Communication arising): Chemokine-receptor genes and AIDS risk. *Nature*, 417, 140.

Raulet, D.H. (2004) Interplay of natural killer cells and their receptors with the adaptive immune response. *Nat Immunol*, 5, 996–1002.

Rosenberg, E.S., Billingsley, J.M., Caliendo, A.M., Boswell, S.L., Sax, P.E., Kalams, S.A., & Walker, B.D. (1997) Vigorous HIV-1-specific CD4$^+$ T cell responses associated with control of viremia. *Science*, 278, 1447–1450.

Sabbe, R., Picchio, G.R., Pastore, C., Chaloin, O., Hartley, O., Offord, R., & Mosier, D.E. (2001) Donor- and ligand-dependent differences in C-C chemokine receptor 5 reexpression. *J Virol*, 75, 661–671.

Saha, K., Bentsman, G., Chess, L., & Volsky, D.J. (1998) Endogenous production of beta-chemokines by CD4$^+$, but not CD8$^+$, T-cell clones correlates with the clinical state of human immunodeficiency virus type 1 (HIV-1)-infected individuals and may be responsible for blocking infection with non-syncytium-inducing HIV-1 in vitro. *J Virol*, 72, 876–881.

Samson, M., Libert, F., Doranz, B.J., Rucker, J., Liesnard, C., Farber, C.M., Saragosti, S., Lapoumeroulie, C., Cognaux, J., Forceille, C., Muyldermans, G., Verhofstede, C., Burtonboy, G., Georges, M., Imai, T., Rana, S., Yi, Y., Smyth, R.J., Collman, R.G., Doms, R.W., Vassart, G., & Parmentier, M. (1996) Resistance to HIV-1 infection in Caucasian individuals bearing mutant alleles of the CCR-5 chemokine receptor gene. *Nature*, 382, 722–725.

Sastry, K., Herman, G.A., Day, L., Deignan, E., Bruns, G., Morton, C.C., & Ezekowitz, R.A. (1989) The human mannose-binding protein gene. Exon structure reveals its evolutionary relationship to a human pulmonary surfactant gene and localization to chromosome 10. *J Exp Med*, 170, 1175–1189.

Scherer, A., Frater, J., Oxenius, A., Agudelo, J., Price, D.A., Gunthard, H.F., Barnardo, M., Perrin, L., Hirschel, B., Phillips, R.E., McLean, A.R., Aebi, C., Battegay, M., Bernasconi, E., Biedermann, K., Bischoff, L., Boni, J., Bosbach, S., Brenner, I., Buchel, I., Bucher, H., Burgisser, P., Cattacin, S., Chapalay, S., Cheseaux, J.J., Cuvit, A.L., Drack, G., Dubs, R., Egger, M., Elzi, L., Erb, P., Fantelli, K., Fischer, M., Flepp, M., Fontana, A., Francioli, P., Francioli-Volz, M.C., Furrer, H., Gorgievski, M., Gremlich, E., Gyr, T., Hirsch, H.H., Hosli, I., Irion, O., Jirasko-

Emmenegger, N., Joller-Jemelka, H.I., Kaiser, L., Kaufmann, G., Keiser, O., Kind, C., Klimkait, T., Knecht, C., Lauper, U., Ledergerber, B., Leuenberger, L., Merk, B., Muller, S., Nadal, D., Oliveira, J., Opravil, M., Ortelli Pin, B., Paccaud, F., Pantaleo, G., Piffaretti, J.C., Reber, M., Reiss, P., Remy, B., Reymond, B., Rickenbach, M., Rudin, C., Russotti, M., Schiffer, V., Schmid, P., Schreyer, A., Schupbach, J., Speck, R., Taffe, P., Tarr, P., Telenti, A., Trkola, A., Vallet, Y., Vanhems, P., Vernazza, P., Weber, R., Wechsler, A., Wunder, D., Wyler-Lazarevitch, C.A., Yeni, P., Yerly, S., Yilmaz, A., & Ziekau, I. (2004) Quantifiable cytotoxic T lymphocyte responses and HLA-related risk of progression to AIDS. *Proc Natl Acad Sci USA*, 101, 12266–12270.

Schwartz, O., Marechal, V., Le Gall, S., Lemonnier, F., & Heard, J.M. (1996) Endocytosis of major histocompatibility complex class I molecules is induced by the HIV-1 Nef protein. *Nat Med*, 2, 338–342.

Sette, A., & Sidney, J. (1999) Nine major HLA class I supertypes account for the vast preponderance of HLA-A and -B polymorphism. *Immunogenetics*, 50, 201–212.

Shields, P.L., & Adams, D.H. (2002) Chemokines and chemokine receptor interactions and functions. In: *Chemokine Receptors and AIDS* (ed. by T.R. O'Brien), pp. 1–30. Marcel Dekker, New York.

Shin, H.D., Winkler, C., Stephens, J.C., Bream, J., Young, H., Goedert, J.J., O'Brien, T.R., Vlahov, D., Buchbinder, S., Giorgi, J., Rinaldo, C., Donfield, S., Willoughby, A., O'Brien, S.J., Smith, M.W. (2000) Genetic restriction of HIV-1 pathogenesis to AIDS by promoter alleles of IL10. *Proc Natl Acad Sci USA*, 97, 14467–14472.

Simmons, G., Clapham, P.R., Picard, L., Offord, R.E., Rosenkilde, M.M., Schwartz, T.W., Buser, R., Wells, T.N.C., & Proudfoot, A.E. (1997) Potent inhibition of HIV-1 infectivity in macrophages and lymphocytes by a novel CCR5 antagonist. *Science*, 276, 276–279.

Smith, M.W., Dean, M., Carrington, M., Winkler, C., Huttley, G.A., Lomb, D.A., Goedert, J.J., O'Brien, T.R., Jacobson, L.P., Kaslow, R.A., Buchbinder, S., Vittinghoff, E., Vlahov, D., Hoots, K., Hilgartner, W., HGDS, MHCS, MACS, SFCC, ALIVE-Study & O'Brien, S.J. (1997) Contrasting genetic influence of CCR2 and CCR5 variants on HIV-1 infection and disease progression. *Science*, 277, 959–965.

Stephens, J.C., Reich, D.E., Goldstein, D.B., Shin, H.D., Smith, M.W., Carrington, M., Winkler, C., Huttley, G.A., Allikmets, R., Schriml, L., Gerrard, B., Malasky, M., Ramos, M.D., Morlot, S., Tzetis, M., Oddoux, C., di Giovine, F.S., Nasioulas, G., Chandler, D., Aseev, M., Hanson, M., Kalaydjieva, L., Glavac, D., Gasparini, P., Dean, M., et al. (1998)

Dating the origin of the CCR5-D32 AIDS-resistance allele by the coalescence of haplotypes. *Am J Hum Genet*, 62, 1507–1515.

Tang, J., Costello, C., Keet, I.P.M., Rivers, C., LeBlanc, S., Karita, E., Allen, S., & Kaslow, R.A. (1999) HLA class I homozygosity accelerates disease progression in human immunodeficiency virus type 1 infection. *AIDS Res Hum Retroviruses*, 15, 317–324.

Tang, J., Penman-Aguilar, A., Lobashevsky, E., Allen, S., Kaslow, R., & Zambia-UAB HIV Research Project (2004) HLA-DRB1 and -DQB1 alleles and haplotypes in Zambian couples and their associations with heterosexual transmission of human immunodeficiency virus type 1. *J Infect Dis*, 189, 1696–1704.

Tang, J., Shelton, B., Makhatadze, N.J., Zhang, Y., Schaen, M., Louie, L., Goedert, J.J., Seaburg, E.C., Margolick, J.B., Mellors, J., & Kaslow, R.A. (2002a) Distribution of chemokine receptor CCR2 and CCR5 genotypes and their relative contribution to human immunodeficiency virus type 1 (HIV-1) seroconversion, early HIV-1 RNA concentration in plasma, and later disease progression. *J Virol*, 76, 662–672.

Tang, J., Tang, S., Lobashevsky, E., Myracle, A.D., Fideli, U., Aldrovandi, G., Allen, S., Musonda, R., & Kaslow, R.A. (2002b) Favorable and unfavorable HLA class I alleles and haplotypes in Zambians predominantly infected with clade C human immunodeficiency virus type 1. *J Virol*, 76, 8276–8284.

Tang, J., Wilson, C.M., Meleth, S., Myracle, A., Lobashevsky, E., Mulligan, M.J., Douglas, S.D., Korber, B., Vermund, S.H., & Kaslow, R.A. (2002c) Host genetic profiles predict virological and immunological control of HIV-1 infection in adolescents. *AIDS*, 16, 2275–2284.

Taylor, M.E., Brickell, P.M., Craig, R.K., & Summerfield, J.A. (1989) Structure and evolutionary origin of the gene encoding a human serum mannose-binding protein. *Biochem J*, 262, 763–771.

Trachtenberg, E., Korber, B., Sollars, C., Kepler, T.B., Hraber, P.T., Hayes, E., Funkhouser, R., Fugate, M., Theiler, J., Hsu, Y.S., Kuntsman, K., Wu, S., Phair, J., Erlich, H., & Wolinsky, S. (2003) Advantage of rare HLA supertype in HIV disease progression. *Nat Med*, 9, 928–935.

Trkola, A., Ketas, T.J., Nagashima, K.A., Zhao, L., Cilliers, T., Morris, L., Moore, J.P., Maddon, P.J., & Olson, W.C. (2001) Potent, broad-spectrum inhibition of human immunodeficiency virus type 1 by the CCR5 monoclonal antibody PRO 140. *J Virol*, 75, 579–588.

Turner, M.W., & Hamvas, R.M. (2000) Mannose-binding lectin: Structure, function, genetics and disease associations. *Rev Immunogenet*, 2, 305–322.

Valdez, H., Purvis, S.F., Lederman, M.M., Fillingame, M., & Zimmerman, P.A. (1999) Association of the CCR5D32 mutation with improved response to antiretroviral therapy. *JAMA*, 282, 734.

Valentin, A., Lu, W.H., Rosati, M., Schneider, R., Albert, J., Karlsson, A., & Pavlakis, G.N. (1998) Dual effect of interleukin 4 on HIV-1 expression—implications for viral phenotypic switch and disease progression. *Proc Natl Acad Sci U S A*, 95, 8886–8891.

van Rij, R.P., Broersen, S., Goudsmit, J., Coutinho, R.A., & Schuitemaker, H. (1998) The role of a stromal cell-derived factor-1 chemokine gene variant in the clinical course of HIV-1 infection. *AIDS*, 12, F85–90.

Vidal, F., Peraire, J., Domingo, P., Broch, M., Cairo, M., Pedrol, E., Montero, M., Vilades, C., Gutierrez, C., Sambeat, M.A., Fontanet, A., Dalmau, D., Deig, E., Knobel, H., Sirvent, J.J., & Richart, C. (2006) Polymorphism of RANTES Chemokine Gene Promoter Is Not Associated With Long-Term Nonprogressive HIV-1 Infection of More Than 16 Years. *J Acquir Immune Defic Syndr*, 41, 17–22.

Vidal, F., Peraire, J., Domingo, P., Broch, M., Knobel, H., Pedrol, E., Dalmau, D., Vilades, C., Sambeat, M.A., Gutierrez, C., & Richart, C. (2005a) Lack of association of SDF-1 3'A variant allele with long-term nonprogressive HIV-1 infection is extended beyond 16 years. *J Acquir Immune Defic Syndr*, 40, 276–279.

Vidal, F., Vilades, C., Domingo, P., Broch, M., Pedrol, E., Dalmau, D., Knobel, H., Peraire, J., Gutierrez, C., Sambeat, M.A., Fontanet, A., Deig, E., Cairo, M., Montero, M., Richart, C., Mallal, S., & Chemokines LTNP Study Group. (2005b) Spanish HIV-1-infected long-term nonprogressors of more than 15 years have an increased frequency of the CX3CR1 249I variant allele. *J Acquir Immune Defic Syndr*, 40, 527–531.

Wang, C., Song, W., Lobashevsky, E., Wilson, C.M., Douglas, S.D., Mytilineos, J., Schoenbaum, E.E., Tang, J., & Kaslow, R.A. (2004) Cytokine and chemokine gene polymorphisms in ethnically diverse North Americans with human immunodeficiency virus type 1 (HIV-1) infection. *J Acquir Immune Defic Syndr*, 35, 446–454.

Wasik, T.J., Jagodzinski, P.P., Hyjek, E.M., Wustner, J., Trinchieri, G., Lischner, H.W., & Kozbor, D. (1997) Diminished HIV-specific CTL activity is associated with lower type 1 and enhanced type 2 responses to HIV-specific peptides during perinatal HIV infection. *J Immunol*, 158, 6029–6036.

Welzel, T.M., Gao, X., Pfeiffer, R.M., Martin, M.P., O'Brien, S.J., Goedert, J.J., Carrington, M., & O'Brien, T.R. (2007) HLA-B Bw4 alleles and HIV-1 transmission in heterosexual couples. *AIDS*, 21, 225–229.

Winkler, C., Modi, W., Smith, M.W., Nelson, G.W., Wu, X., Carrington, M., Dean, M., Honjo, T., Tashiro, K., Yabe, D., Buchbinder, S., Vittinghoff, E., Goedert, J.J., O'Brien, T.R., Jacobson, L.P., Detels, R., Donfield, S., Willoughby, A., Gomperts, E., Vlahov, D., Phair, J., & O'Brien, S.J. (1998) Genetic restriction of AIDS pathogenesis by an SDF-1 chemokine gene variant. ALIVE Study, Hemophilia Growth and Development Study (HGDS), Multicenter AIDS Cohort Study (MACS), Multicenter Hemophilia Cohort Study (MHCS), San Francisco City Cohort (SFCC). *Science*, 279, 389–393.

Wu, L., Paxton, W.A., Kassam, N., Ruffing, N., Rottman, J.B., Sullivan, N., Choe, H., Sodroski, J., Newman, W., Koup, R.A., & Mackay, C.R. (1997) CCR5 levels and expression pattern correlate with infectability by macrophage-tropic HIV-1, in vitro. *J Exp Med*, 185, 1681–1691.

Zou, Y.R., Kottmann, A.H., Kuroda, M., Taniuchi, I., & Littman, D.R. (1998) Function of the chemokine receptor CXCR4 in haematopoiesis and in cerebellar development. *Nature*, 393, 595–599.

20

Human T-Lymphotropic Virus Type 1 (HTLV-1)–Associated Diseases

Charles R. M. Bangham

HTLV-1 causes two distinct types of disease: an aggressive leukemia of CD4$^+$ T-cells, known as adult T-cell leukemia (ATL), and a range of chronic inflammatory diseases, of which HTLV-1–associated myelopathy/tropical spastic paraparesis (HAM/TSP) is the best studied. The risk of inflammatory disease is strongly correlated with the proportion of HTLV-1–infected cells in the blood—the "proviral load," which is stable in each infected person but differs among people by more than 1,000-fold. Because of the high and stable proviral load, the relative lack of immune suppression, and the strong HTLV-1–specific T-cell response, HTLV-1 infection is proving a very useful system to identify and quantify the genetic and cellular determinants of the "efficiency" of the antiviral immune response. This chapter addresses the evidence that genetic factors determine two important measures of the outcome of HTLV-1 infection: the risk of HAM/TSP and the proviral load.

HTLV-1–Associated Myelopathy/Tropical Spastic Paraparesis

Most patients with HAM/TSP originate from areas of endemic HTLV-1 infection: the Caribbean, South America, Central Africa, or southern Japan (Mueller and Blattner 1997, Slattery et al. 1999). HAM/TSP is about twice as common in women as in men. The median age at onset is in the 40s, but the age range is wide, from younger than 10 years to older than 70 years. The lifetime risk of HAM/TSP among HTLV-1–infected people differs among endemic areas, ranging from 0.25% to more than 1%. The lifetime risk of ATL is on the order of 1–5%; ATL and HAM/TSP occur together no more frequently than would be expected by chance.

A patient with HAM/TSP typically presents in middle age with low back pain, frequency or urgency of micturition, and progressive difficulty in walking (Bangham et al. 2000). The chief pathological feature of

HAM/TSP is a patchy mononuclear cell infiltrate (predominantly CD4$^+$ T cells) in the lower cervical and upper thoracic spinal cord, associated with demyelination and neuronal loss (Iwasaki et al. 1992).

The HTLV-1–specific antibody titer in HAM/TSP is frequently very high, not uncommonly reaching 1:256,000. The median proviral load of HTLV-1, that is, the percentage of peripheral blood mononuclear cells (PBMCs) infected with the virus, is about 5% in patients with HAM/TSP, compared with about 0.3% in asymptomatic carriers (Nagai et al. 1998). However, the distribution of proviral load within both HAM/TSP patients and asymptomatic carriers is broad, and the two distributions overlap extensively.

HTLV-1

HTLV-1 is classified as a complex retrovirus, in the genus *Deltaretrovirus* of the subfamily Orthoretrovirinae (Green and Chen 2001). Like other retroviruses, HTLV-1 has a diploid positive-sense RNA genome. HTLV-1 shares with other exogenous retroviruses the structural proteins Gag and Env and the enzymes polymerase, protease, and endonuclease. In addition, there are at least four regulatory proteins coded in the 3′ end of the HTLV-1 genome, known respectively as Tax, Rex, p12 (Rof), and p30 (Tof).

HTLV-1 produces almost no cell-free virus particles *in vivo*: The virus propagates mainly by proliferation of provirus-positive lymphocytes and by direct passage from cell to cell (Cavrois et al. 1996, Igakura et al. 2003, Wodarz et al. 2001). HTLV-1 is transmitted between individuals by three main routes: breast-feeding, sexual contact, and parenteral contact with infected blood, for example, by transfusion or shared hypodermic needles. The virus is virtually confined to T cells *in vivo*: 90–95% of the provirus is present in CD4$^+$ T cells, and 5–10% in CD8$^+$ T cells. There is a degree of preferential infection of HTLV-1–specific T cells, both CD8$^+$ (Hanon et al. 2000) and CD4$^+$ (Goon et al. 2004a).

The cellular immune response to HTLV-1 is characteristically very strong: There are high frequencies of both CD8$^+$ and CD4$^+$ T cells specific to HTLV-1 in patients with HAM/TSP and in asymptomatic carriers (Bangham 2000). The anti–HTLV-1 CD8$^+$ T cells are persistently activated and appear to play a major part in controlling the proviral load (Bangham 2003, Asquith et al. 2005). The frequency of HTLV-1–specific

CD4$^+$ T cells in HAM/TSP is some 10–25 times greater than that in asymptomatic HTLV-1 carriers with a similar proviral load (Goon et al. 2002, 2004); there is less difference in the frequency of specific CD8$^+$ T cells.

The sequence variation observed in HTLV-1 is much less than that observed in HIV-1, both within and between isolates (Daenke et al. 1990, Niewiesk et al. 1994). Although different sequence variants of HTLV-1 are in some cases associated with slightly different risks of HAM/TSP (Furukawa et al. 2000), there is no HTLV-1 sequence that is uniquely associated with neurological disease, and the sequence is frequently identical in asymptomatic carriers and patients with neurological disease (Daenke et al. 1990). Therefore, differences between hosts must explain the development of neurological disease in certain HTLV-1–infected individuals, and such host differences are likely to be genetically determined.

Genetic Determinants of the Outcome of HTLV-1 Infection

Many areas of endemic HTLV-1 infection contain populations of considerable ethnic diversity, in which straightforward genetic association studies are liable to be confounded by genetic stratification. However, the population in the south island of Japan, Kyushu, has been relatively little affected by immigration. A genetic association study has been carried out in the southern prefecture of Kagoshima, with a population of 1.7 million, where the seroprevalence of HTLV-1 in adults is about 8%. In this study, in addition to 94 class I human leukocyte antigen (HLA) and 1 class II HLA genes, more than 60 single nucleotide polymorphisms (SNPs) were examined in more than 40 candidate genes (Jeffery et al. 1999, 2000, Vine et al. 2002).

HLA Class I Genes

Protective HLA Class I Alleles

In a sample of 235 patients with HAM/TSP and 200 asymptomatic HTLV-1 carriers in Kagoshima, southern Japan, HLA-A*02 was present in a significantly lower proportion of patients than carriers (Jeffery et al. 1999; table 20.1). That is, possession of HLA-A*02 appeared to protect against the inflammatory disease HAM/TSP. This result suggested that HLA-A*02$^+$ individuals mount a more effective CD8$^+$ T-cell response to HTLV-1 than HLA-A*02⁻individuals. According to this hypothesis, HLA-A*02⁺ individuals should also have a significantly lower proviral load than those who lack the HLA-A*02⁻allele. The results showed that in asymptomatic carriers, possession of HLA-A*02 was indeed associated with a significantly lower proviral load of HTLV-1, although this effect was not significant in patients with HAM/TSP (Jeffery et al. 2000, Vine et al. 2002). The subtypes of HLA-A*02 present in the Kagoshima cohort were HLA-A*0201, HLA-A*0203, HLA-A*0206, HLA-A*0207 and HLA-A*0210. There was a significant reduction in median proviral load among asymptomatic HTLV-1 carriers associated with HLA-A*0206, whereas the subtypes other than HLA-A*0206 were associated with a lower proviral load among the patients with HAM/TSP (Jeffery et al. 1999). Because of the small number of subjects with each respective HLA-A*02 subtype, it is not clear whether these are real differences in protective effect or merely sampling variation.

The HLA-Cw*08 gene had an effect similar to that of HLA-A*02 (Jeffery et al. 2000, Vine et al. 2002). Possession of either HLA-A*02 or HLA-Cw*08 was associated with a 2-fold reduction in the odds of HAM/TSP and a 3- to 4-fold reduction in the proviral load (Jeffery et al. 2000). These effects were important at the population level: HLA-A*02 prevented 28.2% (± 5.8% standard deviation) of potential cases of HAM/TSP (box 20.1). HLA-Cw*08, whose allele frequency is lower, prevented 12.6% (± 3.7% standard deviation) of potential cases of HAM/TSP.

The protective effects of HLA-A*02 and HLA-Cw*08 appeared to be independent and additive (Jeffery et al. 2000), for the following reasons. First, the two alleles were not in significant linkage disequilibrium in healthy carriers of HTLV-1. Second, HLA-Cw*08 was associated with a significant reduction in the odds of HAM/TSP in HLA-A*02⁻subjects. Third, HLA-Cw*08 was associated with a greater than 3-fold reduction in the median proviral load in both HLA-A*02⁺ and HLA-A*02⁻asymptomatic HTLV-1 carriers.

It is likely that HLA-A*02–restricted and HLA-Cw*08–restricted CD8⁺ T cells reduce the proviral load of HTLV-1 and so reduce the risk of associated inflammatory disease by more efficient (i.e., rapid and sensitive) lysis of HTLV-1–infected lymphocytes in vivo. This proposed mechanism is consistent with the observation that the gene that encodes the dominant CD8⁺ target antigen, Tax, is under positive selection (Niewiesk et al. 1994, Kubota et al. 2007). Recent evidence from experiments on ex vivo cytotoxic T-lymphocyte (CTL) function (Asquith et al. 2005) and CD8⁺ T-cell gene expression (Vine et al. 2004) strongly corroborate the conclusion that a powerful anti–HTLV-1 CTL response reduces the proviral load and hence the risk of HAM/TSP (Bangham and Osame, 2005).

Mathematical explanations have been proposed (Asquith et al. 2000, Nowak and Bangham 1996, Wodarz and Bangham 2000, Wodarz et al. 2001) to reconcile the paradox that individuals with a less efficient CTL response to HTLV-1 have higher frequencies of HTLV-1–specific CTLs in the circulation (Elovaara et al. 1993, Daenke et al. 1996, Jeffery et al. 1999, Goon et al. 2004b). The hypothesis is that the high proviral load observed in a patient with HAM/TSP maintains a high frequency of inefficient HTLV-1–specific CTLs, whereas the efficient CTLs in an asymptomatic carrier

TABLE 20.1. *HLA-A*02 reduces the odds of HTLV-1–associated myelopathy/tropical spastic paraparesis (HAM/TSP).*

Stage of Study	HAM/TSP (n)		HTLV-1 Carrier (n)		χ^{2a}	P-value	Odds Ratio[b]	95% Confidence Interval
	A*02⁺	A*02⁻	A*02⁺	A*02⁻				
1	12	38	32	24	10.6	0.001	0.24	0.10–0.55
2	57	125	68	77	7.6	0.006	0.52	0.33–0.81
All subjects	69	163	100	101	17.3	< 0.0001	0.43	0.29–0.63

A*02⁺ and A*02⁻ denote the presence of absence of the A*02 gene in the subjects studied. In total, 232 HAM/TSP patients and 201 healthy HTLV-1 carriers were studied. Stage of study denotes independent, consecutive case–control studies and do not refer to clinical stage.

[a]With Yates's correction.

[b]Using the approximation of Woolf.

Reproduced from Jeffery et al (1999), by permission of the publishers.

BOX 20.1. The prevented fraction of disease, F_p

To estimate the reduction in the prevalence of a disease that is caused by a protective allele, the appropriate statistic is F_p, the prevented fraction of disease (Jeffery et al 1999). F_p is defined as the proportion of cases of the disease that are prevented by a gene that is present at a specified allele frequency in the population. The more familiar expression for the attributable fraction of disease is appropriate for a susceptibility gene effect but cannot be used to quantify the effect of a protective gene in a population.

F_p denotes the fraction of potential cases of disease D in the population that is prevented by a protective genotype G_1. Consider the 2×2 contingency table:

$$
\begin{array}{ccc}
 & G_1 & G_2 \\
D & a & b \\
H & c & d
\end{array}
$$

where a, b, c, d denote the observed numbers of subjects; D = disease, H = health, G_1 = positive for protective genotype, G_2 = negative for protective genotype. F_p is given by the expression

$$F_p = (1 - R) \times [1 - (dr_1/br_2)]$$

where R = prevalence rate of disease D in the population, $r_1 = a + b$ and $r_2 = c + d$. In the case of HAM/TSP, R is estimated as ~1% of the HTLV-1–infected population. F_p is approximately normally distributed (A. Lloyd and C.R.M.Bangham., unpublished data); the standard deviation is given by the expression

$$SD(F_p) = (1 - R - F_p) \times [(c/dr_2) + (a/br_1)]$$

A full derivation of these formulas is available on request.

---

suppress the proviral load to a lower level at equilibrium (Bangham 2003). Work is now in progress to define this CTL efficiency in molecular, cellular, and mathematical terms (Asquith et al. 2005, 2007).

Although the protective effects of HLA-A*02 and HLA-Cw*08 against HAM/TSP are chiefly accounted for by an associated reduction in the proviral load of HTLV-1, there was a statistically significant additional protective component associated with each of these alleles that remains after the proviral load has been taken into account (Vine et al. 2002). The mechanism of this additional protective effect is unclear.

The Protective Effect of HLA Class I Heterozygosity

The hypothesis that a strong class I HLA-restricted T-cell response is protective in HTLV-1 infection implies that recognition of a greater number of viral epitopes will give better immune control of HTLV-1 replication. This prediction was supported by the observation (Vine et al. 2002) that heterozygosity at HLA class I loci was associated with a significantly lower proviral load of HTLV-1 in patients with HAM/TSP (two-tailed $P = 0.017$) and asymptomatic HTLV-1 carriers (one-tailed $P = 0.039$).

Susceptibility HLA Class I Alleles

In the Kagoshima population study, there was one further class I HLA gene that exerted a statistically significant influence on the outcome of HTLV-1 infection: HLA-B*5401. Whereas HLA-A*02 and HLA-Cw*08 were associated with protection against HAM/TSP and a reduction in proviral load, HLA-B*5401 was associated with an increased odds of HAM/TSP, both in the whole cohort and at a given HTLV-1 proviral load (Jeffery et al. 2000). The susceptibility to HAM/TSP conferred by HLA-B*5401 appeared to override the protection conferred by HLA-A*02 (Jeffery et al. 2000). None of the other alleles examined on this HLA-B*5401–associated haplotype (HLA-A*24, HLA-Cw*01, HLA-DRB1*0405, HLA-DQB1*0401) was significantly associated with HAM/TSP. The population attributable risk of HAM/TSP associated with HLA-B*5401 was 16.8% (95% confidence interval = 8.3–24.4%).

The reason for the increased risk of HAM/TSP associated with HLA-B*5401 is unknown. The HLA-B*5401–containing haplotype is also associated in Japan with two other inflammatory conditions that are unrelated to HTLV-1 infection: hepatitis C virus infection (Kikuchi et al. 1998, Kuzushita et al. 1998) and diffuse panbronchiolitis (Keicho et al. 1998, 2000, Sugiyama et al. 1990). HLA-B*5401 or a closely linked gene may contribute to inflammation in a non-antigen-specific manner.

Frequencies of 45 class I HLA alleles have been reported in samples of patients with HAM/TSP, asymptomatic HTLV-1 carriers, uninfected control subjects, and patients with ATL (Yashiki et al. 2001). In this study, HLA-A*26 was present at a higher allele frequency in ATL patients. However, the observed differences in allele frequency between the groups did not remain significant after correction for multiple comparisons. Yashiki et al. (2001) reproduced the finding of a protective effect of HLA-Cw*08 (Jeffery et al. 2000) ($P = 0.002$).

The same group previously suggested (Kitze et al. 1996) that intrathecal anti–HTLV-1 antibody production was more frequent in patients with HAM/TSP who carried certain HLA haplotypes. However, further data are needed to corroborate this finding, because of the complexity of the haplotype structure of the HLA region (Ahmad et al. 2003).

Additional findings in studies of ATL patients include a comparison of 25 black patients with ATL and 45 ethnically similar controls genotyped for both class I and class II HLA alleles (White et al. 1996); the results suggested an increase in the frequency of HLA-A*36 in the ATL patients (P value after correction for multiple comparisons (P_c) = 0.08). Borducchi et al. (2003) found that HLA-A*02 also gives protection against HTLV-1–associated disease in Brazil. There was a significantly lower frequency of HLA-A*02 in white patients with ATL (15.0% vs. 47.0%) than in the white controls, and a marginally significant ($P < 0.09$) lower frequency of HLA-A*02 in the white patients with HAM/TSP. The Brazilian investigators also found a significantly higher frequency of HLA-A*26 in white patients with ATL than in ethnically matched controls (35.0% vs. 10.3%). This finding recalled an association between HLA-A*26 and ATL in Japan (Sonoda et al. 1996, Yashiki et al. 2001). A*26 was found in 25.0% of 124 ATL patients, compared with 15.1% of 152 asymptomatic HTLV-1 carriers (Yashiki et al. 2001), a statistically significant difference before correction for mul-

tiple comparisons ($P = 0.0026$) but not after (N = 45 alleles typed; $P_c > 0.1$). This apparent association of the same allele with ATL in two different ethnic groups should not be overlooked, although the mechanism by which HLA-A*26 exerts its susceptibility effect is not clear.

Possible Interaction Between HLA Class I Genotype and HTLV-1 Genotype

There is evidence that the risk of HAM/TSP is differentially associated with two sequence variants of HTLV-1 (subgroups A and B of the "cosmopolitan" group of HTLV-1) in Kagoshima (Furukawa et al. 2000). Although the sample size was small, the data suggested that the protection conferred by HLA-A*02 was effective in subjects infected with subgroup B but not in those infected with subgroup A. This may explain the lack of protective effect of HLA-A*02 observed in a population in northern Iran, in which only the subgroup A genotype of HTLV-1 was present (Sabouri et al. 2005). The implication is that full understanding of the role of genetic polymorphisms in determining the outcome of HTLV-1 infection may require genotyping of the virus as well as the host. However, it is highly improbable that the fundamental mechanisms of immune control of HTLV-1 differ between populations.

Conclusion: HLA Class I Genes and HTLV-1 Infection

The influence of genotype on the outcome of HTLV-1 infection will differ among populations because of systematic differences in both the host genetic composition and the prevalent HTLV-1 strains. However, the evidence supports the conclusion that (1) a strong class I MHC-restricted T-cell response to HTLV-1 is beneficial, and (2) therefore, by implication, HTLV-1 is not, as was previously believed, a latent virus but is persistently expressed.

These conclusions suggest that treatment with antiretroviral drugs might be beneficial in HTLV-1–associated diseases. Nucleoside analogues can reduce the proviral load of HTLV-1 (Taylor et al. 1999), but the effectiveness of single drug therapy is limited, as in HIV-1 infection; importantly, no protease inhibitor has been produced that has significant activity against HTLV-1.

A second implication of these results is that boosting the HLA class I–restricted T-cell response to HTLV-1 might reduce the proviral load and therefore reduce the risk of HAM/TSP and other HTLV-1–associated inflammatory diseases. However, it may be possible to boost this response persistently only by persistent stimulation with an exogenously added factor such as antigen. Also, activated CTLs might contribute to the tissue damage that is seen in inflammatory diseases such as HAM/TSP (Biddison et al. 1997).

Class II HLA Alleles

Before the discovery of the influence of class I HLA alleles on the outcome of HTLV-1 infection (Jeffery et al. 1999), a weaker but reproducible association had been found between the class II allele HLA-DRB1*0101 and a higher risk of HAM/TSP (Kitze et al. 1998, Nishimura et al. 1991, Sonoda et al. 1996, Usuku et al. 1990). This association was also reproduced in the Kagoshima population study (Jeffery et al. 1999): possession of HLA-DRB1*0101 was associated with HAM/TSP at a one-tailed probability level ($P = 0.049$). More recently, a similar effect of HLA-DRB1*0101 was observed in a population in northern Iran with endemic HTLV-1 infection (Sabouri et al. 2005). However, the protective effect of HLA-A*02 (see above) abolished the susceptibility effect of HLA-DRB1*0101 (see Jeffery et al. 1999, table 3, p. 3850). Possession of *HLA-DRB1 *0101* was also associated with a significantly lower proviral load of HTLV-1 in the HAM/TSP patients but not in the asymptomatic carriers of HTLV-1 (Jeffery et al. 1999). Because of the strong linkage disequilibrium between HLA-DRB1*0101 and nearby alleles, the observed susceptibility effect cannot be ascribed with certainty to HLA-DRB1*0101 itself. The susceptibility effect associated with HLA-DRB1*0101 is perhaps exerted through an HLA-DRB1*0101-associated haplotype, that is, HLA-B*0702–Cw*0702-DRB1*0101–DQB1*0501. The population attributable risk of HAM/TSP conferred by the HLA-DRB1*0101 haplotype in Kagoshima was 7% in the whole cohort; this fraction rose to 11% in HLA-A*02⁻subjects, and fell to 0.4% in HLA-A*02⁺ subjects (Jeffery et al. 1999). In a logistic regression analysis that included the then known genetic and nongenetic factors that influence the outcome of HTLV-1 infection in Kagoshima, HLA-DRB1*0101 was not a significant predictor of the risk of HAM/TSP (Vine et al. 2002). However, in this analysis the association was maintained between HLA-DRB1*0101 and a lower proviral load in patients with HAM/TSP (Vine et al. 2002). We concluded that the HLA-DRB1*0101–

associated haplotype significantly increases susceptibility to HAM/TSP at a given proviral load in this southern Japanese population but that this effect is weak compared with those of the other factors in the analysis.

The reason for the association between the HLA-DRB1*0101 susceptibility haplotype and HAM/TSP is, as in the great majority of class II MHC–disease associations, unknown. An immunodominant HLA-DRB1*0101–restricted epitope in HTLV-1 Env gp21 has been described in Japan (Kitze et al. 1998). Since patients with HAM/TSP have recently been found to have a 10- to 25-fold higher frequency of HTLV-1–specific CD4⁺ T cells than do asymptomatic HTLV-1 carriers with a similar load (Goon et al. 2002, 2004a), it is possible that HLA-DRB1*0101–restricted HTLV-1–specific T cells, stimulated by the high HTLV-1 antigen load, play a significant part in initiating or perpetuating inflammatory lesions in HAM/TSP. Alternatively, the susceptibility conferred by the HLA-DRB1*0101 haplotype might be independent of HTLV-1 load. If HLA-DRB1*0101⁺ individuals have a lower threshold for HAM/TSP, this could account for the observation of a lower mean proviral load among HLA-DRB1*0101⁺ patients with HAM/TSP than that of HLA-DRB1*0101⁻patients.

Manns et al. (1998) carried out serological typing of class II HLA alleles in 45 asymptomatic carriers of HTLV-1, 49 patients with ATL, 54 patients with HAM/TSP, and 51 seronegative controls in Jamaica. They found an increased frequency of two class alleles in HTLV-1 asymptomatic carriers compared with seronegative controls: DRB1*1501 and DQ1 (DQB1*0501, *0502, *05031, *0602, *0605, *0609). The association with DRB1*1501 did not remain significant after correction for multiple comparisons. The DQ1 association observed was significant ($P = 0.049$) if a correction factor of 5 was used (for five HLA DQ serotypes detected) but not if a correction factor of 20 was used (for all DR and DQ serotypes identified). These researchers also used DNA typing of individual class II HLA alleles and found 35 DRB1 alleles and 13 DQB1 alleles in the study population. They observed a suggestive increase (i.e., not significant after correction) in DQB1*0602 in asymptomatic carriers compared with patients with HAM/TSP (P uncorrected = 0.001). They also found that two *DRB1* alleles were more common in both asymptomatic HTLV-1 carriers and patients with ATL than in patients with HAM/TSP. Although these frequency differences were not significant after correction, the authors pointed out that

DRB1*1501 and DQB1*0602 had also been found at a lower frequency in HAM/TSP patients than in patients with ATL in Japan (Sonoda et al. 1997).

Tumor Necrosis Factor

TNF is a strong candidate gene in HAM/TSP because tumor necrosis factor-α (TNF-α)-producing T cells have been identified in the cerebrospinal fluid in patients with HAM/TSP (Nakamura et al. 1993), in peripheral blood lymphocytes cultured *in vitro* (Nishiura et al. 1996), and in HAM/TSP lesions (Umehara et al. 1994). Furthermore, HTLV-1–specific CD4$^+$ T cells that produce TNF-α were significantly more frequent in HAM/TSP patients than in asymptomatic carriers (Goon et al. 2003). HTLV-1–specific CD8$^+$ T cells also produce TNF-α, as well as other proinflammatory substances (Biddison et al. 1997). HTLV-1 infection of a T cell does not appear to increase TNF-α production directly (Hanon et al. 2001), but antigenic stimulation of the T cells by the abundant HTLV-1 proteins would be sufficient to explain the observed TNF-α production.

In the Kagoshima cohort, nine SNPs were studied in the *TNF* promoter. Six of these SNPs were not informative (i.e., allele frequency <0.1), including the widely studied SNPs at positions−238 and−308. The three informative SNPs were those at nucleotides −1031,−863, and−857 (Vine et al. 2002). Single-factor χ^2 analysis showed a significant association between the−857 T allele and the disease HAM/TSP. However, it had been previously been shown (Jeffery et al. 2000) that this association was attributable to HLA-B*54, which is in strong linkage disequilibrium with TNF−857T in this population. Logistic regression analysis of the three informative *TNF* promoter SNPs showed (Vine et al. 2002) that only one SNP, at nucleotide−863, remained a significant independent predictor of the risk of HAM/TSP after the other factors had been taken into account (see below; table 20.2). This analysis also showed a statistically significant interaction between the TNF−863 SNP and the proviral load of HTLV-1. The TNF−863A$^+$ genotype was associated with an increased risk of HAM/TSP only in individuals with a high proviral load (>3 copies/100 PBMC; see figure 20.1). The TNF−863A$^+$ genotype

TABLE 20.2. Best-fit logistic regression equation for the risk of HTLV-1–associated myelopathy/tropical spastic paraparesis (HAM/TSP) in the Kagoshima HTLV-1–infected cohort ($n = 402$).

Factor, Condition	ln(odds of HAM/TSP)[a] Ratio (P)	Odds
Constant	−1.716	
Age	$-(0.145 \times \text{age}) + (0.003 \times \text{age}^2)$	—[b]
Provirus load	$+0.460 \times \text{load}) + (0.487 \times \text{load}^2)$	—[b]
TNF −863A$^+$	$+3.057-(4.616 \times \text{load})+(1.476 \times \text{load}^2)$	—[b]
SDF-1 +801GA	−0.808	0.45 (.042)
SDF-1 +801AA	−1.689	0.18 (.003)
HLA-A*02$^+$	−0.638	0.53 (.043)[c]
HLA-Cw*08$^+$	−0.894	0.41 (.046)[c]
HTLV-1 subgroup B	−1.587	0.20 (.017)

[a]The natural logarithm of an individual's odds of HAM/TSP in the cohort is calculated as the sum of the components in the central column, contingent on the factors indicated in the left-hand column. Load denotes $\log_{10}$(proviral copy no.)/10^4 PBMCs; age is given in years. HTLV-I subgroups are either A or B. The odds ratio (OR) of developing HAM/TSP conferred by each respective genotype is shown in the right-hand column. This equation correctly classifies 88.0% of patients with HAM/TSP in this Japanese study cohort. The prevalence rate (R) of HAM/TSP in HTLV-1–infected individuals of a given genotype may be calculated as R = H × OR/(1 + OR), where H = prevalence of HAM/TSP in the HTLV-I–infected population and OR = odds ratio of HAM/TSP associated with that genotype. For example, the prevalence of HAM/TSP in HLA-A*02$^+$ individuals in Kagoshima ∼0.01 × (0.53/1.53) ∼0.3%, taking H in Kagoshima ∼1%.

[b]ORs for the continuous variables (age and load) are omitted since their quadratic terms cause the ORs to vary over age and load. Similarly, an OR for TNF −863A is not given as its interaction term with provirus load causes the OR to vary over load; see figure 20.1 for more discussion of this variation.

[c]The HLA class I alleles A*02 and Cw*08 exert their strong effects on the outcome of HTLV-I infection primarily through an effect on provirus load [9, 18]. The 1-tailed P values given here relate to the additional effects of A*02 and Cw*08 after taking into account their effect on load.

Reproduced from Vine et al (2002), by permission of the publishers.

had independently been shown to confer a higher risk of another HTLV-1–associated inflammatory disease, HTLV-1–associated uveitis (HAU; Seki et al. 1999). In neither HAM/TSP nor HAU has a−863A$^+$ genotype been directly shown to be associated with a greater production of TNF-α.

These observations are consistent with a mathematical model that had been proposed (Asquith and Bangham 2000) to reconcile the beneficial and the proinflammatory roles of HTLV-1–specific CD8$^+$ T cells in HAM/TSP. Nishimura et al. (2003) investigated three TNF promoter polymorphisms (−1031, −863,−857) in an independent study in Japan, to test the hypothesis that such polymorphisms affect the proviral load of HTLV-1. No significant effect of these polymorphisms on proviral load was found, consistent with the observations made in the Kagoshima population genetic study (Vine et al. 2002); Nishimura et al. (2003) did not investigate a possible influence of these polymorphisms on the risk of HAM/TSP. These researchers also found no relationship between the outcome of HTLV-1 infection and two polymorphisms in the TNF receptor (TNFR-I,−383A/C; TNFR-II, exon 6 M196R).

Anti–TNF-α antibodies have given great benefit in other inflammatory conditions such as rheumatoid arthritis (Feldmann and Maini 2001) and Crohn's disease (Bondeson and Maini 2001). Serious consideration should be given to treatment with anti–TNF-α antibody of patients with active, progressing HAM/TSP.

CXCL12 (Stromal Cell–Derived Factor 1, SDF-1)

Univariate analysis showed a significantly lower prevalence of HAM/TSP in Kagoshima in individuals with the A allele at nucleotide +801 in the CXCL12 gene product SDF-1 (Vine et al. 2002). This was statistically significant both at the allele level ($P = 0.0021$, uncorrected) and at the genotype level ($P < 0.01$). Although neither result was statistically significant after correction for the number of comparisons made ($N = 58$), logistic regression analysis showed that the +801A allele remained a significant independent predictor of the risk of HAM/TSP in Kagoshima even after the other known predictors had been taken into account (table 20.2). Furthermore, there was an effect of gene dosage: The odds ratio (OR) of HAM/TSP conferred by the +801AA homozygous genotype (AA vs. GG: OR = 0.18; $P = 0.03$) was less than half the OR of HAM/TSP associated with heterozygosity at this site (AG vs. GG; $P = 0.042$). It was concluded that the +801 polymorphism significantly alters the risk of HAM/TSP in the Kagoshima population. This CXCL12 polymorphism had no detectable effect on the proviral load of HTLV-1 either in the whole cohort or in the HAM/TSP patients or asymptomatic carriers alone.

What is the likely role of SDF-1 in the pathogenesis of HAM/TSP? SDF-1 is one of only two chemokines that have been shown to stimulate the movement of

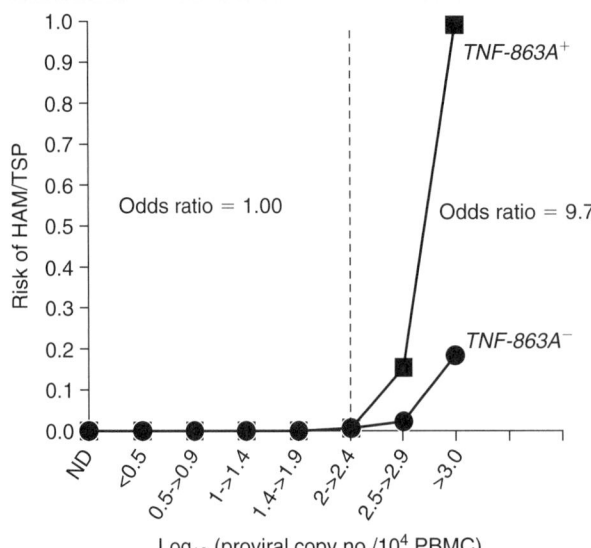

FIGURE 20.1. Interaction between TNF promoter genotype and load of HTLV-1 provirus. The TNF–863A allele increased the risk of HAM/TSP selectively in subjects with a high provirus load. Reproduced from Vine et al. (2002), by permission of the publishers.

resting lymphocytes as well as activated ones (Sallusto et al. 1998). Also, there is evidence that the HTLV-1 Tax protein induces expression of SDF-1 (Arai et al. 1998). Thus, a positive feedback loop may be generated which results in self-perpetuating foci of lymphocytes in, for example, the central nervous system. Activation of these lymphocytes by HTLV-1 proteins acting both as antigens (especially Tax and Env) and as a mitogen (Tax) will then result in production of proinflammatory substances, in addition to SDF-1, which cause bystander damage to nearby cells (Daenke and Bangham 2004, Ijichi et al. 1993). This hypothesis accounts for the influence of polymorphisms in HLA, *TNF* and *CXCL12* on the prevalence of HAM/TSP in the Kagoshima population.

IL15 (Interleukin-15)

The odds of HAM/TSP in the HTLV-1–infected population in Kagoshima were significantly higher in individuals with the +191C allele of *IL15* (Vine et al. 2002), using single-factor analysis ($P = 0.032$). However, in logistic regression analysis this effect was no longer significant after proviral load had been included as a factor. This observation suggests that the effect of the +191C allele is exerted through an effect on proviral load. Across the whole cohort, +191C was associated with a significantly lower proviral load ($P = 0.005$, analysis of covariance).

IL15 is another host cell gene whose expression is induced by HTLV-1 Tax (Azimi et al. 1998), and it has been suggested (Azimi et al. 2001) that interleukin-15, which promotes the survival of memory CD8[+] T cells (Sprent et al. 2000) and natural killer cells (Waldmann and Tagaya 1999), contributes to the high frequency of HTLV-1–specific CD8[+] T cells that is observed. However, in the absence of a comprehensive understanding of the complex dynamics of virus and host cell replication in HTLV-1 infection, the effects of this *IL15* polymorphism are not straightforwardly explained.

IL10 (Interleukin-10)

Sabouri et al. (2004) studied six polymorphisms in the promoter of the *IL10* gene in 280 cases of HAM/TSP and 255 asymptomatic HTLV-1 carriers in the Kagoshima population. Of the four informative SNPs, the one at position−592 had a significant influence on the outcome of HTLV-1 infection. The−592A allele was associated with a significantly lower proviral load in the

whole cohort ($P = 0.004$) and among asymptomatic HTLV-1 carriers ($P = 0.04$). However, this reduction in load, although evident among patients with HAM/TSP, did not reach significance in the patient group. Possession of the A allele was also associated with a significantly lower risk of HAM/TSP in this study cohort ($OR = 0.50$). These effects thus resemble the effects of the protective class I HLA alleles HLA-A*02 and HLA-Cw*08 (see above). Because the IL10−592A allele is present at a high frequency in this population (allele frequency in asymptomatic carriers = 65.3%), its protective effect in HTLV-1 infection is important at the population level: the prevented fraction of disease (F_P) attributable to−592A was 44.7%. The significance of−592A as a predictor of HAM/TSP in a logistic regression analysis appeared to be independent of the effects of HLA-A*02: both alleles remained significant predictors of the risk of HAM/TSP in a logistic progression model. Sabouri et al. (2004) obtained evidence that transcription of the *IL10* promoter was more effectively transactivated by HTLV-1 when the−592C residue (associated with a higher risk of HAM/TSP) was present.

Interleukin-10 (IL-10) is a cytokine that suppresses the production of proinflammatory cytokines by T cells and monocyte/macrophages (Moore et al. 2001). *IL10* promoter polymorphisms have previously been reported to be associated with the outcome of certain other viral infections: Epstein-Barr virus (Helminen et al. 2001), hepatitis B virus (Miyazoe et al. 2002), hepatitis C virus (Yee et al. 2001), and HIV-1 (Shin et al. 2000). In HIV-1 infection, the−592AA genotype was associated with rapid disease progression (Shin et al. 2000), whereas in the Kagoshima population, possession of the−592A allele was associated with protection in HTLV-1 infection.

Since T cells are both the host cell and the chief effector cell in the immune response in HTLV-1 infection, the effects of IL-10 on the risk of HAM/TSP cannot be predicted with certainty. Experimental evidence, preferably from *in vivo* or *ex vivo* sampling of infected humans, is therefore required to identify the mechanism of this observed association.

Nishimura et al. (2003) found no evidence that the IL-10−592 polymorphism influenced the proviral load in a study of 143 asymptomatic HTLV-1 carriers in Kumamoto prefecture, which lies north of Kagoshima in Kyushu, southern Japan. It is possible that the genetic composition of this population differs materially from that of Kagoshima, or that the sample size was too small to detect an effect. The influence of this polymorphism on the risk of HAM/TSP was not studied by Nishimura et al. (2003).

Other Cytokines and Chemokines

Nishimura et al. (2003) found no influence of either the IL-6−634 C/G polymorphism or the IL-1B−511A/C polymorphism on the proviral load of HTLV-1 in 143 asymptomatic carriers in Kumamoto. Suggestive evidence was obtained by Nishimura et al. (2003) of an interaction between a polymorphism in lymphotoxin α (LTα) (Nc01 A/G restriction site polymorphism in intron 1) and a polymorphism in the chemokine gene CCL2 (−2518A/G) in determining the proviral load of HTLV-1 in 143 asymptomatic HTLV-1 carriers in Japan. Individuals who were homozygous (GG) at both of these polymorphic sites had a higher proviral load than other individuals, although this difference was no longer significant after correction for multiple comparisons (uncorrected $P = 0.021$) (Nishimura et al. 2003).

MBL2 (Mannose-Binding Lectin)

Mannose-binding lectin (MBL) is a protein that plays an important part in innate immunity: polymorphisms in the MBL gene have been associated with variation in the outcome of both bacterial and viral infections, including HIV-1 (Garred et al. 1997). Asymptomatic carriers of HTLV-1 who were homozygous for the D allele in the polymorphism in the first exon in MBL (amino acid 54 Gly/Asp) tended to have a lower proviral load of HTLV-1 than other individuals (Nishimura et al. 2003). This difference was statistically significant when uncorrected ($P = 0.008$) but was of marginal significance after correction for multiple comparisons ($P_c = 0.09$).

PRF1 (Perforin 1)

This gene encodes a protein involved in lysis of target cells by the CTL response mechanism. Investigators in Mashhad, an area of endemic HTLV-1 infection in northeastern Iran, studied 60 patients with HAM/TSP, 71 HTLV-1 carriers, and 137 uninfected controls. They observed a higher frequency of the C allele at position +418 (C/T) in patients with HAM/TSP compared with uninfected controls ($P = 0.011$, not $P = 0.005$ as reported) (Rafatpanah et al. 2004). However, there was no significant difference between

HAM/TSP patients and asymptomatic carriers of HTLV-1 in the frequency of either the +418C allele or the CC genotype. Since Vine et al. (2004) have demonstrated an association between a high level of perforin gene expression and a low proviral load of HTLV-1 in both patients with HAM/TSP and asymptomatic carriers, it is an attractive hypothesis that PRF1 +418C is associated with more efficient CTL-mediated lysis of HTLV-1–infected cells in this population. However, this inference remains to be tested.

Vitamin D Receptor

Saito et al. (2005) reported a small but statistically significant protective effect of a polymorphic variant of the vitamin D receptor against HAM/TSP in the Kagoshima population. However, this polymorphism had no detectable effect on the proviral load of HTLV-1, and the interpretation of this finding is not yet clear.

Estimation of the Risk of HAM/TSP and of Proviral Load in Kagoshima

The factors that were found to influence either the prevalence of HAM/TSP or the proviral load of HTLV-1 were analyzed using general linear models and logistic regression (Vine et al. 2002). These techniques allow the inclusion of both categorical parameters (e.g., sex or genotype) and continuous parameters (e.g., age, proviral load) in a single equation.

Table 20.2 shows the best-fit logistic regression equation that was derived from the data in the Kagoshima population study to estimate the odds that an individual in the study cohort has HAM/TSP. Since a case–control design was used in this study, approximately half the subjects in the cohort had HAM/TSP. Therefore, this equation should not be used to estimate the risk of HAM/TSP in an HTLV-1–positive individual drawn at random from the general population in Kagoshima. However, the equation can be used to compare the odds of HAM/TSP between two different individuals of specified age, sex, genotype, and proviral load. For example, a person in Kagoshima with the marker combination TNF−863A$^+$, CXCL12 +801AA, HLA-A*02$^-$, HLA-Cw*08$^+$, infected with subgroup B of the HTLV-1 cosmopolitan group with a load of ~3 copies/100 PBMCs, has a 20-fold greater odds of HAM/TSP than an individual of the same age with the combination TNF−863A$^-$, CXCL12 +801AA, HLA-

A*02$^+$, HLA-Cw*08$^+$ (i.e., differing at *TNF* and *HLA-A*), infected with the same strain of HTLV-1 with a load of 1 copy/100 PBMCs.

Genetic Influence on Susceptibility to Acquisition of HTLV-1 Infection

Most of the clear results obtained to date on the genetic susceptibility in HTLV-1 infection have come from studies of the influence of genetic polymorphisms on the outcome of HTLV-1 infection, that is, the proviral load or the risk of HTLV-1–associated diseases, rather than the possible influence of such polymorphisms on the risk of acquiring HTLV-1 infection. Genes that control only the antigen-specific immune response are unlikely to affect the risk of acquisition of HTLV-1 infection, because the antigen-specific immune response is made only when the infection is already established, and there are few known examples of apparent eradication of HTLV-1 infection (Daenke et al. 1994). But it is possible that polymorphisms in other genes, such as those that control the innate immune response, affect the probability of acquiring HTLV-1. There is a precedent for this in the well-known effect of the polymorphism in CCR5 ($\triangle$32) on the risk of acquiring HIV-1 infection (see chapter 19).

In a population with endemic HTLV-1 infection in French Guiana, a segregation analysis was carried out on 83 families that included 1,638 individuals, of whom 165 or 10.1% were HTLV-1 seropositive (Plancoulaine et al. 2000). This analysis was consistent with the existence of a single Mendelian dominant gene that predisposes to HTLV-1 infection, acting in addition to the expected familial effects on the risk of HTLV-1 infection (mother–offspring, spouse–spouse). This apparent susceptibility locus has now been mapped by a genome-wide linkage analysis to chromosome 6q27 (Plancoulaine et al. 2006). Further work using techniques such as the transmission-disequilibrium test will be required to refine this mapping.

Conclusion

In the Kagoshima study, polymorphic variants at eight loci have so far been reported to affect the outcome of HTLV-1 infection: four HLA loci and *TNF*, two (*IL10* and *IL15*) that encode cytokines, and one (*CXCL12*) that encodes a chemokine. Of these eight, five loci are

in the MHC region. The contribution of each allele to the risk of HAM/TSP has been quantified by logistic regression analysis. In this analysis, the proviral load remains significant as a predictive factor of the risk of HAM/TSP. The working hypothesis is that the proviral load, the strongest single predictor of the risk of HAM/TSP, is determined by the efficiency of the host immune response to HTLV-1—chiefly the CTL response—which in turn varies between individuals because of polymorphisms in certain genes that encode critical proteins in the immune response. If this hypothesis is correct, it should be possible to account for variation between individuals in the proviral load entirely by the host genotype. However, the genetic factors described above account for less than 10% of the observed individual variation in the proviral load (Vine et al. 2002). Presumably, additional important genetic determinants of the outcome of HTLV-1 infection remain to be discovered.

Because HTLV-1 typically causes a stable chronic infection with a high proviral load and a strong, highly focused immune response, HTLV-1 infection has become a useful system to identify and quantify the determinants of the efficiency of the antiviral immune response.

References

Ahmad, T., Neville, M., Marshall, S.E., Armuzzi, A., Mulcahy-Hawes, K., Crawshaw, J., Sato, H., Ling, K.L., Barnardo, M., Goldthorpe, S., Walton, R., Bunce, M., Jewell, D.P., & Welsh, K.I. (2003) Haplotype-specific linkage disequilibrium patterns define the genetic topography of the human MHC. *Hum Mol Genet*, 12, 647–656.

Arai, M., Ohashi, T., Tsukahara, T., Murakami, T., Hori, T., Uchiyama, T., Yamamoto, N., Kannagi, M., & Fujii, M. (1998) Human T-cell leukemia virus type 1 Tax protein induces the expression of lymphocyte chemoattractant SDF-1/PBSF. *Virology*, 241, 298–303.

Asquith, B., & Bangham, C.R. (2000) The role of cytotoxic T lymphocytes in human T-cell lymphotropic virus type 1 infection. *J Theor Biol*, 207, 65–79.

Asquith, B., Hanon, E., Taylor, G.P., & Bangham, C.R. (2000) Is human T-cell lymphotropic virus type I really silent? *Philos Trans R Soc Lond B Biol Sci*, 355, 1013–1019.

Asquith B., Mosley, A.J., Barfield, A., Marshall, S.E., Heaps, A., Goon, P., Hanon, E., Tanaka, Y., Taylor, G.P., & Bangham, C.R.M. 2005. A functional CD8$^+$

cell assay reveals individual variation in CD8[+] cell antiviral efficacy and explains differences in human T-lymphotropic virus type 1 proviral load. *J Gen Virol*, 86, 1515–1523.

Asquith, B., Zhang, Y., Mosley, A. J., de Lara, C. M., Wallace, D. L., Worth, A., Kaftantzi, L., Meekings, K., Griffin, G. E., Tanaka, Y., Tough, D. F., Beverley, P. C., Taylor, G. P., Macallan, D. C., & Bangham, C. R. (2007) In vivo T lymphocyte dynamics in humans and the impact of human T-lymphotropic virus 1 infection. *Proc Natl Acad Sci USA*, 104, 8035–8040.

Azimi, N., Brown, K., Bamford, R.N., Tagaya, Y., Siebenlist, U., & Waldmann, T.A. (1998) Human T cell lymphotropic virus type I Tax protein trans-activates interleukin 15 gene transcription through an NF-kappaB site. *Proc Natl Acad Sci USA*, 95, 2452–2457.

Azimi, N., Nagai, M., Jacobson, S., & Waldmann, T.A. (2001) IL-15 plays a major role in the persistence of Tax-specific CD8 cells in HAM/TSP patients. *Proc Natl Acad Sci USA*, 98, 14559–14564.

Bangham, C.R. (2000) The immune response to HTLV-I. *Curr Opin Immunol*, 12, 397–402.

Bangham, C.R.M. (2003) The immune control and cell to cell spread of HTLV-1. *J Gen Virol* 84, 3177–3189.

Bangham, C.R.M., Nightingale, S., & Osame, M. (2000) HTLV-I and -II and associated diseases. In: *Oxford textbook of medicine* (ed. by D.J. Weatherall et al.). Oxford University Press, Oxford.

Bangham, C.R.M., & Osame, M. (2005) The cellular immune response to HTLV-1. *Oncogene* 24, 6035–6046.

Biddison, W.E., Kubota, R., Kawanishi, T., Taub, D.D., Cruikshank, W.W., Center, D.M., Connor, E.W., Utz, U., & Jacobson, S. (1997) Human T cell leukemia virus type I (HTLV-I)-specific CD8+ CTL clones from patients with HTLV-I-associated neurologic disease secrete proinflammatory cytokines, chemokines, and matrix metalloproteinase. *J Immunol*, 159, 2018–2025.

Bondeson, J., & Maini, R.N. (2001) Tumour necrosis factor as a therapeutic target in rheumatoid arthritis and other chronic inflammatory diseases: the clinical experience with infliximab (REMICADE). *Int J Clin Pract*, 55, 211–216.

Borducchi, D.M., Gerbase-DeLima, M., Morgun, A., Shulzhenko, N., Pombo-de-Oliveira, M.S., Kerbauy, J., & Rodrigues de Oliveira, J.S. (2003) Human leucocyte antigen and human T-cell lymphotropic virus type 1 associated diseases in Brazil. *Br J Haematol*, 123, 954–955.

Cavrois, M., Gessain, A., Wain-Hobson, S., & Wattel, E. (1996) Proliferation of HTLV-1 infected circulating

cells in vivo in all asymptomatic carriers and patients with TSP/HAM. *Oncogene*, 12, 2419–2423.

Daenke, S., & Bangham, C.R. (1994) Do T cells cause HTLV-1-associated disease? A taxing problem. *Clin Exp Immunol*, 96, 179–181.

Daenke, S., Kermode, A.G., Hall, S.E., Taylor, G., Weber, J., Nightingale, S., & Bangham, C.R. (1996) High activated and memory cytotoxic T-cell responses to HTLV-1 in healthy carriers and patients with tropical spastic paraparesis. *Virology*, 217, 139–146.

Daenke, S., Nightingale, S., Cruickshank, J.K., & Bangham, C.R. (1990) Sequence variants of human T-cell lymphotropic virus type I from patients with tropical spastic paraparesis and adult T-cell leukemia do not distinguish neurological from leukemic isolates. *J Virol*, 64, 1278–1282.

Daenke, S., Parker, C.E., Niewiesk, S., Newsom-Davis, J., Nightingale, S., & Bangham, C.R. (1994) Spastic paraparesis in a patient carrying defective human T cell leukemia virus type I (HTLV-I) provirus sequences but lacking a humoral or cytotoxic T cell response to HTLV-I. *J Infect Dis*, 169, 941–943.

Elovaara, I., Koenig, S., Brewah, A.Y., Woods, R.M., Lehky, T., & Jacobson, S. (1993) High human T cell lymphotropic virus type 1 (HTLV-1)-specific precursor cytotoxic T lymphocyte frequencies in patients with HTLV-1-associated neurological disease. *J Exp Med*, 177, 1567–1573.

Feldmann, M., & Maini, R.N. (2001) Anti-TNF alpha therapy of rheumatoid arthritis: what have we learned? *Annu Rev Immunol*, 19, 163–196.

Furukawa, Y., Yamashita, M., Usuku, K., Izumo, S., Nakagawa, M., & Osame, M. (2000) Phylogenetic subgroups of human T cell lymphotropic virus (HTLV) type I in the tax gene and their association with different risks for HTLV-I-associated myelopathy/tropical spastic paraparesis. *J Infect Dis*, 182, 1343–1349.

Garred, P., Madsen, H.O., Balslev, U., Hofmann, B., Pedersen, C., Gerstoft, J., & Svejgaard, A. (1997) Susceptibility to HIV infection and progression of AIDS in relation to variant alleles of mannose-binding lectin. *Lancet*, 349, 236–240.

Goon, P.K., Hanon, E., Igakura, T., Tanaka, Y., Weber, J.N., Taylor, G.P., & Bangham, C.R. (2002) High frequencies of Th1-type CD4(+) T cells specific to HTLV-1 Env and Tax proteins in patients with HTLV-1-associated myelopathy/tropical spastic paraparesis. *Blood*, 99, 3335–3341.

Goon, P.K., Igakura, T., Hanon, E., Mosley, A.J., Asquith, B., Gould, K.G., Taylor, G.P., Weber, J.N., & Bangham, C.R. (2003) High circulating frequencies of tumor necrosis factor alpha- and interleukin-2-secreting human T-lymphotropic virus type 1

(HTLV-1)-specific CD4+ T cells in patients with HTLV-1-associated neurological disease. *J Virol*, 77, 9716–9722.

Goon, P.K., Igakura, T., Hanon, E., Mosley, A.J., Barfield, A., Barnard, A.L., Kaftantzi, L., Tanaka, Y., Taylor, G.P., Weber, J.N., & Bangham, C.R. (2004a) Human T cell lymphotropic virus type I (HTLV-I)-specific CD4+ T cells: immunodominance hierarchy and preferential infection with HTLV-I. *J Immunol*, 172, 1735–1743.

Goon, P.K.C., Biancardi, A., Fast, N., Igakura, T., Hanon, E., Mosley, A., Asquith, B., Gould, K.G., Marshall, S., Taylor, G.P., & Bangham, C.R.M. (2004b) Human T cell lymphotropic virus (HTLV) type-1-specific CD8+ T cells: frequency and immunodominance hierarchy. *J. Infect. Dis.* 189, 2294–2298.

Green, P.L., & Chen, I. S. Y. (2001) Human T lymphotropic viruses types 1 and 2. In: *Fields virology* (edited by D.M. Knipe & P.M. Howley), Vol. 2, pp. 1941–1969. Lippincott Williams and Wilkins, Philadelphia.

Hanon, E., Goon, P., Taylor, G.P., Hasegawa, H., Tanaka, Y., Weber, J.N., & Bangham, C.R. (2001) High production of interferon gamma but not interleukin-2 by human T-lymphotropic virus type I-infected peripheral blood mononuclear cells. *Blood*, 98, 721–726.

Hanon, E., Stinchcombe, J.C., Saito, M., Asquith, B.E., Taylor, G.P., Tanaka, Y., Weber, J.N., Griffiths, G.M., & Bangham, C.R. (2000) Fratricide among CD8(+) T lymphocytes naturally infected with human T cell lymphotropic virus type I. *Immunity*, 13, 657–664.

Helminen, M.E., Kilpinen, S., Virta, M., & Hurme, M. (2001) Susceptibility to primary Epstein-Barr virus infection is associated with interleukin-10 gene promoter polymorphism. *J Infect Dis*, 184, 777–780.

Igakura, T., Stinchcombe, J.C., Goon, P.K., Taylor, G.P., Weber, J.N., Griffiths, G.M., Tanaka, Y., Osame, M., & Bangham, C.R. (2003) Spread of HTLV-I between lymphocytes by virus-induced polarization of the cytoskeleton. *Science*, 299, 1713–1716.

Ijichi, S., Izumo, S., Eiraku, N., Machigashira, K., Kubota, R., Nagai, M., Ikegami, N., Kashio, N., Umehara, F., Maruyama, I., et al. (1993) An autoaggressive process against bystander tissues in HTLV-I-infected individuals: a possible pathomechanism of HAM/TSP. *Med Hypotheses*, 41, 542–547.

Iwasaki, Y., Ohara, Y., Kobayashi, I., & Akizuki, S. (1992) Infiltration of helper/inducer T lymphocytes heralds central nervous system damage in human T-cell leukemia virus infection. *Am J Pathol*, 140, 1003–1008.

Jeffery, K.J., Siddiqui, A.A., Bunce, M., Lloyd, A.L., Vine, A.M., Witkover, A.D., Izumo, S., Usuku, K., Welsh, K.I., Osame, M., & Bangham, C.R. (2000) The in-

fluence of HLA class I alleles and heterozygosity on the outcome of human T cell lymphotropic virus type I infection. *J Immunol*, 165, 7278–7284.

Jeffery, K.J., Usuku, K., Hall, S.E., Matsumoto, W., Taylor, G.P., Procter, J., Bunce, M., Ogg, G.S., Welsh, K.I., Weber, J.N., Lloyd, A.L., Nowak, M.A., Nagai, M., Kodama, D., Izumo, S., Osame, M., & Bangham, C.R. (1999) HLA alleles determine human T-lymphotropic virus-I (HTLV-I) proviral load and the risk of HTLV-I-associated myelopathy. *Proc Natl Acad Sci USA*, 96, 3848–3853.

Keicho, N., Ohashi, J., Tamiya, G., Nakata, K., Taguchi, Y., Azuma, A., Ohishi, N., Emi, M., Park, M.H., Inoko, H., Tokunaga, K., & Kudoh, S. (2000) Fine localization of a major disease-susceptibility locus for diffuse panbronchiolitis. *Am J Hum Genet*, 66, 501–507.

Keicho, N., Tokunaga, K., Nakata, K., Taguchi, Y., Azuma, A., Bannai, M., Emi, M., Ohishi, N., Yazaki, Y., & Kudoh, S. (1998) Contribution of HLA genes to genetic predisposition in diffuse panbronchiolitis. *Am J Respir Crit Care Med*, 158, 846–850.

Kikuchi, I., Ueda, A., Mihara, K., Miyanaga, O., Machidori, H., Ishikawa, E., & Tamura, K. (1998) The effect of HLA alleles on response to interferon therapy in patients with chronic hepatitis C. *Eur J Gastroenterol Hepatol*, 10, 859–863.

Kitze, B., Usuku, K., Yamano, Y., Yashiki, S., Nakamura, M., Fujiyoshi, T., Izumo, S., Osame, M., & Sonoda, S. (1998) Human CD4+ T lymphocytes recognize a highly conserved epitope of human T lymphotropic virus type 1 (HTLV-1) env gp21 restricted by HLA DRB1*0101. *Clin Exp Immunol*, 111, 278–285.

Kitze, B., Usuku, K., Yashiki, S., Ijichi, S., Fujiyoshi, T., Nakamura, M., Izumo, S., Osame, M., & Sonoda, S. (1996) Intrathecal humoral immune response in HAM/TSP in relation to HLA haplotype analysis. *Acta Neurol Scand*, 94, 287–293.

Kubota, R., Hanada, K., Furukawa, Y., Arimura, K., Osame, M., Gojobori, T., & Izumo, S. (2007) Genetic stability of human T lymphotropic virus type I despite antiviral pressures by CTLs. *J Immunol* 178, 5966–5972.

Kuzushita, N., Hayashi, N., Moribe, T., Katayama, K., Kanto, T., Nakatani, S., Kaneshige, T., Tatsumi, T., Ito, A., Mochizuki, K., Sasaki, Y., Kasahara, A., & Hori, M. (1998) Influence of HLA haplotypes on the clinical courses of individuals infected with hepatitis C virus. *Hepatology*, 27, 240–244.

Manns, A., Hanchard, B., Morgan, O.S., Wilks, R., Cranston, B., Nam, J.M., Blank, M., Kuwayama, M., Yashiki, S., Fujiyoshi, T., Blattner, W., & Sonoda, S. (1998) Human leukocyte antigen class II alleles associated with human T-cell lymphotropic virus type I infection and adult T-cell leukemia/lymphoma in a Black population. *J Natl Cancer Inst*, 90, 617–622.

Miyazoe, S., Hamasaki, K., Nakata, K., Kajiya, Y., Kitajima, K., Nakao, K., Daikoku, M., Yatsuhashi, H., Koga, M., Yano, M., & Eguchi, K. (2002) Influence of interleukin-10 gene promoter polymorphisms on disease progression in patients chronically infected with hepatitis B virus. *Am J Gastroenterol*, 97, 2086–2092.

Moore, K.W., de Waal Malefyt, R., Coffman, R.L., & O'Garra, A. (2001) Interleukin-10 and the interleukin-10 receptor. *Annu Rev Immunol*, 19, 683–765.

Mueller, N.E., & Blattner, W.A. (1997) Retroviruses: HTLV. In: *Viral infections of humans: epidemiology and control* (ed. by A.S. Evans & R. Kaslow), pp. 785–813. Plenum Medical Press, New York.

Nagai, M., Usuku, K., Matsumoto, W., Kodama, D., Takenouchi, N., Moritoyo, T., Hashiguchi, S., Ichinose, M., Bangham, C.R., Izumo, S., & Osame, M. (1998) Analysis of HTLV-I proviral load in 202 HAM/TSP patients and 243 asymptomatic HTLV-I carriers: high proviral load strongly predisposes to HAM/TSP. *J Neurovirol*, 4, 586–593.

Nakamura, S., Nagano, I., Yoshioka, M., Shimazaki, S., Onodera, J., & Kogure, K. (1993) Detection of tumor necrosis factor-alpha-positive cells in cerebrospinal fluid of patients with HTLV-I-associated myelopathy. *J Neuroimmunol*, 42, 127–130.

Niewiesk, S., Daenke, S., Parker, C.E., Taylor, G., Weber, J., Nightingale, S., & Bangham, C.R. (1994) The transactivator gene of human T-cell leukemia virus type I is more variable within and between healthy carriers than patients with tropical spastic paraparesis. *J Virol*, 68, 6778–6781.

Nishimura, M., Maeda, M., Yasunaga, J., Kawakami, H., Kaji, R., Adachi, A., Uchiyama, T., & Matsuoka, M. (2003) Influence of cytokine and mannose binding protein gene polymorphisms on human T-cell leukemia virus type I (hTLV-I) provirus load in HTLV-I asymptomatic carriers. *Hum Immunol*, 64, 453–457.

Nishimura, Y., Okubo, R., Minato, S., Itoyama, Y., Goto, I., Mori, M., Hirayama, K., & Sasazuki, T. (1991) A possible association between HLA and HTLV-I-associated myelopathy (HAM) in Japanese. *Tissue Antigens*, 37, 230–231.

Nishiura, Y., Nakamura, T., Ichinose, K., Shirabe, S., Tsujino, A., Goto, H., Furuya, T., & Nagataki, S. (1996) Increased production of inflammatory cytokines in cultured CD4+ cells from patients with HTLV-I-associated myelopathy. *Tohoku J Exp Med*, 179, 227–233.

Nowak, M.A., & Bangham, C.R. (1996) Population dynamics of immune responses to persistent viruses. *Science*, 272, 74–79.

Plancoulaine, S., Gessain, A., Joubert, M., Tortevoye, P., Jeanne, I., Talarmin, A., de The, G., & Abel, L. (2000) Detection of a major gene predisposing to human T lymphotropic virus type I infection in children among an endemic population of African origin. *J Infect Dis*, 182, 405–412.

Plancoulaine, S., Gessain, A., Tortevoye, P., Boland-Auge, A., Vasilescu, A., Matsuda, F., and Abel, L. (2006) A major susceptibility locus for HTLV-1 infection in childhood maps to chromosome 6q27. *Hum Mol Genets*, 15, 3306–3312.

Rafatpanah, H., Pravica, V., Farid, R., Abbaszadegan, R., Tabatabaei, A., Goharjoo, A., Etemadi, M.M., & Hutchinson, I.V. (2004) Association of a novel single nucleotide polymorphism in the human perforin gene with the outcome of HTLV-1 infection in patients from northeast Iran (Mash-had). *Hum Immunol*, 65, 839–846.

Sabouri, A.H., Saito, M., Lloyd, A.L., Vine, A.M., Witkover, A.W., Furukawa, Y., Izumo, S., Arimura, K., Marshall, S.E.F., Usuku, K., Bangham, C.R.M., & Osame, M. (2004) Polymorphism in the IL-10 promoter affects both provirus load and the risk of human T lymphotropic virus type I (HTLV-I)–associated myelopathy/tropical spastic paraparesis. *J Infect Dis*, 190, 1279–1285.

Sabouri, A. H., Saito, M., Usuku, K., Bajestan, S. N., Mahmoudi, M., Forughipour, M., Sabouri, Z., Abbaspour, Z., Goharjoo, M. E., Khayami, E., Hasani, A., Izumo, S., Arimura, K., Farid, R., and Osame, M. (2005) Differences in viral and host genetic risk factors for development of human T-cell lymphotropic virus type 1 (HTLV-1)-associated myelopathy/tropical spastic paraparesis between Iranian and Japanese HTLV-1 infected individuals. *J Gen Virol*, 86, 773–781.

Saito, M., Eiraku, N., Usuku, K., Nobuhara, Y., Matsumoto, W, Kodama, D., Sabouri, A. H., Izumo, S., Arimura, K., and Osame, M. (2005) ApaI polymorphism of vitamin D receptor gene is associated with susceptibility to HTLV-1-associated myelopathy/tropical spastic paraparesis in HTLV-1 infected individuals. *J Neurol Sci*, 232, 29–35.

Sallusto, F., Lanzavecchia, A., & Mackay, C.R. (1998) Chemokines and chemokine receptors in T-cell priming and Th1/Th2-mediated responses. *Immunol Today*, 19, 568–574.

Seki, N., Yamaguchi, K., Yamada, A., Kamizono, S., Sugita, S., Taguchi, C., Matsuoka, M., Matsumoto, H., Nishizaka, S., Itoh, K., & Mochizuki, M. (1999) Polymorphism of the 5'-flanking region of the tumor necrosis factor (TNf)-alpha gene and susceptibility to human T-cell lymphotropic virus type I (HTLV-I) uveitis. *J Infect Dis*, 180, 880–883.

Shin, H.D., Winkler, C., Stephens, J.C., Bream, J., Young, H., Goedert, J.J., O'Brien, T.R., Vlahov, D., Buchbinder, S., Giorgi, J., Rinaldo, C., Donfield, S., Willoughby, A., O'Brien, S.J., & Smith, M.W. (2000) Genetic restriction of HIV-1 pathogenesis to AIDS by promoter alleles of IL10. *Proc Natl Acad Sci USA*, 97, 14467–14472.

Slattery, J.P., Franchini, G., & Gessain, A. (1999) Genomic evolution, patterns of global dissemination, and interspecies transmission of human and simian T-cell leukemia/lymphotropic viruses. *Genome Res*, 9, 525–540.

Sonoda, S., Fujiyoshi, T., & Yashiki, S. (1996) Immunogenetics of HTLV-I/II and associated diseases. *J Acquir Immune Defic Syndr Hum Retrovirol*, 13(suppl 1), S119–S123.

Sonoda, S., Manns, A., Alcalay, D., Jacobson, S., Nikbin, B., Blank, A. et al. (1997) HLA and HTLV. In: *The 12th International Histocompatibility Workshop and Conference Proceedings, Genetic Diversity of HLA: Functional and Medical Implications* (ed. by D. Charron). EDK, Paris.

Sprent, J., Zhang, X., Sun, S., & Tough, D. (2000) T-cell proliferation in vivo and the role of cytokines. *Philos Trans R Soc Lond B Biol Sci*, 355, 317–322.

Sugiyama, Y., Kudoh, S., Maeda, H., Suzaki, H., & Takaku, F. (1990) Analysis of HLA antigens in patients with diffuse panbronchiolitis. *Am Rev Respir Dis*, 141, 1459–1462.

Taylor, G.P., Hall, S.E., Navarrete, S., Michie, C.A., Davis, R., Witkover, A.D., Rossor, M., Nowak, M.A., Rudge, P., Matutes, E., Bangham, C.R., & Weber, J.N. (1999) Effect of lamivudine on human T-cell leukemia virus type 1 (HTLV-1) DNA copy number, T-cell phenotype, and anti-tax cytotoxic T-cell frequency in patients with HTLV-1-associated myelopathy. *J Virol*, 73, 10289–10295.

Umehara, F., Izumo, S., Ronquillo, A.T., Matsumuro, K., Sato, E., & Osame, M. (1994) Cytokine expression in the spinal cord lesions in HTLV-I-associated myelopathy. *J Neuropathol Exp Neurol*, 53, 72–77.

Usuku, K., Nishizawa, M., Matsuki, K., Tokunaga, K., Takahashi, K., Eiraku, N., Suehara, M., Juji, T., Osame, M., & Tabira, T. (1990) Association of a particular amino acid sequence of the HLA-DR beta 1 chain with HTLV-I-associated myelopathy. *Eur J Immunol*, 20, 1603–1606.

Vine, A.M., Heaps, A. G., Kaftantzi, L., Mosley, A., Asquith, B., Witkover, A., Thompson, G., Saito, M., Goon, P.K.C., Carr, L., Martinez-Murillo, F., Taylor, G.P., & Bangham, C.R.M. (2004) The role of CTLs in persistent viral infection: cytolytic gene expression in CD8[+] lymphocytes distinguishes between individuals with a high or low proviral load of HTLV-1. *J Immunol*, 173, 5121–5129.

Vine, A.M., Witkover, A.D., Lloyd, A.L., Jeffery, K.J., Siddiqui, A., Marshall, S.E., Bunce, M., Eiraku, N., Izumo, S., Usuku, K., Osame, M., & Bangham, C.R. (2002) Polygenic control of human T lymphotropic virus type I (HTLV-I) provirus load and the risk of HTLV-I-associated myelopathy/tropical spastic paraparesis. *J Infect Dis*, 186, 932–939.

Waldmann, T.A., & Tagaya, Y. (1999) The multifaceted regulation of interleukin-15 expression and the role of this cytokine in NK cell differentiation and host response to intracellular pathogens. *Annu Rev Immunol*, 17, 19–49.

White, J.D., Johnson, J.A., Nam, J.M., Cranston, B., Hanchard, B., Waldmann, T.A., & Manns, A. (1996) Distribution of human leukocyte antigens in a population of black patients with human T-cell lymphotrophic virus type I-associated adult T-cell leukemia/lymphoma. *Cancer Epidemiol Biomarkers Prev*, 5, 873–877.

Wodarz, D., & Bangham, C.R. (2000) Evolutionary dynamics of HTLV-I. *J Mol Evol*, 50, 448–455.

Wodarz, D., Hall, S.E., Usuku, K., Osame, M., Ogg, G.S., McMichael, A.J., Nowak, M.A., & Bangham, C.R. (2001) Cytotoxic T-cell abundance and virus load in human immunodeficiency virus type 1 and human T-cell leukaemia virus type 1. *Proc R Soc Lond B Biol Sci*, 268, 1215–1221.

Yashiki, S., Fujiyoshi, T., Arima, N., Osame, M., Yoshinaga, M., Nagata, Y., Tara, M., Nomura, K., Utsunomiya, A., Hanada, S., Tajima, K., & Sonoda, S. (2001) HLA-A*26, HLA-B*4002, HLA-B*4006, and HLA-B*4801 alleles predispose to adult T cell leukemia: the limited recognition of HTLV type 1 tax peptide anchor motifs and epitopes to generate anti-HTLV type 1 tax CD8(+) cytotoxic T lymphocytes. *AIDS Res Hum Retroviruses*, 17, 1047–1061.

Yee, L.J., Tang, J., Gibson, A.W., Kimberly, R., Van Leeuwen, D.J., & Kaslow, R.A. (2001) Interleukin 10 polymorphisms as predictors of sustained response in antiviral therapy for chronic hepatitis C infection. *Hepatology*, 33, 708–712.

21

Hepatitis B and Hepatitis C Infection

Leland J. Yee & Mark R. Thursz

Infection with the hepatitis B or hepatitis C viruses may result in a number of different outcomes, ranging from asymptomatic self-limited ("acute") infection to persistent ("chronic") infection with liver cirrhosis, liver failure, or hepatocellular carcinoma. Therapeutic intervention in patients with persistent viral infection may lead to complete resolution of the infection and the associated liver disease, may fail, or may even exacerbate the liver disease. While it is clear that environmental and viral variables play an important role in determining some of these outcomes, it is also evident that host genetic background is a major factor particularly in determining which individuals develop persistent infection.

Hepatitis B Virus Infection

Hepatitis B virus (HBV) is a small partially double-stranded DNA virus of the Hepadnaviridae family (Lee, 1997). Worldwide more than two billion people have been infected with HBV, with 350 million persistently infected. Prevalence is highest in parts of the world such as Asia and sub-Saharan Africa. Approximately 30% of those with persistent infection will die as a result of HBV-induced liver failure or hepatocellular carcinoma. One million deaths annually are attributable to HBV, with the majority occurring in the developing world.

MHC Class II

Self-limiting HBV infection is associated with a vigorous polyclonal and multispecific CD4+ T-helper cell responses, in contrast to the weak responses seen in persistent infection (Ferrari et al., 1990; Chisari and Ferrari, 1995). Therefore, polymorphism in the MHC class II region is a potential explanation for the variation in outcome. Failure of HBV vaccination, defined by an anti-HBs titer < 10 IU/L after three doses of HBsAg vaccination, is thought to arise through a lack of T-cell help for anti-HBs-producing B cells. Therefore, failure to develop anti-HBV immunity following HBV vaccination may also be influenced by MHC class II polymorphism. Vaccine nonresponse is consistently associated with HLA-DRB1*0301 *0401, and *0701 in many populations (see chapter 27).

The results of MHC class II association studies in persistent HBV infection are summarized in table 21.1. The alleles DRB1*1301/2 are consistently associated with resistance to persistent infection in sub-Saharan African, Oriental, and Caucasian populations (Thursz et al., 1995; Höhler et al., 1997; Ahn et al., 2000). HLA-DR7 (DRB1*07−) and HLA-DR3 (DRB1*0301) have been associated with persistent infection (Almarri and Batchelor, 1994; Jiang et al., 2003), and interestingly, the alleles DRB1*0701 and DRB1*0301 have also been associated with failure to respond to HBsAg-based vaccine (Milich and Leroux-Roels, 2003). While this finding needs to be replicated in other populations it

raises two possibilities: (1) T and B cell responses to HBsAg are critical to the development of persistent infection, and (2) individuals who fail to respond to the vaccine may be more susceptible to persistent infection. DRB1*0901, DQA1*0301, DQA1*0501, and DQB1*0301 are consistently associated with persistent HBV infection in different ethnic populations (Ahn et al., 2000; Thio et al., 1999; Meng et al., 2003). Functional analyses of these associations have not been undertaken.

The mechanism(s) underlying the HLA-DRB1*1302 association with resistance to persistent infection is unresolved. Two explanations have been proposed. First, the quality or magnitude of the T-cell response induced by HLA-DRB1*1302 is superior to other alleles. This is supported by work in mice indicating that different H2 backgrounds influence the character and magnitude of the T-cell response to HBV

TABLE 21.1. Studies of HLA class II polymorphism in HBV infection.

Study	Country	Number (Type) of Controls	Specificity	Odds Ratio	P-Value
van Hattum et al. (1987)	Holland	79 (107 SL)	DRw6	0.4	0.02
			DQw1	3.5	0.001
Almarri and Batchelor (1994)	Qatar	34	DR2	0.1	0.013
			DR7	3.73	0.05
Thursz et al. (1995)	Gambia	185 (218 SL)	DRB1*1302	0.53	0.01
		40 (195 SL)	DRB1*1302	0.24	0.01
Höhler et al. (1997)	Germany	70 (24 SL)	DRB1*1301/2	0.12	0.004
Ahn et al. (2000)	Korea	83 (243 SL)	DR13	0.14	0.002
			DR9	3.0	0.001
Thio et al. (1999)	United States (African Americans)	31 (60 SL)	DQA1*0501	2.6	$P = 0.05$
			DQB1*0301	3	$P = 0.01$
			DQA1*0501– DQB1*0301	3	$P = 0.005$
Amarapurpar et al. (2003	India	26 (100 NC)	DRB1*15– –	4	$P = 0.001$
			DRB1*11– –	29.7	$P = 0.00001$
			DRB1*13– –	0	$P = 0.016$
Meng et al. (2003)	China	30 (56 SL)	DRB1*1201	0.07	$P_c = 0.005$
			DRB1*09– –	3.52	$P_c = 0.025$
			DQB1*09– –	3.13	$P_c = 0.05$
Thio et al. (2003)	United States (Caucasian)	194 (342 SL)	DRB1*1302	0.42	$P = 0.03$
Jiang et al. (2003)	China	54 (106 NC)	DRB1*0301	4.2	$P_c = 0.0074$
			DRB1*1101/4	0.06	$P_c = 0.015$
			DQA1*0301	0.35	$P_c = 0.013$
			DQA1*0501	2.87	$P_c = 0.015$
			DQB1*0301	4.1	$P_c = 0.0075$

Abbreviations: SL, self-limiting infection; NC, normal healthy controls; P_c, corrected P value.

antigens. Furthermore CD4[+] T-cell responses in subjects who have recovered from HBV are greater in those who carry the HLA-DRB1*1302 allele (Diepolder, 1998). Alternatively, HLA-DRB1*1302 may present a wider range of epitopes than other alleles. Elution and binding studies suggest that HLA-DRB1*1302 is a relatively promiscuous peptide binder in comparison to other HLA class II molecules (Davenport et al., 1995, 1996). The ability to bind and present a wide range of epitopes is likely to generate a polyclonal and multispecific T-helper cell response, as seen in individuals who spontaneously eliminate the infection. Furthermore, a broad range of potential T-cell epitopes would reduce the opportunity for the virus to evade recognition through sequence variation. The importance of this ability to present a wide range of epitopes is further underlined by the finding that individuals who are heterozygous at MHC class II loci are less likely to develop persistent HBV infection than are homozygous individuals (Thursz et al., 1997).

Tumor Necrosis Factor α

Tumor necrosis factor α (TNF-α) is a proinflammatory cytokine secreted mainly by macrophages that signal through a cell-surface receptor to activate nuclear factor-κB. A model of HBV replication has been established in mice where a dimer of the HBV genome was inserted as a transgene into mice. In this mouse, HBV replication is suppressed or terminated by adoptive transfer of HBV-specific cytotoxic T lymphocytes (CTL; Guidotti et al., 1994, 1996). The number of CTLs required to suppress HBV replication was found to be small relative to the number of infected hepatocytes (100% in the transgenic model). Accordingly, noncytolytic mechanisms were believed to be responsible for controlling viral replication. Antibodies to TNF-α were found to prevent the effects of CTL on HBV replication, whereas infusion of TNF-α mimicked the effect of the CTL (Guidotti et al., 1996). Therefore, it is likely that TNF-α is important in both generating immune and inflammatory responses and in directly activating hepatocyte antiviral processes.

Höhler et al. (1998a,c) reported that possession of the TNFα−238A allele was associated with persistent infection, although these findings have not been replicated amongst Caucasians. However, larger studies that are more comprehensive with respect to the number of polymorphisms examined are needed before conclusions about TNF-α polymorphisms may be drawn. Among Koreans, alleles that are associated with high levels of TNF-α in plasma or increased transcriptional efficiency confer resistance to persistent infection. TNFα−308A allele and HBV persistence ($P = 0.01$), and TNFα−863A with HBV clearance ($P = 0.003$; Kim et al., 2003). These findings are consistent with the role of TNF-α in the noncytolytic control of HBV replication in vivo.

Interleukin-10 Receptor B

The immunomodulatory cytokine interleukin-10 (IL-10) signals its pleiotropic effects through a class II cytokine receptor comprising two subunits: IL-10R1 and IL-10R2 (IL-10RB). The IL10-R1 subunit appears to be specific for the IL-10 ligand, whereas the IL-10R2 participates in ligand binding and signal transduction of IL-10, IL-22, IL-26, IL-28A, IL-28B, and IL-29 (Kotenko et al., 2003).

The IL-10R2 has an extracellular ligand-binding domain, a transmembrane domain, and a cytoplasmic domain that signals via Janus kinase (Jak)1, and tyrosine kinase (Tyk)2, and STAT-1, -3, and -5. IL-10 suppresses the induction and activation of Th1 T-helper cells and suppresses the secretion of IL-1, IL-6, TNF-α, and interferon-γ (IFN-γ). Therefore, it is possible that excess IL-10 or increased signal transduction of IL-10 might suppress the elimination of HBV, leading to persistent HBV infection.

In a cohort of sibling pairs with persistent HBV infection from The Gambia, a genome wide scan has been conducted for susceptibility genes (Frodsham et al., 2006). The initial scan revealed linkage of markers on chromosome 21. Fine-mapping with additional markers revealed a maximum linkage located within a cluster of cytokine receptor genes. Family association studies using the pedigree disequilibrium test (PDT) analysis revealed an *IL10RB* (formerly, *IL10R2*) haplotype that includes the minor allele at both the IL-10R2-K47E and IFNAR2-F8S loci, which conferred resistance to persistent HBV infection.

A systematic exploration of the functional consequences of IL-10R2-K47E demonstrated that the IL10R2*E allele, associated with clearance of the virus, was found to transduce the IL-10 signal more efficiently than the IL-10R2*K allele. This result is counterintuitive because increased IL-10 signaling would be expected to lead to persistent infection. A more plausible explanation would be that increased signal transduction of alternative ligands such as the IL-28A, IL-

28B, and IL-29 cytokines are responsible for the observed linkage and association because these cytokines have antiviral properties (Kotenko et al., 2003).

Interferon-α Receptor 2

Virus infection is usually detected via the Toll-like receptors TLR3, TLR7, or TLR9 (Diebold et al., 2003; Alexopoulou et al., 2001; Hemmi et al., 2000). Ligation of these receptors by their cognate ligands triggers release of type 1 IFNs. IFNs activate a number of innate and adaptive immune responses that block viral replication and eliminate infected cells. Type 1 IFNs use a heterodimeric receptor consisting of an α- and β-chain that signals through Jak1, Tyk2, and STAT-1 and -2 leading to the transcriptional activation of more than 100 genes (Der et al., 1998).

The IFN system is central to the innate response to viral infection and specifically to the outcome of HBV infection. In subjects with persistent HBV infection monocyte production of IFN is reduced in comparison to healthy controls (Ikeda et al., 1986). In addition the cellular response to IFN is inhibited in cells infected with HBV (Foster et al., 1991).

As described above, the IFNAR2-F8S polymorphism was found to be associated with persistent HBV infection using genomewide scanning and family-based association studies. In experiments designed to evaluate the functional consequences of this polymorphism, the IFNAR2*F allele was found to be a more efficient transducer of the IFN signal than was IFNAR2*S. As the IFNAR2*S variant is associated with viral clearance, this result is counterintuitive. Two possible mechanisms may explain this situation. First, when cells receive the IFN signal, they rapidly downregulate IFN receptor expression. It is therefore possible that in the context of a persistent infection the IFNAR2*F allele that appears to be functionally more active *in vitro* is more rapidly inactivated *in vivo* leading to a reduction in the sustained antiviral functions. Second, IFN receptors are expressed on dendritic cells and signaling through these receptors leads to maturation of immature dendritic cells. However, a combination of IFN-α and IL-10 signaling to dendritic cells has been found to generate tolerogenic dendritic cells that express high levels of the cell surface markers ILT3 and ILT4 (Manavalan et al., 2003; Suciu-Foca et al., 2003). These dendritic cells stimulate regulatory T-cell responses rather than Th1 responses. Excess IFN stimulation of dendritic cells through the IFNAR2*F

allele might therefore promote tolerance to HBV antigens and therefore facilitate persistent infection.

Mannose-Binding Lectin

Mannose-binding lectin (MBL) is a calcium-dependent carbohydrate binding protein that is a component of the innate immune system (see chapter 10). MBL is a pathogen-associated molecular pattern recognition receptor in that it binds preferentially to the carbohydrate structures on microbial pathogens including fungi, bacteria, and viruses. MBL activates complement through two MBL associated serine proteases, MASP1 and MASP2. Complement activation leads to lysis of the microorganism or to opsonization and phagocytosis. MBL is produced in the liver and secreted into serum.

The middle surface protein of HBV is glycosylated with a mannose-terminated carbohydrate chain. This theoretically provides a target for MBL although binding has never actually been demonstrated. Because MBL provides early recognition and clearance of invading pathogens, it may theoretically prevent HBV infection or reduce the chance of HBV infection becoming persistent.

Three studies have sought associations of MBL polymorphisms with the outcome of HBV infection. The first published by Thomas et al. (1996) suggested that the codon 52 variant was associated with persistent infection in Caucasians. However, there were only 33 patients with persistent HBV infection and 19 controls with self-limiting HBV infection in this study. A slightly larger study from Germany was unable to replicate these findings (Höhler et al., 1998b). Similarly negative studies have been reported in Vietnamese and Gambian populations (Song et al., 2003; Bellamy et al., 1998). Recently, in a Hong Kong study, genotypes associated with low MBL expression had a dose-dependent correlation with the cirrhosis and hepatocellular carcinoma in progressed HBV carriers (Chong et al., 2005), suggesting that the primary effect of MBL deficiency could be on disease progression in carriers rather than on infection.

The original observation by Thomas et al. (1996) must be treated with caution in view of the size of this study and the failure of other groups to replicate the association. However, the allele frequencies of the *MBL2* polymorphisms vary significantly between ethic groups. The codon 52 variant is rarely or never found in African or Oriental populations, so negative findings in these groups may not be relevant to the Caucasian population.

Hepatitis C Virus Infection

Isolated in 1989, the hepatitis C virus (HCV) accounts for the majority of cases of non-A, non-B hepatitis. HCV is a member of the Flaviviridae family and is the sole member of the genus *Hepacivirus* (Lauer and Walker, 2001). HCV is the leading indication for a liver transplant in the developed world and an important cause of hepatocellular carcinoma.

MHC Class II

Several consistent associations have been observed between MHC alleles and HCV outcomes (Thursz, 2001; Yee, 2004). Perhaps the most interesting and consistent finding has been with respect to the association of the HLA class II allele DQB1*0301 and self-limiting HCV. A number of studies in several populations have reported an association between DQB1*0301 and viral clearance, although one study reported an opposite effect (Wawrzynowicz-Syczewska et al., 2000). Perhaps the most convincing feature of the possible role of DQB1*0301 in self-limiting HCV infection is the fact that this allele, along with different extended haplotypes, has been associated with self-limiting HCV in different populations. A French study found associations between the DRB1*1101-DQA1*0501-DQB1*0301 haplotype and HCV clearance (Alric et al., 1997). A British study found the DRB1*0401-DQA1*03-DQB1*0301 haplotype associated with clearance (Cramp et al., 1998). In Italy, two studies reported an association for DRB1*1104-DQB1*0301 and clearance (Zavaglia et al., 1998; Mangia et al., 1999). The association of the DQB1*0301 allele with self-limiting HCV in the presence of different DRB1 alleles, suggests that this particular allele, rather than the corresponding haplotypes, may play an important role in the natural clearance of HCV viremia (Thursz 2001).

Another allele that is associated HCV clearance is DRB1*1101 (Alric et al., 1997, 2000; Minton et al., 1998; Thursz et al., 1999; Yenigun and Durupinar, 2002). An Italian study found a protective role for the DR5 serogroup against HCV infection (Zavaglia et al., 1996). The molecularly defined DRB1*1100 and DRB1*1200 group of alleles are part of the serologically defined DR5 group. The DRB1*1101 allele is

also associated with susceptibility to vertically transmitted HCV infection (Martinetti et al., 1997).

In a meta-analysis of the effects of DQB1*0301 and DRB1*11 employing molecularly genotyped studies conducted among Caucasians, DQB1*0301 had a relatively strong correlation with self-limiting HCV infection (summary estimates of 3.0 [95% confidence interval, 1.8–4.8] and 2.5 [95% confidence interval, 1.7–3.7], for DQB1*0301 and DRB1*11, respectively; figure 21.1; Yee, 2004).

In contrast, studies of the MHC and the responsiveness to anti-HCV therapy have yielded conflicting results (Gao et al., 2004; Yee, 2004) The HLA-DR4 group was associated with nonresponse in one study (Kikuchi et al., 1998), while another observed the DRB1*0404 allele (a subset of the DR4 serogroup) to be associated with response (Sim et al., 1998). One major explanation for the observed differences between these two studies is that the populations were very different with respect to race. Additionally, the study by Sim et al. (1998) did not take differences in viral genotypes into account.

Studies of the MHC and the progression or severity of HCV have largely been inconsistent. However, there is the suggestion that there might be a trend with DRB1*11 alleles and "less severe" liver disease. Three studies reported associations with normal ALT: DRB1*1104 (OR = 4.82; Asti et al., 1999), DRB1*11 (OR = 2.36; Renou et al., 2002), and DRB1*1101 (OR = 0.3; Kuzushita et al., 1998). Haruna et al. (2000) observed the DRB1*1101 allele to be associated with less piecemeal necrosis, and Hue et al. (2002) reported DRB1*11 to be associated with lower Knodell scores (OR = 0.35). Yasunami et al. (1997) reported an association between DRB1*1101 and lower histological activity index scores. Tillmann et al. (2001) also observed DRB*11 to be lower among cirrhotics (RR = 0.29). Haruna et al. (2000) reported an association of DRB1*1201 with less severe liver disease, as well. It is interesting to note that the DRB1*1100 and DRB1*1200 alleles form the DR5 serogroup.

Tokushige et al. (2003) reported the combination of DRB1*0901 and the TNF-β B1 homozygous genotype to be associated with inactive HCV, while DRB1*0405 along with the TNF-β B2 homozygous genotype was associated with active HCV. The functional significance of these alleles is not currently known. The definition of "less severe disease" in these various studies also varies greatly, ranging from biochemical (i.e., alanine aminotransferase levels) to histologi-

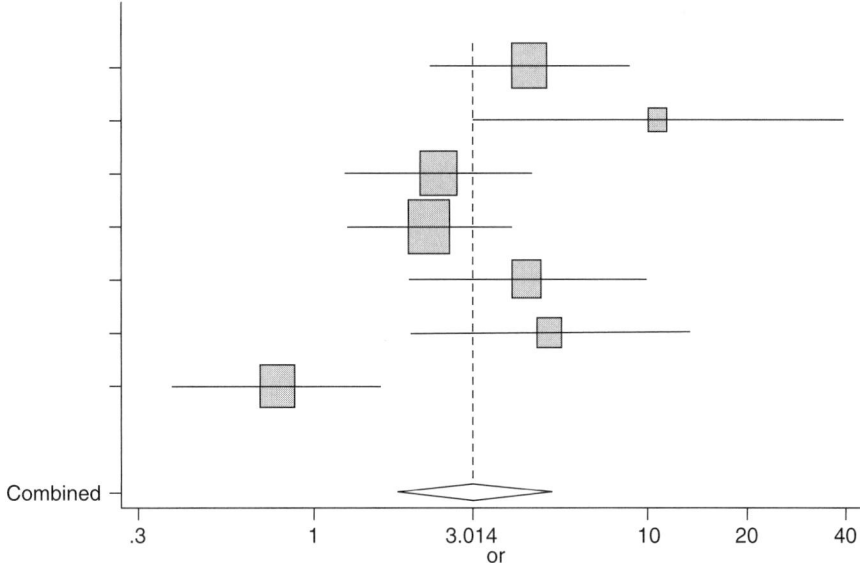

FIGURE 21.1. Meta-analysis of the effects of the DQB1*0301 allele on self-limiting HCV infection among Caucasians. Analysis was restricted to studies employing Caucasian populations and molecular genotyping techniques. A summary estimate (hashed vertical line) of 3.0 (95% confidence interval, 1.8–4.8) was obtained. The sizes of the boxes reflect study size, while the horizontal lines reflect the confidence limits. (From Yee, 2004.)

cal definitions. Future studies are needed to refine these observations. Also, most of these studies did not adjust for potential environmental confounders, such as alcohol use.

Chemokine Receptor 5 Deletion Variant (CCR5-△32)

Chemokines are a superfamily of 8- to 10-kDa proteins that regulate cell migration, adhesion, and activation during inflammatory and immune responses by binding to specific G-protein–coupled cell surface receptors on cells, called chemokine receptors (Tang and Kaslow, 2003). Chemokine receptor 5 (CCR5) is the principal ligand for the chemokines RANTES and the macrophage inflammatory proteins (MIP) MIP-1α and MIP-1β. CCR5 has received much attention in the past few years because it serves as an important co-receptor in HIV-1 entry. Individuals homozygous for a 32-base pair (bp) deletion (CCR5-△32) have extremely high resistance to HIV-1 infection. Homozygosity for this deletion variant occurs in only approximately 1% of Caucasians and is even more uncommon among other racial groups (Deng et al., 1996). While, CCR5-△32's role as a co-receptor for HIV-1 is not immediately rel-

evant to HCV infection, the role of CCR5 as receptor for key immunomodulatory cytokines raises the possibility that variations in CCR5 may affect the immune response to infectious diseases.

Recently, a study conducted among hemophiliacs suggested that homozygosity for CCR5- △32 may confer risk for HCV acquisition. Woitas et al. (2002) reported higher frequencies of homozygous CCR5-△32 among those with HCV mono-infection compared to those with HIV-1 or HIV-1 /HCV co-infection ($P < 0.02$). The frequency of CCR5-△32 was also higher among those with HCV mono-infection (16%) than among healthy controls (8.3%; $P = 0.02$) or those with HIV-1 mono-infection (9.3%; $P = 0.04$). Several other investigators have contended that those results could have arisen entirely from differential selection of the comparison groups. Because CCR5-△32 homozygosity confers a high degree of resistance to HIV-1 infection, individuals carrying this genotype would naturally be underrepresented in a population with HIV-1 infection. Thus, subsequent studies including both subjects with HCV infection alone and subjects with dual (HIV-1/HCV) infection have consistently demonstrated that △32 homozygosity occurs at expected frequencies in those infected only with HCV but at lower frequency among dually infected individuals (Zhang et al., 2003; Klein, 2003; Mangia et al., 2003; Promrat et al., 2003a,b; Wasmuth et al., 2004). Zhang et al. (2003) also examined the distribution of CCR5-$\triangle$32 in a large group of hemophiliacs with HCV and observed that CCR5-$\triangle$32 occurred in this cohort with an overall frequency of about 1%, which is consistent with accepted population frequencies. They also observed 3.4% of HCV-infected but HIV-1 noninfected individuals to be CCR5-$\triangle$32 homozygotes. Only 1 of 13 (7.7%) of CCR5-$\triangle$32 homozygotes was infected with HIV-1, compared to 861 of 1,153 (74.7%) wild-type patients and 142 of 196 (72.4%) CCR5-$\triangle$32 heterozygotes, suggesting that the increased frequency of the homozygous CCR5-$\triangle$32 genotype among HCV-infected but HIV-1 noninfected patients resulted from resistance to HIV-1 infection rather than increased susceptibility to HCV. Klein (2003) also expanded on the possibility that this observation was mainly due to resistance to HIV-1 infection among those with CCR5-$\triangle$32, as well. Mangia et al. (2003) examined 235 Italian chronic HCV patients and 96 healthy controls. They found the only one patient with CCR5-$\triangle$32/$\triangle$32 and 18 patients (7.7%) and 9 healthy controls (9.4%) to be heterozygous. The frequency of the CCR5-$\triangle$32 allele was 4.7% in both HCV patients and controls. One of the larger studies of CCR5-$\triangle$32 polymorphism and HCV involved 417 patients with liver diseases (339 with hepatitis C) and 2,380 blood donors (Promrat et al., 2003a,b) failed to confirm significant differential distribution of CCR5-$\triangle$32 homozygotes. Other studies have failed to find any differences with respect to CCR5-$\triangle$32 and the susceptibility to HCV infection (Wasmuth et al., 2004).

Conflicting observations have been observed with respect to CCR5 variants and HCV therapy. Ahlenstiel et al. (2003) reported that individuals who carried a CCR5-$\triangle$32 allele had lower end-of-treatment response rates than did those who were homozygous for the wild-type CCR5 allele (10.5% vs. 39%; $P = 0.02$). Subsequent multivariable analysis also demonstrated that CCR5-$\triangle$32 carriage was an independent negative predictor of end-of-treatment response in IFN monotherapy ($P = 0.03$). The numbers in this study were small, and it was not a randomized trial. Woitas et al. (2002) reported that CCR5-$\triangle$32 homozygotes had higher HCV RNA levels than did heterozygotes or individuals with the wild type. Dorak et al. (2002) could not replicate this observation. The distribution of the G*2 CCR2–CCR5 haplotype, which exclusively bears

the CCR5-$\triangle$32 deletion, was not associated with any differences in viral load, and the distributions of this haplotype were similar between sustained responders and nonresponders. In addition, the C/G*2 haplotype combination was associated with a marginal decrease in viral load levels ($P = 0.05$) However, Dorak et al. (2002) correlated the homozygous E/E genotype with sustained response to therapy as well as with improved viral dynamics during the course of treatment among individuals with genotype 1 infections. Another study found the 59029A allele, which is an allele of the CCR5-E haplotype, to be associated with sustained response (Promrat et al., 2003a,b). It remains to be seen whether increased expression of CCR5 associated with this promoter profile proves to be of benefit in the context of HCV therapy.

Few studies have examined the role of CCR5 polymorphisms on the progression of HCV. Hellier et al. (2003) found a protective role for CCR5-$\triangle$32 carriage against severe fibrosis ($P = 0.02$) and CCR5-$\triangle$32 homozygotes had milder portal inflammation ($P = 0.01$).

Cytokine Gene Polymorphisms

Interest in the potential role of *IL10* in liver diseases was initiated by a small study examining the role of *IL10* polymorphisms in the initial (week 12) response to anti-HCV therapy. The authors found the *IL10*−592A or−819A alleles, and the corresponding−1082A+−819T+−592A haplotype, to be associated with the initial response to IFN therapy for HCV (Edwards-Smith et al., 1999). A subsequent study examining extended *IL10* haplotypes found that a subset of the−1082A+−819T+−592A haplotype, the *IL10* 108bp10.R+−3575T+−2763C+−1082A+−819T+ −592A extended haplotype to be correlated with sustained response to IFN /ribavirin therapy (Yee et al., 2001). Homozygosity for this extended haplotype was exclusively correlated with sustained response. In another study, the *IL10*−1082G/G genotype, and the *IL10*−1082G+−819C +−592C haplotype were correlated with sustained response (Knapp et al., 2003a). But Vidigal et al. (2002) did not observe any associations with the *IL10* promoter and therapeutic outcome.

Knapp et al. (2003a) found the−592A /−592A genotype to be weakly associated with self-limiting infection ($P = 0.03$), and the−1082G/−1082G genotype was correlated with persistent infection

($P = 0.02$). Vidigal et al. (2002) also reported an association between the–1082G/G genotype and HCV persistence. Functional studies suggesting that the $-1082G$ allele may produce higher levels of IL10, which may in turn compromise the ability of an individual to mount a strong Th1 response, may provide a biological explanation for this observed epidemiological observation (Mosmann, 1994; Eskdale et al., 1998; Edwards-Smith et al., 1999; Reuss et al., 2002)

In a trial of recombinant IL-10 for the treatment of HCV-related cirrhosis, histological improvement was observed, suggesting an important role for IL-10 in liver fibrogenesis (Nelson et al., 2000). Knapp et al. (2003a) observed an association between the low–IL-10–producing genotype $IL10-1082A/A$ and the low–IL-10–producing haplotype combinations IL10−1082A+−819C+−592C/−1082A+−819C+−592C and IL10−1082A+−819T+−592A/−1082A+−819T+−592A with fast fibrosis progression.

Importantly, the *in vivo* functional effects of these polymorphisms have not been fully elucidated. Several studies suggest that specific promoter single nucleotide polymorphisms (SNPs) and haplotypes alter IL-10 production, but *in vitro* production of IL-10 may likely be stimulus and/or cell-line dependent. This may explain, at least in part, the conflicting results presented in functional studies of promoter alleles and IL-10 production. Recent research has also suggested that the expression of *IL10* may be more complicated, with environmental and behavioral factors such as smoking and body mass index affecting IL-10 production (Reuss et al., 2002).

Tumor Necrosis Factor α Polymorphisms

Elevated levels of TNF have been found in the serum as well as the liver of individuals infected with HCV, and individuals with response to IFN have reportedly lower pretreatment levels of TNF mRNA (Larrea et al., 1996; Nelson and Lau, 1997). In spite of the controversies concerning the functional consequences of the polymorphic variants in the *TNF* gene, the biological significance of TNF in the human response to infectious agents is well established.

With respect to self-limiting infection, Höhler et al. (1998c) found an association between the TNF-238A allele and chronicity in an European population. but other studies conducted in Caucasian populations have failed to reproduce this association (Constantini

et al., 2002; Rosen et al., 2002). In contrast, a study conducted in both Caucasian and black individuals found the−863A allele associated with self-limiting HCV infection in blacks only (Thio et al., 2004). Among whites, none of the *TNF* alleles studied was associated with self-limiting infection.

Several studies, conducted among predominantly Caucasian populations, demonstrated a lack of association between *TNF* variants and the response to anti-HCV therapy (Yee et al., 2000; Constantini et al., 2002; Rosen et al., 2002; Schiemann et al., 2003). An additional study conducted in a Taiwanese population also found no association with respect to the response to IFN therapy (Yu et al., 2003).

TNF variants have also been studied with respect to the progression of HCV-related liver disease, and the results have been inconsistent (Yee et al., 2000; Rosen et al., 2002; Tokushige et al., 2003). The functionality of *TNF* variants remains controversial, and these apparent discrepancies may help explain, at least in part, the varied findings (Bayley et al., 2004).

Hemochromatosis Gene Polymorphisms

The hemochromatosis molecule HFE is a MHC I-like molecule that plays an important role in body iron metabolism. HFE knockout animal models exhibit iron overload. In humans HFE is encoded by the *HFE* gene, in which two polymorphisms have attracted much scientific interest. The C282Y polymorphism consists of an amino acid change of a cysteine to a tyrosine at position 282 and is associated with hereditary hemochromatosis. A second polymorphism occurs at position 63 and consists of a change from a histidine to an aspartic acid (H63D). This particular polymorphism is present in a minority of patients, and its exact role in the pathogenesis of hereditary hemochromatosis remains unknown. Of the two polymorphisms, C282Y has been of greater interest, because some individuals with this variant have slightly elevated hepatic iron content, although phenotypic penetrance of this variant is not 100% (Hanson et al., 2001; Pietrangelo 2003).

Iron as a pathogenic co-factor in the progression of HCV-related fibrosis is a topic of interest. Pathological studies of HCV have shown that mild to moderate iron accumulation is common (Saadeh et al., 2001). While the exact mechanisms are not understood, it is plausible that infection with HCV may modify iron trafficking or that the host immune response against HCV may alter liver iron metabolism. It is possible that host genetic differences may contribute, at least in part, to the differences in iron accumulation in HCV-infected livers. disease association studies involving *HFE* polymorphisms have largely been inconclusive (Bataller et al., 2003; Pietrangelo, 2003). Several studies suggested an association between possession of *HFE* variants and increased fibrosis or cirrhosis (Smith et al., 1998; Martinelli et al., 2000; Pirisi et al., 2000; Erhardt et al., 2003), but other studies have found no associations (Knoll et al., 1998; Hezode et al., 1999; Kazemi-Shirazi et al., 1999; Thorburn et al., 2002; Erhardt et al., 2003). Methodological differences (e.g., the use of different histological scoring systems) may contribute to these differing observations.

A few studies have also addressed the potential role of the *HFE* gene variants (Cys282Tyr or His63Asp polymorphisms) and iron levels, rather than histological stage. These studies have yielded inconclusive results, as well (Knoll et al., 1998; Smith et al., 1998; Hezode et al., 1999; Lal et al., 2000). Differences in study design (e.g., whether iron is quantified using serum ferritin levels or iron staining of liver biopsies) further complicate collective interpretation of this literature.

IFN-Stimulated Gene Polymorphisms

The IFN system is an important component of the immune response to infectious agents (figure 21.2). Proteins such as Mx1 (MxA), PKR, and OAS have important antiviral properties. Interactions between HCV and components of the IFN-stimulated genes (e.g., PKR) are important in the resistance of HCV to IFN therapies (Gale et al., 1997).

One European study (Knapp et al., 2003b) examined whether an A → G substitution at position 84 in the 3′ UTR of exon 8 of *OAS1* was correlated with HCV outcomes. The 84-OAS1-G/G genotype was associated with persistent HCV infection: 9% of individuals with self-limiting infection had this genotype, while 18.8% of individuals with persistent HCV had this genotype ($P = 0.01$). The effect was observed mainly among females.

The *PKR* gene also contains a number of polymorphisms that have been explored with respect to HCV infection. A G/T dimorphism at position−180 and a C/T exchange at−168 of the *PKR* gene have been studied. In addition, a short tandem trinucleotide repeat (CGG) is found in exon 1 of the 5′ UTR. Work from our group suggests that the heterozygous−168-PKR-C/T genotype is associated with self-limiting infection ($P = 0.002$), with no associations observed with respect to treatment outcomes. Interestingly, again the effect observed was mainly among females. Individuals with shorter numbers of trinucleotide repeats (<9) in the 5′ UTR region were more frequent among subjects with self-limiting infection ($P = 0.03$) than those with longer repeats (≥ 9). In contrast, patients with two long alleles were found more frequently among those with initial response to IFN ($P = 0.02$), as well as sustained response to IFN ($P = 0.02$). Differential associations by gender were observed for the tandem repeat. Stratification of individuals who had the long/long homozygous genotype suggested that the association with response to therapy was mainly among males and not females.

Polymorphisms at−88 and−123 in the MxA (officially *Mx1*) gene have been more widely studied than OAS and PKR genes in HCV infection. Hijikata et al. (2000) observed the presence of−88MxA-G/G homozygotes to be lower in the sustained type I IFN responders (31%) than in the nonresponders (62%; $P = 0.001$) These effects appeared to be independent of HCV genotype. Suzuki et al. (2004) in an independent Japanese study found a similar association. The−88MxA SNP lies in a region that is highly homologous to the IFN-stimulated response element consensus sequence, with T substitution increasing the homology. Another SNP at position−123 of the MxA gene was subsequently identified (Hijikata et al., 2001). Linkage disequilibrium was observed to be strong between alleles at the two positions, with all individuals who had−88MxA-G also having−123MxA-C, and 73% of those with−88-MxA-T having−123-MxA-A. Homozygosity for−123MxA-C was also correlated with IFN response ($P = 0.003$) (Hijikata et al., 2001). *In vitro* assays to assess the functionality of the−123-MxA-A +−88-MxA-T sequence showed an approximate 4-fold higher activity than the−123-MxA-C +−88-MxA-G haplotype (Hijikata et al., 2001). Knapp et al. (2003b) subsequently reported−88-MxA-G/G genotype associated with HCV persistence ($P = 0.01$), and the−88-MxA-T/T genotype associated with self-limiting HCV ($P = 0.05$). The−88-MxA-G/G genotype was also correlated with nonresponse to IFN monotherapy ($P = 0.02$).

The results observed by both the Japanese and European studies with respect to the response to ther-

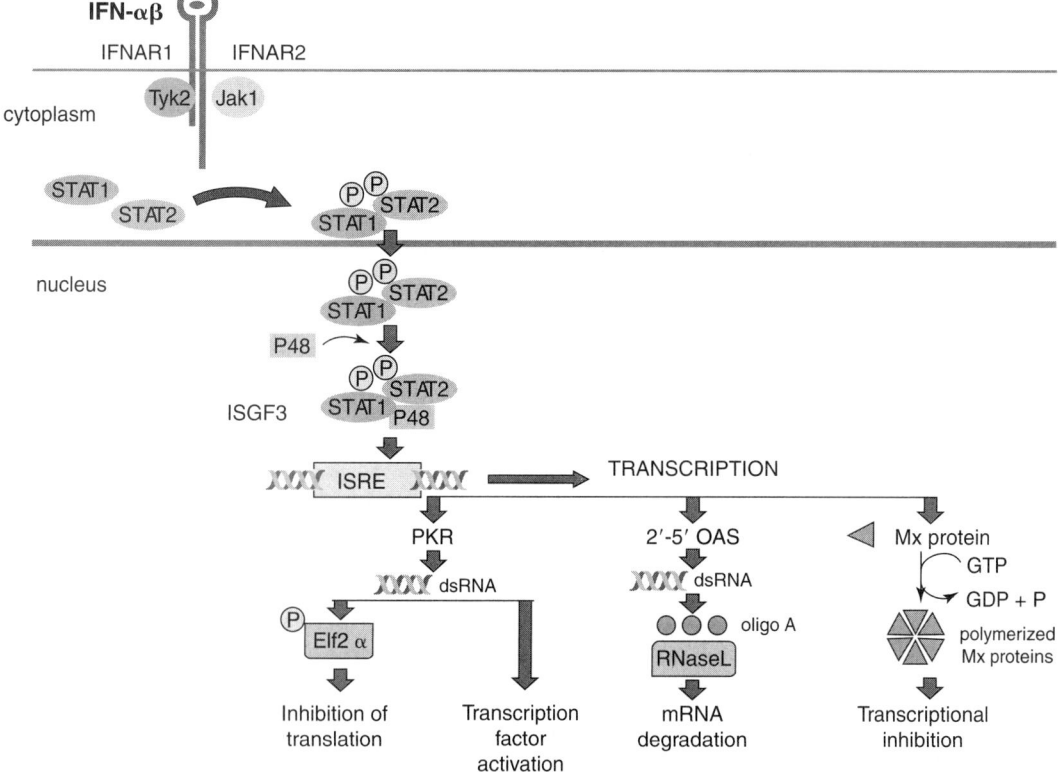

FIGURE 21.2. Schematic diagram of the IFN pathway. Upon binding IFN to the IFN receptor (composed of subunits 1 and 2), the Jak/Stat pathway is activated. Several different proteins with antiviral action including 2′-5′oligoadenylate synthase (OAS), double-stranded RNA-dependent protein kinase (PKR), and myxovirus resistance-1 (Mx1; also called MxA) are induced. In addition, upon binding to double-stranded RNA (dsRNA), OAS catalyzes the formation of 2′-5′–linked oligoadenylate and activates RNAse L, which breaks down viral and cellular RNA. PKR is also activated by dsRNA, which leads to the phosphorylation of its substrate, eIF2, which inhibits the guanosine nucleotide exchange factor, eIF2B, and halts viral replication. PKR may function to shut down protein synthesis following infection of a cell and limit the proliferation of uninfected cells. Interactions between HCV and PKR are believed to be an important mechanism behind the resistance of HCV to IFN therapies. MxA acts selectively against several viruses, although the precise mechanism of its action has not been elucidated. Studies of *in vivo* MxA levels in responders to IFN treatment of HCV have shown greater levels in responders than nonresponders. Similarly, MxA levels have been reported to be significantly increased after initiation of therapy only among responders.

apy are consistent. While Hijikata et al. (2001) demonstrated a beneficial effect of the T allele, Knapp et al. (2003b) observed an opposite effect for the G allele. The T allele appears with much lower frequency in Caucasian populations compared to Japanese populations (14.0% in Caucasians and 29.0% in Japanese), and this may explain why correlations were observed with respect to the G allele and not the T allele in the European study. Taken as a whole, the observations from these two studies are consistent, with each illustrating reciprocal effects.

Factor V Polymorphisms

Tissue injury leads to activation of coagulation pathways and generation of thrombin. Stellate cells are responsible for liver fibrosis. Thrombin is a stellate cell mitogen and thrombin receptors are up-regulated on stellate cells during liver damage (Marra et al., 1995).

A single nucleotide substitution of adenine for guanine at position 1691 results in an amino acid exchange of an glutamine for an arginine at position 506 in the gene that codes for factor V and results in factor V

Leiden (Ridker and Vaughan, 1995). Activated protein C (APC) normally degrades factor V as part of a negative feedback loop, but the factor V Leiden variant leads to APC resistance and thrombophilia. Epidemiological studies support this observation, because the factor V Leiden variant has been associated with an increased risk of thromboembolism (Bertina et al., 1994).

Wright et al. (2003) examined the distribution of coagulation pathway genes and the rate of fibrosis progression (calculated by dividing the fibrosis stage by the estimated duration of infection) among 352 Caucasian Europeans. While they did not observe any patients homozygous for the factor V Leiden variants, the median fibrosis rates were higher among heterozygotes for the factor V Leiden variant (0.37 fibrosis units per year among heterozygotes vs. 0.18 fibrosis units per year for patients with the wild type factor V alleles, $P = 0.004$).

A French study suggested that factor V Leiden may be a risk factor for cirrhosis in chronic HCV (Poujol-Robert et al., 2004a). The researchers measured APC resistance resulting from the factor V Leiden polymorphism using a highly sensitive and specific test for APC resistance in 559 patients with chronic HCV (Bertina et al., 1994), and cirrhosis was highly correlated with APC resistance ($P = 0.003$) (Poujol-Robert et al., 2004a). A further analysis by this group (Poujol-Robert et al., 2004b) highlighted the possible importance of thrombotic risk factors in HCV-related fibrosis, as a majority of 68 patients studied were found to have multiple prothrombotic factors such as protein C deficiency, elevated levels of factor VIII and hyperhomocysteinemia when individuals with extensive fibrosis and cirrhosis were compared to those without. However, it is difficult to determine from this study whether the levels of these parameters are the result of the extensive fibrosis or a biological cause of it.

No studies have addressed whether coagulation pathway polymorphisms are involved with self-limiting HCV infection or the response to therapy. However, given the biological characteristics of the coagulation pathway and its potential role in liver fibrogenesis, it is likely that coagulation pathway polymorphisms are more involved with HCV progression rather than these other outcomes.

Conclusion

Polymorphisms in a number of genes have been demonstrated to influence the outcomes of these two important infections. As the field begins to mature, the quality of published studies has improved and a number of reproducible associations have been established. Identification of genetic factors has revealed a deeper understanding of the biological mechanisms responsible for persistent infection and has provided novel therapeutic opportunities.

References

Ahlenstiel, G., T. Berg, et al. (2003). Effects of the CCR5-delta32 mutation on antiviral treatment in chronic hepatitis C. *J Hepatol* 39.2: 245–52.

Ahn, S. H., et al. (2000) Association between hepatitis B virus infection and HLA-DR type in Korea. *Hepatology* 31.6: 1371–73.

Alexopoulou, L., et al. (2001) Recognition of double-stranded RNA and activation of NF-kappaB by Toll-like receptor 3. *Nature* 413.6857: 732–38.

Almarri, A., and J. R. Batchelor. (1994) HLA and hepatitis B infection. *Lancet* 344.8931: 1194–95.

Alric, L., M. Fort, et al. (2000). Study of host- and virus-related factors associated with spontaneous hepatitis C virus clearance. *Tissue Antigens* 56.2: 154–58.

Alric L, Fort M, Izopet J., et al. (1997). Genes of the major histocompatability complex class II influence outcome of hepatitis C virus infection. *Gastroenterology* 113.5: 1675–81.

Amarapurpar, D.N., N.D. Patel, S.R. Kankonkar. (2003). HLA class II genotyping in chronic hepatitis B infection. *J Assoc Physicians India* 51: 779–81.

Asti, M., M. Martinetti, et al. (1999). Human leukocyte antigen class II and III alleles and severity of hepatitis C virus-related chronic liver disease. *Hepatology* 29.4: 1272–79.

Bataller, R., K. E. North, et al. (2003). Genetic polymorphisms and the progression of liver fibrosis: A critical appraisal. *Hepatology* 37.3: 493–503.

Bayley, J. P., T. H. Ottenhoff, et al. (2004). Is there a future for TNF promoter polymorphisms? *Genes Immun* 55: 315–29.

Bellamy, R., et al. (1998). Mannose binding protein deficiency is not associated with malaria, hepatitis B carriage nor tuberculosis in Africans. *Q J Med* 91.1: 13–18.

Bertina, R. M., B. P. Koeleman, et al. (1994). Mutation in blood coagulation factor V associated with resistance to activated protein C. *Nature* 369.6475: 64–67.

Chisari, F. V., and C. Ferrari. (1995). Hepatitis B immunopathology. *Springer Semin Immunopathol* 17 (2–3): 261–81.

Chong, W. P., Y. F. To, W. K. Ip, et al. (2005). Mannose-binding lectin in chronic hepatitis B virus infection. *Hepatology* 42: 1037–45.

Constantini, P. K., M. Wawrzynowicz-Syczewska, et al. (2002). Interleukin-1, interleukin-10 and tumour necrosis factor-alpha gene polymorphisms in hepatitis C virus infection: An investigation of the relationships with spontaneous viral clearance and response to alpha-interferon therapy. *Liver* 22.5: 404–12.

Cramp, M. E., P. Carucci, et al. (1998). Association between HLA class II genotype and spontaneous clearance of hepatitis C viraemia. *J Hepatol* 29.2: 207–13.

Davenport, M. P., et al. (1995). Naturally processed peptides from two disease-resistance-associated HLA-DR13 alleles show related sequence motifs and the effects of the dimorphism at position 86 of the HLA-DR beta chain. *Proc Natl Acad Sci USA* 92.14: 6567–71.

Davenport, M. P., et al. (1996). Analysis of peptide-binding motifs for two disease associated HLA-DR13 alleles using an M13 phage display library. *Immunology* 88.4: 482–86.

Deng, H., R. Liu, et al. (1996). Identification of a major co-receptor for primary isolates of HIV-1. *Nature* 381.6584: 661–66.

Der, S. D., et al. (1998). Identification of genes differentially regulated by interferon alpha, beta, or gamma using oligonucleotide arrays. *Proc Natl Acad Sci USA* 95.26: 15623–28.

Diebold, S. S., et al. (2003). Viral infection switches non-plasmacytoid dendritic cells into high interferon producers. *Nature* 424.6946: 324–28.

Diepolder, H. M., et al. (1998). A vigorous virus-specific CD4+ T cell response may contribute to the association of HLA-DR13 with viral clearance in hepatitis B. *Clin Exp Immunol* 113.2: 244–51.

Dorak, M. T., G. O. Folayan, et al. (2002). C-C chemokine receptor 2 and C-C chemokine receptor 5 genotypes in patients treated for chronic hepatitis C virus infection. *Immunol Res* 26.1–3: 167–75.

Edwards-Smith, C., et al. (1999). Interleukin-10 promoter polymorphism predicts initial response of chronic hepatitis C to interferon alpha. *Hepatology* 30.2: 526–30.

Erhardt, A., A. Maschner-Olberg, et al. (2003). HFE mutations and chronic hepatitis C: H63D and C282Y heterozygosity are independent risk factors for liver fibrosis and cirrhosis. *J Hepatol* 38.3: 335–42.

Eskdale, J., J. McNicholl, et al. (1998). Interleukin-10 microsatellite polymorphisms and IL-10 locus alleles in rheumatoid arthritis susceptibility. *Lancet* 352: 1282–83.

Ferrari, C., A. Penna, et al. (1990). Cellular immune response to hepatitis B virus-encoded antigens in acute and chronic hepatitis B virus infection. *J Immunol* 145.10: 3442–49.

Foster, G. R., et al. (1991). Expression of the terminal protein region of hepatitis B virus inhibits cellular responses to interferons alpha and gamma and double-stranded RNA. *Proc Natl Acad Sci USA* 88.7: 2888–92.

Frodsham, A.J., L. Zhang, et al. (2006). "Class II cytokine gene clueter is a major locus for hepatitis B persistence." *Proc Natl Acad Sci USA* 103.24: 9148–53.

Gale, M. J., Jr., M. J. Korth, et al. (1997). Evidence that hepatitis C virus resistance to interferon is mediated through repression of the PKR protein kinase by the nonstructural 5A protein. *Virology* 230.2: 217–27.

Gao, B., F. Hong, et al. (2004). Host factors and failure of interferon-alpha treatment in hepatitis C virus. *Hepatology* 39.4: 880–90.

Guidotti, L. G., et al. (1994). Cytotoxic T lymphocytes inhibit hepatitis B virus gene expression by a non-cytolytic mechanism in transgenic mice. *Proc Natl Acad Sci USA* 91: 3764–68.

Guidotti, L. G., et al. (1996). Intracellular inactivation of the hepatitis B virus by cytotoxic T lymphocytes. *Immunity* 4: 25–36.

Hanson, E. H., G. Imperatore, et al. (2001). HFE gene and hereditary hemochromatosis: A HuGE review. Human Genome Epidemiology. *Am J Epidemiol* 154.3: 193–206.

Haruna, Y., T. Miyamoto, et al. (2000). Human leukocyte antigen DRB1 1302 protects against bile duct damage and portal lymphocyte infiltration in patients with chronic hepatitis C. *J Hepatol* 32.5: 837–42.

Hellier, S., A. J. Frodsham, et al. (2003). Association of genetic variants of the chemokine receptor CCR5 and its ligands, RANTES and MCP-2, with outcome of HCV infection. *Hepatology* 38.6: 1468–76.

Hemmi, H., et al. (2000). A Toll-like receptor recognizes bacterial DNA. *Nature* 408.6813: 740–45.

Hezode, C., C. Cazeneuve, et al. (1999). Liver iron accumulation in patients with chronic active hepatitis C: Prevalence and role of hemochromatosis gene mutations and relationship with hepatic histological lesions. *J Hepatol* 31.6: 979–84.

Hijikata, M., S. Mishiro, et al. (2001). Genetic polymorphism of the MxA gene promoter and interferon responsiveness of hepatitis C patients: Revisited by analyzing two SNP sites (-123 and −88) in vivo and in vitro. *Intervirology* 44.6: 379–82.

Hijikata, M., Y. Ohta, and S. Mishiro. (2000). Identification of a single nucleotide polymorphism in the MxA gene promoter (G/T at nt−88) correlated with the response of hepatitis C patients to interferon. *Intervirology* 43: 124–27.

Höhler, T., et al. (1997). HLA-DRBI*1301 and *1302 protect against chronic hepatitis B. *J Hepatol* 26.3: 503–07.

Höhler, T., et al. (1998a). A tumor necrosis factor-alpha (TNF-alpha) promoter polymorphism is associated with chronic hepatitis B infection. *Clin Exp Immunol* 111.3: 579–82.

Höhler, T., et al. (1998b). No association between mannose-binding lectin alleles and susceptibility to chronic hepatitis B virus infection in German patients. *Exp Clin Immunogenet* 15.3: 130–33.

Höhler, T., A. Kruger, et al. (1998c). Tumor necrosis factor-alpha promoter polymorphism at position −238 is associated with chronic active hepatitis C infection. *J Med Virol* 54: 173–77.

Hue, S., P. Cacoub, et al. (2002). Human leukocyte antigen class II alleles may contribute to the severity of hepatitis C virus-related liver disease. *J Infect Dis* 186.1: 106–09.

Ikeda, T., A. M. Lever, and H. C. Thomas. (1986). Evidence for a deficiency of interferon production in patients with chronic hepatitis B virus infection acquired in adult life. *Hepatology* 6.5: 962–65.

Jiang, Y. G., et al. (2003). Association between HLA class II gene and susceptibility or resistance to chronic hepatitis B. *World J Gastroenterol* 9.10: 2221–25.

Kazemi-Shirazi, L., C. Datz, et al. (1999). The relation of iron status and hemochromatosis gene mutations in patients with chronic hepatitis C. *Gastroenterology* 116.1: 127–34.

Kikuchi, I., A. Ueda, et al. (1998). The effect of HLA alleles on response to interferon therapy in patients with chronic hepatitis C. *Eur J Gastroenterol Hepatol* 10.10: 859–63.

Kim, Y. J., et al. (2003). Association of TNF-alpha promoter polymorphisms with the clearance of hepatitis B virus infection. *Hum Mol Genet* 12.19: 2541–46.

Klein, R. (2003). Discussion on frequency of the HIV-protective CC chemokine receptor 5-delta32/delta 32 genotype is increased in hepatitis C. *Gastroenterology* 124: 1558.

Knapp, S., B. J. Hennig, et al. (2003a). Interleukin-10 promoter polymorphisms and the outcome of hepatitis C virus infection. *Immunogenetics* 55.6: 362–69.

Knapp, S., L. J. Yee, et al. (2003b). Polymorphisms in interferon-induced genes and the outcome of hepatitis C virus infection: Roles of MxA, OAS-1 and PKR. *Genes Immun* 4.6: 411–19.

Knoll, A., B. Kreuzpaintner, et al. (1998). Hemochromatosis mutation in hepatitis C: Histopathology. *Gastroenterology* 115.5: 1307–09.

Kotenko, S. V., et al. (2003). IFN-lambdas mediate antiviral protection through a distinct class II cytokine receptor complex. *Nat Immunol* 4, 69–77.

Kuzushita, N., N. Hayashi, et al. (1998). Influence of HLA haplotypes on the clinical courses of individuals infected with hepatitis C virus. *Hepatology* 27: 240–44.

Lal, P., H. Fernandes, et al. (2000). C282Y mutation and hepatic iron status in hepatitis C and cryptogenic cirrhosis. *Arch Pathol Lab Med* 124.11: 1632–35.

Larrea, E., et al. (1996). Tumor necrosis factor alpha gene expression and the response to interferon in chronic hepatitis C. *Hepatology* 23.2: 210–17.

Lauer, G. M., and B. D. Walker (2001). Hepatitis C virus infection. *N Engl J Med* 345.1: 41–52.

Manavalan, J. S., et al. (2003). Generation of tolerogenic antigen presenting cells: Crucial role of inhibitory receptors ILT3 and ILT4. *Hum Immunol* 64.10(suppl): S21.

Lee. W. M. (1997). Hepatitis B virus infection. *N Engl J Med*. 337.24: 1733–45.

Mangia, A., R. Gentile, et al. (1999). HLA class II favors clearance of HCV infection and progression of the chronic liver damage. *J Hepatol* 30.6: 984–89.

Mangia, A., R. Santoro, et al. (2003). HCV chronic infection and CCR5-delta 32/delta 32. *Gastroenterology* 124.3: 868–69.

Marra, F., G. Grandaliano, et al. (1995). Thrombin stimulates proliferation of liver fat-storing cells and expression of monocyte chemotactic protein-1: Potential role in liver injury. *Hepatology* 22.3: 780–87.

Martinelli, A. L., R. F. Franco, et al. (2000). Are haemochromatosis mutations related to the severity of liver disease in hepatitis C virus infection? *Acta Haematol* 102.3: 152–56.

Martinetti, M., I. Pacati, et al. (1997). Critical role of Val/Gly86 HLA-DRB dimorphism in the neonatal resistance or susceptibility to maternal hepatitis C virus infection. *Pediatr Infect Dis J* 16(10): 1001–02.

Meng, X. Q., et al. (2003). Influence of HLA class II molecules on the outcome of hepatitis B virus infection in population of Zhejiang Province in China. *Hepatobiliary Pancreat Dis Int* 2.2: 230–33.

Milich, D. R., and G. G. Leroux-Roels. (2003). Immunogenetics of the response to HBsAg vaccination. *Autoimmun Rev* 2.5: 248–57.

Minton, E. J., D. Smillie, et al. (1998). Association between MHC class II alleles and clearance of circulating hepatitis C virus. *J Infect Dis* 178.1: 39–44.

Mosmann, T. R. (1994). Properties and functions of interleukin-10. *Adv Immunol* 56: 1–26.

Nelson, D. R., and J. Y. Lau (1997). Pathogenesis of hepatocellular damage in chronic hepatitis C virus infection. *Clin Liver Dis* 1.3: 515–28.

Nelson, D. R., G. Y. Lauwers, et al. (2000). Interleukin 10 treatment reduces fibrosis in patients with chronic hepatitis C: A pilot trial of interferon non-responders. *Gastroenterology* 118: 655–60.

Pietrangelo, A. (2003). Hemochromatosis gene modifies course of hepatitis C viral infection. *Gastroenterology* 124.5: 1509–23.

Pirisi, M., C. A. Scott, et al. (2000). Iron deposition and progression of disease in chronic hepatitis C. Role of interface hepatitis, portal inflammation, and HFE missense mutations. *Am J Clin Pathol* 113.4: 546–54.

Poujol-Robert, A., P. Y. Boelle, et al. (2004a). Factor V Leiden as a risk factor for cirrhosis in chronic hepatitis C: Genetic and acquired thrombotic factors in chronic hepatitis C. *Hepatology* 39.4: 1174–75.

Poujol-Robert, A., O. Rosmorduc, et al. (2004b). Genetic and acquired thrombotic factors in chronic hepatitis C. *Am J Gastroenterol* 99.3: 527–31.

Promrat, K., D. H. McDermott, et al. (2003a). Associations of chemokine system polymorphisms with clinical outcomes and treatment responses of chronic hepatitis C. *Gastroenterology* 124.2: 352–60.

Promrat, K., D. H. McDermott, et al. (2003b). Correction: Association of chemokine system polymorphisms with clinical outcomes and treatment responses of chronic hepatitis C. *Gastroenterology* 124.4: 1168.

Renou, C., P. Halfon, et al. (2002). Histological features and HLA class II alleles in hepatitis C virus chronically infected patients with persistently normal alanine aminotransferase levels. *Gut* 51.4: 585–90.

Reuss, E., R. Fimmers, et al. (2002). Differential regulation of interleukin-10 production by genetic and environmental factors—a twin study. *Genes Immun* 3.7: 407–13.

Ridker, P. M., and D. E. Vaughan (1995). Hemostatic factors and the risk of myocardial infarction. *N Engl J Med* 333.6: 389; author reply 389–90.

Rosen, H. R., J. G. McHutchison, et al. (2002). Tumor necrosis factor genetic polymorphisms and response to antiviral therapy in patients with chronic hepatitis C. *Am J Gastroenterol* 97.3: 714–20.

Saadeh, S., G. Cammell, et al. (2001). The role of liver biopsy in chronic hepatitis C. *Hepatology* 33.1: 196–200.

Schiemann, U., J. Glas, et al. (2003). Response to combination therapy with interferon alfa-2a and ribavirin in chronic hepatitis C according to a TNF-alpha promoter polymorphism. *Digestion* 68.1: 1–4.

Sim, H., J. Wojcik, et al. (1998). Response to interferon therapy: Influence of human leucocyte antigen alleles in patients with chronic hepatitis C. *J Viral Hepat* 5.4: 249–53.

Smith, B. C., J. Gorve, et al. (1998). Heterozygosity for hereditary hemochromatosis is associated with more fibrosis in chronic hepatitis C. *Hepatology* 27.6: 1695–9.

Song, le H., et al. (2003). Mannose-binding lectin gene polymorphisms and hepatitis B virus infection in Vietnamese patients. *Mutat Res* 522.1–2: 119–25.

Suciu-Foca, N., J. S. Manavalan, and R. Cortesini. (2003). Generation and function of antigen-specific suppressor and regulatory T cells. *Transpl Immunol* 11.3–4: 235–44.

Suzuki, F., Y. Arase, et al. (2004). Single nucleotide polymorphism of the MxA gene promoter influences the response to interferon monotherapy in patients with hepatitis C viral infection. *J Viral Hepat* 11.3: 271–76.

Tang, J., and R. Kaslow (2003). Polymorphic chemokine receptor and ligand genes in HIV infection. In *Susceptibility to Infectious Diseases: The Importance of Host Genetics* (R. Bellamy, ed.). Cambridge, Cambridge University Press.

Thio, C. L., et al. (1999). Class II HLA alleles and hepatitis B virus persistence in African Americans. *J Infect Dis* 179.4: 1004–06.

Thio, C.L. et al. (2003). Comprehensive analysis of class I and class II HLA antigens and chronic hepatitis B virus infection. *J Virol* 77, 12083–87.

Thio, C. L., J. J. Goedert, et al. (2004). An analysis of tumor necrosis factor alpha gene polymorphisms and haplotypes with natural clearance of hepatitis C virus infection. *Genes Immun* 5.4: 294–300.

Thomas, H. C., et al. (1996) Mutation of gene of mannose-binding protein associated with chronic hepatitis B viral infection. *Lancet* 348.9039: 1417–19.

Thorburn, D., G. Curry, et al. (2002). The role of iron and haemochromatosis gene mutations in the progression of liver disease in chronic hepatitis C. *Gut* 50.2: 248–52.

Thursz, M. (2001). MHC and the viral hepatitides. *Q J Med* 94.6: 287–91.

Thursz, M. R., et al. (1995) Association between an MHC class II allele and clearance of hepatitis B virus in The Gambia. *N Engl J Med* 332: 1065.

Thursz, M. R., et al. (1997) Heterozygote advantage for HLA class-II type in hepatitis B virus infection [letter] [published erratum appears in Nat Genet 1998; 18.1:88]. *Nat Genet* 17.1: 11–12.

Thursz, M., R. Yallop, et al. (1999). Influence of MHC class II genotype on outcome of infection with hepatitis C virus. *Lancet* 354: 2119–24.

Tillmann, H. L., D. F. Chen, et al. (2001). Low frequency of HLA-DRB1*11 in hepatitis C virus induced end stage liver disease. *Gut* 48.5: 714–18.

Tokushige, K., N. Tsuchiya, et al. (2003). Influence of TNF gene polymorphism and HLA-DRB1 haplotype in Japanese patients with chronic liver disease caused by HCV. *Am J Gastroenterol* 98.1: 160–66.

van Hattum, J., et al. (1987) HLA antigens in patients with various courses after hepatitis B virus infection. *Hepatology* 7, 11–14.

Vidigal, P. G., J. J. Germer, et al. (2002). Polymorphisms in the interleukin-10, tumor necrosis factor-alpha, and transforming growth factor-beta1 genes in chronic hepatitis C patients treated with interferon and ribavirin. *J Hepatol* 36.2: 271–77.

Wasmuth, H. E., A. Werth, et al. (2004). CC chemokine receptor 5 delta32 polymorphism in two independent cohorts of hepatitis C virus infected patients without hemophilia. *J Mol Med* 82.1: 64–69.

Wawrzynowicz-Syczewska, M., J. A. Underhill, et al. (2000). HLA class II genotypes associated with chronic hepatitis C virus infection and response to alpha-interferon treatment in Poland. *Liver* 20.3: 234–39.

Woitas, R. P., G. Ahlenstiel, et al. (2002). Frequency of the HIV-protective CC chemokine receptor 5-delta32/delta32 genotype is increased in hepatitis C. *Gastroenterology* 122.7: 1721–28.

Wright, M., R. Goldin, et al. (2003). Factor V Leiden polymorphism and the rate of fibrosis development in chronic hepatitis C virus infection. *Gut* 52.8: 1206–10.

Yasunami, R., T. Miyamoto, et al. (1997). HLA-DRB1 is related to the pathological changes of the liver in chronic hepatitis C. *Hepatol Res* 7: 3–12.

Yee, L. J. (2004). Host genetic determinants in hepatitis C virus infection. *Genes Immun* 5.4: 237–45.

Yee, L. J., J. Tang, et al. (2000). Tumor necrosis factor gene polymorphisms in patients with cirrhosis from chronic hepatitis C virus infection. *Genes Immun* 1.6: 386–90.

Yee, L. J., J. Tang, et al. (2001). Interleukin 10 polymorphisms as predictors of sustained response in antiviral therapy for chronic hepatitis C infection. *Hepatology* 33.3: 708–12.

Yenigun, A., and B. Durupinar (2002). Decreased frequency of the HLA-DRB1*11 allele in patients with chronic hepatitis C virus infection. *J Virol* 76.4: 1787–89.

Yu, M. L., C. Y. Dai, et al. (2003). Tumor necrosis factor alpha promoter polymorphisms at position−308 in Taiwanese chronic hepatitis C patients treated with interferon-alpha. *Antiviral Res* 59.1: 35–40.

Zavaglia, C., C. Bortolon, et al. (1996). HLA typing in chronic type B, D and C hepatitis. *J Hepatol* 24.6: 658–65.

Zavaglia, C., et al. (1998). Association between HLA class II alleles and protection from or susceptibility to chronic hepatitis C. *J Hepatol* 28: 1–7.

Zhang, M., J. J. Goedert, et al. (2003). High frequency of CCR5-delta 32 homozygosity in HCV-infected, HIV-1-uninfected hemophiliacs results from resistance to HIV-1. *Gastroenterology* 124.3: 867–69.

Zhou, G. et al. (2004) Variants in TNFRSF5 locus and association analysis with Hepatitis B virus (HBV) infection. *Hum Mutat* 23.1: 99–100.

22

Tuberculosis, Leprosy, and Other Mycobacterial Diseases

Graham Cooke & Adrian V.S. Hill

Mycobacteria are slow-growing, gram-positive organisms protected by a complex outer cell wall. In common with gram-positive bacteria, this wall contains peptidoglycan (PG). Unlike gram-positive organisms, this PG is linked to arabinogalactan (AG), which in turn is covalently linked to long chain mycolic acids. These and other lipids, including liparabinomannan (LAM), phosphoinositol mannosides found within the cell wall (figure 22.1.) contribute to the organisms' environmental resilience.

Despite similar biochemical characteristics, mycobacteria cause diverse human diseases. *Mycobacterium tuberculosis* alone is responsible for most of the 1.8 million deaths annually attributed to clinical tuberculosis (WHO 2003), while *M. leprae* continues to be responsible for enormous morbidity, causing 700,000 cases of leprosy (WHO 2002) (see table 22.1). Many other mycobacteria are found in environmental sources, including soil and water, and rarely cause disease except in an immunocompromised host. Such immune compromise can be acquired (e.g., due to HIV infection) or genetic. The rare examples of genetic susceptibility to these "atypical" mycobacteria are discussed below and of interest, not only in the treatment of affected individuals but also because the lessons they can teach are relevant to the major mycobacterial killer, tuberculosis.

"Atypical" Mycobacteria and Disease

The study of individuals with disease caused by "atypical" mycobacteria, which are normally commensals, has led to the identification of several mutations within genes known to play an important role in host immunity to intracellular pathogens. In general, genes have been identified by a targeted candidate gene approach (for a comprehensive review, see Ottenhoff et al. 2002b). Genes identified to date all play a role in the type 1 cytokine response, believed to be critical to mycobacterial immunity.

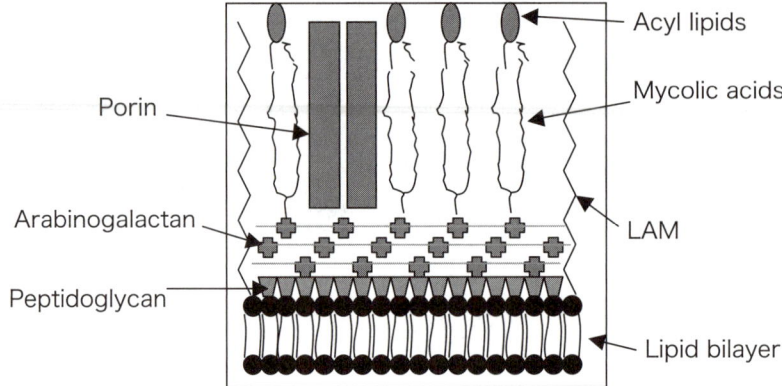

FIGURE 22.1. Schematic representation of the mycobacterial cell wall.

IFNGR1 (6q23–24)

The first family with a single gene defect predisposing to mycobacterial disease was affected by unusual environmental mycobacteria (*M. avium, M. chelonei,* and *M. fortuitum*). Two of the four children of this Maltese family were brothers, with one affected cousin and one other child thought to be a close relation (Levin et al. 1995; Newport et al. 1996). A genomewide scan on this extended pedigree identified linkage to a locus on chromosome 6, a region containing the *IFNGR1* gene encoding a subunit of the interferon-γ (IFN-γ) receptor. A single A → C mutation at position 395 created a stop codon, which truncated the receptor and rendered it undetectable on the surface of lymphocytes from affected individuals. A distinct IFNGR1

mutation was then found in a patient with invasive bacille Calmette-Guerin (BCG) infection (Jouanguy et al. 1996).

Since these discoveries, more than 20 other individuals have been identified with complete IFNGR1 deficiency. The more common form of complete deficiency arises from mutations that truncate the protein before its transmembrane region, effectively excluding it from the cell surface (Ottenhoff et al. 2002a, 2002b). Less commonly, complete functional IFNGR1 deficiency has been observed with mutations that allow the protein expression but remove any IFN-γ responsiveness (Jouanguy et al. 2000; Allende et al. 2001). More frequent than either form of complete deficiency, partial IFNGR1 deficiency has been frequently attributed to deletion within a small genomic region (Jouanguy et al. 1999; Arend et al. 2001). Mutation in this region of exon 6 truncates the protein's cytoplasmic tail, reducing its ability to activate intracellular signaling. The residual ability of the receptors to bind IFN-γ is believed to contribute to a dominant negative effect, and for as yet unknown reasons, these individuals are particularly susceptible to osteomyelitis (Arend et al. 2001).

IFNGR2 (21q22.1-q22.2)

The success in identifying defects in IFNGR1 and an increasing understanding of the importance of IFN-γ signaling in susceptibility to mycobacteria led to interest in *IFNGR2*, the gene encoding the second subunit of the IFN-γ receptor. Three cases are now reported where severe mycobacterial infections are believed to result from IFNGR2 mutation. The first

TABLE 22.1. Mycobacteria.

Organism	Description
M. tuberculosis	Primary cause of tuberculosis
M. bovis	Uncommon cause of tuberculosis in humans
M. africanum	Causes some cases of tuberculosis in Africa
BCG	Developed from passaged *M. bovis* Widely used as a vaccine and rare cause of disease
M. leprae	Causative organism of leprosy
M. avium, kansasii, marinum, ulcerans, malmoense, chelonae, fortuitum, gordonae	"Atypical" mycobacteria that rarely cause disease except in immunocompromised hosts

described was the result of a homozygous dinucleotide deletion, which produces a premature stop codon and results in inability of the protein to locate to the cell surface (Dorman and Holland 1998). More recently a single nucleotide mutation has been identified that produces a partial deficiency in response to IFN (Doffinger et al. 2000).

IL12B (5q31.1-q33.1) and *IL12RB1* (19p13.1)

Interleukin-12 (IL-12) is one of the key mediators of inflammation induced by IFN-γ and closes a feedback loop by stimulating IFN-γ production. Mutation in the subunits making up IL-12 and IL-12 receptor have been well described and produce a similar but distinct phenotype from that seen in IFN-γ pathway mutations. IL-12 is a heterodimer of 40- and 35-kDa subunits. IL-12p40 (IL-12β) deficiency is remarkable as the only familial cytokine deficiency described in humans. Affected individuals with mutation in the *IL12B* gene are usually infected by atypical mycobacteria or salmonellae, which can be fatal (Altare et al. 1998b; Elloumi-Zghal et al. 2002; Picard et al. 2002).

IL-12 receptor deficiencies are more common than *IL12B* mutations, and of the two subunits required for function, only IL-12Rβ1, and not IL-12Rβ2, has been found with functional mutation (Altare et al. 1998a; de Jong et al. 1998). Such mutations are usually recessive and, similarly to those in *IFNGR1*, result from premature stop codons before the transmembrane coding region.

STAT1 (2q32.2–32.3)

Activation of monocytes by IFN-γ leads to a complex cascade of intracellular messaging. STAT1 appears to be a critical molecule in this response. A dominant partial deficiency has recently been described in individuals susceptible to mycobacteria where a germline missense mutation prevents the phosphorylation required to produce a functional dimeric unit (Dupuis et al. 2001).

Atypical Mycobacteria Host Genetics and Susceptibility to *M. Tuberculosis*

There is now some preliminary evidence that the genetic defects described might also predispose to disease caused by *M. tuberculosis* (MTB). Jouanguy et al.

(1997) reported a case of partial IFN-γR1 deficiency in the daughter of consanguineous Portuguese parents. She had not received BCG, but at age 3 she developed cough, fatigue, and anorexia with erythema nodosum and infiltration on her chest X-ray. MTB was not isolated, but a clinical diagnosis was made. As she and her brother had increased susceptibility to other respiratory pathogens, infection with another organism cannot be ruled out. One other individual, whose DNA was not available, was the mother of two children with IFN-γR1 deficiency and is believed to have died after recurrent episodes of pulmonary tuberculosis (Jouanguy et al. 1999, as cited in Dorman and Holland 2000).

Picard et al. (2002) described the daughter of two first cousins in Saudi Arabia with a mutation in IL-12B. She developed BCG adenitis 12 months after BCG vaccination and suffered *Salmonella* gastroenteritis at 15 months. At the age of 2 years 6 months she developed tuberculous lymphadenitis due to MTB. One case in the setting of *IL12RB1* mutation is described by Altare et al. (2001). Two brothers were identified with mutations; the elder brother experienced invasive BCG infection and *Salmonella* infection. His younger brother had no complications from two BCG vaccinations; however, at the age of 18 he did suffer abdominal tuberculosis, proven on culture. More recently, two tuberculosis cases have been described in siblings with *IL12RB1* mutation (Caragol et al. 2003) who appeared to have a severe disease phenotype.

Perhaps surprisingly, therefore, very few cases of tuberculosis are described in the setting of these rare variants, particularly in the setting of *IFNG/IFNGR1/IFNGR2* mutation. One reason for the apparent absence of cases in populations with relatively low incidence of tuberculosis is that an individual is likely to have exposure to environmental mycobacteria long before exposure to MTB and hence is more likely to present with disseminated environmental mycobacterial infection. Also important, however, is a possible dissociation in the important mechanisms protecting from environmental and pathogenic mycobacteria. For *MTB* to have been successful, it is likely to have developed strategies for evading immune defenses that are unlikely to be shared by all mycobacteria. For example, some constitutive components of MTB have been shown to impair signaling pathways of IFN-γ (Ting et al. 1999). Thus, although the study of environmental mycobacteria can inform the study of tuberculosis, mechanisms that are private to MTB will be found only by study of that phenotype.

Tuberculosis

The most common, and most commonly studied, form of tuberculosis is pulmonary disease. Classical pulmonary tuberculosis is characterized by fever, cough, weight loss, and an abnormal chest X-ray. The symptoms of nonpulmonary tuberculosis vary according to the organ(s) affected (commonly lymph nodes, bones, and the central nervous system). Both pulmonary and nonpulmonary forms of disease can mimic other conditions (e.g., bacterial infections, sarcoidosis, or malignancy). Therefore, reliable phenotyping, with proof of the presence of MTB complex, is normally required, and genetic studies will usually only include cases where acid-fast bacilli are seen on microscopy ("smear positive") or where mycobacteria have been cultured from sputum or other fluids ("culture positive").

Despite the complexities of disease pathogenesis, progress has been made in identifying some of the genes involved, in both animals and humans. To date, the greatest success in human studies come from candidate gene association studies, most commonly case–control studies but also family-based association studies. There is a heritable component to cellular proliferative immune responses for some MTB antigens (Jepson et al. 2001). For the immune responses to some antigens (including purified protein derivative, PPD), which show evidence of heritability in twins, the majority of variability is determined by genes outside of the MHC (Jepson et al. 1997). The study of these genes should be rewarding in the search to understand tuberculous immunogenetics. Replicated evidence now exists for the role of human leukocyte antigen (HLA) class II region genes, solute carrier family 11 member 1 (SLC11A1; previously well known as natural resistance-associated macrophage protein 1, NRAMP1), IFNG, and the vitamin D receptor (VDR) in tuberculosis; evidence is accumulating for a number of other genes, including MAL/TIRAP and other genes on the TLR signaling pathways.

Human Leukocyte Antigens

The first and most extensively studied examples of genetic association with human tuberculosis are with genes within the MHC region. Reports of disease association with the class I molecules HLA-A10 and -B8 have not been adequately replicated (Brahmajothi et al. 1991). In contrast, an HLA-DR2 association has been repeatedly detected in India (Singh et al. 1983; Brahmajothi et al. 1991; Ravikumar et al. 1999) and farther afield (Khomenko et al. 1990; Pospelov et al. 1996; Visentainer et al. 1997; Teran-Escandon et al. 1999). Association with other class II alleles, including DQB1 (Ravikumar et al. 1999; Teran-Escandon et al. 1999) and DPB1 (Ravikumar et al. 1999), have not been as consistent in other populations (Hwang et al. 1985; Cox et al. 1988; Hawkins et al. 1988), and linkage disequilibrium between alleles of these three loci has not been thoroughly examined.

The molecular basis for these associations has not been established. A direct relationship between the ability to present pathogen epitopes and disease is supported by the observation that HLA-DRB1 alleles associated with tuberculoid leprosy are more likely to have arginine residues at critical points in the "molecular pocket"–containing antigen (Cox et al. 1988). Alternatively, HLA molecules not directly implicated in disease susceptibility might be in linkage disequilibrium with functional alleles of other immunomodulatory genes in the HLA region, such as a tumor necrosis factor-α (TNF-α) polymorphism previously associated with other infectious diseases, including malaria (McGuire et al. 1994) and leprosy type (Meisner et al. 2001). Negative association studies of TNF polymorphism have been reported in studies from The Gambia (Bellamy 1998), India (Selvaraj et al. 2001), Brazil (Blackwell et al. 1997), and Malawi (Fitness et al. 2004a), but an association has recently been reported from Colombia (Correa et al. 2005).

Candidates from Murine Genetics: SLC11A1 and SP110

SLC11A1 (2q35)

SLC11A1 was one of the first non-HLA genes convincingly implicated in tuberculosis susceptibility. This gene was initially identified after work, particularly by the laboratory of Dr. P. Gros, led to the identification of Nramp1 (or Slc11a1), the murine gene underlying the Bcg susceptibility locus (Vidal et al. 1993; see chapter 13). In mice, this locus controls infection by the intracellular pathogens M. bovis, L. donovani, and S. typhimurium. It has homology to two other molecules Nramp2 and Nramp-rs.

The human homologue, SLC11A1, originally and still more widely known as NRAMP1, is on chromosome 2q35 has 88% similarity to the murine gene (see chapter 13). It has 12 exons encoding a 550 amino acid polypeptide and spans 15 kb of genome (Blackwell et al. 1995). In the first large study of NRAMP1 polymorphism in a West African populations, four variants were identified that were more common in those individuals with disease (Bellamy et al. 1998a). Several subsequent studies detected disease association in the populations of The Gambia (Awomoyi et al. 2002), Guinea-Conakry (Cervino et al. 2000), Korea (Ryu et al. 2000), Japan (Gao et al. 2000), Cambodia (Delgado et al. 2002), and the United States (Ma et al. 2002); another study reports an association with disease severity in Europeans (Soborg et al. 2002). However, not all studies have found positive associations (e.g., Liaw et al. 2002; Soborg et al. 2002; El Baghdadi et al. 2003). Fitness et al. (2004a) added further complexity by finding that the polymorphisms associated with disease in The Gambia (Bellamy et al. 1998a) were not associated in northern Malawi, but another distinct 4-bp insertion deletion polymorphism in the 3′-untranslated region was. Many of these cited studies lacked power to detect the relatively modest effect of NRAMP1 polymorphism, even when present. This modest effect probably also explains the failure to find significant evidence of linkage to NRAMP1 (Shaw et al. 1997; Bellamy et al. 2000), with the exception of one large pedigree where analysis was conditioned on an assigned risk of disease (Greenwood et al. 2000).

Nramp1 is expressed in the phagosomal membrane and is a paralogue of Nramp2, which has been identified as a divalent cation transporter (Fleming et al. 1997). The observation that Nramp2 is mutated in the Belgrade rat (which has a microcytic anemia) suggested that Nramp2 and, by analogy, Nramp1 might have a role in iron transport. There is now some evidence directly supporting this role, including the observation that growth of M. avium in macrophages is inhibited by high iron concentrations (Forbes and Gros 2003; Gomes and Appelberg 1998). It seems possible that Nramp1 is critical to delivering iron into infected phagosomes. Using a Salmonella model of intracellular infection, Gros and colleagues were able to show that iron chelators produced an effect on bacterial growth similar to that seen in Nramp1 knockout mice (Jabado et al. 2003).

Intriguingly, Nramp1 has no effect on murine susceptibility to tuberculosis. Mouse strains homozygous for the resistance allele of Nramp1 are not significantly more resistant to MTB challenge. Nramp1 alleles segregate independently of resistance to MTB in F_2 progeny of homozygous Nramp1 resistant and susceptible mice (Medina and North 1996, 1998; Medina et al. 1996). Using mice with functional deletion of Nramp1, Gros and colleagues were unable to demonstrate an increased resistance to MTB given by low-dose aerosol challenge (North et al. 1999).

SP110 (2q37.1)

Recently fine mapping and positional cloning of a susceptibility gene for tuberculosis in mice, the sst1 locus, led to the isolation of the Ipr-1 gene that encodes a protein that increases macrophage apoptosis and impairs MTB growth in vitro and in vivo (Kramnik et al. 2005; Pan et al. 2005). The human homologue SP110 encodes one of a family of nuclear body proteins and detailed analysis of numerous single nucleotide polymorphisms (SNPs) in this gene in Gambian families has found evidence of association with tuberculosis (Tosh et al. 2006).

Cytokines and Chemokines: IFNG, CCL2, IL8, IL1, IL10

IFNG (12q14)

IFN-γ is a polypeptide of 166 amino acids encoded by the gene IFNG on chromosome 12q14 with four exons. Despite evidence from experiments in ifng and ifngr knockout mice showing a critical role for the IFN-γ pathway in the control of murine tuberculosis (Cooper et al. 1993; Flynn et al. 1993; Huang et al. 1993) and evidence of a role in susceptibility to atypical mycobacteria, the role of IFN-γ in human susceptibility to MTB remains more controversial (Flynn and Chan 2001). For example, IFN-γ alone cannot activate human macrophages to kill MTB, requiring the presence of other, incompletely defined, molecules (Bonecini-Almeida et al. 1998). This, and the fact that many patients with tuberculosis have high levels of IFN-γ at infected sites, has led some authors to suggest that IFN-γ production might be less important than IFN-γ responsiveness in determining disease outcome (Ting et al. 1999).

Four studies have now reported evidence that the A/T polymorphism at the +874 position of the IFNG gene is associated with tuberculous disease (Lio et al. 2002; Lopez-Maderuelo et al. 2003; Rossouw et al.

2003; Tso et al. 2005). The first report, a small Sicilian study (only 45 patients) found the +874TT genotype associated with protection from chronic tuberculosis with a nonsignificant trend toward a protective effect from the +874T allele (Lio et al. 2002). Subsequently, a larger study in the Spanish population demonstrated a strongly significant susceptibility effect for the +874AA genotype. This was supported with evidence that peripheral blood mononuclear cells from individuals with the +874AA genotype, be they cases or controls, produced less IFN-γ when stimulated by PPD (Lopez-Maderuelo et al. 2003).

A study from the colored population of South Africa provided convincing evidence of an association with the +874A/T polymorphism and disease (Rossouw et al. 2003). The +874AA genotype was associated with tuberculous disease in a case–control study and the +874A allele was independently overtransmitted to affected offspring in a family-based study. The polymorphism alters a binding site for the transcription factor NFκB and is therefore likely to influence inflammatory responses (Pravica et al. 2000). Finally a Hong Kong study also found that the +874AA genotype is associated with susceptibility in Chinese (Tso et al. 2005) with an odds ratio of 3.8 for the GG versus AA genotype.

Taken together, these findings probably provide the strongest evidence for a role of any single non-HLA SNP in tuberculosis and provide important evidence that variability in IFN-γ production is likely to play a role in human immunity to MTB. However, a fairly large study from northern Malawi (Fitness et al. 2004a) failed to find association for the +874 genotype with either HIV-1–positive or HIV-1–negative tuberculosis patients.

CCL2 (17q11.2-q12)

In a large Mexican study, a promoter variant of the chemokine (C-C motif) ligand 2 gene (CCL2), encoding a protein known as monocyte chemoattractant protein-1 (MCP-1), was strongly associated with susceptibility to tuberculosis, and in vitro data suggested that monocytes of individuals with the GG susceptibility genotype secreted more MCP-1 and less IL-12p40 in response to MTB (Flores-Villanueva et al. 2005). Analysis of a small Korean population sample supported this association, but studies in Brazil (Jamieson et al. 2004) and West Africa (E. Ling and A.V.S. Hill, unpublished observations) failed to find evidence of association with this SNP.

IL8 (4q13-q21)

Ma et al. (2003) have described association between adult pulmonary tuberculosis in HIV-negative individuals and the−251 promoter polymorphism in both Caucasian and African American populations of Houston, Texas (Ma et al. 2003). The−251AA genotype, previously associated with an increased susceptibility to bronchiolitis, carried an odds ratio for disease greater than 3. In a Gambian study of similar power, no evidence for disease association was found, effectively excluding a major role for IL-8 in that population (Cooke et al. 2004). The role of IL-8 remains to be explored in other populations.

IL1B (2q14)

Three studies have reported weak associations with IL-1 gene cluster polymorphisms, two of them of Gambian populations, but the results differ in the pattern of association (Bellamy et al. 1998c; Wilkinson et al. 1999; Awomoyi et al. 2005).

IL10 (1q31-q32)

Several studies have evaluated IL10 promoter polymorphisms. Probably, the clearest evidence of associations has been of the−592 variant in Korea (Shin et al. 2005). A Cambodian study reported that−1082 variant heterozygotes were susceptible but a surprisingly large number of heterozygotes (>60% in controls) were observed suggesting issues with population stratification (Delgado et al. 2002). Two other large studies of these variants found no association (Bellamy et al. 1998c; Tso et al. 2005).

Receptors: VDR, CR1, CD209, P2RX7, IL12RB1

VDR (12q13.11)

Vitamin D is one of the few agents that can stimulate human cells to kill MTB in vitro (Rook et al. 1986, 1987; Denis 1991). The clinical properties of vitamin D were recognized as long ago as 1850 when Blasius Williams noted that "pure fresh oil from the livers of cod," which are rich in vitamins A and D, "are more beneficial in the treatment of pulmonary consumption than any agent, dietetic, or regimen that has yet been employed" (Dubos and Dubos 1952). Vitamin D is immunomodulatory and, through the vitamin D receptor (VDR), can alter cytokine responses of T cells, including IL-12 (D'Ambrosio et al. 1998) and IFN-γ (Cippitelli and Santoni 1998) by interaction with Stat1. In humans, low vitamin D levels appear to be a risk factor for developing tuberculosis, possibly due to dietary deficiency or reduced sunlight exposure (Strachan et al. 1995). The seasonal changes in vitamin D levels (lower during the dark winter months in the northern hemisphere) are one proposed explanation for the seasonal incidence rates observed for tuberculosis.

There are good reasons to believe that VDR polymorphism might influence an individual's risk of developing tuberculosis. VDR mediates the effects of vitamin D and is found in cells of the monocytic and lymphocytic lineages (Provvedini et al. 1983; Reichel et al. 1987). VDR polymorphism has clinical consequences and been associated with bone mineral density and osteoporosis (Morrison et al. 1992, 1994; Nguyen et al. 1994).

The most frequently studied polymorphisms in VDR are commonly referred to by the restriction enzymes that discriminate them: ApaI (Aa), BsmI (Bb), FokI (Ff), and TaqI (Tt). In a West African case–control study, the "tt" genotype within codon 352 was less frequent in individuals with pulmonary tuberculosis (Bellamy et al. 1999), suggesting a protective effect from disease. In a smaller study within the Gujarati population of West London, there was a trend toward a similar result (Wilkinson et al. 2000). When 25-hydroxycalciferol concentrations were taken into consideration, the tt genotype was again associated with protection from disease. Small studies in India have found an excess of tt individuals among female cases of pulmonary tuberculosis (Selvaraj et al. 2000) and an excess of FF homozygotes amongst patients with spinal tuberculosis (Selvaraj et al. 2004), but a large northern Malawi study and a smaller Peruvian study (Roth et al. 2004) failed to find association.

This heterogeneity may simply reflect lack of definition of the true functional polymorphisms within the gene. Detailed analysis of VDR haplotypes in West Africans provided further evidence of disease association at this locus and suggested that such a variant might lie on a haplotype with FokI F and ApaI A alleles (Bornman 2004). In Peru, a strong association between both F and T genotypes and rate of response to drug treatment was found (Roth et al. 2004). Health prevention strategies using vitamin D have had some benefit in a number of medical conditions but have not been formally tested for tuberculosis. The accumulat-ing genetic data adds to the work suggesting that such a strategy merits evaluation.

CR1 *(1q32)*

On phagocytic cells complement receptor-1 (CD35) encoded by *CR1* mediates the adherence and phagocytosis of complement-opsonized pathogens, and mycobacteria utilize this mechanism to gain entry into macrophages. Homozygosity for a CR1 Q1022H polymorphism was associated with susceptibility to tuberculosis in northern Malawi (Fitness et al. 2004a). The association was observed amongst HIV-negative but not HIV-positive tuberculosis cases.

CD209 *(19p13)*

DC-SIGN, encoded by the *CD209* gene, is a C-type lectin is one of several mycobacterial receptors on macrophages and dendritic cells. Barreiro et al. (2006) reported association of two promoter SNPs with tuberculosis susceptibility in the colored population of Cape Town, South Africa.

P2RX7 *(12q24)*

Lammas et al. (1997) have identified a purinergic-receptor–mediated pathway by which ATP can, *in vitro*, kill both virulent and avirulent environmental mycobacteria. This effect is rapid and more efficient than other mechanisms identified in human cells and results in rapid phagolysosomal fusion within infected cells and hastening microbial degradation (Fairbairn et al. 2001). In a study of the *P2X7* gene, five promoter polymorphisms were screened, and allele C at position–762 of the promoter appeared protective against tuberculosis in The Gambia (Li et al. 2002).

IL12RB1 *(19p13.1)*

IL12RB1 promoter polymorphisms were associated with disease in a study of 98 cases from Japan (Akahoshi et al. 2003). Two haplotypes were identified that differed at three nucleotides. Homozygotes for the haplotype found to reduce IL-12 signaling *in vitro* were significantly more likely to develop disease, possibly because of reduced IFN-γ production.

In contrast to studies on atypical mycobacterial disease, no genetic associations have been found with polymorphisms in the genes for the IFN-γ receptor (Awomoyi et al. 2004).

Innate Immunity: *TIRAP, TLR2, TLR4, MBL2*

TIRAP *(11q24.2)*

TIRAP (or MAL) is one of the four adaptor proteins involved in transmitting signals from toll-like receptors to downstream signaling cascades. Khor et al. (2007) reported a single amino acid change that appeared to act as an inactivating mutation of this gene in Gambians. The less common allele encoding a serine to leucine change at position 180 was associated with resistance to tuberculosis as well as protection from other infectious diseases.

TLR2 *(4q32)* and TLR4 *(9q32-q33)*

TLR2 and TLR4 are the only Toll-like receptors identified able to mediate immune responses induced by ligands within MTB, suggesting these receptors may have a specific role in the immune response to tuberculosis. They are also the two receptors that use the adaptor TIRAP/MAL. There are significant differences in the ligands for each receptor. Ligands identified for TLR2 include AraLAM (Means et al. 1999), dimannosylated phosphatidylinositol (biosynthetic precursor of the larger glycolipid LAM; Jones et al. 2001), and a 19-kDa lipoprotein of MTB (Brightbill et al. 1999). TLR4 mediates cellular activation by an unidentified product of live MTB (Means et al. 2001) and phosphatidylinositol mannosides (Abel et al. 2002; reviewed in Heldwein and Fenton 2002). Data from murine models of *tlr2* knockout and *tlr4* defective mice are conflicting.

Despite considerable interest in Toll-like receptors, there is only one report of TLR2 variation (Ogus et al. 2004) influencing tuberculosis and no evidence to date of disease association within TLR4 (Cooke et al. 2002). The TLR2 +2258A allele, previously reported as reducing TLR2 signaling in response to bacterial peptides (Lorenz et al. 2000), was associated with an increased risk of tuberculosis in a Turkish population. The frequency of +2258A was much lower than in most other populations, suggesting that limited power might make it difficult to replicate these findings.

MBL2 *(10q11.2–21)*

Mannose-binding lectin (MBL), an ancient component of the innate immune system, is a serum lectin with opsonic and complement-activating activity, produced in the liver as part of the acute response to infection (see chapter 10). The association of increased frequency of three polymorphisms within exon 1 of the gene with substantial reductions in circulating levels of MBL has led to speculation that these variants might protect against potentially harmful immune responses. Possibilities include that reduced MBL levels reduce uncontrolled complement activation or that normal levels of MBL might actually facilitate the entry of organisms including MTB into host cells (Garred et al. 1994, 1997).

Three studies have reported association with tuberculosis. High MBL levels are associated with increased susceptibility to tuberculosis in HIV-negative Tanzanians (Garred et al. 1997), and alleles related to reduced MBL levels appeared to protect against tuberculous meningitis in South Africans (Hoal-Van Helden et al. 1999) and Danes (Soborg et al. 2003). However, the evidence also suggests that alleles causing MBL deficiency do not protect from pulmonary disease (Soborg et al. 2003). These studies have tended to be quite small (<100 cases), and in the largest study to date, no significant evidence of association with pulmonary tuberculosis was found in Africans (Bellamy et al. 1998b).

Proteolysis: *UBE3A* (15q11–13)

The *UBE3A* gene has been widely investigated for its role in Prader-Willi syndrome, a condition interesting to geneticists because it demonstrates parental imprinting. The gene lies on chromosome 15q11–13, a region linked to tuberculosis in Gambians (Bellamy et al. 2000). UBE3A, like PARKIN (see below), is a ubiquitin ligase that might play a role in T-cell responses (Oda et al. 1999; Sawabe et al. 2001). Cervino et al. (2002) found association of a 7-bp deletion in *UBE3A* with tuberculosis in Gambians and South Africans. Further work will be needed to understand the how such enzymes might influence disease outcome, but genetic studies to date provide important evidence of a role for this enzyme system against mycobacterial disease in general.

Genomewide Linkage Analysis and Clinical Tuberculosis

The two largest genomewide studies published to date have come from South America and sub-Saharan

Africa. Blackwell and colleagues studied a collection of large pedigrees in Brazil (part of the "Belem" study; Blackwell et al. 1997; Miller et al. 2004). Using different analytical approaches the best evidence for linkage (maximum LOD score = 1.85) was to the region 11q12.3. Combined analysis of leprosy and tuberculosis cases found some evidence for linkage to markers within the region 17q11-q21 (Jamieson et al. 2004). Within this region lie several genes that might influence macrophage-mediated immunity, and although the study did not have sufficient power to identify the precise variants responsible, disease association was found with polymorphisms within four genes (*NOS2A*, *CCL18*, *CCL4*, and *STAT5B*), suggesting one or more of these might influence disease outcome.

Affected sibling pair linkage analysis mapped potential susceptibility loci on chromosome 15q11–13 and Xq27 (Bellamy 2000). Efforts to identify the disease causing alleles within these regions on Xq27 have not yet proved fruitful (Campbell 2001), but there is some evidence that on chromosome 15, the positional candidate gene UBE3A (see above) might be associated with disease (Cervino et al. 2002). Unpublished data on linkage analysis of about 250 affected sibling pairs with tuberculosis from Malawian, South African, and West African families have revealed stronger evidence of linkage to chromosome 20q, and a positional candidate genes analysis suggests association with tuberculosis in these African populations (authors' unpublished observations).

Leprosy

Despite effective therapies and public health control, there are approximately 700,000 new cases of leprosy each year, causing considerable morbidity. Tuberculoid leprosy (TT) is a localized disease characterized by hypopigmented, desensitized skin lesions often with thickening of local nerves. Lepromatous leprosy can affect any organ, but often skin changes, including macules, papules, nodules, or plaques, appear first. Clinical features may fall between these polar types and are associated with different immune responses. TT individuals typically have low bacterial numbers (paucibacillary) and strong type 1 cytokine responses, while lepromatous leprosy has a stronger type 2 response with more bacteria (multibacillary). Individual genes have been implicated both in leprosy susceptibility per se and in the type of leprosy seen.

Candidate Genes Associated with Leprosy and Leprosy Type

HLA Region

There have been many studies of the role of HLA in determining leprosy per se and leprosy type (de Vries et al. 1976, 1980; Fine et al. 1979; van Eden et al. 1980), including some of the earliest examples of family-based association studies. Several reported associations with class I MHC genes are inconsistent and have not been replicated with more accurate molecular techniques (Greiner et al. 1978; Serjeantson 1983; Rani et al. 1992). They could have resulted from linkage disequilibrium to other genes nearby on the genome. One such gene is *MICA*, which acts as a co-stimulatory molecule to activate T-cell responses. The HLA-B46-MICA-5A5 haplotype has been associated with protection from lepromatous leprosy in a Chinese study (Wang et al. 1999).

As with tuberculosis, associations between leprosy and polymorphisms of class II genes have been more consistent. In particular, DQ alleles were associated in India (Rani et al. 1992, 1993), Thailand (Schauf et al. 1985), and Japan (Miyanaga et al. 1981). Associations with DQ alleles have commonly been with the tuberculoid phenotype, whereas DR2 and DR3 alleles have been associated with increased susceptibility to both forms of leprosy (discussed in more detail in Fitness et al. 2002).

Within the class III MHC region lie the genes encoding TNF-α (*TNF*) and lymphotoxin-α (*LTA*, formerly TNF-β). As noted above, TNF-α is an important proinflammatory cytokine. Although polymorphism within the promoter has been studied in detail, the precise functional variants remain controversial. The−308A allele, which is associated with a more vigorous skin reaction to lepromin antigen (Moraes et al. 2001), was associated with protection against leprosy (both tuberculoid and lepromatous) in Brazil (Shaw et al. 2001) but not in Malawi (Fitness et al. 2004b). The neighboring gene, *LTA*, encodes a chemokine implicated in a number of diseases, including myocardial infarction. Haplotypes across *TNF* and *LTA* were associated with disease in Brazil (Shaw et al. 2001), and the precise polymorphisms modifying disease remain uncertain. Recent evidence suggests that linkage disequilibrium with *LTA* promoter polymorphisms might account for some of the effects previously attributed to *TNF* (Knight et al. 2003).

SLC11A1 *(2q35)*

There is less evidence to support a role for *SLC11A1/ NRAMP1* in leprosy when compared to tuberculosis. Polymorphism in this gene appeared to influence susceptibility to leprosy per se in a Vietnamese study (Abel et al. 1995); however, others have failed to confirm this (Shaw et al. 1993; Roger et al. 1997; Roy et al. 1999; Meisner et al. 2001; Fitness et al. 2004b) but have found suggestive association with leprosy type (Meisner et al. 2001) and with the Mitsuda reaction (a delayed hypersensitivity reaction following intradermal injection with *M. leprae* antigen; Alcais et al. 2000).

VDR *(12q13.11)*

The rationale for studying *VDR* in tuberculosis applies equally well to leprosy. Studies of the TaqI polymorphism have found an association with disease type in Bengali Indians (Roy et al. 1999) with tt genotype more common in individuals with tuberculoid leprosy and TT genotype more common among individuals with lepromatous leprosy. In northern Malawi, where tuberculoid leprosy predominates, the tt genotype was also more prevalent in leprosy cases than in controls (Fitness et al. 2004b).

CR1 *(1q32)*

In a case–control study in northern Malawi a variant of the complement receptor-1 (*CR1*) gene was associated with leprosy susceptibility (Fitness et al. 2004a). Homozygotes for the variant K1590E, the change that defines the McCoy b blood group in exon 29 of the gene, were at reduced risk. This is a different variant of *CR1* to that associated with tuberculosis in the same population (Fitness et al. 2004a).

TLR2 *(4q32)*

A novel *TLR2* mutation altering an arginine to tryptophan (R677W) in the receptor was found in Koreans with lepromatous leprosy but not in controls (Kang and Chae 2001). Cell lines transfected with R677W variant are unable to respond to mycobacterial antigen (Bochud et al. 2003), suggesting that impaired signaling through TLR2 can allow *M. leprae* to disseminate widely, perhaps impairing the cellular immune response. This variant has not as yet been identified outside Asia.

Genomewide Linkage Analysis in the Study of Leprosy

To date, genomewide analysis has been more successful in leprosy than any other infectious disease. The first major locus for leprosy susceptibility was found on chromosome 10p13 (Siddiqui et al. 2001) in a study of 185 sibling pairs from Tamil Nadu, India (figure 22.2), and a second locus subsequently found on 20p13 (Tosh et al. 2002). There is now evidence of disease association with *MRC1*, a gene near the center of the region defined by linkage on chromosome 10p13. *MRC1* encodes the macrophage mannose receptor, a calcium-dependent lectin found on dendritic cells that mediates pathogen endocytosis. Terminal mannosyl residues of mycobacterial LAM are recognized by this receptor and correlations have been described between receptor phagocytosis and mycobacterial virulence. One MRC-1 haplotype (Gly396-Ala399-Phe407) is associated with leprosy susceptibility, and one (Ser396-Ala399-Phe407) with resistance. A change in residue 396 seems to alter the receptor structure significantly, although its effect is probably modified by residues in other positions (Tosh et al. unpublished manuscript).

A second study in 197 Vietnamese families found a susceptibility locus on 6q25–26 (Mira et al. 2003). Fine-mapping of this region found a cluster of noncoding SNPs associated with disease and association with leprosy was confirmed in a Brazilian population (Mira et al. 2004). The SNPs lie in a shared promoter region of two genes: *PARK2* and *PACRG*. Which of these is important in leprosy is not known. Both are expressed in Schwann cells and macrophages, the primary host cells of *M. leprae*, as well as many other tissues. *PARK2*, previously associated with early onset Parkinson's disease (Kitada et al. 1998) acts as a ubiquitination E3 ligase, echoing the previous association of *UBE3A* with tuberculosis susceptibility (Cervino et al. 2002) and suggesting it as the stronger biological candidate.

Concluding Remarks

This chapter highlights several genetic associations with mycobacterial disease that contribute to our understanding of disease resistance and immunity. No single gene has been associated with susceptibility to all the mycobacterial phenotypes described here. For example, no mutations in the IFN-γ/IL-12 network have

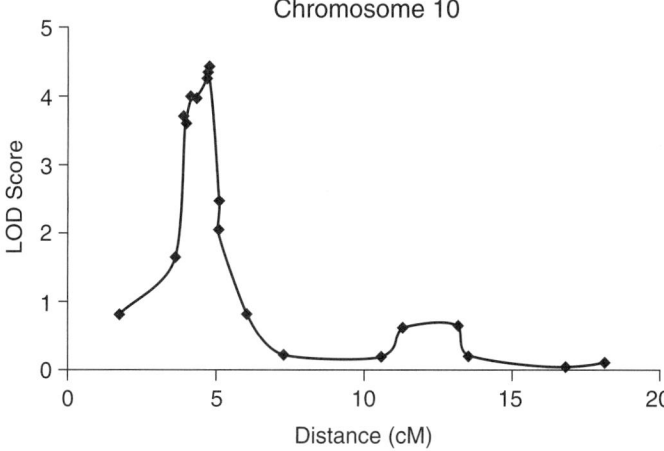

FIGURE 22.2. Linkage peak on chromosome 10p13 identified in a genome scan for susceptibility to leprosy in south Indian affected sibling pairs (Siddiqui et al., 2001). The underlying locus has been identified as the macrophage mannose receptor (Tosh et al., 2008 [in press]).

been associated with leprosy, no TNF polymorphisms associated with tuberculosis, and no *SCL11A1* variant associated with diseases caused by environmental mycobacteria. These differences emphasize the complexity of susceptibility even within a closely related pathogenic species.

To date, the candidate gene approach has been the most successful tool to identify genetic variants associated with disease. Genomewide linkage analysis has had some success in finding genes influencing disease within populations, and this success has been greater in the study of leprosy compared to many other complex diseases, either infectious or otherwise. Why should linkage analysis have been relatively successful in leprosy? It could be chance, but other explanations are possible. Although morbidity from leprosy is severe, mortality is low. Longer survival of patients would enable detrimental polymorphisms to persist at high frequency in the population despite the social stigma of disease. The clear, stable, and readily identifiable phenotype of leprosy has allowed the collection of large family collections with good power to detect population effects.

Polymorphism in genes that differentially influence disease at a population level has had individually modest effects. As the field of complex genetics moves toward large genomewide association studies, it is possible that with the identification of more genes it will be possible to identify individuals with "polygenic immunocompromise" against single diseases. While this goal remains elusive, the study of genetic effects continues to shed light on the pathogenesis of mycobacterial along with other important infectious diseases.

References

Abel B, Thieblemont N, Quesniaux VJ, Brown N, Mpagi J, Miyake K, Bihl F, Ryffel B (2002) Toll-like receptor 4 expression is required to control chronic *Mycobacterium tuberculosis* infection in mice. J Immunol 169:3155–62.

Abel L, Vu DL, Oberti J, Nguyen VT, Van VC, Guilloud-Bataille M, Schurr E, Lagrange PH (1995) Complex segregation analysis of leprosy in southern Vietnam. Genet Epidemiol 12:63–82.

Akahoshi M, Nakashima H, Miyake K, Inoue Y, Shimizu S, Tanaka Y, Okada K, Otsuka T, Harada M (2003) Influence of interleukin-12 receptor beta1 polymorphisms on tuberculosis. Hum Genet 112:237–43.

Alcais A, Sanchez FO, Thuc NV, Lap VD, Oberti J, Lagrange PH, Schurr E, Abel L (2000) Granulomatous reaction to intradermal injection of lepromin (Mitsuda reaction) is linked to the human NRAMP1 gene in Vietnamese leprosy sibships. J Infect Dis 181:302–08.

Allende LM, Lopez-Goyanes A, Paz-Artal E, Corell A, Garcia-Perez MA, Varela P, Scarpellini A, Negreira S, Palenque E, Arnaiz-Villena A (2001) A point mutation in a domain of gamma interferon receptor 1 provokes severe immunodeficiency. Clin Diagn Lab Immunol 8:133–37.

Altare F, Durandy A, Lammas D, Emile JF, Lamhamedi S, Le Deist F, Drysdale P, Jouanguy E, Doffinger R, Bernaudin F, Jeppsson O, Gollob JA, Meinl E, Segal AW, Fischer A, Kumararatne D, Casanova JL (1998a) Impairment of mycobacterial immunity in human interleukin-12 receptor deficiency. Science 280:1432–35.

Altare F, Ensser A, Breiman A, Reichenbach J, Baghdadi JE, Fischer A, Emile JF, Gaillard JL, Meinl E, Casanova JL (2001) Interleukin-12 receptor beta1 deficiency in a patient with abdominal tuberculosis. J Infect Dis 184:231–36.

Altare F, Lammas D, Revy P, Jouanguy E, Doffinger R, Lamhamedi S, Drysdale P, Scheel Toellner D, Girdlestone J, Darbyshire P, Wadhwa M, Dockrell H, Salmon M, Fischer A, Durandy A, Casanova JL, Kumararatne DS (1998b) Inherited interleukin 12 deficiency in a child with bacille Calmette-Guerin and *Salmonella enteritidis* disseminated infection. J Clin Invest 102:2035–40.

Arend SM, Janssen R, Gosen JJ, Waanders H, de Boer T, Ottenhoff TH, van Dissel JT (2001) Multifocal osteomyelitis caused by nontuberculous mycobacteria in patients with a genetic defect of the interferon-gamma receptor. Neth J Med 59:140–51.

Awomoyi AA, Charurat M, Marchant A, Miller EN, Blackwell JM, McAdam KP, Newport MJ. (2005) Polymorphism in IL1B: IL1B-511 association with tuberculosis and decreased lipopolysaccharide-induced IL-1beta in IFN-gamma primed ex-vivo whole blood assay. J Endotoxin Res 11(5):281–86.

Awomoyi AA, Marchant A, Howson JM, McAdam KP, Blackwell JM, Newport MJ (2002) Interleukin-10, polymorphism in SLC11A1 (formerly NRAMP1), and susceptibility to tuberculosis. J Infect Dis 186:1808–14.

Awomoyi AA, Nejentsev S, Richardson A, Hull J, Koch O, Podinovskaia M, Todd JA, McAdam KP, Blackwell JM, Kwiatkowski D, Newport MJ (2004) No association between interferon-gamma receptor-1 gene polymorphism and pulmonary tuberculosis in a Gambian population sample. Thorax 59:291–94.

Barreiro LB, Neyrolles O, Babb CL, Tailleux L, Quach H, McElreavy K, Van Helden PD, Hoal EG, Gicquel B, Quintana-Murci L (2006) Promoter variation in the DC-SIGN-encoding gene CD209 is associated with tuberculosis. PLOS Med. 3(2), e20 doi:10.1371/journal.pmed.0030020.

Bellamy R (1998) Genetic Susceptibility and Resistance to Tuberculosis. Ph.D. thesis. University of Oxford, Oxford.

Bellamy R (2000) Identifying genetic susceptibility factors for tuberculosis in Africans: a combined approach using a candidate gene study and a genome-wide screen. Clin Sci (Colch) 98:245–50.

Bellamy R, Beyers N, McAdam KP, Ruwende C, Gie R, Samaai P, Bester D, Meyer M, Corrah T, Collin M, Camidge DR, Wilkinson D, Hoal-Van Helden E, Whittle HC, Amos W, van Helden P, Hill AV (2000) Genetic susceptibility to tuberculosis in Africans: a genome-wide scan. Proc Natl Acad Sci USA 97: 8005–09

Bellamy R, Ruwende C, Corrah T, McAdam KP, Whittle HC, Hill AV (1998a) Variations in the NRAMP1

gene and susceptibility to tuberculosis in West Africans [see comments]. N Engl J Med 338:640–44.

Bellamy R, Ruwende C, McAdam KP, Thursz M, Sumiya M, Summerfield J, Gilbert SC, Corrah T, Kwiatkowski D, Whittle HC, Hill AV (1998b) Mannose binding protein deficiency is not associated with malaria, hepatitis B carriage nor tuberculosis in Africans. Q J Med 91:13–18.

Bellamy R, Ruwende C, Corrah T, McAdam KP, Whittle HC, Hill AV. (1998c) Assessment of the interleukin 1 gene cluster and other candidate gene polymorphisms in host susceptibility to tuberculosis. Tuber Lung Dis 79:83–89.

Bellamy R, Ruwende C, Corrah T, McAdam KP, Thursz M, Whittle H, Hill AVS (1999) Tuberculosis and chronic hepatitis B virus infection in Africans and variation in the vitamin D receptor gene. J Infect Dis 179:721–24.

Blackwell JM, Barton CH, White JK, Searle S, Baker AM, Williams H, Shaw MA (1995) Genomic organization and sequence of the human NRAMP gene: identification and mapping of a promoter region polymorphism. Mol Med 1:194–205.

Blackwell JM, Black GF, Peacock CS, Miller EN, Sibthorpe D, Gnananandha D, Shaw JJ, Silveira F, Lins-Lainson Z, Ramos F, Collins A, Shaw MA (1997) Immunogenetics of leishmanial and mycobacterial infections: the Belem Family Study. Philos Trans R Soc Lond B Biol Sci 352:1331–45.

Bochud PY, Hawn TR, Aderem A (2003) Cutting edge: a Toll-like receptor 2 polymorphism that is associated with lepromatous leprosy is unable to mediate mycobacterial signaling. J Immunol 170:3451–54.

Bonecini-Almeida MG, Chitale S, Boutsikakis I, Geng J, Doo H, He S, Ho JL (1998) Induction of in vitro human macrophage anti-*Mycobacterium tuberculosis* activity: requirement for IFN-gamma and primed lymphocytes. J Immunol 160:4490–99.

Bornman L, Campbell SJ, Fielding K, Bah B, Sillah J, Gustafson P, Manneh K, Lisse I, Allen A, Sirugo G, Sylla A, Aaby P, McAdam KP, Bah-Sow O, Bennett S, Lienhardt C, Hill AV. (2004) Vitamin D receptor polymorphisms and susceptibility to tuberculosis in West Africa: a case-control and family study. J Infect Dis 190:1631–41.

Brahmajothi V, Pitchappan RM, Kakkanaiah VN, Sashidhar M, Rajaram K, Ramu S, Palanimurugan K, Paramasivan CN, Prabhakar R (1991) Association of pulmonary tuberculosis and HLA in south India. Tubercle 72:123–32.

Brightbill HD, Libraty DH, Krutzik SR, Yang RB, Belisle JT, Bleharski JR, Maitland M, Norgard MV, Plevy SE, Smale ST, Brennan PJ, Bloom BR, Godowski PJ, Modlin RL (1999) Host defense mechanisms triggered by microbial lipoproteins through Toll-like receptors. Science 285:732–36.

Campbell SJ (2001) Genetics of susceptibility to tuberculosis. Ph.D. thesis. Oxford University, Oxford.

Caragol I, Raspall M, Fieschi C, Feinberg J, Larrosa M, Hernandez M, Figueras C, Bertran M, Casanova JL, Espanol T (2003) Clinical Tuberculosis in 2 of 3 siblings with interleukin-12 receptor B1 deficiency. Clin Infect Dis 37:302–06.

Cervino AC, Lakiss S, Sow O, Bellamy R, Beyers N, Hoal-Van Helden E, Van Helden P, McAdam KP, Hill AV (2002) Fine mapping of a putative tuberculosis-susceptibility locus on chromosome 15q11–13 in African families. Hum Mol Genet 11:1599–603.

Cervino AC, Lakiss S, Sow O, Hill AV (2000) Allelic association between the NRAMP1 gene and susceptibility to tuberculosis in Guinea-Conakry. Ann Hum Genet 64:507–12.

Cippitelli M, Santoni A (1998) Vitamin D3: a transcriptional modulator of the interferon-gamma gene. Eur J Immunol 28:3017–30.

Cooke GS, Campbell SJ, Fielding K, Sillah J, Manneh K, Sirugo G, Bennett S, McAdam K, Lienhardt C, Hill AV (2004) Interleukin-8 polymorphism is not associated with pulmonary tuberculosis in The Gambia. J Infect Dis 189:1545–56.

Cooke GS, Segal S, Hill AV (2002) Toll-like receptor 4 polymorphisms and atherogenesis. N Engl J Med 347:1978–80.

Cooper AM, Dalton DK, Stewart TA, Griffin JP, Russell DG, Orme IM (1993) Disseminated tuberculosis in interferon gamma gene-disrupted mice. J Exp Med 178:2243–47.

Correa PA, Gomez LM, Cadena J, Anaya JM (2005) Autoimmunity and tuberculosis. Opposite association with TNF polymorphism. J Rheumatol 32:219–24.

Cox RA, Downs M, Neimes RE, Ognibene AJ, Yamashita TS, Ellner JJ (1988) Immunogenetic analysis of human tuberculosis. J Infect Dis 158:1302–08.

D'Ambrosio D, Cippitelli M, Cocciolo MG, Mazzeo D, Di Lucia P, Lang R, Sinigaglia F, Panina-Bordignon P (1998) Inhibition of IL-12 production by 1,25-dihydroxyvitamin D3: involvement of NF-kappaB downregulation in transcriptional repression of the p40 gene. J Clin Invest 101:252–62.

de Jong R, Altare F, Haagen IA, Elferink DG, Boer T, van Breda Vriesman PJ, Kabel PJ, Draaisma JM, van Dissel JT, Kroon FP, Casanova JL, Ottenhoff TH (1998) Severe mycobacterial and Salmonella infections in interleukin-12 receptor-deficient patients. Science 280:1435–38.

Delgado JC, Baena A, Thim S, Goldfeld AE (2002) Ethnic-specific genetic associations with pulmonary tuberculosis. J Infect Dis 186:1463–68.

Denis M (1991) Killing of Mycobacterium tuberculosis within human monocytes: activation by cytokines and calcitriol. Clin Exp Immunol 84:200–06.

de Vries RR, Fat RF, Nijenhuis LE, van Rood JJ (1976) HLA-linked genetic control of host response to Mycobacterium leprae. Lancet 2:1328–30.

de Vries RR, Mehra NK, Vaidya MC, Gupte MD, Meera Khan P, Van Rood JJ (1980) HLA-linked control of susceptibility to tuberculoid leprosy and association with HLA-DR types. Tissue Antigens 16:294–304.

Doffinger R, Jouanguy E, Dupuis S, Fondaneche MC, Stephan JL, Emile JF, Lamhamedi-Cherradi S, Altare F, Pallier A, Barcenas-Morales G, Meinl E, Krause C, Pestka S, Schreiber RD, Novelli F, Casanova JL (2000) Partial interferon-gamma receptor signaling chain deficiency in a patient with bacille Calmette-Guerin and Mycobacterium abscessus infection. J Infect Dis 181:379–84.

Dorman SE, Holland SM (1998) Mutation in the signal-transducing chain of the interferon-gamma receptor and susceptibility to mycobacterial infection. J Clin Invest 101:2364–69.

Dorman SE, Holland SM (2000) Interferon-gamma and interleukin-12 pathway defects and human disease. Cytokine Growth Factor Rev 11:321–33.

Dubos R, Dubos J (1952) Tuberculosis, Man and Society. Rutgers University Press, New Brunswick, NJ.

Dupuis S, Dargemont C, Fieschi C, Thomassin N, Rosenzweig S, Harris J, Holland SM, Schreiber RD, Casanova JL (2001) Impairment of mycobacterial but not viral immunity by a germline human STAT1 mutation. Science 293:300–03.

El Baghdadi J, Remus N, Benslimane A, El Annaz H, Chentoufi M, Abel L, Schurr E (2003) Variants of the human NRAMP1 gene and susceptibility to tuberculosis in Morocco. Int J Tuberc Lung Dis 7:599–602.

Elloumi-Zghal H, Barbouche MR, Chemli J, Bejaoui M, Harbi A, Snoussi N, Abdelhak S, Dellagi K (2002) Clinical and genetic heterogeneity of inherited autosomal recessive susceptibility to disseminated Mycobacterium bovis bacille calmette-guerin infection. J Infect Dis 185:1468–75.

Fairbairn IP, Stober CB, Kumararatne DS, Lammas DA (2001) ATP-mediated killing of intracellular mycobacteria by macrophages is a P2X(7)-dependent process inducing bacterial death by phagosome-lysosome fusion. J Immunol 167:3300–07.

Fine PE, Wolf E, Pritchard J, Watson B, Bradley DJ, Festenstein H, Chacko CJ (1979) HLA-linked genes and leprosy: a family study in Karigiri, South India. J Infect Dis 140:152–61.

Fitness J, Tosh K, Hill AVS (2002) Genetics of susceptibility to leprosy. Genes Immun 3:441–53.

Fitness J, Floyd S, Warndorff DK, Sichali L, Malema S, Crampin AC, Fine PE, Hill AVS (2004a) Large-scale candidate gene study of tuberculosis susceptibility in the Karonga district of northern Malawi. Am J Trop Med Hyg 71:341–49.

Fitness J, Floyd S, Warndorff DK, Sichali L, Mwaungulu L, Crampin AC, Fine PE, Hill AVS (2004b) Large-scale candidate gene study of leprosy susceptibility in the Karonga district of northern Malawi. Am J Trop Med Hyg 71:330–40.

Fleming MD, Trenor CC, 3rd, Su MA, Foernzler D, Beier DR, Dietrich WF, Andrews NC (1997) Microcytic anaemia mice have a mutation in Nramp2, a candidate iron transporter gene. Nat Genet 16:383–86.

Flores-Villanueva PO, Ruiz-Morales JA, Song CH, Flores LM, Jo EK, Montano M, Barnes PF, Selman M, Granados J. (2005) A functional promoter polymorphism in monocyte chemoattractant protein-1 is associated with increased susceptibility to pulmonary tuberculosis. J Exp Med 202:1649–58.

Flynn JL, Chan J (2001) Immunology of tuberculosis. Annu Rev Immunol 19:93–129.

Flynn JL, Chan J, Triebold KJ, Dalton DK, Stewart TA, Bloom BR (1993) An essential role for interferon gamma in resistance to *Mycobacterium tuberculosis* infection. J Exp Med 178:2249–54.

Forbes JR, Gros P (2003) Iron, manganese, and cobalt transport by Nramp1 (Slc11a1) and Nramp2 (Slc11a2) expressed at the plasma membrane. Blood 102: 1884–92.

Gao PS, Fujishima S, Mao XQ, Remus N, Kanda M, Enomoto T, Dake Y, Bottini N, Tabuchi M, Hasegawa N, Yamaguchi K, Tiemessen C, Hopkin JM, Shirakawa T, Kishi F (2000) Genetic variants of NRAMP1 and active tuberculosis in Japanese populations. International Tuberculosis Genetics Team. Clin Genet 58:74–76.

Garred P, Harboe M, Oettinger T, Koch C, Svejgaard A (1994) Dual role of mannan-binding protein in infections: another case of heterosis? Eur J Immunogenet 21:125–31.

Garred P, Richter C, Andersen AB, Madsen HO, Mtoni I, Svejgaard A, Shao J (1997) Mannan-binding lectin in the sub-Saharan HIV and tuberculosis epidemics. Scand J Immunol 46:204–08.

Gomes MS, Appelberg R (1998) Evidence for a link between iron metabolism and Nramp1 gene function in innate resistance against *Mycobacterium avium*. Immunology 95:165–68.

Greenwood CM, Fujiwara TM, Boothroyd LJ, Miller MA, Frappier D, Fanning EA, Schurr E, Morgan K (2000) Linkage of tuberculosis to chromosome 2q35 loci, including NRAMP1, in a large aboriginal Canadian family. Am J Hum Genet 67:405–16.

Greiner J, Schleiermacher E, Smith T, Lenhard V, Vogel F (1978) The HLA system and leprosy in Thailand. Hum Genet 42:201–13.

Hawkins BR, Higgins DA, Chan SL, Lowrie DD, Mitchison DA, Girling DJ (1988) HLA typing in the Hong Kong Chest Service/British Medical Research Council study of factors associated with the breakdown to active tuberculosis of inactive pulmonary lesions. Am Rev Respir Dis 138:1616–21.

Heldwein KA, Fenton MJ (2002) The role of Toll-like receptors in immunity against mycobacterial infection. Microbes Infect 4:937–44.

Hoal-Van Helden EG, Epstein J, Victor TC, Hon D, Lewis LA, Beyers N, Zurakowski D, Ezekowitz AB, Van Helden PD (1999) Mannose-binding protein B allele confers protection against tuberculous meningitis. Pediatr Res 45:459–64.

Huang S, Hendriks W, Althage A, Hemmi S, Bluethmann H, Kamijo R, Vilcek J, Zinkernagel RM, Aguet M (1993) Immune response in mice that lack the interferon-gamma receptor. Science 259:1742–45.

Hwang CH, Khan S, Ende N, Mangura BT, Reichman LB, Chou J (1985) The HLA-A, -B, and -DR phenotypes and tuberculosis. Am Rev Respir Dis 132:382–85.

Jabado N, Cuellar-Mata P, Grinstein S, Gros P (2003) Iron chelators modulate the fusogenic properties of *Salmonella*-containing phagosomes. Proc Natl Acad Sci USA 100:6127–32.

Jamieson SE, Miller EN, Black GF, Peacock CS, Cordell HJ, Howson JM, Shaw MA, Burgner D, Xu W, Lins-Lainson Z, Shaw JJ, Ramos F, Silveira F, Blackwell JM (2004) Evidence for a cluster of genes on chromosome 17q11-q21 controlling susceptibility to tuberculosis and leprosy in Brazilians. Genes Immun 5:46–57.

Jepson A, Fowler A, Banya W, Singh M, Bennett S, Whittle H, Hill AV (2001) Genetic Regulation of Acquired Immune Responses to Antigens of *Mycobacterium tuberculosis*: a study of twins in West Africa. Infect Immun 69:3989–94.

Jepson A, Sisay-Joof F, Banya W, Hassan-King M, Frodsham A, Bennett S, Hill AV, Whittle H (1997) Genetic linkage of mild malaria to the major histocompatibility complex in Gambian children: study of affected sibling pairs. BMJ 315:96–7.

Jones BW, Means TK, Heldwein KA, Keen MA, Hill PJ, Belisle JT, Fenton MJ (2001) Different Toll-like receptor agonists induce distinct macrophage responses. J Leukoc Biol 69:1036–44.

Jouanguy E, Altare F, Lamhamedi S, Revy P, Emile JF, Newport M, Levin M, Blanche S, Seboun E, Fischer A, Casanova JL (1996) Interferon-gamma-receptor deficiency in an infant with fatal bacille Calmette-Guerin infection. N Engl J Med 335:1956–61.

Jouanguy E, Dupuis S, Pallier A, Doffinger R, Fonda-neche MC, Fieschi C, Lamhamedi-Cherradi S, Al-tare F, Emile JF, Lutz P, Bordigoni P, Cokugras H, Akcakaya N, Landman-Parker J, Donnadieu J, Camcioglu Y, Casanova JL (2000) In a novel form of IFN-gamma receptor 1 deficiency, cell surface re-ceptors fail to bind IFN-gamma. J Clin Invest 105:1429–36.

Jouanguy E, Lamhamedi-Cherradi S, Altare F, Fonda-neche MC, Tuerlinckx D, Blanche S, Emile JF, Gaillard JL, Schreiber R, Levin M, Fischer A, Hivroz C, Casanova JL (1997) Partial interferon-gamma receptor 1 deficiency in a child with tuberculoid bacillus Calmette-Guerin infection and a sibling with clinical tuberculosis. J Clin Invest 100:2658–64.

Jouanguy E, Lamhamedi-Cherradi S, Lammas D, Dor-man SE, Fondaneche MC, Dupuis S, Doffinger R, Altare F, Girdlestone J, Emile JF, Ducoulombier H, Edgar D, Clarke J, Oxelius VA, Brai M, Novelli V, Heyne K, Fischer A, Holland SM, Kumararatne DS, Schreiber RD, Casanova JL (1999) A human IFNGR1 small deletion hotspot associated with dom-inant susceptibility to mycobacterial infection. Nat Genet 21:370–78.

Kang TJ, Chae GT (2001) Detection of Toll-like recep-tor 2 (TLR2) mutation in the lepromatous lep-rosy patients. FEMS Immunol Med Microbiol 31: 53–58.

Khomenko AG, Litvinov VI, Chukanova VP, Pospelov LE (1990) Tuberculosis in patients with various HLA phenotypes. Tubercle 71:187–92.

Khor CC, Chapman SJ, Vannberg FO, Dunne A, Murphy C, Ling EY, Frodsham AJ, Walley AJ, Kyrieleis O, Khan A, Aucan C, Segal S, Moore CE, Knox K, Campbell SJ, Lienhardt C, Scott A, Aaby P, Sow OY, Grignani RT, Sillah J, Sirugo G, Peshu N, Williams TN, Maitland K, Davies RJ, Kwiatkowski DP, Day NP, Yala D, Crook DW, Marsh K, Berkley JA, O'Neill LA, Hill AV. (2007) A Mal functional variant is associated with protection against invasive pneu-mococcal disease, bacteremia, malaria and tubercu-losis. Nat Genet 39:523–28.

Kitada T, Asakawa S, Hattori N, Matsumine H, Yama-mura Y, Minoshima S, Yokochi M, Mizuno Y, Shi-mizu N (1998) Mutations in the parkin gene cause autosomal recessive juvenile parkinsonism. Nature 392:605–08.

Knight JC, Keating BJ, Rockett KA, Kwiatkowski DP (2003) In vivo characterization of regulatory poly-morphisms by allele-specific quantification of RNA polymerase loading. Nat Genet 33:469–75.

Lammas DA, Stober C, Harvey CJ, Kendrick N, Pan-chalingam S, Kumararatne DS (1997) ATP-induced killing of mycobacteria by human macrophages is mediated by purinergic P2Z(P2X7) receptors. Im-munity 7:433–44.

Levin M, Newport MJ, D'Souza S, Kalabalikis P, Brown IN, Lenicker HM, Agius PV, Davies EG, Thrasher A, Klein N, et al. (1995) Familial disseminated atypical mycobacterial infection in childhood: a human my-cobacterial susceptibility gene? Lancet 345:79–83.

Li CM, Campbell SJ, Kumararatne DS, Bellamy R, Ruwende C, McAdam KP, Hill AV, Lammas DA (2002) Association of a polymorphism in the P2X7 gene with tuberculosis in a Gambian population. J Infect Dis 186:1458–62.

Liaw YS, Tsai-Wu JJ, Wu CH, Hung CC, Lee CN, Yang PC, Luh KT, Kuo SH (2002) Variations in the NRAMP1 gene and susceptibility of tuberculosis in Taiwanese. Int J Tuberc Lung Dis 6:454–60.

Lio D, Marino V, Serauto A, Gioia V, Scola L, Crivello A, Forte GI, Colonna-Romano G, Candore G, Caruso C (2002) Genotype frequencies of the +874T→A single nucleotide polymorphism in the first intron of the interferon-gamma gene in a sample of Sicilian patients affected by tuberculosis. Eur J Immunogenet 29:371–74.

Lopez-Maderuelo D, Arnalich F, Serantes R, Gonzalez A, Codoceo R, Madero R, Vazquez JJ, Montiel C (2003) Interferon-gamma and interleukin-10 gene polymorphisms in pulmonary tuberculosis. Am J Respir Crit Care Med 167:970–75.

Lorenz E, Mira JP, Cornish KL, Arbour NC, Schwartz DA (2000) A novel polymorphism in the toll-like recep-tor 2 gene and its potential association with staphy-lococcal infection. Infect Immun 68:6398–401.

Ma X, Dou S, Wright JA, Reich RA, Teeter LD, El Sahly HM, Awe RJ, Musser JM, Graviss EA (2002) 5′ Di-nucleotide repeat polymorphism of NRAMP1 and susceptibility to tuberculosis among Caucasian patients in Houston, Texas. Int J Tuberc Lung Dis 6:818–23.

Ma X, Reich RA, Wright JA, Tooker HR, Teeter LD, Musser JM, Graviss EA (2003) Association between interleukin-8 gene alleles and human susceptibility to tuberculosis disease. J Infect Dis 188:349–55.

McGuire W, Hill AV, Allsopp CE, Greenwood BM, Kwiatkowski D (1994) Variation in the TNF-alpha promoter region associated with susceptibility to ce-rebral malaria. Nature 371:508–10.

Means TK, Jones BW, Schromm AB, Shurtleff BA, Smith JA, Keane J, Golenbock DT, Vogel SN, Fenton MJ (2001) Differential effects of a Toll-like receptor an-tagonist on Mycobacterium tuberculosis-induced macrophage responses. J Immunol 166:4074–82.

Means TK, Lien E, Yoshimura A, Wang S, Golenbock DT, Fenton MJ (1990) The CD14 ligands lipoar-abinomannan and lipopolysaccharide differ in their requirement for Toll-like receptors. J Immunol 163:6748–55.

Medina E, North RJ (1996) Evidence inconsistent with a role for the Bcg gene (Nramp1) in resistance of mice to infection with virulent *Mycobacterium tuberculosis*. J Exp Med 183:1045–51.

Medina E, North RJ (1998) Resistance ranking of some common inbred mouse strains to *Mycobacterium tuberculosis* and relationship to major histocompatibility complex haplotype and Nramp1 genotype. Immunology 93:270–74.

Medina E, Rogerson BJ, North RJ (1996) The Nramp1 antimicrobial resistance gene segregates independently of resistance to virulent *Mycobacterium tuberculosis*. Immunology 88:479–81.

Meisner SJ, Mucklow S, Warner G, Sow SO, Lienhardt C, Hill AVS (2001) Association of NRAMP1 polymorphism with leprosy type but not susceptibility to leprosy per se in West Africans. Amer J Trop Med Hyg. 65:733–35.

Miller EN, Jamieson SE, Joberty C, Fakiola M, Hudson D, Peacock CS, Cordell HJ, Shaw MA, Lins-Lainson Z, Shaw JJ, Ramos F, Silveira F, Blackwell JM (2004) Genome-wide scans for leprosy and tuberculosis susceptibility genes in Brazilians. Genes Immun 5: 63–67.

Mira MT, Alcais A, Nguyen VT, Moraes MO, Di Flumeri C, Vu HT, Mai CP, Nguyen TH, Nguyen NB, Pham XK, Sarno EN, Alter A, Montpetit A, Moraes ME, Moraes JR, Dore C, Gallant CJ, Lepage P, Verner A, Van De Vosse E, Hudson TJ, Abel L, Schurr E (2004) Susceptibility to leprosy is associated with PARK2 and PACRG. Nature 427:636–40.

Mira MT, Alcais A, Van Thuc N, Thai VH, Huong NT, Ba NN, Verner A, Hudson TJ, Abel L, Schurr E (2003) Chromosome 6q25 is linked to susceptibility to leprosy in a Vietnamese population. Nat Genet 33:412–15.

Miyanaga K, Juji T, Maeda H, Nakajima S, Kobayashi S (1981) Tuberculoid leprosy and HLA in Japanese. Tissue Antigens 18:331–34.

Moraes MO, Duppre NC, Suffys PN, Santos AR, Almeida AS, Nery JA, Sampaio EP, Sarno EN (2001) Tumor necrosis factor-alpha promoter polymorphism TNF2 is associated with a stronger delayed-type hypersensitivity reaction in the skin of borderline tuberculoid leprosy patients. Immunogenetics 53:45–47.

Morrison NA, Yeoman R, Kelly PJ, Eisman JA (1992) Contribution of trans-acting factor alleles to normal physiological variability: vitamin D receptor gene polymorphism and circulating osteocalcin. Proc Natl Acad Sci USA 89:6665–69.

Morrison NA, Qi JC, Tokita A, Kelly PJ, Crofts L, Nguyen TV, Sambrook PN, Eisman JA (1994) Prediction of

bone density from vitamin D receptor alleles. Nature 367:284–87.

Newport MJ, Huxley CM, Huston S, Hawrylowicz CM, Oostra BA, Williamson R, Levin M (1996) A mutation in the interferon-gamma-receptor gene and susceptibility to mycobacterial infection. N Engl J Med 335:1941–49.

Nguyen TV, Kelly PJ, Morrison NA, Sambrook PN, Eisman JA (1994) Vitamin D receptor genotypes in osteoporosis. Lancet 344:1580–81.

North RJ, LaCourse R, Ryan L, Gros P (1999) Consequence of Nramp1 deletion to *Mycobacterium tuberculosis* infection in mice. Infect Immun 67: 5811–14.

Oda H, Kumar S, Howley PM (1999) Regulation of the Src family tyrosine kinase Blk through E6AP-mediated ubiquitination. Proc Natl Acad Sci USA 96: 9557–62.

Ogus AC, Yoldas B, Ozdemir T, Uguz A, Olcen S, Keser I, Coskun M, Cilli A, Yegin O (2004) The Arg753Gln polymorphism of the human toll-like receptor 2 gene in tuberculosis disease. Eur Respir J 23:219–23.

Ottenhoff TH, Verreck FA, Lichtenauer-Kaligis EG, Hoeve MA, Sanal O, Van Dissel JT (2002a) Erratum: Genetics, cytokines and human infectious disease: lessons from weakly pathogenic mycobacteria and salmonellae. Nat Genet 32:331.

Ottenhoff TH, Verreck FA, Lichtenauer-Kaligis EG, Hoeve MA, Sanal O, van Dissel JT (2002b) Genetics, cytokines and human infectious disease: lessons from weakly pathogenic mycobacteria and salmonellae. Nat Genet 32:97–105.

Pan H, Yan BS, Rojas M, Shebzukhov YV, Zhou H, Kobzik L, Higgins DE, Daly MJ, Bloom BR, Kramnik I (2005) Ipr1 gene mediates innate immunity to tuberculosis. Nature 434:767–72.

Picard C, Fieschi C, Altare F, Al-Jumaah S, Al-Hajjar S, Feinberg J, Dupuis S, Soudais C, Al-Mohsen IZ, Genin E, Lammas D, Kumararatne DS, Leclerc T, Rafii A, Frayha H, Murugasu B, Wah LB, Sinniah R, Loubser M, Okamoto E, Al-Ghonaium A, Tufenkeji H, Abel L, Casanova JL (2002) Inherited interleukin-12 deficiency: IL12B genotype and clinical phenotype of 13 patients from six kindreds. Am J Hum Genet 70:336–48.

Pospelov LE, Matrakshin AG, Chernousova LN, Tsoi KN, Afanasjev KI, Rubtsova GA, Yeremeyev VV (1996) Association of various genetic markers with tuberculosis and other lung diseases in Tuvinian children. Tuber Lung Dis 77:77–80.

Pravica V, Perrey C, Stevens A, Lee JH, Hutchinson IV (2000) A single nucleotide polymorphism in the first intron of the human IFN-gamma gene: absolute correlation with a polymorphic CA microsatellite marker of high IFN-gamma production. Hum Immunol 61:863–66.

Provvedini DM, Tsoukas CD, Deftos LJ, Manolagas SC (1983) 1,25-Dihydroxyvitamin D3 receptors in human leukocytes. Science 221:1181–83.

Rani R, Fernandez-Vina MA, Zaheer SA, Beena KR, Stastny P (1993) Study of HLA class II alleles by PCR oligotyping in leprosy patients from north India. Tissue Antigens 42:133–37.

Rani R, Zaheer SA, Mukherjee R (1992) Do human leukocyte antigens have a role to play in differential manifestation of multibacillary leprosy: a study on multibacillary leprosy patients from north India. Tissue Antigens 40:124–27.

Ravikumar M, Dheenadhayalan V, Rajaram K, Lakshmi SS, Kumaran PP, Paramasivan CN, Balakrishnan K, Pitchappan RM (1999) Associations of HLA-DRB1, DQB1 and DPB1 alleles with pulmonary tuberculosis in south India. Tuber Lung Dis 79:309–17.

Reichel H, Koeffler HP, Tobler A, Norman AW (1987) 1 alpha,25-Dihydroxyvitamin D3 inhibits gamma-interferon synthesis by normal human peripheral blood lymphocytes. Proc Natl Acad Sci USA 84: 3385–89.

Roger M, Levee G, Chanteau S, Gicquel B, Schurr E (1997) No evidence for linkage between leprosy susceptibility and the human natural resistance-associated macrophage protein 1 (NRAMP1) gene in French Polynesia. Int J Lepr Other Mycobact Dis 65:197–202.

Rook GA, Steele J, Fraher L, Barker S, Karmali R, O'Riordan J, Stanford J (1986) Vitamin D3, gamma interferon, and control of proliferation of *Mycobacterium tuberculosis* by human monocytes. Immunology 57:159–63.

Rook GA, Taverne J, Leveton C, Steele J (1987) The role of gamma-interferon, vitamin D3 metabolites and tumour necrosis factor in the pathogenesis of tuberculosis. Immunology 62:229–34.

Rossouw M, Nel HJ, Cooke GS, van Helden PD, Hoal EG (2003) Association between tuberculosis and a polymorphic NFkappaB binding site in the interferon gamma gene. Lancet 361:1871–72.

Roth DE, Soto G, Arenas F, Bautista CT, Ortiz J, Rodriguez R, Cabrera L, Gilman RH. (2004) Association between vitamin D receptor gene polymorphisms and response to treatment of pulmonary tuberculosis. J Infect Dis 190:920–27.

Roy S, Frodsham A, Saha B, Hazra SK, Mascie-Taylor CG, Hill AV (1999) Association of vitamin D receptor genotype with leprosy type. J Infect Dis 179: 187–91.

Ryu S, Park YK, Bai GH, Kim SJ, Park SN, Kang S (2000) 3'UTR polymorphisms in the NRAMP1 gene are associated with susceptibility to tuberculosis in Koreans. Int J Tuberc Lung Dis 4:577–80.

Sawabe T, Horiuchi T, Nakamura M, Tsukamoto H, Nakahara K, Harashima SI, Tsuchiya T, Nakano S (2001) Defect of lck in a patient with common variable immunodeficiency. Int J Mol Med 7:609–14.

Schauf V, Ryan S, Scollard D, Jonasson O, Brown A, Nelson K, Smith T, Vithayasai V (1985) Leprosy associated with HLA-DR2 and DQw1 in the population of northern Thailand. Tissue Antigens 26: 243–47.

Selvaraj P, Kurian SM, Chandra G, Reetha AM, Charles N, Narayanan PR (2004) Vitamin D receptor gene variants of BsmI, ApaI, TaqI, and FokI polymorphisms in spinal tuberculosis. Clin Genet 65:73–76.

Selvaraj P, Narayanan PR, Reetha AM (2000) Association of vitamin D receptor genotypes with the susceptibility to pulmonary tuberculosis in female patients and resistance in female contacts. Indian J Med Res 111:172–79.

Selvaraj P, Sriram U, Mathan Kurian S, Reetha AM, Narayanan PR. (2001) Tumour necrosis factor alpha (-238 and -308) and beta gene polymorphisms in pulmonary tuberculosis: haplotype analysis with HLA-A, B and DR genes. Tuberculosis (Edinb) 81(5–6):335–41.

Serjeantson SW (1983) HLA and susceptibility to leprosy. Immunol Rev 70:89–112.

Shaw MA, Atkinson S, Dockrell H, Hussain R, Lins-Lainson Z, Shaw J, Ramos F, Silveira F, Mehdi SQ, Kaukab F, et al. (1993) An RFLP map for 2q33-q37 from multicase mycobacterial and leishmanial disease families: no evidence for an Lsh/Ity/Bcg gene homologue influencing susceptibility to leprosy. Ann Hum Genet 57(pt 4):251–71.

Shaw MA, Collins A, Peacock CS, Miller EN, Black GF, Sibthorpe D, Lins-Lainson Z, Shaw JJ, Ramos F, Silveira F, Blackwell JM (1997) Evidence that genetic susceptibility to mycobacterium tuberculosis in a Brazilian population is under oligogenic control: linkage study of the candidate genes NRAMP1 and TNFa. Tubercle Lung Dis 78:35–45.

Shaw MA, Donaldson IJ, Collins A, Peacock CS, Lins-Lainson Z, Shaw JJ, Ramos F, Silveira F, Blackwell JM (2001) Association and linkage of leprosy phenotypes with HLA class II and tumour necrosis factor genes. Genes Immun 2:196–204.

Shin HD, Park BL, Kim YH, Cheong HS, Lee IH, Park SK (2005) Common interleukin 10 polymorphism associated with decreased risk of tuberculosis. Exp Mol Me. 37(2):128–32.

Siddiqui MR, Meisner S, Tosh K, Balakrishnan K, Ghei S, Fisher SE, Golding M, Shanker Narayan NP, Sitaraman T, Sengupta U, Pitchappan R, Hill AV

(2001) A major susceptibility locus for leprosy in India maps to chromosome 10p13. Nat Genet 27: 439–41.

Singh SP, Mehra NK, Dingley HB, Pande JN, Vaidya MC (1983) Human leukocyte antigen (HLA)-linked control of susceptibility to pulmonary tuberculosis and association with HLA-DR types. J Infect Dis 148: 676–81.

Soborg C, Andersen AB, Madsen HO, Kok-Jensen A, Skinhoj P, Garred P (2002) Natural resistance-associated macrophage protein 1 polymorphisms are associated with microscopy-positive tuberculosis. J Infect Dis 186:517–21.

Soborg C, Madsen HO, Andersen AB, Lillebaek T, Kok-Jensen A, Garred P (2003) Mannose-binding lectin polymorphisms in clinical tuberculosis. J Infect Dis 188:777–82.

Strachan DP, Powell KJ, Thaker A, Millard FJ, Maxwell JD (1995) Vegetarian diet as a risk factor for tuberculosis in immigrant south London Asians. Thorax 50:175–80.

Teran-Escandon D, Teran-Ortiz L, Camarena-Olvera A, Gonzalez-Avila G, Vaca-Marin MA, Granados J, Selman M (1999) Human leukocyte antigen-associated susceptibility to pulmonary tuberculosis: molecular analysis of class II alleles by DNA amplification and oligonucleotide hybridization in Mexican patients. Chest 115:428–33.

Ting LM, Kim AC, Cattamanchi A, Ernst JD (1999) *Mycobacterium tuberculosis* inhibits IFN-gamma transcriptional responses without inhibiting activation of STAT1. J Immunol 163:3898–906.

Tosh K, Vannberg F, Gochhait S, Frodsham AJ, Malhotra D, Fletcher H, Meisner S, Shaw JM, Roy S, Cardon L, Drickamer K, Taylor M, Fitness J, Floyd S, Fine P, Bamezai RNK, Pitchappan K, Hill AV. The macrophage mannose receptor is a major susceptibility locus for leprosy in India. (unpublished manuscript)

Tosh K, Meisner S, Siddiqui MR, Balakrishnan K, Ghei S, Golding M, Sengupta U, Pitchappan RM, Hill AV (2002) A region of chromosome 20 is linked to leprosy susceptibility in a South Indian population. J Infect Dis 186:1190–93.

Tosh, K, Campbell, SJ, Fielding, K, Sillah, J, Bah, B, Gustafson, P, Manneh, K, Lisse, I, Sirugo, G, Bennett, S, Aaby, P, McAdam, KP, Bah-Sow, O, Lienhardt, C, Kramnik, I, Hill, AV (2006) Variants in the SP110 gene are associated with genetic susceptibility to tuberculosis in West Africa. Proc Nat Acad Sci 103:10364–68.

Tso HW, Ip WK, Chong WP, Tam CM, Chiang AK, Lau YL. (2005) Association of interferon gamma and interleukin 10 genes with tuberculosis in Hong Kong Chinese. Genes Immun 6:358–63.

van Eden W, de Vries RR, Mehra NK, Vaidya MC, D'Amaro J, van Rood JJ (1980) HLA segregation of tuberculoid leprosy: confirmation of the DR2 marker. J Infect Dis 141:693–701.

Vidal SM, Malo D, Vogan K, Skamene E, Gros P (1993) Natural resistance to infection with intracellular parasites: isolation of a candidate for BCG. Cell 73:469–85.

Visentainer JE, Tsuneto LT, Serra MF, Peixoto PR, Petzl-Erler ML (1997) Association of leprosy with HLA-DR2 in a southern Brazilian population. Braz J Med Biol Res 30:51–59.

Wang LM, Kimura A, Satoh M, Mineshita S (1999) HLA linked with leprosy in southern China: HLA-linked resistance alleles to leprosy. Int J Lepr Other Mycobact Dis 67:403–08.

WHO (2002) Leprosy. Wkly Epidemiol Rec 77:1–8.

WHO (2003) Global Tuberculosis Control: Surveillance, Planning, Financing. WHO Report 2003. World Health Organization, Geneva.

Wilkinson RJ, Llewelyn M, Toossi Z, Patel P, Pasvol G, Lalvani A, Wright D, Latif M, Davidson RN (2000) Influence of vitamin D deficiency and vitamin D receptor polymorphisms on tuberculosis among Gujarati Asians in west London: a case-control study [see comments]. Lancet 355:618–21.

Wilkinson RJ, Patel P, Llewelyn M, Hirsch CS, Pasvol G, Snounou G, Davidson RN, Toossi Z. (1999) Influence of polymorphism in the genes for the interleukin (IL)-1 receptor antagonist and IL-1beta on tuberculosis. J Exp Med 189:1863–74.

23

Diseases Due to Encapsulated Bacteria

Malak Kotb

In addition to epidemiological and socioeconomic differences that influence susceptibility to certain bacterial infections, host genetic variability contributes importantly to the substantial differences in their occurrence and course. The same bacteria cause a spectrum of clinical manifestations from asymptomatic infection in some to fatal disease in others. Studying the immune response and differences in genetic makeup of susceptible and resistant individuals can provide insight into disease mechanisms and a deeper understanding of the network of interactive pathways that lead either to eradication of infection or to serious host-mediated pathological consequences. This knowledge can guide the development of diagnostic and therapeutic advances.

Inasmuch as the immune response plays a pivotal role in infectious diseases, it is not surprising that, among the genetic susceptibility loci implicated in bacterial pathogenesis to date, the majority regulate and/or mediate host immunity. Although potential contributions of pathways with no direct relation to the immune response cannot be ignored, far less is known of them at this point. Although information is accumulating on many types of bacterial infections, this chapter concentrates on immunogenetic associations with selected gram-positive and gram-negative encapsulated bacteria.

Genetic Associations with Encapsulated Bacteria

Encapsulated bacteria cause some of the most common and often the most deadly diseases in humans. Among them are *Streptococcus pyogenes*, *Streptococcus pneumoniae*, *Staphylococcus aureus*, *Hemophilus influenzae*, *Klebsiella pneumoniae*, *Neisseria meningitidis*, *Bacillus anthracis*, and *Bordetella pertussis*. These microorganisms produce a variety of syndromes whose detailed clinical and epidemiological characteristics are beyond the scope of this chapter. They include genital and other mucocutaneous inflammatory responses, upper and lower respiratory infection with pneumonia, localized abscesses, meningitis, postinfectious rheumatic fever and glomerulonephritis, and disseminated infection with bacteremia and sepsis. Table 23.1 broadly summarizes some of the genetic associations with these bacterial infections. Much of the remainder of the chapter presents a more in-depth discussion of susceptibility to infections leading to starkly different outcomes in genetically distinct hosts: S. pyogenes and B. anthracis as representatives of gram-positive encapsulated bacteria and N. meningitidis as a representative of gram-negative encapsulated bacteria.

Conditions Caused by *S. Pyogenes* (Group A Streptococcus) Infection

Group A streptococci (GAS) are extremely contagious human pathogens that can cause a broad range of diseases due directly to replication and spread of the pathogen, often into normally sterile sites (figure 23.1) (Cunningham, 2000). The severe forms of acute suppurative invasive GAS infections were noted more than 150 years ago and became a major concern with the high fatality rates during epidemics of the early twentieth century. The incidence of complicated GAS infections, including acute rheumatic fever (ARF), declined for several decades after the 1920s, but severe invasive GAS disease resurged in the early 1980s (Cone et al., 1987; Low et al., 1997; Stevens et al., 1989), manifesting as either mild bacteremia, erysipelas, and cellulitis or as very severe illnesses such as pneumonia, streptococcal toxic shock syndrome (STSS), and necrotizing fasciitis (NF), also known as the flesh-eating disease (Davies et al., 1996; Eriksson et al., 1998; Working Group on Severe Streptococcal Infections, 1993; Kaul et al., 1997; Kotb et al., 2002; Low et al., 1997; Muller et al., 2003; Vlaminckx et al., 2004).

GAS can also produce postinfectious nonsuppurative (often considered "autoimmune") conditions that may affect the heart, kidney, skin, joints, and central nervous system (Cunningham, 2000, 2003; Stollerman, 2001, 2002). These include ARF, acute glomerulonephritis (AGN), carditis, neurological disorders (Loiselle and Singer, 2001; Nordstrand et al., 1999; Stollerman, 2002), and poststreptococcal reactive arthritis (PRSA) (Deighton, 1993; Jansen et al., 2005). While most patients recover with no complications, others suffer chronic and debilitating sequelae such as rheumatic heart disease (RHD), renal failure,

Sydenham chorea–associated obsessive-compulsive symptoms, parkinsonian features, or exacerbated pediatric autoimmune neuropsychiatric disorders (PANDAS) (Ashabr et al., 2005; Ben-Pazi et al., 2003; Dale, 2005; Kurlan and Kaplan, 2004; Maia et al., 2005; Snider and Swedo, 2003). Certain individuals develop skin conditions, including psoriasis (Bisno and Stevens, 1996).

The seriousness of severe GAS infections (e.g., STSS, NF, ARF, RHD, and AGN) as a major global health threat is underscored by recent estimates of 1.8 million new cases and at least 517,000 deaths each year (Carapetis et al., 2005).

Diagnosis

Guidelines for the diagnosis of GAS diseases, including streptococcal pharyngitis (Pechère and Kaplan, 2004), invasive GAS infections (Working Group on Severe Streptococcal Infections, 1993; Kotb et al., 2002; Louie et al., 1998; Muller et al., 2003), and the above-enumerated post-GAS infection complications (Cunningham, 2000) have been established and are periodically updated.

Following the resurgence of severe invasive GAS infections in the 1980s, new guidelines were developed for the diagnosis of STSS, NF, mild bacteremia, and cellulitis (Davies et al., 1996; Working Group on Severe Streptococcal Infections, 1993; Kaul et al., 1997; Kotb et al., 2002; Louie et al., 1998; Low et al., 1997; Muller et al., 2003; Vlaminckx et al., 2004). The clinical diagnosis of STSS requires the isolation of GAS from a normally sterile site in a patient who is hypotensive and has two or more of the following: renal impairment; coagulopathy; liver dysfunction; acute respiratory distress syndrome; a generalized erythematous macular rash; soft-tissue necrosis, including NF or myositis; or gangrene (Antibiotic Subcommittee at Mount Sinai Hospital 1998; Working Group on Severe Streptococcal Infections, 1993). Severe systemic disease (SSD) is a subclassification of STSS that emphasizes the severity of the immune response in STSS and requires the presence of hypotension and multiple organ failure (MOF) (Kotb et al., 2002).

Nonsuppurative complications accompany or follow ARF during the early weeks after an initial GAS infection. The reason for this lag period between GAS infection and the onset of ARF remains unknown. In different times and places, ARF has been either under- or overdiagnosed, and although the Jones cri-

TABLE 23.1. Genetic Variations Affecting the Outcomes of Encapsulated Bacteria

Bacteria	Gene, Region (NCBI ID)	Variants	Effect	References
Neisseria meningitidis	FCGR2A, 1q23 (2212) ± FCGR3B, 1q23 (2215) FCGR3A, 1q23 (2214)	+131R/R genotype ± NA2/NA2 +158F/F genotype	Severe forms of meningococcal disease (also to a wide variety of encapsulated bacteria)	(Domingo et al., 2002, 2004; Fijen et al., 2000; van der Pol and van de Winkel, 1998; van der Pol et al., 2001)
	CFP (properdin), Xp11.3-p11.23 (5199) ± Certain complement component genes	Total or partial deficiency (X-linked)	Impaired clearance and predisposition to fulminant meningococcal disease	(Fremeaux-Bacchi et al., 1995; Rameix-Welti et al., 2005)
	SERPINE1 (plasminogen-activator-inhibitor-1, PAI-1), 7q21.3-q22 (5054)	+4G/G genotype	Higher plasma PAI-1; increased risk for vascular complications and death from sepsis (independent of meningitis)	(Emonts et al., 2003; Geishofer et al., 2005; Haralambous et al., 2003; Hermans and Hazelzet, 2005; Hermans et al., 1999)
	ACE (angiotensin I converting enzyme), 17q23.3 (1636)	Deletion (D) vs. insertion (I), DD genotype	Increased illness severity in meningococcal disease	(Harding et al., 2002)
	TAFI (thrombin-activable fibrinolysis inhibitor), 13q14.11 (1361)	+325I homozygosity	Increased illness severity in meningococcal disease	(Kremer Hovinga et al., 2004)
	IL1RN, 2q14.2 (3557)	A2 and +2018 polymorphism	Poor outcome and higher mortality	(Read et al., 2000)
	IL6, 7p21 (3569) IL10, 1q31-q32 (3568)	−174G/G genotype −1082A/A genotype	Reduced survival	(Balding et al., 2003)
	TLR4, 9q32-q33 (7099)	Increased frequency of rare, mis-sense mutations	Increased risk of invasive disease in infancy and meningococcal disease in adult white population	(Faber et al., 2006; Smirnova et al., 2003)
	TLR2, 4q32 (7097)	+1752 C/T	Increased risk of meningococcal disease	
	MBP (mannose-binding protein), 18q23 (4155)	Codon 52 mutation, codon 54 homozygosity, codon 57 mutation	Increased risk of sepsis	(Hibberd et al., 1999; Vermont et al., 2002)
Streptococcus pneumoniae	FCGR2A, 1q23 (2212)	+131R/R and 131R/H genotype	Increased risk	(Domingo et al., 2002, 2004; Fijen et al., 2000; van der Pol and van de Winkel, 1998; van der Pol et al., 2001)
	IGHG2 (G2m), 14q32.33 (3501) IL10, 1q31-q32 (3586)	n/n genotype −1082G allele	Protective for sepsis in children, including those with C2 deficiency Increased risk of sepsis	(Jonsson et al., 2006) (Schaaf et al., 2003)
Klebsiella pneumoniae	LTA (TNFβ, lymphotoxin-α), 6p21.3 (4049) HSPA1B (heat-shock protein 70-2) 6p21.3 (3304)	+250A/A genotype +1267 polymorphism	Increased risk for septic shock Increased risk for septic shock Predictor of septic shock	(Waterer et al., 2003; Waterer and Wunderink, 2003)
Haemophilus influenzae type b S. pyogenes	IGHG2 (G2m), 14q32.33 (3501)	Absence of n allele	Increased risk	(Ambrosino et al., 1985; Goddard et al., 1996)

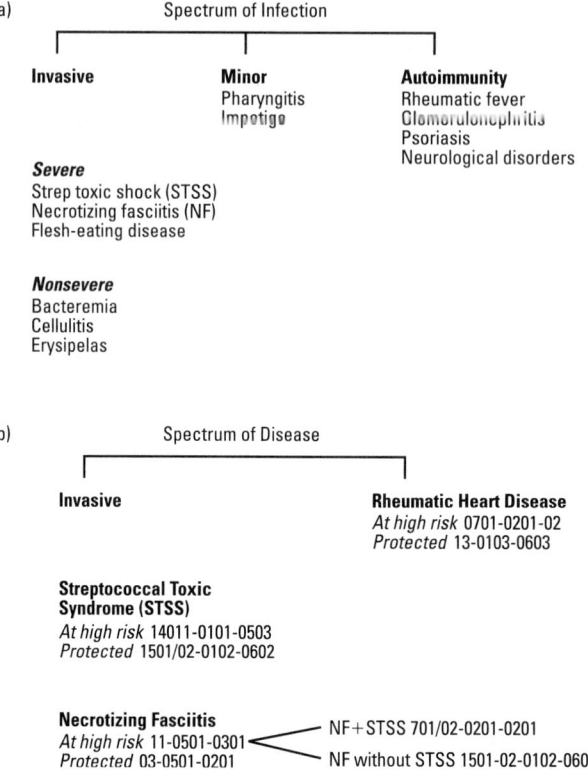

FIGURE 23.1. Human diseases caused by *Streptococcus pyogenes* and their distinctive HLA class II associations. (a) The wide spectrum of infection. (b) HLA class II haplotypes reported in association with clinically distinct sequelae of disease. Numbers in sequence represent haplotypes composed of DRB1*x-DQA1*y-DQB1*z. (Adapted from Kotb et al., *Nat Med*, 2002, 8:1398–1404.)

teria (Jones, 1944, 1951) remain the standard for the diagnosis of unambiguous cases of ARF (carditis, polyarthritis, or chorea), recent updates have included subtle manifestations such as subcutaneous nodules and erythema marginatum and have improved the diagnosis of recurrent disease (Baddour et al., 2005; Dajani et al., 1992; Kadir et al., 2004; Kaufhold et al., 1992; Markowitz and Gerber, 1995; Newburger et al., 2004; Stollerman, 2001). Updated approaches have been published for the diagnostic evaluation of PRSA (Jansen et al., 2005) and PANDAS (Dale, 2005; Kurlan and Kaplan, 2004; Snider and Swedo, 2003; Swedo et al., 1998), and for RHD, the chronic complication of ARF that remains the leading cause of heart disease in children and young adults in India, the Middle East, sub-Saharan Africa, and Latin America. Most individuals who develop acute rheumatic carditis during ARF experience progressive autoimmune phenomena leading to mitral valve disease (MVD) and/or multivalvular lesions (Ayoub, 1995; Kaplan, 1993; Markowitz and Gerber, 1987; Stollerman, 1997).

The reasons that some people develop STSS and NF during an invasive infection and others experience chronic autoimmune diseases following an ARF attack are not fully understood, but host immunogenetic factors appear to play a prominent role in determining susceptibility. One major pitfall in the study of genetic associations with the outcomes of GAS infection has been the tendency to combine patients with distinct clinical manifestations in a single analysis simply because their diseases had a similar etiology. For example, aggregating ARF patients with carditis, arthritis, or Sydenham chorea, or grouping patients with invasive GAS disease regardless of whether they have STSS, NF, or mild cellulitis, could well mask a genetic association with any one of the specific clinical conditions. While certain genetically mediated responses may be common to the GAS that causes these syndromes, the clinical entities are distinctive enough to warrant separate analysis. An equally compelling argument for insisting on homogeneity in case study definitions is that different GAS strains, including those belonging to the same serotype, can possess both common and distinct bacterial virulence components that may interact differently with individual host immune cells and tissues.

Pathogen

GAS bacteria are classified primarily according to the serotype of their surface M-protein; more than 100 M serotypes are currently recognized (Cunningham, 2000; Duarte et al., 2005; Facklam et al., 2002). Bessen and Fischetti (1990) have recognized two broad classes (I and II) based on immunodeterminants contained within the conserved region (C repeat domain) of the M-protein. Whereas some believe that the different autoimmune sequelae of GAS infection are caused by distinct serotypes or classes, others argue against this notion (Bessen et al., 1989, 1995, 1996; Dinkla et al., 2003; Hassell et al., 2004; Johnson et al., 2002; Kaufhold et al., 1992; Martin, 1997; Stollerman, 1991; Talkington et al., 1993). A similar argument is ongoing for the association between certain serotypes and invasive GAS diseases (Chaussee et al., 1996; Ho et al., 2003). While these issues remain unresolved, discoveries using modern biotechnological and bioinformatic tools have reinforced the common theme that considerable variation exists in the virulence components within a serotype. A good example is the striking difference in virulence and persistence between two subclones of the M1 serotype as a result of horizontal transfer of virulence genes mediated by phages as well as by recombination events (Aziz et al., 2005; Banks et al., 2002; Sumby et al., 2005). Conversely, strong evidence that the same strain can cause very different clinical manifestations in different people (Chatellier et al., 2000; Johnson et al., 2002; Kotb et al., 2002) underscores the critical role of host factors in modulating the outcome of GAS infections and provides an impetus to search for the genetic basis of these differences.

GAS possesses a large repertoire of virulence factors; some are surface associated, and others are secreted. These factors can be functionally subclassified into mediators of bacterial adhesion and invasion, evasion of host defenses, inflammation, or toxic destruction, but some of them may have overlapping roles in modulating host defenses (Bisno et al., 2003; Chhatwal and McMillan, 2005; Cunningham, 2000; Kreikemeyer et al., 2003; Norrby-Teglund and Kotb, 2000).

Genetic Determinants

As emphasized above, those investigating genetic association studies of bacterial infections with very different manifestations must carefully define the clinical outcome of interest, specify the diagnostic correlates, and establish enrollment criteria. In intermittent or chronic conditions punctuated exacerbations and recurrences, detailed clinical history is of the utmost importance. This is illustrated by studies of genetic determinants of severe manifestations of invasive GAS disease (STSS and NF) and of RHD as one of the most severe chronic sequelae of ARF.

Host Determinants in Severe Invasive GAS Disease (STSS and NF)

Among the large repertoire of virulence factors elaborated by GAS, the secreted streptococcal pyrogenic exotoxins, which belong to the family of microbial superantigens (SAgs), are pivotal contributors to the pathogenesis of STSS, SSD, and NF (Kotb 1992; 1995; 1998; Lungstras-Bufler et al., 2004). Individuals can be accurately classified by laboratory assay as high or low responders to the GAS SAgs. Patients who developed STSS and SSD during the acute infection produced significantly higher levels of inflammatory cytokines compared with patients who had less severe invasive disease. Then, during convalescence, the severe cases continued to be significantly associated with higher proliferative and inflammatory cytokine responses to the same GAS SAgs they encountered during the acute infection, whereas the mild invasive cases continued to be associated with low responses (Kotb et al., 2002; Norrby-Teglund et al., 2000; Norrby-Teglund and Kotb, 2000).

Although a number of distinct GAS strains have been isolated from invasive GAS infections, one particular M1T1 serotype has disseminated globally and persisted as the most frequently isolated strain for more than 25 years (Chatellier et al., 2000; Cleary et al., 1998). This clonal M1 strain can cause STSS, NF, or nonsevere invasive disease (Chatellier et al., 2000; Kotb et al., 2002), and host factors must be key in determining the outcome of the invasive infection.

HLA Class II Associations in STSS and NF

That human leukocyte antigen (HLA) class II molecules are receptors for GAS SAgs, and their allelic variations affect the presentation of a given SAg (Cole et al., 1997; Herman et al., 1990; Wen et al., 1995), provided the rationale for examining their association with the outcomes of SAg-mediated GAS disease. The distribution of HLA-DRB1, -DQA1, and -DQB1 alleles and haplotypes among invasive cases, recruited through active surveillance of all invasive GAS infections in Ontario, was determined (Kotb et al., 2002). Confounding factors, such as age and underlying disease, that may lead to misclassification of severe invasive cases were clearly defined and patients with these conditions were excluded in the final analysis. The DRB1*1501–DQB1*0602 haplotype conferred strong protection against STSS, while the DRB1*14–DQB1*0503 haplotype increased the risk. Among those with soft-tissue infections, the DRB1*03–DQB1*0201 haplotype was significantly associated with protection from NF, and the DRB1*11–DQB1*0301 haplotype showed a trend toward an association with risk for NF among invasive cases without STSS compared with healthy controls. The presence of the DRB1*1501–DQB1*0602 haplotype in NF cases protected them from developing a combination of STSS plus NF, the deadliest form of invasive disease (Kotb et al., 2002, 2003). These associations highlight the complex genetic susceptibility to the different manifestations of GAS infection.

The contribution of HLA class II polymorphism to GAS-associated syndromes may be disproportional because of their dual role in presenting conventional and superantigens. SAgs are bifunctional protein toxins that elicit highly potent immune responses because of the unconventional way by which they interact with the HLA molecules on antigen-presenting cells (APCs: B cells, monocytes, and dendritic cells) and with immune receptors on T cells. Unlike normal antigens, SAgs are able to bind directly to specific $V\beta$ elements within the T-cell receptor (TCR) β-chain, as well as to the MHC class II molecules (see chapter 5). The simultaneous binding of SAgs to APCs and T cells promotes efficient exchange of activation signals between these cells. This efficient activation coupled with the relatively less restricted binding of the SAgs to the TCR compared with conventional antigen binding (Kotb, 1992; 1995; White et al., 1989) results in activation of a high proportion of T cells (5–40%) and release of ex-

cessive levels of inflammatory cytokines. The magnitude of cytokine responses to SAgs is controlled to a great extent by the specificity of the class II allele presenting the SAg(s) to the T cells (Kotb, 2004).

Pathogenesis: STSS and NF

Individuals who lack protective antibodies mediating opsonization of bacteria or neutralization of the SAgs are at relatively high risk of bacterial invasion of a normally sterile site (Basma et al., 1999; Norrby-Teglund et al., 1996). Such invasion initiates the production of virulence factors that interact with the host innate and adaptive immune system. As in most infections, a balanced and controlled response that can eradicate the infection is usually associated with uncomplicated, relatively nonsevere invasive disease manifested by cellulitis or mild bacteremia. However, a robust and uncontrolled inflammatory response can cause substantial damage to the host with the possible development of STSS and/or NF (Davies et al., 1996; Working Group on Severe Streptococcal Infections, 1993; Low et al., 1997; Stevens et al., 1989).

Consistent with the HLA studies summarized above, in vitro responses of healthy individuals and recovered patients with different HLA types to mixtures of SAgs produced by the widely disseminated M1T1 GAS strain showed that those who had the protective DRB1*1501–DQB1*0602 haplotype mounted much reduced cytokine and proliferative responses to the GAS SAgs compared with those who carried the high-risk DRB1*14–DQB1*0503 or DRB1*07–DQB1*0201 haplotypes (Kotb et al., 2002) and compared with individuals who carried neutral haplotypes (neither associated with protection nor high risk of STSS). Furthermore, the presence of the protective haplotype in heterozygotes actually suppressed the response to the SAgs presented by the neutral or the high risk alleles. Work is now under way to clarify the molecular events initiated through the presentation of specific SAgs by specific alleles.

Animal Studies

Several studies have shown that mice are less sensitive to SAg-induced septic shock than humans or other primates. Induction of SAg-mediated toxic shock in mice with a native murine genome requires conditioning with D-galactosamine or lipopolysaccharide (LPS) to potentiate the biological activity of the SAgs in these animals (Miethke et al., 1992[1], 1993; Unnikrishnan et al., 2002; Welcher et al., 2002). In contrast, HLA-transgenic mice have proven quite informative for studying SAg-mediated diseases *in vivo* because SAgs are presented better by the human HLA class II than by the mouse class II molecules. This is particularly true for streptococcal SAgs. Interestingly, mouse models of STSS support the protective effect of the DRB1*15 and DQB1*06 alleles (Welcher et al., 2002; Nooh, 2007). In these studies, mice carrying those protective alleles survived longer and mounted significantly lower inflammatory responses than mice carrying neutral class II alleles (e.g., DR4/DQ8 mice). Further support for the findings in human population studies may be forthcoming from studies of HLA-transgenic mice expressing alleles on haplotypes associated with high risk for STSS and/or NF. A better understanding of the mechanism by which certain HLA class II genes encode susceptibility or protection from disease should help direct the development of targeted vaccines and the testing of treatment for STSS against different genetic backgrounds.

Intervention

Antibodies that neutralize the action of the streptococcal SAgs as well as those that can promote the opsonization of the bacteria can protect against invasive GAS disease. Pooled immunoglobulin preparations containing high titers of these protective antibodies, formulated for intravenous administration (IVIG), have shown great benefit as an adjunct to antimicrobial therapy. The IVIG is believed not only to neutralize the biological activity of the SAgs but also to modulate the host immune response and halt the progress of SSD (Kaul et al., 1999; Norrby-Teglund et al., 2003a, 2003b). Although the IVIG treatment is remarkably effective, it is expensive, and not all patients with invasive disease may require it. One strategy may be to determine the HLA class II profile and administer IVIG immediately to those with the high-risk alleles, while postponing treatment of those with neutral or favorable haplotypes until their condition starts to deteriorate.

Genetic Determinants in Rheumatic Heart Disease

Studies conducted by several groups around the world have reported associations of RHD with HLA class II loci (Guedez et al., 1999), albeit with considerable inconsistency in the specific effects of the alleles or

haplotypes. Inaccurate serological HLA typing used during these earlier studies probably led to mistyping. An earlier U.S. study that detected an association with HLA-DR4 serologically later failed to confirm the finding by molecular typing of the same patients. Discrepancies across ethnically distinct populations could also have resulted from differences in linkage disequilibrium (Fernandez-Viña et al., 1991). Certain of these studies may have failed to separate the various outcomes of ARF, to accurately diagnose rheumatic carditis, or to differentiate between subcategories of RHD for analysis (Guedez et al., 1999). The fraction of ARF cases with carditis can vary from 30% to 90% in different geographically areas (Chun et al., 1987; Gharib, 1969; Kotby et al., 1996; Luc et al., 1979; Majeed et al., 1986; Sanyal et al., 1982). The majority of ARF cases with carditis develop progressive RHD, but the pattern of valve damage in RHD patients can vary greatly, suggesting different pathological pathways (Al-Sekait et al., 1990; Feinstein et al., 1964; Lue et al., 1979; Majeed et al., 1986; Sanyal and Abu-Melha, 1988; Sanyal et al., 1982; Tompkins et al., 1972).

On the other hand, restriction of eligible subjects to those who developed post-ARF MVD has revealed a more consistent association of DRB1*0701–DQA1*0201 with increased risk for MVD in RHD. The same HLA class II associations have been detected in a number studies where (1) cases were confined to RHD excluding ARF without carditis or (2) the majority of cases analyzed had MVD reported (Guilherme et al., 1991; Weidebach et al., 1994; Debaz et al., 1996; Koyanagi et al., 1996; Maharaj et al., 1987; Ozkan et al., 1993; Stanevicha et al., 2003; Visentainer et al., 2000). Different associations were found in Mexican and Indian populations (Hernandez-Pacheco et al., 2003). The DR16-DQA1*0501–DQB1*0301 haplotype was associated with RHD susceptibility in the Mexican Mestizo population. This discrepant association may have been due to the ethnic differences or to misclassifcation of cases. With the advent of advanced molecular tools, it may be possible to identify immune correlates or other molecular markers that can help confirm the diagnosis of acute rheumatic carditis that so often results in debilitating RHD.

Pathogenesis

Despite considerable effort to unravel the molecular basis for the association between the DRB1*0701–DQA1*0201 haplotype and the increased risk of RHD noted above, promising clues remain relatively sparse. The presence of epitopes in several streptococcal proteins (including the surface M-protein) that cross-react with components of heart protein supports the molecular mimicry theory of RHD. Mimicry between a number of streptococcal components and cardiac proteins has been shown to trigger humoral and cellular reactions in the host (Ayoub, 1995; Beachey et al., 1990; Cunningham, 2000; Zabriskie et al., 1970). However, the relevance of these specific reactions to disease pathogenesis has not been demonstrated definitively. Heart cross-reactive autoantibodies in sera of RHD patients have been reported, but the level of autoantibodies often shows little correlation with clinical and/or histopathological manifestations of the disease. Furthermore, the same antibodies have also been found in the sera of many patients with streptococcal pharyngitis but no evidence of rheumatic fever or cardiac injury.

On the other hand, evidence has been mounting that T-cell immunity, including heart-reactive cytotoxic T lymphocytes circulating in patients with active rheumatic carditis, mediates the pathogenesis of RHD (Ayoub et al., 2000; Cunningham, 2004; Friedman et al., 1971; Hutto and Ayoub, 1980). Guilherme et al. (1995, 2001, 2005) generated T-cell clones from the valvular tissues of RHD patients and demonstrated that these clones were responsive to specific epitopes of serotype 5 M-protein. T-cell clones derived from human mitral and aortic valvular tissues preferentially responded to a streptococcal M5 peptide (81–96: DKLKQQRDTLSTQKET). Thus, structural mimicry between the streptococcal M-protein and cardiac proteins can elicit both humoral and T-cell autoimmunity. Of particular relevance is the finding that the T cells from DRB1*0701-bearing individuals mounted the strongest response to the M5 (81–96) peptide (Guilherme and Kalil, 2002).

The target autoantigen(s) that seems to be preferentially presented by DRB1*0701 remains unidentified. Cunningham (2004) provided strong evidence that cardiac myosin is a target autoantigen for autoimmune T cells in both rheumatic carditis and myocarditis (Cunningham, 2004). This finding was followed by the discovery of a putative 50- to 54-kDa myocardial autoantigenic protein that was preferentially recognized by RHD patients (El-Demellawy et al., 1997). Unstimulated cells from approximately 40% of RHD patients tested proliferated in response to this protein, and *ex vivo* stimulation of peripheral mononuclear cells with opsonized GAS increased the proportion of the RHD patients responding to 90%. None of the control subjects, including healthy subjects and cardiac patients with non-RHD, recognized this protein even after stimulation with the opsonized GAS. Any of several candidate proteins, including the cellular filament protein vimentin, may be responsible for this phenomenon; work now under way may clarify the target(s) of this response (El-Demellawy et al., 1997; Guilherme and Kalil, 2002).

Animal Studies

Although there is no ideal model for RHD because humans are the natural host for GAS, several attempts have been made to generate an animal model (Unny and Middlebrooks, 1983). Recently, BALB/c mice were induced to develop cross-reactive T cells primed against cardiac myosin following immunization with streptococcal M-protein peptides containing cardiac myosin homologies (Cunningham, 2004; Galvin et al., 2002; Quinn et al., 2001). In a Lewis rat model, the same investigators demonstrated that 50% of the rats immunized with rM6 streptococcal protein developed valvulitis and myocarditis, and that rat T-cell lines specific to the cardiac myosin-like sequences of streptococcal M-protein migrated to the valves after passive transfer of the M-protein–specific T-cell lines. Thus, HLA-transgenic mice carrying RHD susceptibility alleles may be useful as a model for the disorder. These mice, although not currently widely available, will soon be offered to investigators who are interested in dissecting the genetic and molecular basis of RHD.

Conditions Caused by *Bacillus anthracis* Infection

The intentional exposure of the U.S. population to anthrax in 2001 revealed a serious lack of preparedness for natural or deliberate biological threats from emerging and reemerging pathogens. The U.S. Public Health Service identified at least 19 dangerous organisms that have the potential for use as bioterrorism weapons or have recently emerged as deadly pathogens, for which neither accurate rapid diagnosis nor optimally effective treatments or vaccines exist. Encapsulated *B. anthracis* is high on the list of select agents. Until the limitation in quantities of medication and stockpiles of vaccine can be overcome, distribution of those limited quantities will likely depend on the ability to assess exposed individuals for their risk of severe illness and to deliver available drugs and vaccines preferentially to them.

Anthrax is rare in general human population. Cutaneous disease is the most common form of anthrax and is usually contracted from *B. anthracis* spores. These spores are environmentally resistant and highly stable, entering the body through skin abrasions from anthrax-infected animals or anthrax-contaminated animal products, including fibers, hide, and feces. Gastrointestinal anthrax can be contracted through ingestion of *B. anthracis*–contaminated feed. When intentionally dispersed, the spores can cause skin (cutaneous), lung (inhalation or pulmonary), or intestinal (ingestion) anthrax.

Diagnosis

The onset of illness usually occurs within a week of exposure but can take as long as six or seven weeks to develop. Inhalation anthrax can cause pneumonia and death within 1–4 days of onset. Because patients usually cough infected blood, they can easily spread the disease to others. In 1979, an accidental aerosolized release of anthrax spores from a military microbiology facility in the former Soviet Union resulted in at least 79 cases and 68 deaths. Of particular interest here is why 14% of those who inhaled the anthrax did not die.

Pathogen

The organisms are encapsulated, gram-positive, spore-forming bacteria that have a unique capsule consisting of D-glutamic acid, which protects it from phagocytic cells. The encapsulated, toxinogenic strains are highly virulent, particularly when dispersed in an aerosol formulation. Following inhalation of as few as 8,000–10,000 spores, fatality within hours is high. The virulent strains produce two deadly catalytic toxins, lethal toxin (LT) and edema toxin, and can induce severe systemic illness. Because of the stability of the bacterial spores and the high case fatality ratio, aerosolized anthrax has been attractive as a potential biological weapon for almost 80 years.

Genetic Determinants

No systematic study has identified the basis for interindividual variation in susceptibility to the severe forms of anthrax or in the response to the current vaccine, and because human disease is rare, investigation of genetic susceptibility to inhalation anthrax in humans has been lacking.

Several murine studies have investigated the role of certain immune response genes in the susceptibility to and outcome of anthrax (Chaudry et al., 2002). Various inbred mouse strains showed dramatic differences with respect to their susceptibility (time to death) to infection with the virulent, encapsulated Vollum 1B strain of *B. anthracis* (Welkos et al., 1986). More recently, investigators reported that mouse susceptibility to anthrax LT may be influenced by genetic factors besides those controlling macrophage sensitivity (Moayeri et al., 2004). Others studied a panel of interval-specific, recombinant-congenic lines carrying various segments of central mouse chromosome 11 derived from LT-resistant DBA/2 mice on the LT-susceptible BALB/c background; they reported that mortality appeared to be controlled by three linked quantitative trait loci (QTLs) in those segments: *Ltxs1*, *Ltxs2*, and *Ltxs3* (McAllister et al., 2003). Further mapping confirmed the association of a dominant susceptibility phenotype with the *Ltxs1* region (Roberts et al., 1998; Watters and Dietrich, 2001) and narrowed down the susceptibility factors to 19 candidate genes, of which the most likely is *Kif1C* (Watters and Dietrich, 2001). This gene encodes a ubiquitously expressed kinesin-like motor protein that carries molecules along cellular microtubules (Dorner et al., 1998) and, in humans, is involved in retrograde transport of vesicles from the Golgi apparatus to the endoplasmic reticulum (Chaudry et al., 2002). Polymorphisms in the *Kif1C* gene may alter the ability of the protein to protect the macrophage from the anthrax toxin.

A second likely candidate gene within *Ltxs3* is *Nos2*, which encodes the inducible nitric oxide synthase. Suggested involvement of *Nos2* is interesting because knockout mice have been shown to succumb to infection with anthrax spores sooner than their wild-type parental mice (Kalns et al., 2002). Another attractive candidate gene within *Ltxs3* is the *Tnfaip1* that encodes a tumor necrosis factor (TNF)-induced protein (McAllister et al., 2003).

Pathogenesis

From animal studies it is has been surmised that anthrax spores are phagocytosed by macrophages and transported to the regional lymph nodes, where they germinate and multiply within the macrophages, express toxins, stimulate cytokine responses, and kill the macrophage, whereupon they are released into the bloodstream and eventually cause severe sepsis. Germination of the spores and toxin production by the bacteria appear to be triggered by host signals (Mock and Fouet, 2001; Mock and Mignot, 2003). Variation in host signals may be a factor that can either enhance or suppress bacterial spore germination and vegetative growth inside the macrophage.

B. anthracis and its toxins can cause SSD with vascular leakage, edema, and thrombosis and in most cases results in death of the host (Hanna, 1999; Ireland and Hanna, 2002; Starnbach and Collier, 2003). The bacteria produce several toxins, including its major lethal toxin (LT), which consists of a metalloprotease called lethal factor (LF) and protective antigen (PA). PA binds to cell receptors and translocates LF into the host cells (Agrawal and Pulendran, 2004; Fouet and Mesnage, 2002; Lacy and Collier, 2002; Mock and Fouet, 2001; Mock and Mignot, 2003). Once in the cytosol, high doses of LF are cytolytic leading to apoptosis, while low doses induce inflammatory cytokine production. LF cleaves and inactivates most members of protein kinase-kinases (MAPKKs or MEKs) (Pellizzari et al., 1999; Vitale et al., 1998). Inactivation of these molecules can lead to apoptosis, necrosis, multisystem dysfunction, and death (Agrawal and Pulendran, 2004; Moayeri et al., 2004; Starnbach and Collier, 2003). LF also activates interleukin-1β (IL-1β) β-converting enzyme/caspase-1 (ICE) promoting increased release of IL-1β and IL-18 and contributing to the systemic effects of the toxin (Cordoba-Rodriguez et al., 2004). Through inhibition of p38 MAPK phosphorylation by LF, low doses of LF may block the activity of specific hormone receptors, including the glucocorticoid receptor, a key mediator of immune response (Webster et al., 2003, 2004).

PA also binds to edema factor (EF) to generate edema toxin, which is a calmodulin-dependent adenylate cyclase that converts intracellular ATP into cAMP (Hoover et al., 1994). The increase in cAMP stimulates chemotaxis of human neutrophils, incapacitates phagocytes, and interrupts cytokine pathways (Hoover et al., 1994; O'Brien et al., 1985; Wade et al., 1985). Thus, both LF and EF play a major role in the pathogenesis of B. anthracis infection.

Animal Studies

Strong immune responses are triggered in both the early and late phases of the infection. However, there is an unclear correlation between mouse macrophage sensitivity to LF and susceptibility to anthrax infection. Effects of the purified toxins may not represent events that take place after exposure to anthrax spores. In relevant models of infection with anthrax spores, there is robust production of cytokines such as TNF and IL-6 (Pickering et al., 2004), and in vitro studies showed that in addition to TNF and IL-6, human dendritic cells produced the cytokines IL-1β, IL-8, and IL-12. On the other hand, genetic knockouts of the TNF receptor 1, IL-1 receptor, and inducible NOS did not protect mice from anthrax infection (Kalns et al., 2002). Thus, additional cellular pathways might be involved.

Intervention

Although prompt treatment with high doses of antibiotics such as ciprofloxacin, penicillin, doxycycline, and fluoroquinolones can be effective in treating some presymptomatic cases, particularly when administered within hours of exposure, inhalation anthrax can be refractory to antibiotic treatment. However, current stockpiles are limited, and the available vaccine, produced from an attenuated strain of B. anthracis, has a 93% efficacy and troublesome side effects in some individuals. Newer vaccine formulations are in development or at various stages of completion of phase II trials, but the profile of their effectiveness and side effects remain to be documented.

Conditions from *N. Meningitidis* Infection

N. meningitidis infections can manifest in a broad spectrum of disease. The bacteria often colonize the nasopharynx asymptomatically or elicit a mild upper respiratory tract infection, but in susceptible children and adults, they cause potentially fatal meningitis and sepsis (Vermont et al., 2002). The relatively high prevalence of carriage (10–45%), largely confined to the nasopharynx, contrasts sharply with the low incidence of invasive disease (1–6%, depending on age as well as geographic and probably racial/genetic factors). As with invasive S. pyogenes infections, the influence of host genetic variation on the outcome of infection with the same strain is evident in the dramatic differences among individuals—from mild, self-limiting disease to meningococcal bacteremia and death within hours of onset despite extensive treatment to chronic meningococcemia.

Diagnosis

Patients may present with clinically mild bacteremia or chronic meningococcemia, or disease progresses to severe and potentially fatal toxic shock. The bacteria can also cross the blood–brain barrier to infect the central nervous system and cause meningitis. Other manifestations include respiratory tract disease, meningococcemia (purpura fulminans and Waterhouse-Friderichsen syndrome), and a wide variety of syndromes that include conjunctivitis, otitis media, epiglottitis, arthritis, urethritis, and pericarditis (Rosenstein et al., 2001; Schmidtt and Hensel, 2004). Both bacterial variation and host genetic diversity are likely to contribute interactively to this wide spectrum of diseases.

Pathogen

N. meningitidis is a human-specific, commensal, intracellular gram-negative diplococcus bacteria that normally resides in the nasopharynx. Serogroups are classified by differences in their capsular polysaccharides. Among the dozen or so serogroups, those designated A, B, and C are most commonly associated with clinically significant infection, although their relative prevalence varies in different geographical areas around the world and/or for distinct ethnic and racial populations. Interestingly, the bacteria can undergo extensive genetic diversification primarily via horizontal gene transfer and recombination, resulting in exchange of microbial genetic material that may even result in serotype switching (Schmidtt and Hensel, 2004).

Major virulence components include a capsule, pili, iron-acquisition factors, outer membrane adhesin proteins (Opa and Opc), porins, and a mechanism for release of endotoxin (Nassif et al., 1999). Adherence and colonization of the bacteria on mucosal surfaces are primarily mediated by type IV pili, which bind to the CD46 receptor on epithelial as well as other nucleated cells. Opa and Opc then bind to their respective receptors: CD66 and a heparan sulfate proteoglycan receptor (Kallstrom et al., 1997). Opc, which interacts with host proteoglycan and vitronectin, is also believed to contribute to pathogenesis. In addition, pathogenic Neisseria species express outer membrane protein receptors that are specific for scavenging human transferrin, lactoferrin, hemoglobin, and hemoglobin–haptoglobin complexes to acquire iron from the host (Vermont et al., 2002). The bacteria are very rich in LPS, which elicits potent inflammatory responses and mediators. N. meningitidis is also capable of eliciting inflammatory responses via a Toll-like receptor (TLR2) in the absence of LPS.

Genetic Determinants

The different disease outcomes of N. meningitidis infection have been associated with genetic polymorphisms in Fc receptors, IgG allotypes, innate complement proteins, plasminogen activator inhibitor type 1 (PAI1), IL-1, IL-10, TNF, LPS-binding receptors or proteins, and hemostatic proteins (Emonts et al., 2003; McNicholl and Cuenco, 1999; Vermont et al., 2002). The strongest support for genetically mediated variation in susceptibility to invasive infection seems to be with allelic variants of three of those factors: FcγRIIa, complement, and IL-1.

Polymorphism of the Fcγ Receptors

Inefficient variants of Fcγ seem to play an important role in susceptibility to meningococcal sepsis. The FcγRIIa (CD32) receptor on dendritic and other immunoactive cells is the only Fc receptor that binds IgG2, which is of particular importance in host defense against encapsulated bacteria. FcγRIIa has two allotypic forms, arising from a single point mutation in exon 4 of the gene (FCGR2A), which changes the amino acid at position 131 from histidine (H) to arginine (R). The resulting allelic variants of FcγRIIa, +131R and +131H, differ strikingly in their efficiency of interaction with IgG2 and IgG3 subclasses; FcγRIIa +131R is inefficient in binding these IgG subclasses, and polymorphonuclear leukocytes from individuals with this variant phagocytose IgG2-opsonized N. meningitidis serogroup B less effectively than those from individuals with the +131H allele (Bredius et al., 1994). Among patients with meningococcal infection, fulminant meningococcal disease and meningococcemia without meningitis were significantly more common in those with the +131R variant (Domingo et al., 2004). For more on Fcγ receptors, see chapter 9.

Complement Deficiencies

Defects in the alternative and/or lectin-specific pathways of complement activation have been associated with susceptibility to invasive and severe forms of N. meningitidis infections. Two specific defects in complement activity, one involving properdin and the other the mannose-binding lectin (MBL) receptor, have been associated with increased risk for meningococcal disease (Spath et al., 1999; Fremeaux-Bacchi et al., 1995). Properdin is a positive regulator of the alternative pathway, and it optimizes the amplification of the complement cascade initiated by either the classical or the lectin pathways (Fredrikson et al., 1996). Genetic variants of the properdin gene (CFP) located on chromosome X can prevent protein expression, cause low expression, or result in loss of function (Linton and Morgan, 1999; Bathum et al., 2006). They increase the risk of disease in patients infected with N. meningitidis (Linton and Morgan, 1999). The negative effects of properdin deficiency on meningococcal disease are exaggerated when combined with other immune deficiencies, most notably those affecting MBL levels, antibody allotypes, and protein C (Bathum et al., 2006). Similarly, polymorphisms resulting in MBL deficiency have detrimental effects on meningococcal disease in infants older than 24 months, but the combination of MBL deficiency and any of several other immune deficiencies is a poor prognostic marker for severe disease in older patients. For more on MBL and complement deficiencies, see chapters 10 and 11.

Plasminogen Activator Inhibitor 1

Plasminogen activator inhibitor 1 (PAI-1) is a 50-kDa glycoprotein of the serine protease inhibitor (SERPIN) family. It inhibits plasminogen activator and blocks fibrinolysis (Brandtzaeg et al., 1990). At high levels, PAI-1 contributes to the pathogenesis of severe meningococcal sepsis by impacting fibrin deposition, impairing endothelial function and contributing to intravascular fibrin deposition and coagulopathy (Aird, 2001). High levels of PAI-1 have been found in severe meningococcal disease and correlate with poor prognosis (Brandtzaeg et al., 1990). The amount of PAI-1 produced is governed by an insertion/deletion single nucleotide polymorphism (SNP) located at position–675 relative to the transcription initiation site. This SNP consisting of either four or five guanine bases (4G/5G) plays an important role in regulating PAI-1 gene expression. The 4G/4G homozygotes produce more PAI-1 than do individuals with either of the other two genotypes (4G/5G or 5G/5G) (Dahmer et al., 2005; Dawson et al., 1999; Hermans and Hazelzet, 2005; Hermans et al., 1999; Westendorp et al., 1999). Further, these 4G/4G homozygotes are at an increased risk of developing vascular complications and dying from meningococcal disease (Dawson et al., 1999; Haralambous et al., 2003).

Cytokines and TLR

The role of polymorphisms in TNF, IL1, and IL10 genes in meningococcal disease is not as convincingly demonstrated as for those genes mentioned above. One study in pediatric patients suggested an association between a particular TNF allele (TNF2; TNF-308A) and decreased disease severity (Nadel et al., 1996), but this conclusion was not substantiated in two other studies and needs to be revisited in a larger population with more attention to possible effects of other genetic variations in linkage disequilibrium with this TNF allele. Similar uncertainties regarding the role of TLR4 polymorphisms exist despite its role in mediating the bacterial LPS effects. By contrast, associations with IL1 and IL10 polymorphisms are more convincing. Serum levels of IL-1β and IL-1 receptor antagonist (IL-1RN) are elevated in patients with meningococcal disease and appear to be higher in those with more severe disease (van Deuren et al., 1997). A comprehensive study found significant association between fatal outcome and the IL1B–511C/T variant, and an apparently interactive combination of IL1B–511C/T and another SNP (IL1RN +2018C/T) significantly increased the risk for death from the invasive infections, with mortality rates of up to 42% (Read et al., 2000). Finally, elevated levels of IL-10 have been associated with risk for fatal disease, and interactions between IL10–1082 polymorphism and the FCGR2A +131R/H allelic variants may reflect the location of genes on the long arm of chromosome 1 (Emonts et al., 2003; van der Pol et al., 2001).

Pathogenesis

N. meningitidis can asymptomatically reside in the nasopharynx; however, in susceptible individuals, pathogenic strains of the bacteria can evade host defenses and invade through the mucosal epithelium and, in relatively rare cases, gain access to the bloodstream causing severe sepsis, or cross the blood–brain barrier to elicit meningitis (Rosenstein et al., 2001; Schmidtt and Hensel, 2004; Vermont et al., 2002). In the absence of an effective protective immunity that can opsonize or neutralize the bacteria, the invasive bacteria release massive amounts of LPS, which elicits potent inflammatory cascades that, in the susceptible host, can lead to hypotension, MOF, and shock. Indeed, several inflammatory cytokines, including TNF-α, IL-1, IL-6, IL-8, interferon-γ, and IL-1RN, are elevated in patients with severe meningococcemia (van Deuren et al., 1995).

Animal Models

Several animal models have been developed to study of *N. meningitidis* (Perera et al., 2006; Yi et al., 2003). To generate these models, mice need to be treated with human transferrin, which constitutes an essential source of iron for these bacteria, or express transgenic human CD46, which binds to the bacterial type IV pili and mediates pathogenesis (Johansson et al., 2005). Despite the availability of these models, in-depth animal studies investigating the influence of host genetic variations on disease course and severity are lacking.

Intervention

Several vaccines are being used to prevent the infection, and intervention measures are primarily focused on antibiotic treatment, usually with penicillin G, one of two cephalosporins, or ampicillin, alone or in specific combinations. In severe acute disease, the administration of pressors, oxygen supplementation, and inotropic drugs such as epinephrine, norepinephrine, dopamine, and dobutamine can be beneficial. However, the morbidity and mortality rates associated with meningococcal disease remain quite high, even among patients who receive early antibiotic treatment (Kirsch et al., 1996; Kirsch and Giroir, 2000). Novel approaches aimed at modulating pathological immune responses during the severe infections are being tested. Drugs that target LPS effects and/or modulate cytokines to control inflammatory cascades have shown promise.

Based on findings that patients with severe meningococcemia have reduced levels of protein C as a result of the potent inflammatory response, clinical trials have been initiated using activated recombinant protein C, which acts as anticoagulant and has antiinflammatory activities (Alberio et al., 2001). In addition, a limited number of clinical trials have shown promising results with the administration of tissue plasminogen activator and antithrombin III infusion (Singh and Arrieta, 2004).

Conclusions and Prospects

New molecular targets, new tools, and new animal models will continue to expand our understanding of these bacterial infections. In the case of anthrax, *Kif1C*

may play a key role. *In vitro* studies using macrophages from individuals with different allelic variants may be useful in determining whether this gene modulates human macrophage sensitivity to LT. Screening individuals who have been exposed to virulent *B. anthracis* but developed disease of different severity may reveal how *KIF1C* or other variants affect outcomes. Evaluation of the impact of ethnicity and other potential confounding factors (e.g., age, preexisting conditions, time of intervention relative to time of exposure) must be taken into account. Another promising tool to test the effects of human genetic variations *in vivo* include the recently improved fully humanized mouse model of engrafted hematopoietic stem cells (Shultz et al., 2005) and recombinant inbred strains generated by the International Collaborative Cross Consortium (Churchill et al., 2004). Investigating one gene at time can be informative but at the same time may miss genes that may not have individually strong effects. By tracking the various QTLs that modulate susceptibility to an infection in a population of genetically diverse yet stable and genetically characterized mouse populations, one can identify gene networks and interactive pathways involved in disease susceptibility and pathogenesis (Peirce et al., 2004; Williams et al., 2001, 2004).

Understanding the genetics of host resistance and susceptibility to these pathogens can provide important clues into the interactions between these bacteria and their host, reveal critical virulence factors of the organism, expose host interactive pathways involved in pathogenesis, and help identify specific host defense mechanisms to which the pathogen is exceptionally sensitive. This knowledge is critical to the development of effective disease intervention measures.

References

Agrawal, A., Pulendran, B. (2004) Anthrax lethal toxin: A weapon of multisystem destruction. *Cell Mol Life Sci*, 61, 2859–2865.

Aird, W. (2001) Vascular bed-specific hemostasis: Role of endothelium in sepsis pathogenesis. *Crit Care Med*, 29, S28–S35.

Alberio, L., Lammle, B., Esmon, C. (2001) Protein C replacement in severe meningococcemia: Rationale and clinical experience. *Clin Infect Dis.* 32, 1338–1134.

Al-Sekait, M.A., Al-Swilem, A.R.A., Tahir, M. (1990) Rheumatic heart disease in school children from

Al-Medina Al-Mounawarrah district, Saudi Arabia. *Ann Saudi Med*, 10, 590–592.

Ambrosino, D.M., et al. (1985). Correlation between G2m(n) immunoglobulin allotype and human antibody response and susceptibility to polysaccharide encapsulated bacteria. *J Clin Invest*, 75, 1935–1942.

Antibiotic Subcommittee at Mount Sinai Hospital. (1998) Guidelines for the Treatment of Necrotizing Fasciitis (NF) and Streptococcal Toxic Shock Syndrome (STSS). Available at www.microbiology.mtsinai.on .ca/protocols/pdf/k5a.pdf

Asbahr, F.R., Garvey, M.A., Snider, L.A., Zanetta, D.M., Elkis, H., Swedo, S.E. (2005) Obsessive-compulsive symptoms among patients with Sydenham chorea. *Biol Psychiatry*, 57, 1073–1076.

Ayoub, E. (1995) Acute rheumatic fever. In Emmanouilides, G.C., Riemenschneider, T.A., Allen, H.D., Gutgesell, H.P. (eds.), *Heart disease in infants, children, and adolescents*. Williams & Wilkins, Baltimore, MD, pp. 1400–1416.

Ayoub, E.M., Kotb, M., Cunningham, M.W. (2000) Rheumatic fever pathogenesis. In Stevens, D.L., and Kaplan, E.L. (eds.), *Streptococcal infections*. Oxford University Press, New York, pp. 102–132.

Aziz, R.K., Edwards, R.A., Taylor, W.W., Low, D.E., McGeer, A., Kotb, M. (2005) Mosaic prophages with horizontally acquired genes account for the emergence and diversification of the globally disseminated M1T1 clone of *Streptococcus pyogenes*. *J Bacteriol*, 187, 3311–3318.

Baddour, L.M., et al. (2005) Infective endocarditis: Diagnosis, antimicrobial therapy, and management of complications: A statement for healthcare professionals from the Committee on Rheumatic Fever, Endocarditis, and Kawasaki Disease, Council on Cardiovascular Disease in the Young, and the Councils on Clinical Cardiology, Stroke, and Cardiovascular Surgery and Anesthesia, American Heart Association: Endorsed by the Infectious Diseases Society of America. *Circulation*, 111, e394–e434.

Balding, J., et al. (2003) Genomic polymorphic profiles in an Irish population with meningococcaemia: is it possible to predict severity and outcome of disease? *Genes Immun*, 4, 533–540.

Banks, D.J., Beres, S.B., Musser, J.M. (2002) The fundamental contribution of phages to GAS evolution, genome diversification and strain emergence. *Trends Microbiol*, 10, 515–521.

Basma, H., Norrby-Teglund, A., Guedez, Y., McGeer, A., Low, D.E., El-Ahmedy, O., Schwartz, B., Kotb, M. (1999) Risk factors in the pathogenesis of invasive group A streptococcal infections: Role of protective humoral immunity. *Infect Immun*, 67, 1871–1877.

Bathum, L., Hansen, H., Teisner, B., Koch, C., Garred, P, Rasmussen, K., Wang, P. (2006) Association between combined properdin and mannose-binding lectin deficiency and infection with Neisseria meningitidis. *Mol Immunol*, 43, 473–479.

Beachey, E., Majumdar G, Tomai M, Kotb M. (1990) Molecular aspects of autoimmune responses to streptococcal M proteins. In Gallin, F. (ed.), *Advances in host defense mechanisms*. Raven Press, New York, pp. 83–95.

Ben-Pazi, H., Livne, A., Shapira, Y., Dale, R.C. (2003) Parkinsonian features after streptococcal pharyngitis. *J Pediatr*, 143, 267–269.

Bessen, D.E., Fischetti, V.A. (1990) Differentiation between two biologically distinct classes of group A streptococci by limited substitutions of amino acids within the shared region of M protein-like molecules. *J Exp Med*, 172, 1757–1764.

Bessen, D.E., Jones, K.F., Fischetti, V.A. (1989) Evidence for two distinct classes of streptococcal M protein and their relationship to rheumatic fever. *J Exp Med*, 169, 269–283.

Bessen, D.E., Sotir, C.M., Readdy, T.L., Hollingshead, S.K. (1996) Genetic correlates of throat and skin isolates of group A streptococci. *J Infect Dis*, 173, 896–900.

Bisno, A.L., Stevens, D.L. (1996) Streptococcal infections of skin and soft tissues. *N Engl J Med*, 334, 240–245.

Bessen, D.E., Veasy, L.G., Hill, H.R., Augustine, N.H., Fischetti, V.A. (1995) Serologic evidence for a class I group A streptococcal infection among rheumatic fever patients. *J Infect Dis*, 172, 1608–1611.

Bisno, A.L., Brito, M.O., Collins, C.M. (2003) Molecular basis of group A streptococcal virulence. *Lancet Infect Dis*, 3, 191–200.

Brandtzaeg. P., Joø, GB., Brusletto, B., Kierulf, P. (1990) Plasminogen activator inhibitor 1 and 2, alpha-2-antiplasmin, plasminogen, and endotoxin levels in systemic meningococcal disease. *Thromb Res*, 57(2), 271–8.

Bredius, R., Derkx, B., Fijen, C., de Wit, T., De Haas, M., Weening, R., van de Winkel, J., Out, T. (1994) Fc gamma receptor IIa (CD32) polymorphism in fulminant meningococcal septic shock in children. *J Infect Dis*, 170, 848–853.

Carapetis, J.R., Steer, A.C., Mulholland, E.K., Weber, M. (2005) The global burden of group A streptococcal diseases. *Lancet Infect Dis*, 5, 685–694.

Chatellier, S., Ihendyane, N., Kansal, R.G., Khambaty, F., Basma, H., Norrby-Teglund, A., Low, D.E., McGeer, A., Kotb, M. (2000) Genetic relatedness superantigen expression in group A streptococcus serotype M1 isolates from patients with severe and nonsevere invasive diseases. *Infect Immun*, 68, 3523–3534.

Chaudry, G.J., Moayeri, M., Liu, S., Leppla, S.H. (2002) Quickening the pace of anthrax research: Three advances point towards possible therapies. *Trends Microbiol*, 10, 58–62.

Chaussee, M.S., Liu, J., Stevens, D.L., Ferretti, J.J. (1996) Genetic and phenotypic diversity among isolates of *Streptococcus pyogenes* from invasive infections. *J Infect Dis*, 173, 901–908.

Chhatwal, G.S., McMillan, D.J. (2005) Uncovering the mysteries of invasive streptococcal diseases. *Trends Mol Med*, 11, 152–155.

Chun, L.T., Reddy, V., Yamamoto, L.G. (1987) Rheumatic fever in children and adolescents in Hawaii. *Pediatrics*, 79, 549–552.

Churchill, G.A., et al. (2004) The Collaborative Cross, a community resource for the genetic analysis of complex traits. *Nat Genet*, 36, 1133–1137.

Cleary, P.P., LaPenta, D., Vessela, R., Lam, H., Cue, D. (1998) A globally disseminated M1 subclone of group A streptococci differs from other subclones by 70 kilobases of prophage DNA and capacity for high-frequency intracellular invasion. *Infect Immun*, 66, 5592–5597.

Cole, B.C., Sawitzke, A.D., Ahmed, E.A., Atkin, C.L., David, C.S. (1997) Allelic polymorphisms at the H-2A and HLA-DQ loci influence the response of murine lymphocytes to the *Mycoplasma arthritidis* superantigen MAM. *Infect Immun*, 65, 4190–4198.

Cone, L.A., Woodard, D.R., Schlievert, P.M., Tomory, G.S. (1987) Clinical and bacteriologic observations of a toxic shock-like syndrome due to *Streptococcus pyogenes*. *N Engl J Med*, 317, 146–149.

Cordoba-Rodriguez, R., Fang, H., Lankford, C.S., Frucht, D.M. (2004) Anthrax lethal toxin rapidly activates caspase-1/ICE and induces extracellular release of interleukin (IL)-1beta and IL-18. *J Biol Chem*, 279, 20563–20566.

Cunningham, M.W. (2000) Pathogenesis of group A streptococcal infections. *Clin Microbiol Rev*, 13, 470–511.

Cunningham, M.W. (2003) Autoimmunity and molecular mimicry in the pathogenesis of post-streptococcal heart disease. *Front Biosci*, 8, s533–s543.

Cunningham, M.W. (2004) T cell mimicry in inflammatory heart disease. *Mol Immunol*, 40, 1121–1127.

Dahmer, M.K., Randolph, A., Vitali, S., Quasney, M.W. (2005) Genetic polymorphisms in sepsis. *Pediatr Crit Care Med*, 6, S61–S73.

Dajani, A.S., et al. (1992) Guidelines for the diagnosis of rheumatic fever. Jones criteria, 1992 update. Special Writing Group of the Committee on Rheumatic Fever, Endocarditis, and Kawasaki Disease of the Council on Cardiovascular Disease in the Young of the American Heart Association. *JAMA*, 268, 2069–2073.

Dale, R.C. (2005) Post-streptococcal autoimmune disorders of the central nervous system. *Dev Med Child Neurol*, 47, 785–791.

Davies, H.D., McGeer, A., Schwartz, B., Green, K., Cann, D., Simor, A.E., Low, D.E. (1996) Invasive group A streptococcal infections in Ontario, Canada. Ontario Group A Streptococcal Study Group. *N Engl J Med*, 335, 547–554.

Dawson, S.J., Fey, R.E., McNulty, C.A. (1999) Meningococcal disease in siblings caused by rifampicin sensitive and rifampicin resistant strains. *Commun Dis Public Health*, 2, 215–216.

Debaz, H., Olivo, A., Perez-Luque, E., Vasquez-Garcia, M.N., Burguete, A., Chavez-Negrete, A., Velasco, C., Arguero, R., Gorodeszky, C. (1996) DNA Analysis of class II alleles in rheumatic heart disease in Mexicans. *Hum Immunol*, 49(1 suppl), 63.

Deighton, C. (1993) Beta haemolytic streptococci and reactive arthritis in adults. *Ann Rheum Dis*, 52, 475–482.

Dinkla, K., Rohde, M., Jansen, W.T., Kaplan, E.L., Chhatwal, G.S., Talay, S.R. (2003) Rheumatic fever-associated *Streptococcus pyogenes* isolates aggregate collagen. *J Clin Invest*, 111, 1905–1912.

Domingo, P., et al. (2002) Associations between Fc gamma receptor IIA polymorphisms and the risk and prognosis of meningococcal disease. *Am J Med*, 112, 19–25.

Domingo, P., et al. (2004) Relevance of genetically determined host factors to the prognosis of meningococcal disease. *Eur J Clin Microbiol Infect Dis*, 23, 634–637.

Dorner, C., Ciossek, T., Muller, S., Moller, P.H., Ullrich, A., Lammers, R. (1998) Characterization of KIF1C, a new kinesin-like protein involved in vesicle transport from the Golgi apparatus to the endoplasmic reticulum. *J Biol Chem*, 273, 20267–20275.

Duarte, R.S., Barros, R.R., Facklam, R.R., Teixeira, L.M. (2005) Phenotypic and genotypic characteristics of *Streptococcus* porcinus isolated from human sources. *J Clin Microbiol*, 43, 4592–4601.

El-Demellawy, M., El-Ridi, R., Guirguis, N.I., Abdel Alim, M., Kotby, A., Kotb, M. (1997) Preferential recognition of human myocardial antigens by T lymphocytes from rheumatic heart disease patients. *Infect Immun*, 65, 2197–2205.

Emonts, M., Hazelzet, J.A., de Groot, R., Hermans, P.W. (2003) Host genetic determinants of *Neisseria meningitidis* infections. *Lancet Infect Dis*, 3, 565–577.

Eriksson, B.K., Andersson, J., Holm, S.E., Norgren, M. (1998) Epidemiological and clinical aspects of invasive group A streptococcal infections and the streptococcal toxic shock syndrome. *Clin Infect Dis*, 27, 1428–1436.

Faber, J., et al. (2006) Human Toll-like receptor 4 mutations are associated with susceptibility to invasive meningococcal disease in infancy. *Pediatr Infect Dis J*, 25 80–81.

Facklam, R.F., Martin, D.R., Lovgren, M., Johnson, D.R., Efstratiou, A., Thompson, T.A., Gowan, S., Kriz, P., Tyrrell, G.J., Kaplan, E., Beall, B. (2002) Extension of the Lancefield classification for group A streptococci by addition of 22 new M protein gene sequence types from clinical isolates: emm103 to emm124. *Clin Infect Dis*, 34, 28–38.

Feinstein, A.R., Wood, H.F., Spagnuolo, M., Taranta, A., Jonas, S., Kleinberg, E., Tursky, E. (1964) Rheumatic fever in children and adolescents. *Ann Intern Med*, 60, 87–126.

Fernandez-Viña, M.A., Gao, X., Moraes, M.E., Moraes, J.R., Salatiel, I., Miller, S., Tsai, J., Sun, Y., An, J., Layrisse, Z., Gazit, E., Brautbar, C., Stastny, P. (1991) Alleles at four HLA class II loci determined by oligonucleotide hybridization and their associations in five ethnic groups. *Immunogenetics*, 34, 299–312.

Fijen, C.A., et al. (2000) The role of Fegamma receptor polymorphisms and C3 in the immune defence against Neisseria meningitidis in complement-deficient individuals. *Clin Exp Immunol*, 120, 338–345.

Fouet, A., Mesnage, S. (2002) *Bacillus anthracis* cell envelope components. *Curr Top Microbiol Immunol*, 271, 87–113.

Fredrikson, G.N., Westberg, J., Kuijper, E.J., Tijssen, C.C., Sjöholm, A.G., Uhlén, M., Truedsson, L. (1996) Molecular characterization of properdin deficiency type III: dysfunction produced by a single point mutation in exon 9 of the structural gene causing a tyrosine to aspartic acid interchange. *J Immunol*, 157, 3666–3671.

Fremeaux-Bacchi, V., Le Coustumier, A., Blouin, J., Kazatchkine, M., Weiss, L. (1995) Partial properdin deficiency revealed by a septicemia caused by *Neisseria meningitidis*. *Presse Med ks*, 24(28), 1305–1307.

Friedman, I., Laufer, A., Ron, N., Davies, A.M. (1971) Experimental myocarditis: *In vitro* and *in vivo* studies of lymphocytes sensitized to heart extracts and group A streptococci. *Immunology*, 20, 225–232.

Galvin, J.E., Hemric, M.E., Kosanke, S.D., Factor, S.M., Quinn, A., Cunningham, M.W. (2002) Induction of myocarditis and valvulitis in lewis rats by different epitopes of cardiac myosin and its implications in rheumatic carditis. *Am J Pathol*, 160, 297–306.

Geishofer, G., et al. (2005). 4G/5G promoter polymorphism in the plasminogen-activator-inhibitor-1 gene in children with systemic meningococcaemia. *Eur J Pediatr*, 164, 486–490.

Gharib, R. (1969) Acute rheumatic fever in Shiraz, Iran. Its prevalence and characteristics in two socioeconomic groups. *Am J Dis Child*, 118, 694–699.

Goddard, E.A., Beatty, D.W., Hoffman, E.B. (1996) Immunoglobulin allotypes and genetic susceptibility to invasive Haemophilus influenzae type b and Staphylococcus aureus infections in South African children. *Pediatr Infect Dis J*, 15, 419–424.

Guedez, Y., Kotby, A., El-Demellawy, M., Galal, A., Thomson, G., Zaher, S., Kassem, S., Kotb, M. (1999) HLA class II associations with rheumatic heart disease are more evident and consistent among clinically homogeneous patients. *Circulation*, 99, 2784–2790.

Guilherme, L., Cunha-Neto, E., Coelho, V., et al. (1995) Human heart-infiltrating T cell clones from rheumatic heart disease recognize both streptococcal and cardiac proteins. *Circulation*, 92, 415–420.

Guilherme, L., Fae, K., Oshiro, S.E., Kalil, J. (2005) Molecular pathogenesis of rheumatic fever and rheumatic heart disease. *Expert Rev Mol Med*, 7, 1–15.

Guilherme, L., Kalil, J. (2002) Rheumatic fever: The T cell response leading to autoimmune aggression in the heart. *Autoimmun Rev*, 1, 261–266.

Guilherme, L., Oshiro, S.E., Fae, K.C., Cunha-Neto, E., Renesto, G., Goldberg, A.C., Tanaka, A.C., Pomerantzeff, P.M., Kiss, M.H., Silva, C., Guzman, F., Patarroyo, M.E., Southwood, S., Sette, A., Kalil, J. (2001) T-cell reactivity against streptococcal antigens in the periphery mirrors reactivity of heart-infiltrating T lymphocytes in rheumatic heart disease patients. *Infect Immun*, 69, 5345–5351.

Guilherme, L., Weidebach, W., Kiss, M.H., Snitcowsky, R., Khalil, J. (1991) Association of human leukocyte class II antigens with rheumatic heart disease in Brazilian population. *Circulation*, 83, 1995–1998.

Hanna, P. (1999) Lethal toxin actions and their consequences. *J Appl Microbiol*, 87, 285–287.

Haralambous, E., Hibberd, M., Hermans, P., Ninis, N., Nadel, S., Levin, M. (2003) Role of functional plasminogen-activator-inhibitor-1 4G/5G promoter polymorphism in susceptibility, severity, and outcome of meningococcal disease in Caucasian children. *Crit Care Med*, 31(12), 2788–2793.

Harding, D., et al. (2002) Severity of meningococcal disease in children and the angiotensin-converting enzyme insertion/deletion polymorphism. *Am J Respir Crit Care Med*, 165, 1103–1106.

Hassell, M., Fagan, P., Carson, P., Currie, B.J. (2004) Streptococcal necrotising fasciitis from diverse strains of *Streptococcus pyogenes* in tropical northern Australia: Case series and comparison with the literature. *BMC Infect Dis*, 4, 60.

Herman, A., Croteau, G., Sekaly, R.P., Kappler, J., Marrack, P. (1990) HLA-DR alleles differ in their ability to present staphylococcal enterotoxins to T cells. *J Exp Med*, 172, 709–717.

Hermans, P.W., Hazelzet, J.A. (2005) Plasminogen activator inhibitor type 1 gene polymorphism and sepsis. *Clin Infect Dis*, 41(suppl 7), S453–S458.

Hermans, P.W., Hibberd, M.L., Booy, R., Daramola, O., Hazelzet, J.A., de Groot, R., Levin, M. (1999) 4G/5G promoter polymorphism in the plasminogen-activator-inhibitor-1 gene and outcome of meningococcal disease. Meningococcal Research Group. *Lancet*, 354, 556–560.

Hernandez-Pacheco, G., Aguilar-Garcia, J., Flores-Dominguez, C., Rodriguez-Perez, J.M., Perez-Hernandez, N., Alvarez-Leon, E., Reyes, P.A., Vargas-Alarcon, G. (2003) MHC class II alleles in Mexican patients with rheumatic heart disease. *Int J Cardiol*, 92, 49–54.

Hibberd, M.L., et al. (1999) Association of variants of the gene for mannose-binding lectin with susceptibility to meningococcal disease. Meningococcal Research Group. *Lancet*, 353, 1049–1053.

Ho, P.L., Johnson, D.R., Yue, A.W., Tsang, D.N., Que, T.L., Beall, B., Kaplan, E.L. (2003) Epidemiologic analysis of invasive and noninvasive group a streptococcal isolates in Hong Kong. *J Clin Microbiol*, 41, 937–942.

Hoover, D.L., Friedlander, A.M., Rogers, L.C., Yoon, I.K., Warren, R.L., Cross, A.S. (1994) Anthrax edema toxin differentially regulates lipopolysaccharide-induced monocyte production of tumor necrosis factor alpha and interleukin-6 by increasing intracellular cyclic AMP. *Infect Immun*, 62, 4432–4439.

Hutto, J., Ayoub, E.M. (1980) Cytotoxicity of lymphocytes from patients with rheumatic carditis to cardiac cells in vitro. In Read, S.E., Zabriskie, J.B. (eds.), *Streptococcal disease and immune response*. Academic Press, New York, pp. 733–738.

Ireland, J.A.W., Hanna, P.C. (2002) Macrophage-enhanced germination of *Bacillus anthracis* endospores requires gerS. *Infect Immun*, 70, 5870–5872.

Jansen, T.L., Efde, M., Spoorenberg, A. (2005) Post-streptococcal reactive arthritis (PSRA): A plea for diagnostic criteria. *Rheumatology (Oxford)*, 44, 136; author reply 136–137.

Johansson, L., Rytkonen, A., Wan, H., Bergman, P., Plant, L., Agerberth, B., Hokfelt, T., Jonsson, A.B. (2005) Human-like immune responses in CD46 transgenic mice. *J Immunol*, 175, 433–440.

Johnson, D.R., Wotton, J.T., Shet, A., Kaplan, E.L. (2002) A comparison of group A streptococci from invasive and uncomplicated infections: Are virulent clones responsible for serious streptococcal infections? *J Infect Dis*, 185, 1586–1595.

Jones, T. (1944) The diagnosis of rheumatic fever. *JAMA*, 126, 481.

Jones, T.D. (1951) VI. Rheumatic fever and rheumatic heart disease. *R I Med J*, 34, 22; passim.

Jonsson, G., et al. (2006) Homozygosity for the IgG2 subclass allotype G2M(n) protects against severe infection in hereditary C2 deficiency. *J Immunol*, 177, 722–728.

Kadir, I.S., Barker, T.A., Clarke, B., Denley, H., Grotte, G.J. (2004) Recurrent acute rheumatic fever: A forgotten diagnosis? *Ann Thorac Surg*, 78, 699–701.

Kallstrom, H., Liszewski, M., Atkinson, J., Jonsson, A. (1997) Membrane cofactor protein (MCP or CD46) is a cellular pilus receptor for pathogenic *Neisseria*. *Mol Microbiol*, 25, 639–647.

Kalns, J., Scruggs, J., Millenbaugh, N., Vivekananda, J., Shealy, D., Eggers, J., Kiel, J. (2002) TNF receptor 1, IL-1 receptor, and iNOS genetic knockout mice are not protected from anthrax infection. *Biochem Biophys Res Commun*, 292, 41–44.

Kaplan, E.L. (1993) Global assessment of rheumatic fever and rheumatic heart disease at the close of the century. Influences and dynamics of populations and pathogens: A failure to realize prevention? *Circulation*, 88, 1964–1972.

Kaufhold, A., Podbielski, A., Kuhnemund, O., Lutticken, R. (1992) Infections by *Streptococcus pyogenes*: New aspects of diagnosis, epidemiology, clinical practice, and therapy. *Immun Infekt*, 20, 192–199.

Kaul, R., McGeer, A., Low, D.E., Green, K., Schwartz, B. (1997) Population-based surveillance for group A streptococcal necrotizing fasciitis: Clinical features, prognostic indicators, and microbiologic analysis of seventy-seven cases. Ontario Group A Streptococcal Study. *Am J Med*, 103, 18–24.

Kaul, R., McGeer, A., Norrby-Teglund, A., Kotb, M., Schwartz, B., O'Rourke, K., Talbot, J., Low, D.E. (1999) Intravenous immunoglobulin therapy for streptococcal toxic shock syndrome—a comparative observational study. The Canadian Streptococcal Study Group. *Clin Infect Dis*, 28, 800–807.

Kirsch, E.A., Giroir, B.P. (2000) Improving the outcome of septic shock in children. *Curr Opin Infect Dis*, 13, 253–258.

Kirsch, E.A., Barton, R.P., Kitchen, L., Giroir, B.P. (1996) Pathophysiology, treatment and outcome of meningococcemia: A review and recent experience. *Pediatr Infect Dis J*, 15, 967–978; quiz 979.

Kotb, M. (1992) Role of superantigens in the pathogenesis of infectious diseases and their sequelae. *Curr Opin Infect Dis*, 5, 364.

Kotb, M. (1995) Bacterial exotoxins as superantigens. *Clin Microbiol Rev*, 8, 411–426.

Kotb, M. (1998) Superantigens of gram-positive bacteria: Structure-function analyses and their implications for biological activity. *Curr Opin Microbiol*, 1, 56–65.

Kotb, M. (2004) Genetics of susceptibility to infectious diseases. *ASM News*, 70(10), 457–463.

Kotb, M., Norrby-Teglund, A., McGeer, A., El-Sherbini, H., Dorak, M.T., Khurshid, A., Green, K., Peeples, J., Wade, J., Thomson, G., Schwartz, B., Low, D.E. (2002) An immunogenetic and molecular basis for differences in outcomes of invasive group A streptococcal infections. *Nat Med*, 8, 1398–1404.

Kotb, M., Norrby-Teglund, A., McGeer, A., Green, K., Low, D.E. (2003) Association of human leukocyte antigen with outcomes of infectious diseases: The streptococcal experience. *Scand J Infect Dis*, 35, 665–669.

Kotby, A.A., El-Monim, M.T.A., Hassan, A.S. (1996) Assessment of rheumatic fever and rheumatic heart disease in the Children's Hospital of Ain Shams University from 1981–1995. *Egypt J Pediatr*, 13, 183–205.

Koyanagi, T., Koga, Y., Nishi, H., Toshima, H., Sasazuki, T., Imaizumi, T., Kimura, A. (1996) DNA typing of HLA class II genes in Japanese patients with rheumatic heart disease. *J Mol Cell Cardiol*, 28, 1349–1353.

Kreikemeyer, B., McIver, K.S., Podbielski, A. (2003) Virulence factor regulation and regulatory networks in *Streptococcus pyogenes* and their impact on pathogen-host interactions. *Trends Microbiol*, 11, 224–232.

Kremer Hovinga, J.A., et al. (2004) A functional single nucleotide polymorphism in the thrombin-activatable fibrinolysis inhibitor (TAFI) gene associates with outcome of meningococcal disease. *J Thromb Haemost*, 2, 54–57.

Kurlan, R., Kaplan, E.L. (2004) The pediatric autoimmune neuropsychiatric disorders associated with streptococcal infection (PANDAS) etiology for tics and obsessive-compulsive symptoms: Hypothesis or entity? Practical considerations for the clinician. *Pediatrics*, 113, 883–886.

Lacy, D.B., Collier, R.J. (2002) Structure and function of anthrax toxin. *Curr Top Microbiol Immunol*, 271, 61–85.

Linton, S.M., Morgan, B.P. (1999) Properdin deficiency and meningococcal disease—identifying those most at risk. *Clin Exp Immunol*, 118, 189–191.

Loiselle, C.R., Singer, H.S. (2001) Genetics of childhood disorders: XXXI. Autoimmune disorders, part 4: Is Sydenham chorea an autoimmune disorder? *J Am Acad Child Adolesc Psychiatry*, 40, 1234–1236.

Louie, L., Simor, A.E., Louie, M., McGeer, A., Low, D.E. (1998) Diagnosis of group A streptococcal necrotizing fasciitis by using PCR to amplify the streptococcal pyrogenic exotoxin B gene. *J Clin Microbiol*, 36, 1769–1771.

Low, D.E., Schwartz, B., McGeer, A. (1997) *The Reemergence of Severe Group A Streptococcal Disease: An Evolutionary Perspetive.* American Society for Microbiology Press, Washington, DC.

Lue, H.-C., Chen, C.-L., Wei, H., Okuni, M., Mabilangan, L.M., Dharmasakti, D., Hanafiah, A. (1979) The natural history of rheumatic fever and rheumatic heart disease in the Orient. *Jap Heart J*, 20, 237–252.

Lungstras-Bufler, K., Bufler, P., Abdullah, R., Rutherford, C., Endres, S., Abraham, E., Dinarello, C.A., Rodriguez, R.M. (2004) High cytokine levels at admission are associated with fatal outcome in patients with necrotizing fasciitis. *Eur Cytokine Netw*, 15, 135–138.

Maharaj, B., Hammond, M.G., Appadoo, B., Leary, W.P., Phil, D., Pudifin, D.J. (1987) HLA-A,B,DR, and DQ antigens in black patients with severe chronic rheumatic heart disease. *Circulation*, 76, 259–261.

Maia, D.P., Teixeira, A.L., Jr., Quintao Cunningham, M.C., Cardoso, F. (2005) Obsessive compulsive behavior, hyperactivity, and attention deficit disorder in Sydenham chorea. *Neurology*, 64, 1799–1801.

Majeed, H.A., Yousof, A.M., Khuffash, F.A., Yusuf, A.R., Farwana, S., Khan, N. (1986) The natural history of acute rheumatic fever in Kuwait: A prospective six year follow-up report. *J Chron Dis*, 39, 361–369.

Markowitz, M., Gerber, M.A. (1987) Rheumatic fever: Recent outbreaks of an old disease. *Conn Med*, 51, 229–233.

Markowitz, M., Gerber, M.A. (1995) The Jones criteria for guidance in the diagnosis of rheumatic fever. Another perspective. *Arch Pediatr Adolesc Med*, 149, 725–726.

Martin, D.R. (1997) Rheumatogenic and nephritogenic group A streptococci. Myth or reality? An opening lecture. *Adv Exp Med Biol*, 418, 21–27.

McAllister, R.D., Singh, Y., du Bois, W.D., Potter, M., Boehm, T., Meeker, N.D., Fillmore, P.D., Anderson, L.M., Poynter, M.E., Teuscher, C. (2003) Susceptibility to anthrax lethal toxin is controlled by three linked quantitative trait loci. *Am J Pathol*, 163, 1735–1741.

McNicholl, J.M., Cuenco, K.T. (1999) Host genes and infectious diseases. HIV, other pathogens, and a public health perspective. *Am J Prev Med*, 16, 141–154.

Miethke, T., Duschek, K., Wahl, C., Heeg, K., Wagner, H. (1993) Pathogenesis of the toxic shock syndrome: T cell mediated lethal shock caused by the superantigen TSST-1. *Eur J Immunol*, 23, 1494–1500.

Miethke, T., Wahl, C., Heeg, K., Echtenacher, B., Krammer, P.H., Wagner, H. (1992) T cell-mediated lethal shock triggered in mice by the superantigen staphylococcal enterotoxin B: Critical role of tumor necrosis factor. *J Exp Med*, 175, 91–98.

Moayeri, M., Martinez, N.W., Wiggins, J., Young, H.A., Leppla, S.H. (2004) Mouse susceptibility to anthrax lethal toxin is influenced by genetic factors in addition to those controlling macrophage sensitivity. *Infect Immun*, 72, 4439–4447.

Mock, M., Fouet, A. (2001) Anthrax. *Annu Rev Microbiol*, 55, 647–671.

Mock, M., Mignot, T. (2003) Anthrax toxins and the host: A story of intimacy. *Cell Microbiol*, 5, 15–23.

Muller, M.P., Low, D.E., Green, K.A., Simor, A.E., Loeb, M., Gregson, D., McGeer, A. (2003) Clinical and epidemiologic features of group a streptococcal pneumonia in Ontario, Canada. *Arch Intern Med*, 163, 467–472.

Nadel, S., Newport, M.J., Booy, R., Levin, M. (1996) Variation in the tumor necrosis factor-alpha gene promoter region may be associated with death from meningococcal disease. *J Infect Dis*, 174, 878–880.

Nassif, X., Pujol, C., Morand, P., Eugene, E. (1999) Interactions of pathogenic *Neisseria* with host cells. Is it possible to assemble the puzzle? *Mol Microbiol*, 32, 1124–3112.

Newburger, J.W., Takahashi, M., Gerber, M.A., Gewitz, M.H., Tani, L.Y., Burns, J.C., Shulman, S.T., Bolger, A.F., Ferrieri, P., Baltimore, R.S., Wilson, W.R., Baddour, L.M., Levison, M.E., Pallasch, T.J., Falace, D.A., Taubert, K.A. (2004) Diagnosis, treatment, and long-term management of Kawasaki disease: A statement for health professionals from the Committee on Rheumatic Fever, Endocarditis, and Kawasaki Disease, Council on Cardiovascular Disease in the Young, American Heart Association. *Pediatrics*, 114, 1708–1733.

Nooh, M.M., El-Gengehi, N., Kansal, R., David, C.S., Kotb, M. (2007). Evidence for a direct role of HLA class II allelic variation in potentiating the outcome of invasive streptococcal infection. *J Immunol*, 178, 3076–3083.

Nordstrand, A., Norgren, M., Holm, S.E. (1999) Pathogenic mechanism of acute post-streptococcal glomerulonephritis. *Scand J Infect Dis*, 31, 523–537.

Norrby-Teglund, A., Chatellier, S., Low, D.E., McGeer, A., Green, K., Kotb, M. (2000) Host variation in cytokine responses to superantigens determine the severity of invasive group A streptococcal infection. *Eur J Immunol*, 30, 3247–3255.

Norrby-Teglund, A., Ihendyane, N., Darenberg, J. (2003a) Intravenous immunoglobulin adjunctive therapy in sepsis, with special emphasis on severe invasive group A streptococcal infections. *Scand J Infect Dis*, 35, 683–689.

Norrby-Teglund, A., Kaul, R., Low, D.E., McGeer, A., Newton, D.W., Andersson, J., Andersson, U., Kotb, M. (1996) Plasma from patients with severe invasive group A streptococcal infections treated with normal polyspecific IgG inhibits streptococcal superantigen-induced T cell proliferation and cytokine production. *J Immunol*, 156, 3057–3064.

Norrby-Teglund, A., Kotb, M. (2000) Host-microbe interactions in the pathogenesis of invasive group A streptococcal infections. *J Med Microbiol*, 49, 849–852.

Norrby-Teglund, A., Norrby, S.R., and Low, D.E. (2003b) The treatment of severe group A streptococcal infections. *Curr Infect Dis Rep*, 5, 28–37.

O'Brien, J., Friedlander, A., Dreier, T., Ezzell, J., Leppla, S. (1985) Effects of anthrax toxin components on human neutrophils. *Infect Immun*, 47, 306–310.

Ozkan, M., Carin, M., Sonmez, G., Senocak, M., Ozdemir, M., Yakut, C. (1993) HLA antigens in Turkish race with rheumatic heart disease. *Circulation*, 87, 1974–1978.

Pechère, J., Kaplan, E.E. (2004) Streptococcal pharyngitis. *Issues Infect Dis*, 3, 1–12.

Peirce, J.L., Lu, L., Gu, J., Silver, L.M., Williams, R.W. (2004) A new set of BXD recombinant inbred lines from advanced intercross populations in mice. *BMC Genet*, 5, 7.

Pellizzari, R., Guidi-Rontani, C., Vitale, G., Mock, M., Montecucco, C. (1999) Anthrax lethal factor cleaves MKK3 in macrophages and inhibits the LPS/IFNgamma-induced release of NO and TNFalpha. *FEBS Lett*, 462, 199–204.

Perera, Y., Cobas, K., Garrido, Y., Nazabal, C., Brown, E., Pajon, R. (2006) Determination of human transferrin concentrations in mouse models of neisserial infection. *J Immunol Methods*, 311, 153–163.

Pickering, A.K., Osorio, M., Lee, G.M., Grippe, V.K., Bray, M., Merkel, T.J. (2004) Cytokine response to infection with *Bacillus anthracis* spores. *Infect Immun*, 72, 6382–6389.

Quinn, A., Kosanke, S., Fischetti, V.A., Factor, S.M., Cunningham, M.W. (2001) Induction of autoimmune valvular heart disease by recombinant streptococcal m protein. *Infect Immun*, 69, 4072–4078.

Rameix-Welti, M.A., et al. (2005) [Neisseria meningitidis infection: clinical critera oriented toward a deficiency in the proteins of the complement]. *Presse Med*, 34, 425–430.

Read, R.C., Camp, N.J., di Giovine, F.S., Borrow, R., Kaczmarski, E.B., Chaudhary, A.G., Fox, A.J., Duff, G.W. (2000) An interleukin-1 genotype is associated with fatal outcome of meningococcal disease. *J Infect Dis*, 182, 1557–1560.

Roberts, J.E., Watters, J.W., Ballard, J.D., Dietrich, W.F. (1998) Ltx1, a mouse locus that influences the susceptibility of macrophages to cytolysis caused by intoxication with *Bacillus anthracis* lethal factor, maps to chromosome 11. *Mol Microbiol*, 29, 581–591.

Rosenstein, N.E., Perkins, B., Stephens, D., Popovic, T., Hughes, J. (2001) Meningococcal disease. *N Engl J Med*, 344, 1378–1388.

Sanyal, S.K., Abu-Melha, A. (1988) Acute rheumatic fever and its sequelae during childhood: Current concensus and controversies. *Ann Saudi Med*, 8, 362–372.

Sanyal, S.K., Berry, A.M., Duggal, S., Hooja, V., Ghosh, S. (1982) Sequelae of the initial attack of acute rheumatic fever in children from North India. *Circulation*, 65, 375–379.

Schaaf, B.M., et al. (2003). Pneumococcal septic shock is associated with the interleukin-10-182 gene promoter polymorphism. *Am J Respir Crit Care Med*, 168, 476–480.

Schmidtt, H., Hensel, M. (2004) Pathogenicity islands in bacterial pathogenesis. *Clin Microbiol Rev*, 17, 14–56.

Shultz, L.D., Lyons, B.L., Burzenski, L.M., Gott, B., Chen, X., Chaleff, S., Kotb, M., Gillies, S.D., King, M., Mangada, J., Greiner, D.L., Handgretinger, R. (2005) Human lymphoid and myeloid cell development in NOD/LtSz-scid IL2R gamma null mice engrafted with mobilized human hemopoietic stem cells. *J Immunol*, 174, 6477–6489.

Singh, J., Arrieta, A.C. (2004) Management of meningococcemia. *Indian J Pediatr*, 71, 909–913.

Smirnova, I., et al. (2003) Assay of locus-specific genetic load implicates rare Toll-like receptor 4 mutations in meningococcal susceptibility. *Proc Natl Acad Sci USA*, 100, 6075–6080.

Snider, L.A., Swedo, S.E. (2003) Post-streptococcal autoimmune disorders of the central nervous system. *Curr Opin Neurol*, 16, 359–365.

Spath, P.J., Sjoholm, A.G., Fredrikson, G.N., Misiano, G., et al. (1999) Properdin deficiency in a large Swiss family; identification of a stop codon in the properdin gene, and association of meningococcal disease with lack of the IgG2 allotype marker G2m(n). *Clin Exp Immunol*, 118, 278–284(7)

Stanevicha, V., Eglite, J., Sochnevs, A., Gardovska, D., Zavadska, D., Shantere, R. (2003) HLA class II associations with rheumatic heart disease among clinically homogeneous patients in children in Latvia. *Arthritis Res Ther*, 5, R340–R346.

Starnbach, M.N., Collier, R.J. (2003) Anthrax delivers a lethal blow to host immunity. *Nat Med*, 9, 996–997.

Stevens, D.L., Tanner, M.H., Winship, J., Swarts, R., Ries, K., Schlievert, P.M., Kaplan, E. (1989) Severe group A streptococcal infections associated with a toxic shock-like syndrome and scarlet fever toxin. *N Engl J Med*, 321, 1.

Stollerman, G.H. (1991) Rheumatogenic streptococci and autoimmunity. *Clin Immunol Immunopathol*, 61, 131–142.

Stollerman, G.H. (1997) Rheumatic fever. *Lancet*, 349, 935–942.

Stollerman, G.H. (2001) Rheumatic fever in the 21st century. *Clin Infect Dis*, 33, 806–814.

Stollerman, G.H. (2002) Current issues in the prevention of rheumatic fever. *Minerva Med*, 93, 371–387.

Sumby, P., et al. (2005) Evolutionary origin and emergence of a highly successful clone of serotype M1 group A *Streptococcus* involved multiple horizontal gene transfer events. *J Infect Dis*, 192, 771–782.

Swedo, S.E., Leonard, H.L., Garvey, M., Mittleman, B., Allen, A.J., Perlmutter, S., Lougee, L., Dow, S., Zamkoff, J., Dubbert, B.K. (1998) Pediatric autoimmune neuropsychiatric disorders associated with streptococcal infections: Clinical description of the first 50 cases. *Am J Psychiatry*, 155, 264–271.

Talkington, D.F., Schwartz, B., Black, C.M., Todd, J.K., Elliott, J., Breiman, R.F., Facklam, R.R. (1993) Association of phenotypic and genotypic characteristics of invasive *Streptococcus pyogenes* isolates with clinical components of streptococcal toxic shock syndrome. *Infect Immun*, 61, 3369–3374.

Tompkins, D.G., Boxerbaum, B., Liebman, J. (1972) Long-term prognosis of rheumatic fever patients receiving regular intramuscular benzathine penicillin. *Circulation*, 45, 543–551.

Unnikrishnan, M., Altmann, D.M., Proft, T., Wahid, F., Cohen, J., Fraser, J.D., Sriskandan, S. (2002) The bacterial superantigen streptococcal mitogenic exotoxin Z is the major immunoactive agent of *Streptococcus pyogenes*. *J Immunol*, 169, 2561–2569.

Unny, S.K., Middlebrooks, B.L. (1983) Streptococcal rheumatic carditis. *Microbiol Rev*, 47, 97–120.

van der Pol, W.L., Huizinga, T.W., Vidarsson, G., van der Linden, M.W., Jansen, M.D., Keijsers, V., de Straat, F.G., Westerdaal, N.A., de Winkel, J.G., Westendorp, R.G. (2001) Relevance of Fcgamma receptor and interleukin-10 polymorphisms for meningococcal disease. *J Infect Dis*, 184, 1548–1555.

van der Pol, W., van de Winkel, J.G. (1998) IgG receptor polymorphisms: risk factors for disease. *Immunogenetics*, 48, 222–232.

van Deuren, M., van der Ven-Jongekrijg, J., Bartelink, A.K., van Dalen, R., Sauerwein, R.W., van der Meer, J.W. (1995) Correlation between proinflammatory cytokines and antiinflammatory mediators and the severity of disease in meningococcal infections. *J Infect Dis*, 172, 433–439.

van Deuren, M., van der Ven-Jongekrijg, J., Vannie, E., et al. (1997) The pattern of interleukin-1beta (IL-1β) and its modulating agents IL-1 receptor antagonist and IL-1 soluble receptor type II in acute meningococcal infections. *Blood*, 90, 1101–1108.

Vermont, C.L., Groot, R., Hazelzet, J.A. (2002) Bench-to-bedside review: Genetic influences on meningococcal disease. *Crit Care*, 6, 60–65.

Visentainer, J.E., Pereira, F.C., Dalalio, M.M., Tsuneto, L.T., Donadio, P.R., Moliterno, R.A. (2000) Association of HLA-DR7 with rheumatic fever in the Brazilian population. *J Rheumatol*, 27, 1518–1520.

Vitale, G., Pellizzari, R., Recchi, C., Napolitani, G., Mock, M., Montecucco, C. (1998) Anthrax lethal factor cleaves the N-terminus of MAPKKs and induces tyrosine/threonine phosphorylation of MAPKs in cultured macrophages. *Biochem Biophys Res Commun*, 248, 706–711.

Vlaminckx, B., van Pelt, W., Schouls, L., van Silfhout, A., Elzenaar, C., Mascini, E., Verhoef, J., Schellekens, J. (2004) Epidemiological features of invasive and noninvasive group A streptococcal disease in the Netherlands, 1992–1996. *Eur J Clin Microbiol Infect Dis*, 23, 434–444.

Wade, B.H., Wright, G.G., Hewlett, E.L., Leppla, S.H., Mandell, G.L. (1985) Anthrax toxin components stimulate chemotaxis of human polymorphonuclear neutrophils. *Proc Soc Exp Biol Med*, 179, 159–162.

Waterer, G.W., Eibahlawan, L., et al. (2003) Heat shock protein 70-2+1267 AA homozygotes have an increased risk of septic shock in adults with community-acquired pneumonia. *Crit Care Med*, 31, 1367–1372.

Waterer, G.W., Wunderink, R.G. (2003) Science review: genetic variability in the systemic inflammatory response. *Crit Care*, 7, 308–314.

Watters, J.W., Dietrich, W.F. (2001) Genetic, physical, and transcript map of the Ltxs1 region of mouse chromosome 11. *Genomics*, 73, 223–231.

Webster, J.I., Moayeri, M., Sternberg, E.M. (2004) Novel repression of the glucocorticoid receptor by anthrax lethal toxin. *Ann N Y Acad Sci*, 1024, 9–23.

Webster, J.I., Tonelli, L.H., Moayeri, M., Simons, S.S., Jr., Leppla, S.H., Sternberg, E.M. (2003) Anthrax lethal factor represses glucocorticoid and progesterone receptor activity. *Proc Natl Acad Sci USA*, 100, 5706–5711.

Weidebach, W., Goldberg, A.C., Chiarella, J.M., Guilherme, L., Snitcowsky, R., Pileggi, F., Khalil, J. (1994) HLA class II antigens in rheumatic fever: Analysis of the DR locus by restriction fragment-length polymorphism and oligotyping. *Hum Immunol*, 40, 253–258.

Welcher, B.C., Carra, J.H., DaSilva, L., Hanson, J., David, C.S., Aman, M.J., Bavari, S. (2002) Lethal shock induced by streptococcal pyrogenic exotoxin A in mice transgenic for human leukocyte antigen-DQ8 and human CD4 receptors: Implications for development of vaccines and therapeutics. *J Infect Dis*, 186, 501–510.

Welkos, S.L., Keener, T.J., Gibbs, P.H. (1986) Differences in susceptibility of inbred mice to *Bacillus anthracis*. *Infect Immun*, 51, 795–800.

Wen, R., Blackman, M.A., Woodland, D.L. (1995) Variable influence of MHC polymorphism on the recognition of bacterial superantigens by T cells. *J Immunol*, 155, 1884–1892.

Westendorp, R., Hottenga, J., Slagboom, P. (1999) Variation in plasminogen-activator-inhibitor-1 gene and risk of meningococcal septic shock. *Lancet*, 354, 561–563.

White, J., Herman, A., Pullen, A.M., Kubo, R., Kappler, J.W., Marrack, P. (1989) The V beta-specific superantigen staphylococcal enterotoxin B: Stimulation of mature T cells and clonal deletion in neonatal mice. *Cell*, 56, 27–35.

Williams, R.W., Bennett, B., Lu, L., Gu, J., DeFries, J.C., Carosone-Link, P.J., Rikke, B.A., Belknap, J.K., Johnson, T.E. (2004) Genetic structure of the LXS panel of recombinant inbred mouse strains: A powerful resource for complex trait analysis. *Mamm Genome*, 15, 637–647.

Williams, R.W., Gu, J., Qi, S., Lu, L. (2001) The genetic structure of recombinant inbred mice: High-resolution consensus maps for complex trait analysis. *Genome Biol*, 2: RESEARCH 46.1–46.18.

Working Group on Severe Streptococcal Infections. (1993) Defining the group A streptococcal toxic shock syndrome. Rationale and consensus definition. *JAMA*, 269, 390–391.

Yi, K., Stephens, D.S., Stojiljkovic, I. (2003) Development and evaluation of an improved mouse model of meningococcal colonization. *Infect Immun*, 71, 1849–1855.

Zabriskie, J.B., Hsu, K.C., Seegal, B.C. (1970) Heart-reactive antibody associated with rheumatic fever: Characterization and diagnostic significance. *Clin Exp Immunol*, 7, 147–159.

24

Malaria

*Dominic P. Kwiatkowski & Gaia Luoni**

Each year, malaria kills more than a million children in Africa alone and is a significant cause of illness and poverty in hundreds of millions of people worldwide. Of the four species of malaria parasite that infect humans, *Plasmodium falciparum* is the most virulent, accounting for almost all deaths due to malaria, and has a remarkable ability to develop resistance against commonly used antimalarial drugs. Despite initiatives such as the World Health Organization's Roll Back Malaria campaign, there is no evidence that the global malaria problem is coming under control. Promising results from recent malaria vaccine trials have given an important boost to vaccine developers (Alonso et al. 2005), but we still have a very long way to go before we have a vaccine—or any other intervention—that is capable of achieving a radical reduction in the global burden of malaria.

A practical reason for understanding the human genetic factors that determine resistance to malaria is that they may provide vital clues about molecular mechanisms of disease and immunity that are central to the development of an effective vaccine. For example, we have only a vague understanding of the molecular mechanisms by which malaria parasites invade erythrocytes, or the immunological mechanisms that are critical for clearing malaria parasites from the bloodstream. Genetic findings may offer radical new insights into those questions. The discovery that Duffy blood group–negative individuals are resistant to infection with *Plasmodium vivax* was the vital clue in understanding how this species of parasite invades erythrocytes and has led to the development of a *P. vivax* vaccine that is now undergoing testing (discussed below). One of the many practical reasons for investing in large-scale epidemiological studies of malaria is to gain similar clues about the molecular mechanisms by which *P. falciparum* invades erythrocytes, and other

*Deceased.

aspects of protective immunity that could be crucial for vaccine development.

Geneticists are particularly interested in malaria for another reason: It is the strongest known environmental force for evolutionary pressure on the human genome, responsible for the most common human Mendelian disorders: α- and β-thalassemia, sickle cell disease, G6PD deficiency, and various other erythrocyte defects (see chapter 8). If a genetic variant confers a significant degree of protection against death from malaria, then there is a good chance that it will undergo positive selection in regions where malaria is a major public health problem. That includes most of sub-Saharan Africa and large parts of the Indian subcontinent, Southeast Asia, and South America, and in the relatively recent past it also included parts of Europe. Thus, many human populations carry malaria resistance genes because their ancestors were exposed to malaria—including groups such as African Americans who have not been exposed to malaria for many generations—and this may be an important factor in susceptibility to contemporary diseases, in addition to the hemoglobinopathies and erythrocyte disorders. Many scientists suspect—although it has yet to be proved—that the historical influence of malaria on polymorphisms of immune and inflammatory genes may be a significant factor in the etiology of common diseases of affluent Western societies.

Variation at the Level of Population, Ethnic Group, and Family

The clinical pattern of malaria differs between populations. This is mostly due to differences in climate and other environmental factors that determine the level of malaria transmission, but there is also a significant genetic influence. Most of the population of sub-Saharan Africa is resistant to infection with *P. vivax* because of a single nucleotide polymorphism (SNP) of the *FY* gene that is rarely found in other populations and appears to have arisen through recent positive selection (Hamblin and Di Rienzo 2000). This suppresses expression of the Duffy blood group antigen on erythrocytes (Tournamille et al. 1995) and thereby prevents erythrocyte invasion by this species of parasite (Miller et al. 1976). It is possible that human genetic factors are responsible for other geographic differences, such as the rarity of certain clinical complications of *P. falciparum* infec-

tion (e.g., renal failure, pulmonary edema, and jaundice) in Africa compared to South Asia.

Differences in resistance to malaria have been observed between ethnic groups who live in the same geographical region. The best documented example is the Fulani of Burkina Faso, who have a lower prevalence of malaria parasitemia and fewer clinical attacks of malaria than other ethnic groups who live in closely neighboring villages (Modiano et al. 1996). Detailed epidemiological investigations strongly suggest that this due to genetic rather than cultural or environmental factors. Intriguingly, the Fulani have higher levels of antimalarial antibodies than do their neighbors (Modiano et al. 1998, 1999), and they have a lower frequency of protective globin variants and other classical malaria resistance factors (Modiano et al. 2001a). This suggests that they may possess a novel genetic resistance factor that affects the antibody response to infection, and there is preliminary evidence that variation in the region of the interleukin *IL4* gene may be responsible (Luoni et al. 2001).

The heritability of malaria is not easy to estimate due to practical obstacles. For example, to assess resistance to severe malaria, it would be necessary to ascertain whether malaria was responsible for previous episodes of severe illness and death within the family, and that is difficult since detailed medical records are rarely available in the communities that are most afflicted by malaria. An alternative strategy is to conduct longitudinal studies of quantitative traits such as malaria infection intensity or the frequency of malaria fever episodes. Such studies are epidemiologically demanding and require frequent monitoring, since infection intensity varies greatly over time within a single individual and is greatly affected by age and environment.

However, there have been some successes. A study in Kenyan children, using pedigree-based genetic variance component analysis, determined that genetic factors explained 24% of the total variation in mild malaria fever episodes and 25% of the total variation in hospital admissions due to malaria, while household effects accounted for 29% and 14%, respectively (Mackinnon et al. 2005). Only 2% of the total variation was explained by the hemoglobin S gene, implying that many other genetic factors may remain to be discovered. A longitudinal study of Gambian twins showed that susceptibility to malaria fever episodes is partly determined by genetic factors (Jepson et al. 1995) with linkage to the MHC region on chromosome 6 (Jepson et al. 1997). Longitudinal family studies of infection intensity in Cameroon and Burkina Faso indicate that complex genetic factors are involved (Garcia et al. 1998a; Rihet et al. 1998a) and that there is linkage to MHC and the 5q31–33 region (Garcia et al. 1998b; Rihet et al. 1998b; Flori et al. 2003a). Familial segregation analysis of immunological responses to malaria antigens in Papua New Guinea has suggested that Mendelian effects might govern specific antigen responses, but the overall picture is complex (Stirnadel et al. 1999a, 2000a, 2000b).

Genes Implicated in Resistance and Susceptibility to Malaria

Hemoglobin Genes

Globin and other red cell genes implicated in malaria resistance are discussed elsewhere (chapter 8) but, for completeness, are also summarized here. Adult hemoglobin, HbA, is a tetramer consisting of heme plus two α-globin chains (encoded by the almost identical *HBA1* and *HBA2* genes) and two β-globin chains (encoded by *HBB*). The selective pressure of malaria has been responsible for a remarkable variety of functional variants of these three genes.

HBB *(β-Globin)*

Hemoglobin S (HbS) results from a glutamic acid to valine substitution at codon 6 of the β-globin chain. HbS homozygotes have sickle cell disease, a debilitating and often fatal disorder caused by the red cell deformities that result from this structural defect, particularly at low oxygen concentrations. Heterozygotes, who do not generally have any clinical abnormality, have about 10-fold protection from life-threatening forms of malaria and somewhat lower levels of protection against milder forms of the disease (Allison 1954; Gilles et al. 1967; Hill et al. 1991; Allen et al. 1992; Stirnadel et al. 1999b). The trade-off between risk and benefit acts to maintain the HbS polymorphism at allele frequencies of around 10% in many parts of Africa, despite the grave consequences of the homozygous state. This is the most striking example of heterozygote advantage in human population genetics.

HbC is a different structural variant encoded by the same region of the *HBB* gene, where lysine replaces glutamic acid at codon 6. It is found in several parts of West Africa but is less common than HbS. HbC ho-

mozygotes have a relatively mild hemolytic anemia; that is, it is a much less damaging phenotype than sickle cell disease. Heterozygotes do not experience a significant reduction in hemoglobin levels (Diallo et al. 2004). Several recent studies have shown that both HbC heterozygotes and homozygotes are protected against clinical episodes of malaria (Agarwal et al. 2000; Modiano et al. 2001b; Rihet et al. 2004).

HbE is yet another structural variant of the *HBB* gene, a glutamic acid → lysine substitution at codon 26. It is extremely common in Southeast Asia, with carrier rates of 50% in some places, and homozygotes generally have symptomless anemia. In heterozygotes it seems that *P. falciparum* can only invade a fraction of erythrocytes, and it has been proposed that this acts to protect against high parasitemia and thus severe disease (Chotivanich et al. 2002). Analysis of haplotype structure suggests that the mutation is relatively recent and has risen rapidly in allele frequency (Ohashi et al. 2004).

HBA1/HBA2 *(α-Globin)*

The thalassemias are a group of genetic disorders due to defective production of α- or β-globin chains, arising from a diverse set of deletions and other disruptions of the globin gene clusters on chromosomes 11 and 16. The clinical phenotypes are complex, but broadly speaking, the homozygous state results in severe disease or is fatal, while heterozygotes are healthy apart from mild anemia. An exception to this general rule is α+ thalassemia, which occurs when either the HBA1 or the HBA2 gene is disrupted but not both, such that some α globin production is possible: α+ thalassemia homozygotes are only mildly anemic.

The thalassemias are the commonest Mendelian diseases of humans and are believed to have resulted from evolutionary selection by malaria, because their global distribution corresponds so closely to the regions that have historically been exposed to malaria, including the Mediterranean and the Middle East, as well as Africa, the Indian subcontinent, and Southeast Asia. In a detailed population genetic survey of Melanesia it was found that the frequency of α+ thalassemia varied according to both altitude and latitude, in a manner that was highly correlated with malaria endemicity (Flint et al. 1986).

Although population genetic findings strongly suggest that common forms of thalassemia have resulted from natural selection by malaria, direct evidence of a malaria-protective effect has only recently become apparent. In Kenyan children, both heterozygous and homozygous α+ thalassemia appears to be protective against severe malaria (Williams et al. 2005b), and a study of Ghanaian children found that heterozygotes were protected (Mockenhaupt et al. 2004). A case–control study in Papua New Guinea found that the risk of severe malaria was reduced by 60% in α+ thalassemia homozygotes and by a smaller amount in heterozygotes, but curiously, a similar effect was seen in other childhood infectious diseases (Allen et al. 1997). To complicate matters, in Vanuatu it has been observed that young children with α+ thalassemia have a significantly higher incidence of malaria than do nonthalassemic children (Williams et al. 1996). Since most of the increased incidence was found in young children infected with P. vivax rather than P. falciparum, the researchers propose that if young children are highly exposed to the relatively benign parasite P. vivax, they may be protected against severe disease caused by P. falciparum.

A recent study in Kenyan children came up with the remarkable recent finding that both sickle cell trait and

α+ thalassemia were protective when individually present, but not when present in combination (figure 24.1) (Williams et al. 2005a). Although the small sample size did not allow conclusive inferences, these findings are strongly suggestive of negative epistasis, that is, some conflict in the biological mechanisms by which sickle cell trait and α+ thalassemia confer protection. The researchers suggest that this might explain why α+ thalassemia in Africa has failed to achieve the very high allele frequencies found in parts of Asia.

Erythrocyte Surface Molecules

As noted in the introductory remarks, genetic variation in erythrocyte surface proteins is particularly interesting to vaccine developers because it may provide important clues about how we might be able to prevent parasites from invading red cells.

FY (Duffy Antigen/Chemokine Receptor)

The glycoprotein Duffy antigen, encoded by the FY gene, is expressed on the surface of erythrocytes in most

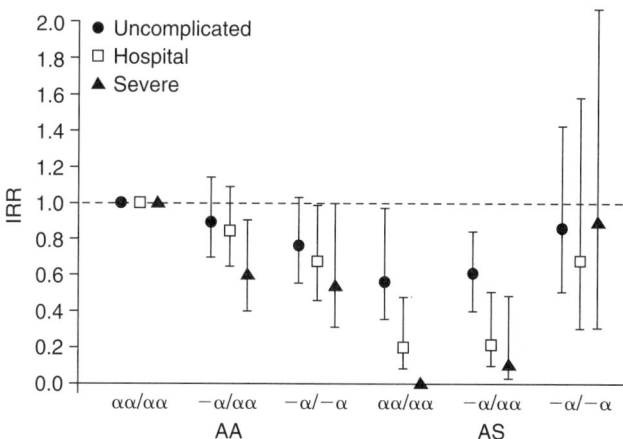

FIGURE 24.1. Incidence of *P. falciparum* malaria in Kenyan children with sickle cell trait (AS) and/or α+ thalassemia in the homozygous (−α/−α) or heterozygous (−α/αα) form. The incidence is expressed as a risk ratio (IRR) with reference to the values observed in children who carry neither sickle cell hemoglobin nor α+ thalassemia. Different severities of malaria are represented by closed circles (uncomplicated malaria fever), open squares (malaria requiring hospital admission), and closed triangles (severe malaria). Note that both sickle cell trait and α+ thalassemia are protective when individually present, but not when present in combination. From Williams et al. (2005a).

people except sub-Saharan Africa populations and their descendents. It is also expressed on various other cell types where it functions as a chemokine receptor. Its three common alleles are denoted FY*A, FY*B, and FY*O. The FY*O allele corresponds to the absence of the Duffy antigen on red blood cells and is defined by a SNP in the FY promoter region, which disrupts a binding site for the transcription factor GATA-1 (Allen et al. 1997). It was discovered almost 30 years that P. vivax requires the Duffy antigen to invade red blood cells (Miller et al. 1976), and this led to the biochemical and molecular biological characterization of a parasite molecule, P. vivax Duffy binding protein, that is critical for erythrocyte invasion (Chitnis and Miller 1994). This, in turn, has led to the development of a candidate vaccine against P. vivax (Yazdani et al. 2004) that is now undergoing clinical trials.

SLC4A1 *(Erythrocyte Band 3 Protein)*

SLC4A1 (also known as CD233 or erythrocyte band 3 protein) is an anion exchanger in the erythrocyte membrane, acting as a chloride/bicarbonate exchanger involved in transporting carbon dioxide from tissues to the lungs. Its correct conformation depends on its association with glycophorin A (see below). There are many different SLC4A1 mutations, some of which cause hereditary spherocytosis. Southeast Asian ovalocytosis occurs in heterozygotes for a 27-bp deletion in SLC4A1. Studies in Papua New Guinea (Cattani et al. 1987) and in Malaya (Foo et al. 1992) have found reduced malaria infection in individuals with ovalocytosis. In an area of Papua New Guinea where 9% of normal individuals have ovalocytosis, two independent studies have found it to be protective against cerebral malaria (Genton et al. 1995; Allen et al. 1999). The mechanism of this protective effect is not well understood; it may be due to inhibition of parasite invasion or growth, but it may also be due to an effect on parasite sequestration, as erythrocyte band 3 protein appears to be involved in the cytoadherence of parasitized erythrocytes to vascular endothelium.

GYPA *and* GYPB *(Glycophorins A and B)*

Glycophorins A and B, encoded by the homologous genes GYPA and GYPC, are major sialoglycoproteins of the erythrocyte membrane, which carries the antigenic determinants for various blood groups. Human erythrocytes that are genetically deficient in glyco-

phorin A or B show resistance to invasion by P. falciparum (Facer 1983). Specific sialic acid residues on the glycophorin A molecule are recognized by a Duffy-binding-like domain of P. falciparum erythrocyte-binding antigen 175 (Orlandi et al. 1992; Mayor et al. 2004). Analyses of GYPA and GYPB sequence variation among primates and human show evidence of strong evolutionary selection (Baum et al. 2002; Wang et al. 2003). It has also been noted that the highest rate of nonsynonymous polymorphism observed in the genome of P. falciparum is in EBA-175, suggesting that both the parasite ligand and the host receptor are engaged in an ongoing evolutionary battle (Wang et al. 2003).

GYPC *(Glycophorin C)*

Glycophorin C (encoded by GYPC) is a minor component of the erythrocyte membrane that is important for the mechanical stability of red cells. P. falciparum erythrocyte-binding antigen 140 (EBA140) binds to glycophorin C. A deletion of GYPC exon 3 is responsible for Gerbich blood group negativity and is found at frequencies approaching 50% in coastal areas of Papua New Guinea. It has been found that, in individuals who are Gerbich negative, EBA140 does not bind to glycophorin C, and P. falciparum invasion is blocked (Maier et al. 2003). Curiously, epidemiological studies in Papua New Guinea have so far failed to find evidence that this GYPC deletion affects malaria infection, but there may be effects on clinical severity which has not yet been studied in detail (Patel et al. 2001, 2004).

Other Erythrocyte-Related Proteins

G6PD *(Glucose-6-Phosphate Dehydrogenase)*

The G6PD gene on chromosome X encodes glucose-6-phosphate dehydrogenase, an enzyme that acts to produce NADPH, which is a key electron donor in defense against oxidizing agents. G6PD shows huge genetic diversity, causing wide variation in enzyme activity that can lead to hemolytic anemia. Common forms of G6PD deficiency are believed to have arisen as a result of evolutionary selection by malaria, because of their geographical distribution both at the global and at the local level (Ganczakowski et al. 1995). Different methods of haplotype analysis agree that the G6PD locus has undergone recent evolutionary selection (Tishkoff et al. 2001; Sabeti et al. 2002b). Studies of G6PD enzyme phenotype (Gilles et al. 1967) and of a common underlying mutation in African children (Ruwende et al. 1995) have confirmed that that G6PD deficiency confers protection against severe malaria in both hemizygous males and heterozygous females. This is thought to be because parasite replication is diminished in G6PD-deficient erythrocytes (Luzzatto et al. 1969), although it appears that the parasite is capable of evading this host-protective mechanism by synthesizing its own form of G6PD (Usanga and Luzzatto 1985).

HP (Haptoglobin)

Haptoglobin, encoded by the *HP* gene, is a protein found in plasma. It is mentioned here, although it is not an erythrocyte protein, because one of its major functions is to bind free hemoglobin, thus preventing hemoglobin-induced oxidative tissue damage. Studies in Sudan and Ghana have found an association between the haptoglobin 1–1 phenotype (determined by electrophoresis of sera) and susceptibility to severe *P. falciparum* malaria (Elagib et al. 1998; Quaye et al. 2000), and this is consistent with experiments in mice which showed that *HP* gene knockout led to greater parasite burden (Hunt et al. 2001). However a DNA-based study of haptoglobin polymorphisms in The Gambia failed to identify a significant association with disease susceptibility (Aucan et al. 2002).

Adhesion Molecules

Parasite sequestration in small blood vessels is central to the pathogenesis of severe malaria. It is caused by the ability of parasitized erythrocytes to bind to host adhesion molecules that are expressed on endothelium, platelets, and other erythrocytes. These binding properties are largely due to a parasite protein called *P. falciparum* erythrocyte membrane protein-1 (PfEMP-1) encoded by the *var* gene family, so called because each parasite contains multiple copies that are highly variable and is able to switch expression among them. Four well-characterized human adhesion molecules serve as receptors for different forms of PfEMP1.

ICAM1 (Intercellular Adhesion Molecule-1)

Intercellular adhesion molecule-1, also known as CD54, is encoded by the *ICAM1* gene. The molecule is expressed on endothelial cells and cells of the immune system and normally binds to integrins that are expressed by leukocytes. It is a strong binding receptor for some isolates of *P. falciparum* (Berendt et al. 1989). This binding is reduced by an N-terminal domain polymorphism found at high frequency in African populations (Fernandez-Reyes et al. 1997). This polymorphism would be expected to reduce susceptibility to severe malaria, and that is what was found in a study in Gabon (Kun et al. 1999), but a study in Kenya found the opposite (Fernandez-Reyes et al. 1997) and another in The Gambia found no significant association (Bellamy et al. 1998a).

CD36 (CD36 Antigen)

CD36 antigen, encoded by the *CD36* gene, is a surface glycoprotein that acts as a receptor for various molecules, including collagen, thrombospondin, anionic phospholipids, and long–chain fatty acids. It is highly expressed on the platelet surface and is also found on endothelial and dendritic cells. It serves as an endothelial binding receptor for many isolates of *P. falciparum* (Barnwell et al. 1989). It also allows parasites to bind dendritic cells and to suppress their ability to present parasite antigens (Urban et al. 1999, 2001). A range of *CD36* polymorphisms have been described in West African and Southeast Asian populations where malaria is endemic (Aitman et al. 2000; Omi et al. 2003), but the results of disease association studies are perplexing. A study that used both Gambian and Kenyan case–control samples found that homozygotes for the CD36 +1264G allele (a non-sense mutation) were susceptible to cerebral malaria (Aitman et al. 2000), while a study that looked at the same allele in Kenya alone found that heterozygosity was associated with protection against severe malaria (Pain et al. 2001). In Thailand, the +1264G allele was absent or very rare, but a dinucleotide repeat sequence in intron 3 implicated in alternative splicing was associated with protection against cerebral malaria (Omi et al. 2003).

CR1 (Complement Receptor 1)

CR1 encodes an erythrocyte membrane glycoprotein (also found on some dendritic cells) that acts as receptor for complement components C3b and C4b and regulates the activity of the complement cascade. CR1 is a binding receptor for some *P. falciparum* isolates and accounts for the phenomenon known as rosetting, where a parasitized erythrocyte binds to other erythrocytes (Rowe et al. 1997). Early work on *CR1* polymorphisms in The Gambia, including studies of the Knops blood group system, found no evidence of an association with disease severity (Bellamy et al. 1998a; Zimmerman et al. 2003), while a study based on restriction fragment length polymorphisms in Thailand found evidence of increased susceptibility to severe malaria among homozygotes for an allele that was associated with reduced expression of CR1 on erythrocytes (Nagayasu et al. 2001). More recently, a study in malaria-endemic regions of Papua New Guinea found that up to 80% of the population had erythrocyte CR1 deficiency, which was associated both with polymorphisms in the CR1 gene and, intriguingly, with the α+ thalassemia common in this population. In a case–control analysis, CR1 polymorphisms and α-thalassemia were independently associated with resistance to severe malaria (Cockburn et al. 2004).

PECAM1 *(Platelet-Endothelial Cell Adhesion Molecule)*

Platelet-endothelial cell adhesion molecule, also known as CD31, is a member of the immunoglobulin superfamily that is expressed on platelets, various leukocyte subsets, and endothelial cells. This endothelial binding receptor for *P. falciparum* (Treutiger et al. 1997) has a common coding variant (Leu > Val at codon 125) that showed no significant association with severe malaria in case–control studies in Papua New Guinea and Kenya (Casals-Pascual et al. 2001). A study from Thailand has reported a *PECAM1* haplotype that is more common in cerebral malaria compared to other forms of severe malaria (Kikuchi et al. 2001).

Mediators of Innate Immunity

TNF *(Tumor Necrosis Factor)*

Tumor necrosis factor (TNF) is a pro-inflammatory cytokine that is critical for innate immunity against malaria parasites but has also been implicated in the pathogenesis of severe malaria (reviewed in Kwiatkowski 1999). The *TNF* locus is at the centre of the linkage peaks identified in longitudinal family studies of malaria episodes in The Gambia and Burkina Faso (Jepson et al. 1997; Flori et al. 2003b). Several *TNF* promoter polymorphisms have been independently associated with severe malaria. Gambian children who are homozygous for the TNF-308A allele have in-

creased susceptibility to cerebral malaria (McGuire et al. 1994), and in Gabon those who carried this allele were more likely to experience symptomatic reinfections with *P. falciparum* (Meyer et al. 2002). Among other investigations of the TNF-308A allele in malaria endemic areas, a study in Sri Lanka found that carriers had increased risk of severe infectious diseases in general (Wattavidanage et al. 1999), and a study in Kenya found that carriers had an increase in infant mortality and malaria morbidity (Aidoo et al. 2001). The TNF−376A allele, which acts to recruit the transcription factor OCT-1, has been associated with susceptibility to cerebral malaria (Knight et al. 1999). The TNF-238A allele has been associated with susceptibility to severe malarial anemia in The Gambia (McGuire et al. 1999). The functional role of TNF-308 and other *TNF* polymorphisms has generated controversy that remains unresolved (Abraham and Kroeger 1999; Knight et al. 2003; Bayley et al. 2004). *TNF* resides in the MHC class III region, one densely packed with interesting immunologically active genes showing complex patterns of linkage disequilibrium in extended haplotypes (Ackerman et al. 2003). It is not unlikely that the reported *TNF* associations are simply markers for neighboring functional polymorphisms.

NOS2A *(Inducible Nitric Oxide Synthase)*

Nitric oxide is a reactive free radical of great interest in malaria research because it kills parasites but can also perturb immune function and neurotransmission (reviewed in Clark et al. 2004). The latter property suggests a potential role in cerebral malaria. The NOS2A gene encodes an inducible nitric oxide synthase. The NOS2A-954C allele has been associated with high baseline nitric oxide synthase (NOS) activity in cells from Gabonese individuals, and in this population it has been associated with protection from severe malaria and resistance to reinfection (Kun et al. 1998, 2001). Gambian and Tanzanian studies found no association with this SNP allele (Levesque et al. 1999; Burgner et al. 2003). The NOS2A-1173T allele has been associated with increased fasting concentrations of an nitric oxide metabolite in urine and plasma of Tanzanian children; it is associated with protection from symptomatic malaria in Tanzania and with protection from severe malarial anemia in Kenya (Hobbs et al. 2002). This allele was not associated with severe malaria in the Gambia, where an NOS2 microsatellite polymorphism has been associated with susceptibility to fatal malaria, and a haplotype uniquely defined by the NOS2A-1659T allele was associated with cerebral malaria by both transmission disequilibrium test and case–control analysis (Burgner et al. 1998, 2003).

IFNGR1 *(Interferon-γ Receptor, α-Chain)*

IFNGR1 encodes the ligand-binding chain of the heterodimeric interferon-γ (IFN-γ) receptor. There is copious evidence that IFN-γ is a critical mediator of immunity to malaria, but is also implicated in the pathogenesis of severe malarial disease (reviewed in Stevenson and Riley 2004). In a case–control study of the Mandinka, the major Gambian ethnic group, heterozygotes for the IFNGR1–56 polymorphism were protected against cerebral malaria (Koch et al. 2002). Reporter gene analysis suggests that the minor allele acts to reduce levels of *IFNGR1* gene expression (Juliger et al. 2003).

IFNAR1 *(Interferon-α Receptor 1)*

This gene encodes a type I membrane protein, one of the two chains of a receptor for IFN-α and IFN-β. In a murine malaria model it has been observed that IFN-α inhibits parasite development within erythrocytes (Vigario et al. 2001). A Gambian case–control study found two *IFNAR1* SNPs that were associated with protection against severe malaria, and a resistance haplotype was identified (Aucan et al. 2003).

IL12B *(Interleukin-12 p40)*

This gene encodes a subunit of interleukin-12, a cytokine produced by activated macrophages that is essential for the development of Th1 cells. Homozygosity for an *IL12B* promoter polymorphism was associated with both decreased cellular production of nitric oxide in blood samples and with fatality in Tanzanian children with cerebral malaria. However, the same investigators could not reproduce the latter association in Kenyan children with severe malaria (Morahan et al. 2002).

IL1A *and* IL1B *(Interleukin-1α and -1β)*

The interleukin-1 family of cytokines, produced mainly by macrophages, are important mediators of fever and the inflammatory response to infection. In a Gambian case–control study, one SNP in *IL1A* and another in *IL1B* showed a marginal association with susceptibility to malaria, but the effect was small (Walley et al. 2004).

MBL2 *(Mannose-Binding Lectin)*

MBL2 encodes a serum mannose-binding lectin (MBL), also known as protein C. It recognizes mannose and N-acetylglucosamine on bacterial pathogens and can activate the classical complement pathway. *MBL2* polymorphisms have been associated with susceptibility to various infectious diseases, possibly including malaria. A study in Gabon found that children patients with severe malaria had a lower serum MBL levels than did those with mild malaria and that mutations in codons 54 and 57 of *MBL2* (which lead to low protein levels) were present at higher frequency in those with severe malaria (Luty et al. 1998). However, a study in The Gambia found no evidence that these alleles were associated with susceptibility to severe malaria (Bellamy et al. 1998b).

Mechanisms of Acquired Immunity

HLA-B *(Major Histocompatibility Complex, Class I, B)*

HLA-B encodes an MHC class I heavy chain that forms a heterodimer with β2-microglobulin to make up the HLA-B antigen presentation complex. Hundreds of HLA-B alleles have been described. The HLA-B*53 allele, which is much more common in West Africa than elsewhere in the world, is associated with a significant reduction in life-threatening complications of malaria in the Gambian population (Hill et al. 1991). This implies that MHC class I–dependent cytotoxic T-lymphocyte (CTL) mechanisms afford a significant degree of immunological protection, and since MHC class I is expressed by liver cells but not by erythrocytes, this observation has bolstered efforts to develop a liver-stage malaria vaccine. Analysis of peptides that bind to HLA-B*53 provides a way of screening for T-cell epitopes that may be effective targets for vaccine development (Hill et al. 1992). However, the parasite may be rapidly evolving to evade the host antigen presentation system. A study of a single fragment of the *P. falciparum* circumsporozoite protein found that the Gambian parasite population expressed four common variants, of which only two (cp26 and cp29) bound to HLA-B*35 and were therefore potential targets for CTL attack in HLA-B*35+ individuals. *In vitro*, although both cp26 and cp29 acted as effective targets for CTLs when expressed on their own, each variant acted to suppress the CTL response to the other variant (Gilbert et al. 1998). Moreover, when malaria parasites were recovered from the blood of infected individuals, the frequency of mixed infections with parasites expressing cp26 and cp29 was much greater than would be predicted from the individual frequencies of each variant. This seems to be an example of immunological antagonism, whereby the CTL response to one peptide fragment may be inhibited by a similar but nonidentical fragment. The parasite may exploit this strategy of expressing antagonistic CTL epitopes as a mechanism of immune evasion.

HLA-DRB1 *(Major Histocompatibility Complex, Class II, DRβ1)*

HLA-DRB1 encodes an HLA class II β-chain, which forms a heterodimer with an α-chain (DRA) to make up the HLA-DR antigen presenting complex. DRB1 is expressed on B lymphocytes, dendritic cells, and macrophages; it presents peptides derived from extracellular proteins and is crucial for stimulating antibody production. The DRB1*1302–DQB1*0501 haplotype has been associated with protection from severe malaria in The Gambia (Hill et al. 1991). A longitudinal cohort study of children in The Gambia found that malaria attack rates were associated with the overall MHC class II distribution, but individual DR-DQ haplotype associations were not conclusively identified (Bennett et al. 1993).

IL4 *(Interleukin-4)*

Interleukin-4, produced by activated T cells, is important for the proliferation and differentiation of antibody-producing B cells. A study of *IL4* was carried out in the Fulani of Burkina Faso, who are more resistant to malaria attacks than neighboring ethnic groups, and who also have higher levels of antimalarial antibodies. The IL4–524 T allele occurred at high frequency and was associated with elevated antibody levels against malaria antigens, raising the possibility that this might be a factor in their increased resistance to malaria (Luoni et al. 2001).

TNFSF5 *(CD40 Ligand)*

TNFSF5, so called because it is a member of the TNF superfamily, encodes a glycoprotein that is expressed on T cells, known as CD40 ligand. By engaging CD40 on the B-cell surface, it regulates B-cell function, particularly immunoglobulin class switching, and rare coding mutations in CD40L can lead to life-threatening immunodeficiency. In a Gambian case–control study, a significant reduction in risk for severe malaria (odds ratio = 0.52, P = 0.002) was associated with males hemizygous for the *TNFSF5*−726C allele, and this was confirmed by transmission disequilibrium test (TDT) analysis in affected families. A similar but nonsignificant trend was found in females (Sabeti et al. 2002a). Long-range haplotype analysis of this allele suggest that it has recently undergone positive evolutionary selection (Sabeti et al. 2002b).

FCGR2A *(Low-affinity IIa Receptor for Fc Fragment of IgG)*

Receptors for the Fc portion of IgG are present on many leukocytes, and they are essential in removing antigen–antibody complexes from the circulation. *In vitro* studies indicate that IgG1 and IgG3, but not IgG2, are essential for inhibition of *P. falciparum* by antibody-dependent cellular mechanisms. An amino acid substitution of His to Arg at codon 131 of *FCGR2A* results in failure to bind to IgG2, and has been associated with protection against high levels of *P. falciparum* parasitemia in Kenya (Shi et al. 2001). Consistent with this observation, studies in Thailand and The Gambia found that homozygotes for the 131His genotype are susceptible to cerebral malaria (Omi et al. 2002; Cooke et al. 2003). In the Thai study, the *FCGR2A* association with severe malaria involved interaction with a polymorphism of the *FCGR3B* gene.

Conclusion

The International.HapMap Project has paved the way for genetic association analysis to be conducted at the level of the whole genome (Altshuler et al. 2005). Malaria is a strong candidate for this approach, as the chances of detecting association are favored by the fact that malaria resistance alleles tend to rise to high frequency in malaria endemic regions and to maintain haplotypic relationships over large genomic regions due to recent positive selection (Sabeti et al. 2002b; Ohashi et al. 2004; Altshuler et al. 2005; Hanchard et al. 2006). Genetic studies of malaria have already yielded results of practical importance for disease prevention: The observation of resistance to infection with *P. vivax* in Duffy antigen–negative individuals provided the fundamental clue needed to clone a parasite ligand that is vital for erythrocyte invasion and that represents a candidate vaccine against this species of parasite.

To screen the whole genome for most common forms of variation is estimated to require genotyping of approximately 1.5 million SNPs in an African population, compared to roughly 0.6 million in populations of European ancestry (Altshuler et al. 2005). Analysis of different populations is needed for a number of reasons: to achieve the large sample sizes needed to detect modest effects while correcting for multiple comparisons, to authenticate positive findings, to pinpoint functional polymorphisms by analysis of different haplotypes, and to start to understand gene–environment interactions. A global network of malaria researchers is now working toward these goals (see www.malariagen.net). Large-scale genomic epidemiology may teach us about molecular mechanisms of protective immunity that provide vital clues in the development of an effective malaria vaccine.

References

Abraham LJ, Kroeger KM (1999) Impact of the -308 TNF promoter polymorphism on the transcriptional regulation of the TNF gene: relevance to disease. J Leukoc Biol 66:562–566.

Ackerman HC, Ribas G, Jallow M, Mott R, Neville M, Sisay-Joof F, Pinder M, Campbell RD, Kwiatkowski DP (2003) Complex haplotypic structure of the central MHC region flanking TNF in a West African population. Genes Immun 4:476–486.

Agarwal A, Guindo A, Cissoko Y, Taylor JG, Coulibaly D, Kone A, Kayentao K, Djimde A, Plowe CV, Doumbo O, Wellems TE, Diallo D (2000) Hemoglobin C associated with protection from severe malaria in the Dogon of Mali, a West African population with a low prevalence of hemoglobin S. Blood 96:2358–2363.

Aidoo M, McElroy PD, Kolczak MS, Terlouw DJ, ter Kuile FO, Nahlen B, Lal AA, Udhayakumar V (2001) Tumor necrosis factor-alpha promoter variant 2 (TNF2) is associated with pre-term delivery, infant mortality, and malaria morbidity in western Kenya: Asembo Bay Cohort Project IX. Genet Epidemiol 21:201–211.

Aitman TJ, Cooper LD, Norsworthy PJ, Wahid FN, Gray JK, Curtis BR, McKeigue PM, Kwiatkowski D, Greenwood BM, Snow RW, Hill AV, Scott J (2000) Malaria susceptibility and CD36 mutation. Nature 405:1015–1016.

Allen SJ, Bennett S, Riley EM, Rowe PA, Jakobsen PH, O'Donnell A, Greenwood BM (1992) Morbidity from malaria and immune responses to defined Plasmodium falciparum antigens in children with sickle cell trait in The Gambia. Trans R Soc Trop Med Hyg 86:494–498.

Allen SJ, O'Donnell A, Alexander ND, Alpers MP, Peto TE, Clegg JB, Weatherall DJ (1997) alpha+-thalassemia protects children against disease caused by other infections as well as malaria. Proc Natl Acad Sci USA 94:14736–14741.

Allen SJ, O'Donnell A, Alexander ND, Mgone CS, Peto TE, Clegg JB, Alpers MP, Weatherall DJ (1999) Prevention of cerebral malaria in children in Papua New Guinea by southeast Asian ovalocytosis band 3. Am J Trop Med Hyg 60:1056–1060.

Allison AC (1954) Protection afforded by sickle-cell trait against subtertian malareal infection. Br Med J 4857:290–294.

Alonso PL, Sacarlal J, Aponte JJ, Leach A, Macete E, Aide P, Sigauque B, Milman J, Mandomando I, Bassat Q, Guinovart C, Espasa M, Corachan S, Lievens M, Navia MM, Dubois MC, Menendez C, Dubovsky F, Cohen J, Thompson R, Ballou WR (2005) Duration of protection with RTS,S/AS02A malaria vaccine in prevention of Plasmodium falciparum disease in Mozambican children: single-blind extended follow-up of a randomised controlled trial. Lancet 366: 2012–2018.

Altshuler D, Brooks LD, Chakravarti A, Collins FS, Daly MJ, Donnelly P (2005) A haplotype map of the human genome. Nature 437:1299–1320.

Aucan C, Walley AJ, Greenwood BM, Hill AV (2002) Haptoglobin genotypes are not associated with resistance to severe malaria in The Gambia. Trans R Soc Trop Med Hyg 96:327–328.

Aucan C, Walley AJ, Hennig BJ, Fitness J, Frodsham A, Zhang L, Kwiatkowski D, Hill AV (2003) Interferon-alpha receptor-1 (IFNAR1) variants are associated with protection against cerebral malaria in The Gambia. Genes Immun 4:275–282.

Barnwell JW, Asch AS, Nachman RL, Yamaya M, Aikawa M, Ingravallo P (1989) A human 88-kD membrane glycoprotein (CD36) functions in vitro as a receptor for a cytoadherence ligand on Plasmodium falciparum-infected erythrocytes. J Clin Invest 84:765–772.

Baum J, Ward RH, Conway DJ (2002) Natural selection on the erythrocyte surface. Mol Biol Evol 19:223–229.

Bayley JP, Ottenhoff TH, Verweij CL (2004) Is there a future for TNF promoter polymorphisms? Genes Immun 5:315–329.

Bellamy R, Kwiatkowski D, Hill AV (1998a) Absence of an association between intercellular adhesion molecule

1, complement receptor 1 and interleukin 1 receptor antagonist gene polymorphisms and severe malaria in a West African population. Trans R Soc Trop Med Hyg 92:312–316.

Bellamy R, Ruwende C, McAdam KP, Thursz M, Sumiya M, Summerfield J, Gilbert SC, Corrah T, Kwiatkowski D, Whittle HC, Hill AV (1998b) Mannose binding protein deficiency is not associated with malaria, hepatitis B carriage nor tuberculosis in Africans. Q J Med 91:13–18.

Bennett S, Allen SJ, Olerup O, Jackson DJ, Wheeler JG, Rowe PA, Riley EM, Greenwood BM (1993) Human leucocyte antigen (HLA) and malaria morbidity in a Gambian community. Trans R Soc Trop Med Hyg 87:286–287.

Berendt AR, Simmons DL, Tansey J, Newbold CI, Marsh K (1989) Intercellular adhesion molecule-1 is an endothelial cell adhesion receptor for *Plasmodium falciparum*. Nature 341:57–59.

Burgner D, Usen S, Rockett K, Jallow M, Ackerman H, Cervino A, Pinder M, Kwiatkowski DP (2003) Nucleotide and haplotypic diversity of the NOS2A promoter region and its relationship to cerebral malaria. Hum Genet 112:379–386.

Burgner D, Xu W, Rockett K, Gravenor M, Charles IG, Hill AV, Kwiatkowski D (1998) Inducible nitric oxide synthase polymorphism and fatal cerebral malaria. Lancet 352:1193–1194.

Casals-Pascual C, Allen S, Allen A, Kai O, Lowe B, Pain A, Roberts DJ (2001) Short report: codon 125 polymorphism of CD31 and susceptibility to malaria. Am J Trop Med Hyg 65:736–737.

Cattani JA, Gibson FD, Alpers MP, Crane GG (1987) Hereditary ovalocytosis and reduced susceptibility to malaria in Papua New Guinea. Trans R Soc Trop Med Hyg 81:705–709.

Chitnis CE, Miller LH (1994) Identification of the erythrocyte binding domains of *Plasmodium vivax* and *Plasmodium knowlesi* proteins involved in erythrocyte invasion. J Exp Med 180:497–506.

Chotivanich K, Udomsangpetch R, Pattanapanyasat K, Chierakul W, Simpson J, Looareesuwan S, White N (2002) Hemoglobin E: a balanced polymorphism protective against high parasitemias and thus severe *P falciparum* malaria. Blood 100:1172–1176.

Clark IA, Alleva LM, Mills AC, Cowden WB (2004) Pathogenesis of malaria and clinically similar conditions. Clin Microbiol Rev 17:509–539.

Cockburn IA, Mackinnon MJ, O'Donnell A, Allen SJ, Moulds JM, Baisor M, Bockarie M, Reeder JC, Rowe JA (2004) A human complement receptor 1 polymorphism that reduces *Plasmodium falciparum* rosetting confers protection against severe malaria. Proc Natl Acad Sci USA 101:272–277.

Cooke GS, Aucan C, Walley AJ, Segal S, Greenwood BM, Kwiatkowski DP, Hill AV (2003) Association of Fcgamma receptor IIa (CD32) polymorphism with severe malaria in West Africa. Am J Trop Med Hyg 69:565–568.

Diallo DA, Doumbo OK, Dicko A, Guindo A, Coulibaly D, Kayentao K, Djimde AA, Thera MA, Fairhurst RM, Plowe CV, Wellems TE (2004) A comparison of anemia in hemoglobin C and normal hemoglobin A children with *Plasmodium falciparum* malaria. Acta Trop 90:295–299.

Elagib AA, Kider AO, Akerstrom B, Elbashir MI (1998) Association of the haptoglobin phenotype (1–1) with *falciparum* malaria in Sudan. Trans R Soc Trop Med Hyg 92:309–311.

Facer CA (1983) Merozoites of *P. falciparum* require glycophorin for invasion into red cells. Bull Soc Pathol Exot Filiales 76:463–469.

Fernandez-Reyes D, Craig AG, Kyes SA, Peshu N, Snow RW, Berendt AR, Marsh K, Newbold CI (1997) A high frequency African coding polymorphism in the N-terminal domain of ICAM-1 predisposing to cerebral malaria in Kenya. Hum Mol Genet 6:1357–1360.

Flint J, Hill AV, Bowden DK, Oppenheimer SJ, Sill PR, Serjeantson SW, Bana-Koiri J, Bhatia K, Alpers MP, Boyce AJ, et al. (1986) High frequencies of alpha-thalassaemia are the result of natural selection by malaria. Nature 321:744–750.

Flori L, Kumulungui B, Aucan C, Esnault C, Traore AS, Fumoux F, Rihet P (2003a) Linkage and association between *Plasmodium falciparum* blood infection levels and chromosome 5q31-q33. Genes Immun 4:265–268.

Flori L, Sawadogo S, Esnault C, Delahaye NF, Fumoux F, Rihet P (2003b) Linkage of mild malaria to the major histocompatibility complex in families living in Burkina Faso. Hum Mol Genet 12:375–378.

Foo LC, Rekhraj V, Chiang GL, Mak JW (1992) Ovalocytosis protects against severe malaria parasitemia in the Malayan aborigines. Am J Trop Med Hyg 47:271–275.

Ganczakowski M, Town M, Bowden DK, Vulliamy TJ, Kaneko A, Clegg JB, Weatherall DJ, Luzzatto L (1995) Multiple glucose 6-phosphate dehydrogenase-deficient variants correlate with malaria endemicity in the Vanuatu archipelago (southwestern Pacific). Am J Hum Genet 56:294–301.

Garcia A, Cot M, Chippaux JP, Ranque S, Feingold J, Demenais F, Abel L (1998a) Genetic control of blood infection levels in human malaria: evidence for a complex genetic model. Am J Trop Med Hyg 58:480–488.

Garcia A, Marquet S, Bucheton B, Hillaire D, Cot M, Fievet N, Dessein AJ, Abel L (1998b) Linkage analysis of blood *Plasmodium falciparum* levels: interest of the 5q31-q33 chromosome region. Am J Trop Med Hyg 58:705–709.

Genton B, al-Yaman F, Mgone CS, Alexander N, Paniu MM, Alpers MP, Mokela D (1995) Ovalocytosis and cerebral malaria. Nature 378:564–565.

Gilbert SC, Plebanski M, Gupta S, Morris J, Cox M, Aidoo M, Kwiatkowski D, Greenwood BM, Whittle HC, Hill AV (1998) Association of malaria parasite population structure, HLA, and immunological antagonism. Science 279:1173–1177.

Gilles HM, Fletcher KA, Hendrickse RG, Lindner R, Reddy S, Allan N (1967) Glucose-6-phosphate-dehydrogenase deficiency, sickling, and malaria in African children in south western Nigeria. Lancet 1:138–140.

Hamblin MT, Di Rienzo A (2000) Detection of the signature of natural selection in humans: evidence from the Duffy blood group locus. Am J Hum Genet 66:1669–1679.

Hanchard NA, Rockett KA, Spencer C, Coop G, Pinder M, Jallow M, Kimber M, McVean G, Mott R, Kwiatkowski DP (2006) Screening for recently selected alleles by analysis of human haplotype similarity. Am J Hum Genet 78:153–159.

Hill AV, Allsopp CE, Kwiatkowski D, Anstey NM, Twumasi P, Rowe PA, Bennett S, Brewster D, McMichael AJ, Greenwood BM (1991) Common west African HLA antigens are associated with protection from severe malaria. Nature 352:595–600.

Hill AV, Elvin J, Willis AC, Aidoo M, Allsopp CE, Gotch FM, Gao XM, Takiguchi M, Greenwood BM, Townsend AR, et al. (1992) Molecular analysis of the association of HLA-B53 and resistance to severe malaria. Nature 360:434–439.

Hobbs MR, Udhayakumar V, Levesque MC, Booth J, Roberts JM, Tkachuk AN, Pole A, Coon H, Kariuki S, Nahlen BL, Mwaikambo ED, Lal AL, Granger DL, Anstey NM, Weinberg JB (2002) A new NOS2 promoter polymorphism associated with increased nitric oxide production and protection from severe malaria in Tanzanian and Kenyan children. Lancet 360:1468–1475.

Hunt NH, Driussi C, Sai-Kiang L (2001) Haptoglobin and malaria. Redox Rep 6:389–392.

Jepson AP, Banya WA, Sisay-Joof F, Hassan-King M, Bennett S, Whittle HC (1995) Genetic regulation of fever in *Plasmodium falciparum* malaria in Gambian twin children. J Infect Dis 172:316–319.

Jepson A, Sisay-Joof F, Banya W, Hassan-King M, Frodsham A, Bennett S, Hill AV, Whittle H (1997) Genetic linkage of mild malaria to the major histocompatibility complex in Gambian children: study of affected sibling pairs. BMJ 315:96–97.

Juliger S, Bongartz M, Luty AJ, Kremsner PG, Kun JF (2003) Functional analysis of a promoter variant of the gene encoding the interferon-gamma receptor chain I. Immunogenetics 54:675–680.

Kikuchi M, Looareesuwan S, Ubalee R, Tasanor O, Suzuki F, Wattanagoon Y, Na-Bangchang K, Kimura A, Aikawa M, Hirayama K (2001) Association of adhesion molecule PECAM-1/CD31 polymorphism with susceptibility to cerebral malaria in Thais. Parasitol Int 50:235–239.

Knight JC, Keating BJ, Rockett KA, Kwiatkowski DP (2003) In vivo characterization of regulatory polymorphisms by allele-specific quantification of RNA polymerase loading. Nat Genet 33:469–475.

Knight JC, Udalova I, Hill AV, Greenwood BM, Peshu N, Marsh K, Kwiatkowski D (1999) A polymorphism that affects OCT-1 binding to the TNF promoter region is associated with severe malaria. Nat Genet 22:145–150.

Koch O, Awomoyi A, Usen S, Jallow M, Richardson A, Hull J, Pinder M, Newport M, Kwiatkowski D (2002) IFNGR1 gene promoter polymorphisms and susceptibility to cerebral malaria. J Infect Dis 185:1684–1687.

Kun JF, Klabunde J, Lell B, Luckner D, Alpers M, May J, Meyer C, Kremsner PG (1999) Association of the ICAM-1Kilifi mutation with protection against severe malaria in Lambarene, Gabon. Am J Trop Med Hyg 61:776–779.

Kun JF, Mordmuller B, Lell B, Lehman LG, Luckner D, Kremsner PG (1998) Polymorphism in promoter region of inducible nitric oxide synthase gene and protection against malaria. Lancet 351:265–266.

Kun JF, Mordmuller B, Perkins DJ, May J, Mercereau-Puijalon O, Alpers M, Weinberg JB, Kremsner PG (2001) Nitric oxide synthase 2(Lambarene) (G-954C), increased nitric oxide production, and protection against malaria. J Infect Dis 184:330–336.

Kwiatkowski D (1999) Inflammatory processes in the pathogenesis of malaria. In: Wahlgen M, Perlmann P (eds), Malaria: molecular and clinical aspects, pp 329–362. Harwood Academic Publishers, Amsterdam.

Levesque MC, Hobbs MR, Anstey NM, Vaughn TN, Chancellor JA, Pole A, Perkins DJ, Misukonis MA, Chanock SJ, Granger DL, Weinberg JB (1999) Nitric oxide synthase type 2 promoter polymorphisms, nitric oxide production, and disease severity in Tanzanian children with malaria. J Infect Dis 180:1994–2002.

Luoni G, Verra F, Arca B, Sirima BS, Troye-Blomberg M, Coluzzi M, Kwiatkowski D, Modiano D (2001) Antimalarial antibody levels and IL4 polymorphism in the Fulani of West Africa. Genes Immun 2:411–414.

Luty AJ, Kun JF, Kremsner PG (1998) Mannose-binding lectin plasma levels and gene polymorphisms in *Plasmodium falciparum* malaria. J Infect Dis 178: 1221–1224.

Luzzatto L, Usanga FA, Reddy S (1969) Glucose-6-phosphate dehydrogenase deficient red cells: resistance to infection by malarial parasites. Science 164:839–842.

Mackinnon MJ, Mwangi TW, Snow RW, Marsh K, Williams TN (2005) Heritability of Malaria in Africa. PLoS Med 2:e340.

Maier AG, Duraisingh MT, Reeder JC, Patel SS, Kazura JW, Zimmerman PA, Cowman AF (2003) *Plasmodium falciparum* erythrocyte invasion through glycophorin C and selection for Gerbich negativity in human populations. Nat Med 9:87–92.

Mayor A, Bir N, Sawhney R, Singh S, Pattnaik P, Singh SK, Sharma A, Chitnis CE (2005) Receptor-binding residues lie in central regions of Duffy-binding-like domains involved in red cell invasion and cytoadherence by malaria parasites. Blood 105:2557–2563

McGuire W, Hill AV, Allsopp CE, Greenwood BM, Kwiatkowski D (1994) Variation in the TNF-alpha promoter region associated with susceptibility to cerebral malaria. Nature 371:508–510.

McGuire W, Knight JC, Hill AV, Allsopp CE, Greenwood BM, Kwiatkowski D (1999) Severe malarial anemia and cerebral malaria are associated with different tumor necrosis factor promoter alleles. J Infect Dis 179:287–290.

Meyer CG, May J, Luty AJ, Lell B, Kremsner PG (2002) TNFalpha-308A associated with shorter intervals of *Plasmodium falciparum* reinfections. Tissue Antigens 59:287–292.

Miller LH, Mason SJ, Clyde DF, McGinniss MH (1976) The resistance factor to *Plasmodium vivax* in blacks: the Duffy-blood-group genotype, FyFy. N Engl J Med 295:302–304.

Mockenhaupt FP, Ehrhardt S, Gellert S, Otchwemah RN, Dietz E, Anemana SD, Bienzle U (2004) Alpha(+)-thalassemia protects African children from severe malaria. Blood 104:2003–2006.

Modiano D, Chiucchiuini A, Petrarca V, Sirima BS, Luoni G, Perlmann H, Esposito F, Coluzzi M (1998) Humoral response to *Plasmodium falciparum* Pf155/ring-infected erythrocyte surface antigen and Pf332 in three sympatric ethnic groups of Burkina Faso. Am J Trop Med Hyg 58:220–224.

Modiano D, Chiucchiuini A, Petrarca V, Sirima BS, Luoni G, Roggero MA, Corradin G, Coluzzi M, Esposito F (1999) Interethnic differences in the humoral response to non-repetitive regions of the *Plasmodium falciparum* circumsporozoite protein. Am J Trop Med Hyg 61:663–667.

Modiano D, Luoni G, Sirima BS, Lanfrancotti A, Petrarca V, Cruciani F, Simpore J, Ciminelli BM, Foglietta E, Grisanti P, Bianco I, Modiano G, Coluzzi M (2001a) The lower susceptibility to *Plasmodium falciparum* malaria of Fulani of Burkina Faso (West Africa) is associated with low frequencies of classic malaria-resistance genes. Trans R Soc Trop Med Hyg 95:149–152.

Modiano D, Luoni G, Sirima BS, Simpore J, Verra F, Konate A, Rastrelli E, Olivieri A, Calissano C, Paganotti GM, D'Urbano L, Sanou I, Sawadogo A, Modiano G, Coluzzi M (2001b) Haemoglobin C protects against clinical *Plasmodium falciparum* malaria. Nature 414:305–308.

Modiano D, Petrarca V, Sirima BS, Nebie I, Diallo D, Esposito F, Coluzzi M (1996) Different response to *Plasmodium falciparum* malaria in West African sympatric ethnic groups. Proc Natl Acad Sci USA 93:13206–13211.

Morahan G, Boutlis CS, Huang D, Pain A, Saunders JR, Hobbs MR, Granger DL, Weinberg JB, Peshu N, Mwaikambo ED, Marsh K, Roberts DJ, Anstey NM (2002) A promoter polymorphism in the gene encoding interleukin-12 p40 (IL12B) is associated with mortality from cerebral malaria and with reduced nitric oxide production. Genes Immun 3: 414–418.

Nagayasu E, Ito M, Akaki M, Nakano Y, Kimura M, Looareesuwan S, Aikawa M (2001) CR1 density polymorphism on erythrocytes of *falciparum* malaria patients in Thailand. Am J Trop Med Hyg 64:1–5.

Ohashi J, Naka I, Patarapotikul J, Hananantachai H, Brittenham G, Looareesuwan S, Clark AG, Tokunaga K (2004) Extended linkage disequilibrium surrounding the hemoglobin E variant due to malarial selection. Am J Hum Genet 74:1198–1208.

Omi K, Ohashi J, Patarapotikul J, Hananantachai H, Naka I, Looareesuwan S, Tokunaga K (2002) Fcgamma receptor IIA and IIIB polymorphisms are associated with susceptibility to cerebral malaria. Parasitol Int 51:361–366.

Omi K, Ohashi J, Patarapotikul J, Hananantachai H, Naka I, Looareesuwan S, Tokunaga K (2003) CD36 polymorphism is associated with protection from cerebral malaria. Am J Hum Genet 72:364–374.

Orlandi PA, Klotz FW, Haynes JD (1992) A malaria invasion receptor, the 175-kilodalton erythrocyte binding antigen of *Plasmodium falciparum* recognizes the terminal Neu5Ac(alpha 2–3)Gal-sequences of glycophorin A. J Cell Biol 116:901–909.

Pain A, Urban BC, Kai O, Casals-Pascual C, Shafi J, Marsh K, Roberts DJ (2001) A non-sense mutation in Cd36 gene is associated with protection from severe malaria. Lancet 357:1502–1503.

Patel SS, King CL, Mgone CS, Kazura JW, Zimmerman PA (2004) Glycophorin C (Gerbich antigen blood group) and band 3 polymorphisms in two malaria holoendemic regions of Papua New Guinea. Am J Hematol 75:1–5.

Patel SS, Mehlotra RK, Kastens W, Mgone CS, Kazura JW, Zimmerman PA (2001) The association of the glycophorin C exon 3 deletion with ovalocytosis and malaria susceptibility in the Wosera, Papua New Guinea. Blood 98:3489–3491.

Quaye IK, Ekuban FA, Goka BQ, Adabayeri V, Kurtzhals JA, Gyan B, Ankrah NA, Hviid L, Akanmori BD (2000) Haptoglobin 1–1 is associated with susceptibility to severe *Plasmodium falciparum* malaria. Trans R Soc Trop Med Hyg 94:216–219.

Rihet P, Abel L, Traore Y, Traore-Leroux T, Aucan C, Fumoux F (1998a) Human malaria: segregation analysis of blood infection levels in a suburban area and a rural area in Burkina Faso. Genet Epidemiol 15:435–450.

Rihet P, Flori L, Tall F, Traore AS, Fumoux F (2004) Hemoglobin C is associated with reduced *Plasmodium falciparum* parasitemia and low risk of mild malaria attack. Hum Mol Genet 13:1–6.

Rihet P, Traore Y, Abel L, Aucan C, Traore-Leroux T, Fumoux F (1998b) Malaria in humans: *Plasmodium falciparum* blood infection levels are linked to chromosome 5q31-q33. Am J Hum Genet 63:498–505.

Rowe JA, Moulds JM, Newbold CI, Miller LH (1997) *P. falciparum* rosetting mediated by a parasite-variant erythrocyte membrane protein and complement-receptor 1. Nature 388:292–295.

Ruwende C, Khoo SC, Snow RW, Yates SN, Kwiatkowski D, Gupta S, Warn P, Allsopp CE, Gilbert SC, Peschu N, et al. (1995) Natural selection of hemi- and heterozygotes for G6PD deficiency in Africa by resistance to severe malaria. Nature 376:246–249.

Sabeti PC, Reich DE, Higgins JM, Levine HZ, Richter DJ, Schaffner SF, Gabriel SB, Platko JV, Patterson NJ, McDonald GJ, Ackerman HC, Campbell SJ, Altshuler D, Cooper R, Kwiatkowski D, Ward R, Lander ES (2002b) Detecting recent positive selection in the human genome from haplotype structure. Nature 419:832–837.

Sabeti P, Usen S, Farhadian S, Jallow M, Doherty T, Newport M, Pinder M, Ward R, Kwiatkowski D (2002a) CD40L association with protection from severe malaria. Genes Immun 3:286–291.

Shi YP, Nahlen BL, Kariuki S, Urdahl KB, McElroy PD, Roberts JM, Lal AA (2001) Fcgamma receptor IIa (CD32) polymorphism is associated with protection of infants against high-density *Plasmodium falciparum* infection. VII. Asembo Bay Cohort Project. J Infect Dis 184:107–111.

Stevenson MM, Riley EM (2004) Innate immunity to malaria. Nat Rev Immunol 4:169–180.

Stirnadel HA, Beck HP, Alpers MP, Smith TA (1999a) Heritability and segregation analysis of immune responses to specific malaria antigens in Papua New Guinea. Genet Epidemiol 17:16–34.

Stirnadel HA, Stockle M, Felger I, Smith T, Tanner M, Beck HP (1999b) Malaria infection and morbidity in infants in relation to genetic polymorphisms in Tanzania. Trop Med Int Health 4:187–193.

Stirnadel HA, Al-Yaman F, Genton B, Alpers MP, Smith TA (2000a) Assessment of different sources of variation in the antibody responses to specific malaria antigens in children in Papua New Guinea. Int J Epidemiol 29:579–586.

Stirnadel HA, Beck HP, Alpers MP, Smith TA (2000b) Genetic analysis of IgG subclass responses against RESA and MSP2 of *Plasmodium falciparum* in adults in Papua New Guinea. Epidemiol Infect 124:153–162.

Tishkoff SA, Varkonyi R, Cahinhinan N, Abbes S, Argyropoulos G, Destro-Bisol G, Drousiotou A, Dangerfield B, Lefranc G, Loiselet J, Piro A, Stoneking M, Tagarelli A, Tagarelli G, Touma EH, Williams SM, Clark AG (2001) Haplotype diversity and linkage disequilibrium at human G6PD: recent origin of alleles that confer malarial resistance. Science 293:455–462.

Tournamille C, Colin Y, Cartron JP, Le Van Kim C (1995) Disruption of a GATA motif in the Duffy gene promoter abolishes erythroid gene expression in Duffy-negative individuals. Nat Genet 10:224–228.

Treutiger CJ, Heddini A, Fernandez V, Muller WA, Wahlgren M (1997) PECAM-1/CD31, an endothelial receptor for binding *Plasmodium falciparum*-infected erythrocytes. Nat Med 3:1405–1408.

Urban BC, Ferguson DJ, Pain A, Willcox N, Plebanski M, Austyn JM, Roberts DJ (1999) *Plasmodium falciparum*-infected erythrocytes modulate the maturation of dendritic cells. Nature 400:73–77.

Urban BC, Willcox N, Roberts DJ (2001) A role for CD36 in the regulation of dendritic cell function. Proc Natl Acad Sci U S A 98:8750–8755.

Usanga EA, Luzzatto L (1985) Adaptation of *Plasmodium falciparum* to glucose 6-phosphate dehydrogenase-deficient host red cells by production of parasite-encoded enzyme. Nature 313:793–795.

Vigario AM, Belnoue E, Cumano A, Marussig M, Miltgen F, Landau I, Mazier D, Gresser I, Renia L (2001) Inhibition of Plasmodium yoelii blood-stage malaria by interferon alpha through the inhibition of the production of its target cell, the reticulocyte. Blood 97:3966–3971.

Walley AJ, Aucan C, Kwiatkowski D, Hill AV (2004) Interleukin-1 gene cluster polymorphisms and susceptibility to clinical malaria in a Gambian case-control study. Eur J Hum Genet 12:132–138.

Wang HY, Tang H, Shen CK, Wu CI (2003) Rapidly evolving genes in human. I. The glycophorins and their possible role in evading malaria parasites. Mol Biol Evol 20:1795–1804.

Wattavidanage J, Carter R, Perera KL, Munasingha A, Bandara S, McGuinness D, Wickramasinghe AR, Alles HK, Mendis KN, Premawansa S (1999) TNFalpha*2 marks high risk of severe disease during *Plasmodium falciparum* malaria and other infections in Sri Lankans. Clin Exp Immunol 115:350–355.

Williams TN, Maitland K, Bennett S, Ganczakowski M, Peto TE, Newbold CI, Bowden DK, Weatherall DJ, Clegg JB (1996) High incidence of malaria in alpha-thalassaemic children. Nature 383:522–525.

Williams TN, Mwangi TW, Wambua S, Peto TE, Weatherall DJ, Gupta S, Recker M, Penman BS, Uyoga S, Macharia A, Mwacharo JK, Snow RW, Marsh K (2005a) Negative epistasis between the malaria-protective effects of alpha+-thalassemia and the sickle cell trait. Nat Genet 37:1253–1257.

Williams TN, Wambua S, Uyoga S, Macharia A, Mwacharo JK, Newton CR, Maitland K (2005b) Both heterozygous and homozygous {alpha}+thalassemia protect against severe and fatal *Plasmodium falciparum* malaria on the coast of Kenya. Blood 106:368–371.

Yazdani SS, Shakri AR, Mukherjee P, Baniwal SK, Chitnis CE (2004) Evaluation of immune responses elicited in mice against a recombinant malaria vaccine based on *Plasmodium vivax* Duffy binding protein. Vaccine 22:3727–3737.

Zimmerman PA, Fitness J, Moulds JM, McNamara DT, Kasehagen LJ, Rowe JA, Hill AV (2003) CR1 Knops blood group alleles are not associated with severe malaria in the Gambia. Genes Immun 4:368–373.

25

Leishmaniasis

Alain Dessein

The Pathogens, the Diseases, and Their Relationships

The different forms of leishmaniasis are caused by the protozoan *Leishmania*, belonging to the order Kinetoplastida, family Trypanosomatidae (Lainson 1987). *Leishmania* is injected in vertebrate epidermis and dermis by female sand flies (phlebotomes) when they take their blood meal. These organisms can parasitize a wide range of vertebrate hosts, from lizards to humans. *Leishmania* is an obligate intracellular parasite that develops inside macrophage phagolysosomes. These parasites have evolved sophisticated strategies to evade destruction by a phagocytic cell that is well suited for killing microorganisms (reviewed in Olivier et al. 2005).

Leishmania causes a broad range of clinical disease in humans: simple skin ulcers, disfiguring lesions of the face, or visceral disease leading to patient death. Leishmaniasis involving superficial tissues is referred to as to cutaneous leishmaniasis (CL), and leishmaniasis caused by high levels of parasite multiplication in deep organs such as spleen and liver is referred to as visceral leishmaniasis (VL) or kala azar (KA).

CL and VL/KA are caused by different *Leishmania* species that are characterized by their respective insect vectors, geographic distributions, and pathological effects in humans. That classification is further supported by molecular markers, originally isoenzymes and more recently polymorphic DNA sequences. Based on these characteristics, *Leishmania* classification has been divided into old-world species found in the Mediterranean basin, East Africa, Middle East, and Asia, and new-world species in Central and South America.

CL is subdivided into localized CL (LCL), diffuse CL (DCL), and mucocutaneous CL (MCL). LCL refers to a few well-delimited ulcers; MCL is a severe chronic inflammation of the mucocutaneous tissues of the face with progressive destruction of palatine and nasal septum. DCL is characterized by a large number of acneiform and papular skin lesions, with very few or no parasites in the skin tissue. The host genetic background and immune response are likely critical to the arrest of the infection at the asymptomatic stage or its evolution into one of the CL forms.

Many strains of both new- and old-world *Leishmania* species can cause CL with characteristic clinical manifestations, but only certain new-world species can cause severe MCL. In contrast, diversity of VL strains is quite limited. Eventually, CL strains can cause visceral disease in certain individuals, and VL strains have also been reported to cause cutaneous lesions in certain individuals. The post-KA dermal leishmaniasis (PKDL) that develops in 20–30% of KA subjects several months after pentamidine treatment of KA is an example of cutaneous manifestations caused by VL strains (*L. donovani*, *L. infantum*).

Diagnosis of CL or VL (KA)

Diagnosis of CL is based on clinical examination (ulcers) and a positive delayed-type hypersensitivity reaction to *Leishmania* antigen (leishmanin skin test); eventually, parasite forms can be visualized on a biopsy taken from the peripherae of the lesion. Diagnosis of KA relies on clinical examination (fever, splenomegaly, anemia, lymphadenopathy) and the demonstration of the parasite, either by microscopic examination or by PCR, in bone marrow or inguinal lymph node.

Genetic Determinants of CL

Observations made in immunological studies of *Leishmania* infections are essential to the design and to the interpretation of genetic studies; this chapter summarizes immunological observations in experimental animals and in humans that could be directly relevant to the genetics of leishmaniasis.

Immunology of Human CL Infection

In humans living in North Africa, Iran, or Afghanistan, *L. major* causes cutaneous lesions that heal spontaneously in most subjects and usually confer long-lasting immunity. The cytokine secretion profile of *Leishmania*-stimulated peripheral blood morphonuclear cells (PBMCs) from subjects with nonhealing lesions (>2 years) was comparable to that of susceptible BALB/c mice (see below): they produced low amounts of interferon-γ (IFN-γ) and high amounts of interleukin-4 (IL-4) (Ajdary et al. 2000). PBMCs of subjects with active but healing lesions produced as much IFN-γ as did those of subjects who recovered from infection and produced little IL-4, such as resistant C57BL/7 mice. IFN-γ, IL-1, IL-12p40, tumor necrosis factor (TNF), transforming growth factor-β (TGF-β), and IL-10 mRNA were detected in the lesions of healing subjects, whereas IL-4 transcripts were only found in a few biopsies (Louzir et al. 1998). Healing of lesions was associated with elevated IFN-γ and low IL-4. However, large numbers of parasites were observed in lesions in the presence of IFN-γ transcripts, indicating that the effects of IFN-γ may have been partly neutralized by cytokines with anti-inflammatory properties like IL-10. The parasite must prevent macrophage activation and the release of IL-12 as well as the production of reactive oxygen intermediates (ROI) and reactive nitrogen intermediates (RNI). Macrophages parasitized by *L. donovani* fail to up-regulate MHC class II antigens and co-stimulatory molecules and do not produce inflammatory cytokines such as IL-1, IL-12; they do, however, produce TNF (Gorak et al. 1998). *Leishmania* has several ways to prevent macrophage activation and to actively inhibit it. *Leishmania* generates macrophage protein tyrosine phosphatases that cause selective dephosphorylation of tyrosyl residues and inhibition of JAK and MAPK signaling pathways, thus blocking signal transmission from IFN-γ receptor (Blanchette et al. 1999). In addition, the parasite causes proteasome-mediated degradation (Forget et al. 2005) of STAT-1, which is required for IFN-γ signal transduction and induction of IL-12Rβ2.

TGF-β and IL-10 are most likely responsible for such neutralization: IL-10 inhibits the production of RNI by IFN-γ–activated macrophages (Gazzinelli et al. 1992; Vieth et al. 1994), reduces the production of IL-12 and TNF (de Waal Malefyt et al. 1991; Fiorentino et al. 1991a,b) by activated macrophages, and deviates the T-helper (Th) response toward a Th2 response by acting on co-stimulatory molecules of antigen-presenting cells (Ding et al. 1993). TGF-β is also a potent inhibitor of T-cell–mediated immune responses (Bright et al. 1997; Kehrl et al. 1986; Schmitt et al. 1994); it inhibits macrophage microbicidal activity while enhancing parasite multiplication and virulence (Barral et al. 1993; Barral-Netto and Barral 1994). TGF-β synergizes with IL-10 and IL-4 to inhibit macrophage microbicidal activity (Oswald et al. 1992). Anti–TGF-β promotes healing in BALB/c mice infections with *L. major* (Li et al. 1999).

Although subjects with *L. braziliensis* infection mount a good delayed type hypersensitivity (DTH) response to *Leishmania* antigens, most lesions do not heal without treatment. The nonhealer phenotype is associated with production of a mixed Th1/Th2 cytokine response, with a predominant Th1 (IFN-γ, TNF) cytokine production pattern in MCL and Th2 (IL-4) pattern in DCL (Caceres-Dittmar et al. 1993). Similar findings were reported in LCL caused by *L. mexicana*: IFN-γ, TNF, IL-1, IL-10, and TGF-β are present in all lesions (Melby et al. 1994). Thus, failure of IFN-γ to provide protection in *L. mexicana* LCL again suggests neutralization by IL-10 and/or TGF-β consistent with the increase of IL-10 and TGF-β in late lesions (Melby et al. 1994). The role of IL-4 in LCL is not understood since there is no clear deviation of the Th immune response toward Th2 in LCL; IL-4 (and not IL-5), however, is associated with DCL (Caceres-Dittmar et al. 1993), which is also associated with lower IFN-γ and TNF production than LCL (Turetz et al. 2002). Compared with LCL subjects, those with MCL show enhanced Th1 cytokine production (IFN-γ and TNF) (Bacellar et al. 2002), and their PBMCs produce less IL-10, respond less to IL-10 and TGF-β (Bacellar et al. 2002), and show lower IL-10 receptor expression (Faria et al. 2005). Thus, the current view is that MCL is the consequence of a strong Th1 (IFN-γ and TNF) inflammatory response to *Leishmania* due to insufficient control by IL-10 and TGF-β of the collateral damage caused by the inflammatory response as in various other pathologies caused by chronic inflammatory stimuli (O'Garra et al. 2004)

Immunology of Experimental CL Infection

Experimental studies have been performed on congenic inbred strain of mice, especially on C57BL/6 and BALB/c mice. The injection of metacyclic promastigotes of *L. major* in footpad causes a small lesion that heals within 8–12 weeks in C57BL/6 mice and leaves the animal resistant to reinfection; BALB/c mice do not control the lesion and are not immune to reinfection (Handman et al. 1979).

Acquired resistance to *L. major* requires a Th1-type immune response (C57BL/7 mice) and production of IFN-γ by CD4$^+$ (Liew 1989; Locksley and Scott 1991) and CD8$^+$ T lymphocytes (Muller et al. 1991). IFN-γ is critical to protection against *L. major* (Belosevic et al. 1989; Sadick et al. 1986; Swihart et al. 1995; Wang

et al. 1994) by enhancing the production by macrophages of RNI toxic for *Leishmania* (Assreuy et al. 1994; Green et al. 1991). Full protection, however, requires TNF (Wilhelm et al. 2001). Natural killer (NK) cells that release IFN-γ early in the infection are critical in linking innate and acquired immunity against *L. major* (Scharton and Scott 1993).

Inhibition of IFN-γ or alterations of IFN-γ receptors (Belosevic et al. 1989, Swihart et al. 1995) abolish resistance of C57BL/6 mice. Injections of IL-4 (Chatelain et al. 1992) or constitutive IL-4 expression (Leal et al. 1993) redirects the immune response of C57BL/6 mice toward Th2 and results in progression of *L. major* infection. Nevertheless, murine cutaneous disease can be exacerbated by injection of *L. major*–specific Th1 clones (Titus et al. 1991), and this has implications for MCL. In susceptible BALB/c mice, *Leishmania* stimulates the early production of a Th2 (IL-4, IL-13) response (Heinzel et al. 1991, Launois et al. 1995); administration of anti–IL-4 antiserum to these mice causes healing or disease attenuation (Sadick et al. 1990), and interfering with Th2 development early in infection has the same effects (Corry et al. 1994, Heinzel and Rerko 1999). Double knockout IL4−/−IL13−/−(Matthews et al. 2000) BALB/c or IL4R−/−(Mohrs et al. 1999, Noben-Trauth et al. 1999) BALB/c mice heal spontaneously. Healing is variable in IL4−/−mice, and the healing is more dramatic in IL4R−/−(Mohrs et al. 1999; Noben-Trauth et al. 1999) than in IL4−/−or IL13−/−mice, suggesting synergies between IL-4 and IL-13. Overexpression of IL-13 or IL-4 causes suppression of IL-12 and IFN-γ in C57BL/6 mice and renders them susceptible (Matthews et al. 2000). In addition to its effects on Th1 differentiation, IL-4 abrogates macrophage activation by IFN-γ (Liew et al. 1989). IL-12 is essential in the induction of an anti-*Leishmania* Th1 response (Heinzel et al. 1993; Sypek et al. 1993); however, early IL-12 response has not been observed in all resistant strains of mice (Reiner et al. 1994; Scharton-Kersten et al. 1995), and IL-12 protective effects may not all depend on IFN-γ ?(Heinzel et al. 1993), because anti–IL-4 and anti–IFN-γ (Sadick et al. 1990)–treated mice show some resistance, and IL-4 produced early in the infection in BALB/c mice and downregulated IL-12Rβ2, contributing to unresponsiveness to IL-12 (Himmelrich et al. 1998).

Recent work, however, has revealed some heterogeneity among *L. major* strains: growth of certain substrains in IL4R−/−BALB/c mice and restoration of protection with anti–IL-10R injections or by knocking out *IL10* (IL10–/–IL4R–/–mice) (Noben-Trauth et al. 2003). Furthermore, an *L. major* strain (Sd strain) isolated from a patient with nonhealing lesions was shown to grow well in C57BL/6 mice mounting a normal Th1 response. Protection was partially restored in IL10–/–C57BL/6 mice or in CD25$^+$ cell–depleted animals (Anderson et al. 2005). Furthermore, resistant mice harboring a transgene encoding IL-10 are less resistant to common *L. major* strains, and *L. major*–infected C57BL/6 mice injected with anti–IL-10R antibody achieved sterile cure (Belkaid et al. 2001). In short, IL-10 appears to abrogate protection conferred by Th1 cytokines.

Thus, both IL-10 and TGF-β play key roles in regulating the anti-*Leishmania* immune response by limiting both collateral damage due to extreme inflammation and parasite destruction. Many cells, monocytes, B cells, dendritic cells (DCs), Th2 cells, and even Th1 cells can produce IL-10 and TGF-β; these cytokines are likely produced by more than one cell type involved in the infection (Moore et al. 1993). Recent studies have emphasized that IL-10–producing CD4$^+$CD25$^+$ T-regulatory cells regulate the immune response in *L. major*–and *L. amazonensis*–infected mice (Ji et al. 2005) and that these TGF-β–secreting CD24$^+$CD45$^+$ cells can be generated by *in vitro* exposure of PBMCs from subjects who are not immune to *L. guyanensis* antigens (Kariminia et al. 2005). More work is needed to evaluate the role of CD4$^+$CD25$^+$ T-regulatory cells in the control of infection and disease. Interestingly, however, their elimination allowed total clearance of *L. major* infection in mice (Belkaid et al. 2002), supporting the view that IL-10–producing T–regulatory cells may play an important role in maintaining immunity to reinfection.

Immunogenetic Determinants of Human CL Infection

Several researchers have reported a family clustering of CL cases that suggests a hereditary component in disease, although it is impossible to rule out family concentration due to heavy environmental exposure since transmission is often very focal. Nevertheless, immunological studies have identified resistant families living in close proximity with others who were heavily affected. Segregation analysis was used to detect a major genetic effect.

In populations infected by *L. peruviana* (Shaw et al. 1995), a two-locus model best explained the distribution of severe (as opposed to resistant) individuals in 636 nuclear families. The model included a recessive gene and a modifier gene. Working in a population that recently migrated to an endemic area of *L. braziliensis*, Dedet and colleagues measured the time elapsed between arrival in the endemic region and the onset of the lesion. Evidence for a recessive major gene controlling the onset of the primary cutaneous lesion in new migrants was obtained (Alcais et al. 1997). There was no evidence for a genetic control of CL in the native population that had been living in the region for several generations. No confirmation of the existence of these loci by linkage studies has been reported.

Studies of association with human leukocyte antigen (HLA) markers have yielded positive associations between HLA-Cw7 and LCL (*L. braziliensis*) (Barbier et al. 1987) in French Guiana, between HLA-DQw3 and HLA-Bw22 and LCL in families of Venezuela (Lara et al. 1991), and between DRB1*0407, DPA1*0401, and DPB1*0101 and LCL caused by *L. mexicana* in Mexico (Olivo-Diaz et al. 2004) (table 25.1). Mucosal lesions were associated with a decreased frequency of HLA-DR2 and an increased frequency of HLA-DQw3 (Petzl-Erler et al. 1991). Thus, several studies point to a role for HLA class II alleles in susceptibility to LCL and MCL; such results are remarkable in contrast to the lack of associations between VL and HLA loci (see below).

TNF is produced in MCL lesions, suggesting that it could contribute to the deleterious Th1-mediated inflammation in MCL patients (see above). This hypothesis is supported by the report of an association between allele TNF-308A and a 3.2-fold increase of the risk of MCL in a Venezuelan population infected by *L. braziliensis*. Furthermore, a 7.5-fold higher risk of MCL was reported for subjects carrying a high-producing allele of the lymphotoxin gene *LT* (Cabrera et al. 1995). The effects of the *TNF* and *LT* alleles were apparently independent of each other and also independent of polymorphisms in the closely linked MHC class II gene cluster. The functional effects of these polymorphisms on gene transcription and TNF or LT production are still being debated, and other polymorphisms in the same or adjacent genes may actually be responsible for the observed effects. Nevertheless, this and observations that TNF is elevated in the serum of MCL patient lend strong support to the view that TNF contributes to the exaggerated Th1 response in MCL.

More recently we have demonstrated that the C allele of IL10–819 C/T was associated with an in-

TABLE 25.1. Genes and genetic loci linked or associated with human susceptibility to leishmaniasis: localized cutaneous (LCL), mucocutaneous (MCL), or visceral (KA).

Disease/Leishmania Strain	Region (Gene)	Allele	Population	Reference
LCL				
L. braziliensis	HLA	Cw7	Guiana	Barbier et al (1987)
L. braziliensis	HLA	DQw3, Bw22	Venezuela	Lara et al (1991)
L. mexicana	HLA	DRB1, DPA1, DPB1	Mexico	Olivo-Diaz et al (2004)
MCL				
L. braziliensis	HLA	DR2, DQw3	Brazil	Petzl-Erler et al (1991)
L. braziliensis	TNF (7124)	−308A	Venezuela	Cabrera et al (1995)
L. braziliensis	LTA (4049)	SNP in intron 2	Venezuela	Cabrera et al (1995)
KA				
L. donovani	22q12		Sudan	Bucheton et al (2003a)
L. donovani	SLC11A1 (6556)		Sudan	Bucheton et al (2003b)
L. donovani	SLC11A1 (6556)		Sudan	Mohamed et al (2003)
L. donovani	IL4 (3565)	IL4RP2	Sudan	Mohamed et al (2003)

creased risk of cutaneous lesions in *L. braziliensis* infections (A. Salhi, unpublished observations). The C/C genotype was associated with increased IL-10 production and the sequence of the -819 C and T alleles bound different nuclear factors in the EMSA. This result, together with observations in experimental models, demonstrates that IL-10 plays a significant role in the control of skin lesions in human infected by *L. braziliensis*.

Immunogenetic Determinants of Experimental CL Infection

Mouse inbred strains can be classified as resistant, intermediate, susceptible, and very susceptible to *L. major* infection (Bradley 1987; Bradley and Kirkley 1977; Bradley et al. 1979; Kellina 1973). BALB/c mice are susceptible and allow parasite metastasis and visceralization, DBA/2 is intermediate, and C57BL/6 C3H, AKR, and CBA are resistant. DBA/2 mice that are susceptible to *L. major* are resistant to *L. mexicana* (Perez et al. 1978, 1979); BALB/c is highly susceptible to both *L. major* and *L. tropica*, but the latter causes smaller lesions in mice. This indicates strain-specific genetic factors and probably polygenic control of lesion size. Analysis of the segregation of the susceptibility trait in F_1 and F_2 progenies in various combinations of resistant and susceptible mice showed a control of cutaneous lesions by several loci referred as to *Scl*

(susceptibility to CL) (Bradley and Kirkley 1977). *Scl-1* was described as controlling lesions caused by *L. major*; *Scl-1* and *Scl-2* (Roberts et al. 1990) control lesions caused by *L. mexicana*. In addition, the locus *H-11* first described in the control of visceralizing *Leishmania* strains was also shown to control cutaneous lesions caused by *L. major* (Blackwell et al. 1985). *Scl* loci do not influence infections by KA strains. However, genetic loci (*Lsh*, *H-2*, and *H-11*) that control visceralization of KA strains influence the visceralization of CL strains in deep organs of mice, such as spleen and liver (Blackwell et al. 1985; Roberts et al. 1989). In humans, CL strains do not normally visceralize.

Scl-1 was mapped to (mouse) chromosome 8, and several groups have confirmed the effects of the H-2 locus (Blackwell 1986; Howard et al. 1980; Mitchell et al. 1981). The early *L. major* lesion expansion locus (*Scl-1*) was located on chromosome 11, and the study also suggested an additional locus on chromosome 11 controlling infection (Roberts et al. 1993). In a subsequent study, a nonparametric quantitative trait locus (QTL) analysis showed linkage of lesion score severity to a chromosome 9 locus and to a region including the MHC locus on chromosome 17 (Roberts et al. 1997); this study failed, however, to detect linkage to chromosome 11. Interestingly, the chromosome 9 locus overlies the IL-10 receptor gene, and H2 is right at the QTL peak on chromosome 17. The same group also reported a susceptibility locus close to CD40 on chromosome X, the effect of which depended on chromosome 17 alleles on and epistatic interactions between the loci on chromosomes 17 and 9 (Roberts et al. 1999).

Multiple additional loci showed a high frequency of heterozygosity in resistant backcrossed mice (Beebe et al. 1997). Various combinations of alleles could confer resistance, and no single locus was required. In an attempt to confirm these loci by transmission disequilibrium testing, only the loci on mouse chromosomes 6, 11, and 15 reached a suggestive level of linkage. However, when tested as pairs of candidate loci, other loci showed linkage, suggesting interaction between one or more loci to produce measurable effects. Finally, single congenic lines were derived with single or paired candidate loci, confirming the presence of resistance genes on chromosomes 6 and 11 and suggesting additional resistance loci on other chromosomes (Beebe et al. 1999).

Another group of investigators (Gorham et al. 1996) has attempted to identify the genes controlling IL-12 responsiveness in crosses that eliminated genetic diversity linked to antigen recognition/presentation. A single locus was mapped to chromosome 11 in the region spanning the Th2 cytokine locus (Il4, 5, 13) along with Il9, Irf1 and Il12b (a gene known to encode natural killer cell stimulatory factor, IL-12p40). That locus determined the maintenance of responsiveness to IL-12 by CD4$^+$ (OVA TcR) T lymphocytes in culture.

Demant and colleagues have created recombinant lines (referred as to RC lines), congenic strains each carrying a different random set of 12.5% of the genes from a resistant (STS/A) strain on a BALB/c background (Demant and Hart 1986; Moen et al. 1991). The analysis of different clinical phenotypes (lesion, hepatomegaly, splenomegaly) and serum immunological parameters (including IgE) in F_2 of BALB/c × resistant RC indicated that clinical and immunological phenotypes were determined by at least five additional loci (Lipoldova et al. 2000). Skin lesions were found to be influenced by two loci, and a third locus was associated with splenomegaly and hepatomegaly and IgE levels (Badalova et al. 2002; Lipoldova et al. 2002). Other loci controlling serum levels of cytokines were also reported. The presence of a locus on chromosome 11 (Scl1) was not confirmed. In a second study, these researchers mapped three additional loci: one for skin lesions and two others for hepatosplenomegaly (Vladimirov et al. 2003).

In summary, various loci have been reported to control of clinical and immunological phenotypes in

L. major infections in mice. No specific genes controlling any phenotypes have been identified yet in these genetic regions. Whether these genetic loci will be the same in infections with more pathogenic Leishmania strains is unclear.

Genetic Determinants of KA

Immunology of Human KA Infection

Most immunological studies on human KA have been performed on subjects infected with L. chagasi in Brazil and with L. donovani in Sudan. Patients with acute KA due to L. chagasi exhibit a marked depression of cellular immunity, a low reactivity in blastogenesis assays against Leishmania antigen, a low production of IL-2 and of Th1 cytokines IFN-γ and IL-12. These patients, unlike CL patients, fail to mount a delayed-type hypersensitivity reaction to parasite antigen. In contrast, IL-10 and IL-4 are up-regulated (Carvalho et al. 1985; Ghalib et al. 1995), and KA patients exhibit high serum levels of parasite-specific antibodies, TNF (Barral-Netto et al. 1991), and IL-6. Recovery after treatment is associated with a return to a normal immune response, including the production of IFN-γ by PBMCs and a positive leishmanin skin test. That IFN-γ plays a key role in protection is also indicated by patient improvement after a treatment combining IFN-γ and meglumine antimoniate (Badaro et al. 1990). Evidence for a role of T cells in suppressing the immune response of PBMC during acute disease has been presented (Carvalho et al. 1989). Studies with KA patients infected with L. donovani in Sudan (Karp et al. 1993) have detected high levels of IFN-γ and IL-10 transcripts in bone marrow aspirate; IFN-γ was not, however, detected in culture of Leishmania antigen–stimulated PBMCs from the patients. The resolution of disease was associated with a decrease of IL-10 transcripts (Karp et al. 1993) and addition of anti–IL-10 in cultures of PBMCs from KA patients enhanced IFN-γ production (Ghalib et al. 1995), indicating that IL-10 may contribute to the suppression of the Th1 response. Similar observations on IL-10 were reported in L. chagasi infections (Bacellar et al. 1996). Most interesting, the addition of IL-12 restores IFN-γ production and increases NK cytotoxic activity in PBMC of KA subjects (L. chagasi (Bacellar et al. 1996) or L. donovani (Ghalib et al. 1995), indicating that the inhibition of IL-12 production is likely crucial in the suppression of the immune response in KA patients. Thus, studies conducted on both *L. donovani* and *L. chagasi* infections strongly suggest that IL-10 and IL-12 play opposite crucial roles in immunity to infection by KA *Leishmania* strains. IL-10 could also play an important role in influencing the cutaneous lesions observed in 20–30% of subjects weeks or months after the completion of pentamidine treatment. PKDL is an inflammatory reaction directed against the parasite in the skin that shows infiltration by CD3$^+$ lymphocytes and production of IL-10 and IFN-γ. IL-10 appears to be the most prominent cytokine, and IL-4 transcripts are also found in some lesions (Ismail et al. 1999).

Immunology of Experimental KA Infection

The initial site of parasite multiplication of KA *Leishmania* strains in deep organs is the liver, while the spleen allows the long-term persistence of the parasite. Such a tissue pattern is probably relevant to the early hepatic stage of human KA and to the persistence of the parasite after chemotherapy in human KA. *L. donovani* is first ingested by liver Kupffer cells, where they multiply. Kupffer cells are permissive for *Leishmania* since they do not produce ROI and do not respond to IFN-γ *Leishmania* overgrowth is likely controlled by Th cells recruiting, and activating monocytes, eosinophils and neutrophils during the first four weeks of infection. Resolution of the infection after four weeks probably requires lysis of infected Kupffer cells by cytolytic cells either the CD8$^+$ T cells that are present in large number in the tissue at this time or other killing cells activated by CD8$^+$ T-cell secretory products (McElrath et al. 1988).

Mouse capacity to control *L. donovani* infection correlates with the capacity of T cells to secrete macrophage activating cytokines and with the development of IFN-γ and IL-12 responses (Murray et al. 1982, 1987). Local production of IFN-γ in *L. chagasi*–infected BALB/c mice inversely correlates with parasite multiplication: A low production of IFN-γ in liver granulomas is associated with parasite multiplication in liver; large amounts of IFN-γ are produced in the spleen, where parasite multiplication is controlled (Wilson et al. 1996). IFN-γ increases the production of ROI and RNI via NADPH oxidase and iNOS pathways and is critical in the induction of the Th1 response. ROI and RNI act together in the killing of the parasite in the early phase of the infection and also in regulating monocyte recruitment in parasitized tissues. RNI alone are required for the control of the late phase of infection (Murray and Nathan 1999): ROI-but not RNI-deficient mice fully control parasite multiplication, and granulomas show no evidence of activity against the parasite in RNI deficient mice (Murray and Nathan 1999).

*IL12−/−*C57BL/6 mice display higher parasite load in both liver and spleen (Satoskar et al. 2000), and this effect correlates with less inflammation and disorganized granuloma. Splenocytes from *IL12−/−* animals produce less IFN-γ and more IL-4. Repeated injections of IL-12 reduce liver parasite burden in "susceptible" BALB/c mice; this effect was dependent on CD4$^+$CD8$^+$ T cells, IFN-γ, IL-2, and TNF (Murray and Hariprashad 1995); conversely, IL-12 neutralization in BALB/c causes delayed resolution of parasite load, transient reduction in hepatic and splenic IFN-γ/TNF-producing cells, decreased NOS2 transcription, and suppressed granuloma formation (Engwerda et al. 1998). *L. donovani* inhibits IL-12 production in macrophage but not in DCs, suggesting that DC together with NK cells are probably critical in the induction of the Th1 response early in the infection (Gorak et al. 1998).

Susceptibility or relapse after treatment is not associated with marked Th2 response. Unlike CL infections, IL-4 is not critical in experimental infections by KA strains (Kaye and Bancroft 1992; Kaye et al. 1991; Miralles et al. 1994): Injections of anti–IL-4 antibodies or disruption of IL-4 does not accelerate the resolution of the infection (Satoskar et al. 1995). TNF produced by macrophages early in the infection (Gorak et al. 1998) is critical in protection against *L. donovani*. TNF-deficient mice (Murray et al. 2000) or anti-TNF–treated mice (Tumang et al. 1994) show a marked increase in parasite liver burden. The granulomatous reaction is aggravated in the late stage of the infection in TNF−/−mice, causing severe inflammation, widespread tissue necrosis, and death by 10 weeks (Murray et al. 2000). This differs from the reduced inflammation and the granuloma disorganization observed in IL-12– and IFN-γ–deficient mice (see below), in which pathology is decreased. LT−/−mice also show increased susceptibility to infection but acquire resistance later, clear the parasite, and survive. The effects of TNF deficiency are due to the many pleiotropic properties of these cytokines on macrophage microbicidal capacity, tissue remodeling, and modulation of signals that determine leukocyte migration and positioning in tissues (reviewed in (Kaye et al. 2004).

TNF decreases CCL21 and CCL19 from periarteriolar lymphoid sheath cells causing mislocalization of DCs expressing CCR7. Furthermore, CCR7/CCL21 guide T cell exit from the skin and entry into afferent lymphatics (Bromley et al. 2005). DC migration is also probably further impaired by IL-10 that reduces CCR7 expression on DC. The inhibition of CCR7 expression on DC caused by TNF-induced IL-10 increases mouse susceptibility to infection by *L. donovani* (Ato et al. 2002).

Treatment with anti–IL-10 antibody does not affect IFN-γ in granuloma but increases IFN-γ in splenocyte culture (Wilson et al. 1996), indicating that suppression of IFN-γ in liver is probably not mediated by IL-10. IL-10 may play a more important role in the control of *L. donovani* infections since IL-10−/−BALB/c mice efficiently control parasite multiplication both in spleen and liver. Enhanced protection is associated with increased nitric oxide and IFN-γ production (Murphy et al. 2001).

TGF-β levels are high in hepatic granuloma from *L. chagasi*–infected BALB/c mice but low in granuloma from resistant C3H mice and overexpressing TGF-β decreased resistance of C3H mice. Thus, TGF-β is likely mediating suppression of IFN-γ in *L. chagasi*–infected livers (Wilson et al. 1998).

Genetic Determinants of Experimental Infections by KA Strains

As discussed above, Bradley, Blackwell, and collaborators (Blackwell 1986; Bradley 1987; Bradley and Kirkley 1977; Bradley et al. 1979) have analyzed the genetic basis of resistance/susceptibility to *Leishmania* infections of mouse congenic lines. Segregation of the phenotype "parasite burden at 15 days," in the progeny of a cross of resistant x susceptible animals showed control by a single locus *Lsh* that was mapped on mouse chromosome 1. Further studies identified two additional loci (H-2 and H-11) that are involved later in the infection (Blackwell et al. 1980, 1983, 1985). The analysis could not dissociate *Lsh* from two other loci controlling susceptibility to certain mycobacterium (locus *Bcg*) and Salmonella (locus *Ity*) infections. The fact that these pathogens reside in macrophage phagosome and neutralize macrophage anti-microbicidal activity suggested that the loci *Ity Lsh* and *Bcg* could be a single locus of control of pathogens developing in the phagolysosome. Positional cloning identified *Nramp1* (now *Slc11a1*) as a possible candidate for the control of

infection, and nucleotide sequence analysis showed that a single mutation (a G to A substitution at nucleotide position 783) resulted in the non-conservative replacement of Gly^{105} to Asp^{105} within the second transmembrane domain of the Nramp1 protein. The association was found in 20 resistant and 7 susceptible mouse strains (reviewed in Malo et al. 1994). Gene disruption (Vidal et al. 1995) and the use of transgenic (Govoni et al. 1996) established that *Slc11a1* (*Nramp1*) was indeed Bcg/Lsh /Ity. *Slc11a1* encodes a 90–100 KDa integral membrane protein containing 12 hydrophobic transmembrane regions and a heavily glycosylated extracellular loop. The Nramp1 protein is expressed in late endosome and lysosome membranes in macrophages. The function of the Nramp1 protein is still the subject of debate (Wyllie et al. 2002; see chapter 13 in this volume).

Immunogenetic Determinants of Human VL

Studies conducted in populations exposed to *L. donovani* in Sudan (Bucheton et al. 2002) and *L. chagasi* in Brazil (Cabello et al. 1995) have shown that KA is concentrated in certain families. A segregation analysis in Brazil (Peacock et al. 2001) indicated that KA was determined by a major genetic locus. To date, the presence of this locus has not been confirmed by linkage analysis. A study in a population of Sudan infected by *L. donovani* showed that polygenic control was more likely than control by a single locus in KA caused by *L. donovani* (Bucheton et al. 2003a). Higher prevalence of KA cases in certain ethnic groups (Bucheton et al. 2002, Ibrahim et al. 1999) living in the same geographic area including in the same village is also suggestive of a hereditary component since these studies show that exposure to *Leishmania* is comparable between ethnic groups (Bucheton et al. 2002).

Various studies that have tested association or linkage between HLA and KA in *L. chagasi* (Peacock et al. 2002), *L. infantum* (Meddeb-Garnaoui et al. 2001), and *L. donovani* (Bucheton et al. 2003b; Singh et al. 1997) infections have failed to detect effects of these genes.

Two recent studies in Sudan have analyzed the control of KA in endemic populations. The first study was carried out during an outbreak of *L. donovani* in a village of the Ethiopian–Sudanese border (SH et al. 2002). Although >90% of the villagers showed immunological evidence of infection, only 30% developed visceral disease. Phenotypes were defined by clinical and parasitological examination. Certain families and certain ethnic groups were more affected than others. An attempt to demonstrate that this familial/ethnic component was due to a major genetic effect by segregation analysis was unsuccessful. A linkage study that tested linkage with a few genetic regions found no linkage with regions containing the HLA/TNF (MHC), IFN-γ (12q15), IFN-γ receptor (6q23-q24), or Th2 cytokine (5q32-q33) locus (Bucheton et al. 2003b). However, linkage (LOD score = 1.32, $p = 0.007$) with a 5′ polymorphism in SLC11A1 (the human gene for Nramp1, mapped to 2q35) was observed (Bucheton et al. 2003b).

A genomewide scan performed on 169 affected children (63 families) uncovered a locus on chromosome 22q12 (LOD = 3.5, $p = 3 \times 10^{-5}$ in all patients; LOD = 3.9, $p = 10^{-5}$ in patients affected early in the outbreak) and possibly a second nearby genetic locus controlling susceptibility to KA (Bucheton et al. 2003a). Based on the size of the study sample, the contribution of the 22q12 locus to the control of VL is likely to be important.

Another study was also carried out in an area of eastern Sudan, 70 km away from the above-described population (Ibrahim et al. 1999). VL phenotypes were defined by clinical and immunological evaluation. Higher susceptibility in certain ethnic groups was also observed. This study replicated the linkage observed by Bucheton et al. (2003b) with polymorphisms in SLC11A1 and demonstrated that the main effect was contributed by a single nucleotide polymorphism (SNP) in intron 4 (Mohamed et al. 2004). These polymorphisms had tentatively been associated with susceptibility to tuberculosis (see chapter 22 in this volume). Since the extent of linkage disequilibrium upstream the promoter region has not been determined, a polymorphism outside the tested region could be responsible for the observed association. However, this is unlikely given the large body of literature on the role of the SLC11A1 ortholog in both mouse and human susceptibility to intracellular pathogens, including L. donovani. Thus, these results indicate a contribution of SLC11A1 to the susceptibility to KA in Sudanese subjects (Aringa and Massalit, which are close ethnic groups). The same group also reported a linkage of VL with two SNPs in IL4 (best LOD = 1.8, $p = 0.002$) that was confirmed by transmission disequilibrium test (TDT) and case–(pseudo)control analysis ($p = 0.008$) (Mohamed et al. 2003). Thus, VL is likely associated with a polymorphism in IL4 or a gene close to it.

Finally, the same study showed weak linkage of polymorphisms in IFNGR1 (LOD = 0.7, $p = 0.03$) with PKDL. An association analysis using the TDT also provided consistent results (Mohamed et al. 2003). The suggestive linkage of PKDL with IFNGR1 is interesting since the latter locus has been linked to control of susceptibility to severe schistosomiasis and to atypical disseminated mycobacteria infections.

Conclusions

The Leishmania genus consists of a large variety of genetically different parasites that cause different cutaneous and visceral diseases. For each Leishmania species, molecular epidemiological and immunological investigation has shown intraspecies heterogeneity that is associated with different virulence. Such large Leishmania heterogeneity in endemic populations contrasts with the relative homogeneity in schistosomes and could complicate the search for human genes involved in susceptibility. Human geneticists are now awaiting the identification of susceptibility genes in experimental models of infections. In no other infectious disease than leishmaniasis do investigators have more excellent experimental work to stimulate and guide human studies. In this regard, the lessons from the story of SLC11A1 (NRAMP1) continue to stimulate human and mouse geneticists working on leishmaniasis.

Finally, Leishmania species cause severe diseases, and populations fear infection by parasites such as L. braziliensis or L. donovani. Leishmaniasis has considerable social and medical impact, and it is urgent to develop effective, nontoxic, and inexpensive treatments against these diseases. Immunogenetic research will facilitate the identification of new targets for chemotherapy and vaccination. Drugs targeted at host genetic defects are less likely than pathogen-targeted drugs to generate resistant parasites. Genetic studies will also allow the identification of subjects at high risk of severe disease. Such subjects will benefit from targeted prophylactic measures; their careful, separate evaluation in drug and vaccine trials will also be informative.

References

Ajdary, S., Alimohammadian, M.H., Eslami, M.B., Kemp, K., & Kharazmi, A. (2000) Comparison of the immune profile of nonhealing cutaneous leishmaniasis patients with those with active lesions and those who have recovered from infection. *Infect Immun,* 68, 1760–1764.

Alcais, A., Abel, L., David, C., Torrez, M.E., Flandre, P., & Dedet, J.P. (1997) Evidence for a major gene controlling susceptibility to tegumentary leishmaniasis in a recently exposed Bolivian population. *Am J Hum Genet,* 61, 968–979.

Anderson, C.F., Mendez, S., & Sacks, D.L. (2005) Non-healing infection despite Th1 polarization produced by a strain of *Leishmania major* in C57BL/6 mice. *J Immunol,* 174, 2934–2941.

Assreuy, J., Cunha, F.Q., Epperlein, M., Noronha-Dutra, A., O'Donnell, C.A., Liew, F.Y., & Moncada, S. (1994) Production of nitric oxide and superoxide by activated macrophages and killing of *Leishmania major. Eur J Immunol,* 24, 672–676.

Ato, M., Stager, S., Engwerda, C.R. & Kaye, P.M. (2002) Defective CCR7 expression on dendritic cells contributes to the development of visceral leishmaniasis. *Nat Immunol* 3, 1185–1191.

Bacellar, O., Brodskyn, C., Guerreiro, J., Barral-Netto, M., Costa, C.H., Coffman, R.L., Johnson, W.D., & Carvalho, E.M. (1996) Interleukin-12 restores interferon-gamma production and cytotoxic responses in visceral leishmaniasis. *J Infect Dis,* 173, 1515–1518.

Bacellar, O., Lessa, H., Schriefer, A., Machado, P., Ribeiro de Jesus, A., Dutra, W.O., Gollob, K.J., & Carvalho, E.M. (2002) Up-regulation of Th1-type responses in mucosal leishmaniasis patients. *Infect Immun,* 70, 6734–6740.

Badalova, J., Svobodova, M., Havelkova, H., Vladimirov, V., Vojtiskova, J., Engova, J., Pilcik, T., Volf, P., Demant, P., & Lipoldova, M. (2002) Separation and mapping of multiple genes that control IgE level in *Leishmania major* infected mice. *Genes Immun,* 3, 187–195.

Badaro, R., Falcoff, E., Badaro, F.S., Carvalho, E.M., Pedral-Sampaio, D., Barral, A., Carvalho, J.S., Barral-Netto, M., Brandely, M., Silva, L., et al. (1990) Treatment of visceral leishmaniasis with pentavalent antimony and interferon gamma. *N Engl J Med,* 322, 16–21.

Barbier, D., Demenais, F., Lefait, J.F., David, B., Blanc, M., Hors, J., & Feingold, N. (1987) Susceptibility to human cutaneous leishmaniasis and HLA, Gm, Km markers. *Tissue Antigens,* 30, 63–67.

Barral, A., Barral-Netto, M., Yong, E.C., Brownell, C.E., Twardzik, D.R., & Reed, S.G. (1993) Transforming growth factor beta as a virulence mechanism for *Leishmania braziliensis. Proc Natl Acad Sci USA,* 90, 3442–3446.

Barral-Netto, M., & Barral, A. (1994) Transforming growth factor-beta in tegumentary leishmaniasis. *Braz J Med Biol Res,* 27, 1–9.

Barral-Netto, M., Badaro, R., Barral, A., Almeida, R.P., Santos, S.B., Badaro, F., Pedral-Sampaio, D., Carvalho, E.M., Falcoff, E., & Falcoff, R. (1991) Tumor necrosis factor (cachectin) in human visceral leishmaniasis. *J Infect Dis,* 163, 853–857.

Beebe, A.M., Cua, D.J., & Coffman, R.L. (1999) Genetic control of T helper subset differentiation in *Leishmania major* infection of mice. *Microbes Infect,* 1, 89–94.

Beebe, A.M., Mauze, S., Schork, N.J., & Coffman, R.L. (1997) Serial backcross mapping of multiple loci associated with resistance to *Leishmania major* in mice. *Immunity,* 6, 551–557.

Belkaid, Y., Hoffmann, K.F., Mendez, S., Kamhawi, S., Udey, M.C., Wynn, T.A., & Sacks, D.L. (2001) The role of interleukin (IL)-10 in the persistence of *Leishmania major* in the skin after healing and the therapeutic potential of anti-IL-10 receptor antibody for sterile cure. *J Exp Med,* 194, 1497–1506.

Belkaid, Y., Piccirillo, C.A., Mendez, S., Shevach, E.M., & Sacks, D.L. (2002) CD4+CD25+ regulatory T cells control *Leishmania major* persistence and immunity. *Nature,* 420, 502–507.

Belosevic, M., Finbloom, D.S., Van Der Meide, P.H., Slayter, M.V., & Nacy, C.A. (1989) Administration of monoclonal anti-IFN-gamma antibodies in vivo abrogates natural resistance of C3H/HeN mice to infection with *Leishmania major. J Immunol,* 143, 266–274.

Blackwell, J., Freeman, J., & Bradley, D. (1980) Influence of H-2 complex on acquired resistance to *Leishmania donovani* infection in mice. *Nature,* 283, 72–74.

Blackwell, J.M. (1983) Regulation of *Leishmania* populations within the host. V. Resistance to *L. donovani* in wild mice. *J Trop Med Hyg,* 86, 17–22.

Blackwell, J.M. (1986) *Different host genes recognize and control infection with taxonomically distinct* Leishmania *species.* Institut Méditerranéen d'Études Épidémiologiques et Écologiques, Montpellier.

Blackwell, J.M., Hale, C., Roberts, M.B., Ulczak, O.M., Liew, F.Y., & Howard, J.G. (1985) An H-11-linked gene has a parallel effect on *Leishmania major* and L. *donovani* infections in mice. *Immunogenetics,* 21, 385–395.

Blanchette, J., Racette, N., Faure, R., Siminovitch, K.A., & Olivier, M. (1999) *Leishmania*-induced increases in activation of macrophage SHP-1 tyrosine phosphatase are associated with impaired IFN-gamma-triggered JAK2 activation. *Eur J Immunol,* 29, 3737–3744.

Bradley, D.J. (1987) Genetics of susceptibility and resistance in the vertebrate host. In: *The Leishmaniases in Biology and Medicine* (ed. by W. Peters & R. Killick-Kendrick), vol. 2. Academic Press, London.

Bradley, D.J., & Kirkley, J. (1977) Regulation of *Leishmania* populations within the host. I. The variable course of *Leishmania donovani* infections in mice. *Clin Exp Immunol*, 30, 119–129.

Bradley, D.J., Taylor, B.A., Blackwell, J., Evans, E.P., & Freeman, J. (1979) Regulation of *Leishmania* populations within the host. III. Mapping of the locus controlling susceptibility to visceral leishmaniasis in the mouse. *Clin Exp Immunol*, 37, 7–14.

Bright, J.J., Kerr, L.D., & Sriram, S. (1997) TGF-beta inhibits IL-2-induced tyrosine phosphorylation and activation of Jak-1 and Stat 5 in T lymphocytes. *J Immunol*, 159, 175–183.

Bromley, S.K., Thomas, S.Y. & Luster, A.D. (2005) Chemokine receptor CCR7 guides T cell exit from peripheral tissues and entry into afferent lymphatics. *Nat Immunol* 6, 895–901.

Bucheton, B., Abel, L., El-Safi, S., Kheir, M.M., Pavek, S., Lemainque, A., & Dessein, A.J. (2003a) A major susceptibility locus on chromosome 22q12 plays a critical role in the control of kala-azar. *Am J Hum Genet*, 73, 1052–1060.

Bucheton, B., Abel, L., Kheir, M.M., Mirgani, A., El-Safi, S.H., Chevillard, C., & Dessein, A. (2003b) Genetic control of visceral leishmaniasis in a Sudanese population: candidate gene testing indicates a linkage to the NRAMP1 region. *Genes Immun*, 4, 104–109.

Bucheton, B., Kheir, M.M., El-Safi, S.H., Hammad, A., Mergani, A., Mary, C., Abel, L., & Dessein, A. (2002) The interplay between environmental and host factors during an outbreak of visceral leishmaniasis in eastern Sudan. *Microbes Infect*, 4, 1449–1457.

Cabello, P.H., Lima, A.M., Azevedo, E.S., & Krieger, H. (1995) Familial aggregation of *Leishmania chagasi* infection in northeastern Brazil. *Am J Trop Med Hyg*, 52, 364–365.

Cabrera, M., Shaw, M.A., Sharples, C., Williams, H., Castes, M., Convit, J., & Blackwell, J.M. (1995) Polymorphism in tumor necrosis factor genes associated with mucocutaneous leishmaniasis. *J Exp Med*, 182, 1259–1264.

Caceres-Dittmar, G., Tapia, F.J., Sanchez, M.A., Yamamura, M., Uyemura, K., Modlin, R.L., Bloom, B.R., & Convit, J. (1993) Determination of the cytokine profile in American cutaneous leishmaniasis using the polymerase chain reaction. *Clin Exp Immunol*, 91, 500–505.

Carvalho, E.M., Bacellar, O., Barral, A., Badaro, R., & Johnson, W.D., Jr. (1989) Antigen-specific immunosuppression in visceral leishmaniasis is cell mediated. *J Clin Invest*, 83, 860–864.

Carvalho, E.M., Badaro, R., Reed, S.G., Jones, T.C., & Johnson, W.D., Jr. (1985) Absence of gamma interferon and interleukin 2 production during active visceral leishmaniasis. *J Clin Invest*, 76, 2066–2069.

Chatelain, R., Varkila, K., & Coffman, R.L. (1992) IL-4 induces a Th2 response in *Leishmania major*-infected mice. *J Immunol*, 148, 1182–1187.

Corry, D.B., Reiner, S.L., Linsley, P.S., & Locksley, R.M. (1994) Differential effects of blockade of CD28-B7 on the development of Th1 or Th2 effector cells in experimental leishmaniasis. *J Immunol*, 153, 4142–4148.

Demant, P., & Hart, A.A. (1986) Recombinant congenic strains—a new tool for analyzing genetic traits determined by more than one gene. *Immunogenetics*, 24, 416–422.

de Waal Malefyt, R., Abrams, J., Bennett, B., Figdor, C.G., & de Vries, J.E. (1991) Interleukin 10(IL-10) inhibits cytokine synthesis by human monocytes: an autoregulatory role of IL-10 produced by monocytes. *J Exp Med*, 174, 1209–1220.

Ding, L., Linsley, P.S., Huang, L.Y., Germain, R.N., & Shevach, E.M. (1993) IL-10 inhibits macrophage costimulatory activity by selectively inhibiting the up-regulation of B7 expression. *J Immunol*, 151, 1224–1234.

Engwerda, C.R., Murphy, M.L., Cotterell, S.E., Smelt, S.C., & Kaye, P.M. (1998) Neutralization of IL-12 demonstrates the existence of discrete organ-specific phases in the control of *Leishmania donovani*. *Eur J Immunol*, 28, 669–680.

Faria, D.R., Gollob, K.J., Barbosa, J., Jr., Schriefer, A., Machado, P.R., Lessa, H., Carvalho, L.P., Romano-Silva, M.A., de Jesus, A.R., Carvalho, E.M., & Dutra, W.O. (2005) Decreased in situ expression of interleukin-10 receptor is correlated with the exacerbated inflammatory and cytotoxic responses observed in mucosal leishmaniasis. *Infect Immun*, 73, 7853–7859.

Fiorentino, D.F., Zlotnik, A., Mosmann, T.R., Howard, M., & O'Garra, A. (1991a) IL-10 inhibits cytokine production by activated macrophages. *J Immunol*, 147, 3815–3822.

Fiorentino, D.F., Zlotnik, A., Vieira, P., Mosmann, T.R., Howard, M., Moore, K.W., & O'Garra, A. (1991b) IL-10 acts on the antigen-presenting cell to inhibit cytokine production by Th1 cells. *J Immunol*, 146, 3444–3451.

Forget, G., Gregory, D.J., & Olivier, M. (2005) Proteasome-mediated degradation of STAT1alpha following infection of macrophages with *Leishmania donovani*. *J Biol Chem*, 280, 30542–30549.

Gazzinelli, R.T., Oswald, I.P., James, S.L., & Sher, A. (1992) IL-10 inhibits parasite killing and nitrogen oxide production by IFN-gamma-activated macrophages. *J Immunol*, 148, 1792–1796.

Ghalib, H.W., Whittle, J.A., Kubin, M., Hashim, F.A., el-Hassan, A.M., Grabstein, K.H., Trinchieri, G., & Reed, S.G. (1995) IL-12 enhances Th1-type responses in human *Leishmania donovani* infections. *J Immunol*, **154**, 4623–4629.

Gorak, P.M., Engwerda, C.R., & Kaye, P.M. (1998) Dendritic cells, but not macrophages, produce IL-12 immediately following *Leishmania donovani* infection. *Eur J Immunol*, **28**, 687–695.

Gorham, J.D., Guler, M.L., Steen, R.G., Mackey, A.J., Daly, M.J., Frederick, K., Dietrich, W.F., & Murphy, K.M. (1996) Genetic mapping of a murine locus controlling development of T helper 1/T helper 2 type responses. *Proc Natl Acad Sci USA*, **93**, 12467–12472.

Govoni, G., Vidal, S., Gauthier, S., Skamene, E., Malo, D., & Gros, P. (1996) The Bcg/Ity/Lsh locus: genetic transfer of resistance to infections in C57BL/6J mice transgenic for the Nramp1 Gly169 allele. *Infect Immun*, **64**, 2923–2929.

Green, S.J., Nacy, C.A., & Meltzer, M.S. (1991) Cytokine-induced synthesis of nitrogen oxides in macrophages: a protective host response to *Leishmania* and other intracellular pathogens. *J Leukoc Biol*, **50**, 93–103.

Handman, E., Ceredig, R., & Mitchell, G.F. (1979) Murine cutaneous leishmaniasis: disease patterns in intact and nude mice of various genotypes and examination of some differences between normal and infected macrophages. *Aust J Exp Biol Med Sci*, **57**, 9–29.

Heinzel, F.P., & Rerko, R.M. (1999) Cure of progressive murine leishmaniasis: interleukin 4 dominance is abolished by transient CD4(+) T cell depletion and T helper cell type 1-selective cytokine therapy. *J Exp Med*, **189**, 1895–1906.

Heinzel, F.P., Sadick, M.D., Mutha, S.S., & Locksley, R.M. (1991) Production of interferon gamma, interleukin 2, interleukin 4, and interleukin 10 by CD4+ lymphocytes in vivo during healing and progressive murine leishmaniasis. *Proc Natl Acad Sci USA*, **88**, 7011–7015.

Heinzel, F.P., Schoenhaut, D.S., Rerko, R.M., Rosser, L.E., & Gately, M.K. (1993) Recombinant interleukin 12 cures mice infected with *Leishmania major*. *J Exp Med*, **177**, 1505–1509.

Himmelrich, H., Parra-Lopez, C., Tacchini-Cottier, F., Louis, J.A., & Launois, P. (1998) The IL-4 rapidly produced in BALB/c mice after infection with *Leishmania major* down-regulates IL-12 receptor beta 2-chain expression on CD4+ T cells resulting in a state of unresponsiveness to IL-12. *J Immunol*, **161**, 6156–6163.

Howard, J.G., Hale, C., & Liew, F.Y. (1980) Genetically determined susceptibility to *Leishmania tropica* infection is expressed by haematopoietic donor cells in mouse radiation chimaeras. *Nature*, **288**, 161–162.

Ibrahim, M.E., Lambson, B., Yousif, A.O., Deifalla, N.S., Alnaiem, D.A., Ismail, A., Yousif, H., Ghalib, H.W., Khalil, E.A., Kadaro, A., Barker, D.C., & El Hassan, A.M. (1999) Kala-azar in a high transmission focus: an ethnic and geographic dimension. *Am J Trop Med Hyg*, **61**, 941–944.

Ismail, A., El Hassan, A.M., Kemp, K., Gasim, S., Kadaru, A.E., Moller, T., Kharazmi, A., & Theander, T.G. (1999) Immunopathology of post kala-azar dermal leishmaniasis (PKDL): T-cell phenotypes and cytokine profile. *J Pathol*, **189**, 615–622.

Ji, J., Masterson, J., Sun, J., & Soong, L. (2005) CD4+CD25+ regulatory T cells restrain pathogenic responses during *Leishmania amazonensis* infection. *J Immunol*, **174**, 7147–7153.

Kariminia, A., Bourreau, E., Pascalis, H., Couppie, P., Sainte-Marie, D., Tacchini-Cottier, F., & Launois, P. (2005) Transforming growth factor beta 1 production by CD4+ CD25+ regulatory T cells in peripheral blood mononuclear cells from healthy subjects stimulated with *Leishmania guyanensis*. *Infect Immun*, **73**, 5908–5914.

Karp, C.L., el-Safi, S.H., Wynn, T.A., Satti, M.M., Kordofani, A.M., Hashim, F.A., Hag-Ali, M., Neva, F.A., Nutman, T.B., & Sacks, D.L. (1993) In vivo cytokine profiles in patients with kala-azar. Marked elevation of both interleukin-10 and interferon-gamma. *J Clin Invest*, **91**, 1644–1648.

Kaye, P.M., & Bancroft, G.J. (1992) *Leishmania donovani* infection in scid mice: lack of tissue response and in vivo macrophage activation correlates with failure to trigger natural killer cell-derived gamma interferon production in vitro. *Infect Immun*, **60**, 4335–4342.

Kaye, P.M., Curry, A.J., & Blackwell, J.M. (1991) Differential production of Th1- and Th2-derived cytokines does not determine the genetically controlled or vaccine-induced rate of cure in murine visceral leishmaniasis. *J Immunol*, **146**, 2763–2770.

Kaye, P.M., Svensson, M., Ato, M., Maroof, A., Polley, R., Stager, S., Zubairi, S., & Engwerda, C.R. (2004) The immunopathology of experimental visceral leishmaniasis. *Immunol Rev*, **201**, 239–253.

Kehrl, J.H., Wakefield, L.M., Roberts, A.B., Jakowlew, S., Alvarez-Mon, M., Derynck, R., Sporn, M.B., & Fauci, A.S. (1986) Production of transforming growth factor beta by human T lymphocytes and its potential role in the regulation of T cell growth. *J Exp Med*, **163**, 1037–1050.

Kellina, O.I. (1973) [Differences in the sensitivity of inbred mice of different lines to *Leishmania tropica* major]. *Med Parazitol (Mosk)*, **42**, 279–285.

Lainson, R, & Shaw, J.J. (1987) Evolution, classification and geographical distribution. In: *The Leishmaniases in Biology and Medicine* (ed. by R. Killick-Kendricks & W. Peters), vol. 1, pp. 1–120. Academic Press, London.

Lara, M.L., Layrisse, Z., Scorza, J.V., Garcia, E., Stoikow, Z., Granados, J., & Bias, W. (1991) Immunogenetics of human American cutaneous leishmaniasis. Study of HLA haplotypes in 24 families from Venezuela. *Hum Immunol*, **30**, 129–135.

Launois, P., Ohteki, T., Swihart, K., MacDonald, H.R., & Louis, J.A. (1995) In susceptible mice, *Leishmania major* induce very rapid interleukin-4 production by CD4+ T cells which are NK1.1. *Eur J Immunol*, **25**, 3298–3307.

Leal, L.M., Moss, D.W., Kuhn, R., Muller, W., & Liew, F.Y. (1993) Interleukin-4 transgenic mice of resistant background are susceptible to *Leishmania major* infection. *Eur J Immunol*, **23**, 566–569.

Li, J., Hunter, C.A., & Farrell, J.P. (1999) Anti-TGF-beta treatment promotes rapid healing of *Leishmania major* infection in mice by enhancing in vivo nitric oxide production. *J Immunol*, **162**, 974–979.

Liew, F.Y. (1989) Functional heterogeneity of CD4+ T cells in leishmaniasis. *Immunol Today*, **10**, 40–45.

Liew, F.Y., Millott, S., Li, Y., Lelchuk, R., Chan, W.L., & Ziltener, H. (1989) Macrophage activation by interferon-gamma from host-protective T cells is inhibited by interleukin (IL)3 and IL4 produced by disease-promoting T cells in leishmaniasis. *Eur J Immunol*, **19**, 1227–1232.

Lipoldova, M., Svobodova, M., Havelkova, H., Krulova, M., Badalova, J., Nohynkova, E., Hart, A.A., Schlegel, D., Volf, P., & Demant, P. (2002) Mouse genetic model for clinical and immunological heterogeneity of leishmaniasis. *Immunogenetics*, **54**, 174–183.

Lipoldova, M., Svobodova, M., Krulova, M., Havelkova, H., Badalova, J., Nohynkova, E., Holan, V., Hart, A.A., Volf, P., & Demant, P. (2000) Susceptibility to *Leishmania major* infection in mice: multiple loci and heterogeneity of immunopathological phenotypes. *Genes Immun*, **1**, 200–206.

Locksley, R.M., & Scott, P. (1991) Helper T-cell subsets in mouse leishmaniasis: induction, expansion and effector function. *Immunol Today*, **12**, A58–61.

Louzir, H., Melby, P.C., Ben Salah, A., Marrakchi, H., Aoun, K., Ben Ismail, R., & Dellagi, K. (1998) Immunologic determinants of disease evolution in localized cutaneous leishmaniasis due to *Leishmania major*. *J Infect Dis*, **177**, 1687–1695.

Malo, D., Vogan, K., Vidal, S., Hu, J., Cellier, M., Schurr, E., Fuks, A., Bumstead, N., Morgan, K., & Gros, P. (1994) Haplotype mapping and sequence analysis of the mouse Nramp gene predict susceptibility to infection with intracellular parasites. *Genomics*, **23**, 51–61.

Matthews, D.J., Emson, C.L., McKenzie, G.J., Jolin, H.E., Blackwell, J.M., & McKenzie, A.N. (2000) IL-13 is a susceptibility factor for *Leishmania major* infection. *J Immunol*, **164**, 1458–1462.

McElrath, M.J., Murray, H.W., & Cohn, Z.A. (1988) The dynamics of granuloma formation in experimental visceral leishmaniasis. *J Exp Med*, **167**, 1927–1937.

Meddeb-Garnaoui, A., Gritli, S., Garbouj, S., Ben Fadhel, M., El Kares, R., Mansour, L., Kaabi, B., Chouchane, L., Ben Salah, A., & Dellagi, K. (2001) Association analysis of HLA-class II and class III gene polymorphisms in the susceptibility to mediterranean visceral leishmaniasis. *Hum Immunol*, **62**, 509–517.

Melby, P.C., Andrade-Narvaez, F.J., Darnell, B.J., Valencia-Pacheco, G., Tryon, V.V., & Palomo-Cetina, A. (1994) Increased expression of proinflammatory cytokines in chronic lesions of human cutaneous leishmaniasis. *Infect Immun*, **62**, 837–842.

Miralles, G.D., Stoeckle, M.Y., McDermott, D.F., Finkelman, F.D., & Murray, H.W. (1994) Th1 and Th2 cell-associated cytokines in experimental visceral leishmaniasis. *Infect Immun*, **62**, 1058–1063.

Mitchell, G.F., Curtis, J.M., & Handman, E. (1981) Resistance to cutaneous leishmaniasis in genetically susceptible BALB/c mice. *Aust J Exp Biol Med Sci*, **59**, 555–565.

Moen, C.J., van der Valk, M.A., Snoek, M., van Zutphen, B.F., von Deimling, O., Hart, A.A., & Demant, P. (1991) The recombinant congenic strains—a novel genetic tool applied to the study of colon tumor development in the mouse. *Mamm Genome*, **1**, 217–227.

Mohamed, H.S., Ibrahim, M.E., Miller, E.N., Peacock, C.S., Khalil, E.A., Cordell, H.J., Howson, J.M., El Hassan, A.M., Bereir, R.E., & Blackwell, J.M. (2003) Genetic susceptibility to visceral leishmaniasis in The Sudan: linkage and association with IL4 and IFNGR1. *Genes Immun*, **4**, 351–355.

Mohamed, H.S., Ibrahim, M.E., Miller, E.N., White, J.K., Cordell, H.J., Howson, J.M., Peacock, C.S., Khalil, E.A., El Hassan, A.M., & Blackwell, J.M. (2004) SLC11A1 (formerly NRAMP1) and susceptibility to visceral leishmaniasis in The Sudan. *Eur J Hum Genet*, **12**, 66–74.

Mohrs, M., Ledermann, B., Kohler, G., Dorfmuller, A., Gessner, A., & Brombacher, F. (1999) Differences between IL-4- and IL-4 receptor alpha-deficient mice in chronic leishmaniasis reveal a protective role for IL-13 receptor signaling. *J Immunol*, **162**, 7302–7308.

Moore, K.W., O'Garra, A., de Waal Malefyt, R., Vieira, P., & Mosmann, T.R. (1993) Interleukin-10. *Annu Rev Immunol*, **11**, 165–190.

Muller, I., Pedrazzini, T., Kropf, P., Louis, J., & Milon, G. (1991) Establishment of resistance to *Leishmania major* infection in susceptible BALB/c mice requires parasite-specific CD8+ T cells. *Int Immunol*, **3**, 587–597.

Murphy, M.L., Wille, U., Villegas, E.N., Hunter, C.A., & Farrell, J.P. (2001) IL-10 mediates susceptibility to *Leishmania donovani* infection. *Eur J Immunol*, **31**, 2848–2856.

Murray, H.W., & Hariprashad, J. (1995) Interleukin 12 is effective treatment for an established systemic intracellular infection: experimental visceral leishmaniasis. *J Exp Med*, **181**, 387–391.

Murray, H.W., Jungbluth, A., Ritter, E., Montelibano, C., & Marino, M.W. (2000) Visceral leishmaniasis in mice devoid of tumor necrosis factor and response to treatment. *Infect Immun*, **68**, 6289–6293.

Murray, H.W., Masur, H., & Keithly, J.S. (1982) Cell-mediated immune response in experimental visceral leishmaniasis. I. Correlation between resistance to *Leishmania donovani* and lymphokine-generating capacity. *J Immunol*, **129**, 344–350.

Murray, H.W., & Nathan, C.F. (1999) Macrophage microbicidal mechanisms in vivo: reactive nitrogen versus oxygen intermediates in the killing of intracellular visceral *Leishmania donovani*. *J Exp Med*, **189**, 741–746.

Murray, H.W., Stern, J.J., Welte, K., Rubin, B.Y., Carriero, S.M., & Nathan, C.F. (1987) Experimental visceral leishmaniasis: production of interleukin 2 and interferon-gamma, tissue immune reaction, and response to treatment with interleukin 2 and interferon-gamma. *J Immunol*, **138**, 2290–2297.

Noben-Trauth, N., Lira, R., Nagase, H., Paul, W.E., & Sacks, D.L. (2003) The relative contribution of IL-4 receptor signaling and IL-10 to susceptibility to *Leishmania major*. *J Immunol*, **170**, 5152–5158.

Noben-Trauth, N., Paul, W.E., & Sacks, D.L. (1999) IL-4- and IL-4 receptor-deficient BALB/c mice reveal differences in susceptibility to *Leishmania major* parasite substrains. *J Immunol*, **162**, 6132–6140.

O'Garra, A., Vieira, P.L., Vieira, P., & Goldfeld, A.E. (2004) IL-10-producing and naturally occurring CD4+ Tregs: limiting collateral damage. *J Clin Invest*, **114**, 1372–1378.

Olivier, M., Gregory, D.J., & Forget, G. (2005) Subversion mechanisms by which *Leishmania* parasites can escape the host immune response: a signaling point of view. *Clin Microbiol Rev*, **18**, 293–305.

Olivo-Diaz, A., Debaz, H., Alaez, C., Islas, V.J., Perez-Perez, H., Hobart, O., & Gorodezky, C. (2004) Role of HLA class II alleles in susceptibility to and protection from localized cutaneous leishmaniasis. *Hum Immunol*, **65**, 255–261.

Oswald, I.P., Gazzinelli, R.T., Sher, A., & James, S.L. (1992) IL-10 synergizes with IL-4 and transforming growth factor-beta to inhibit macrophage cytotoxic activity. *J Immunol*, **148**, 3578–3582.

Peacock, C.S., Collins, A., Shaw, M.A., Silveira, F., Costa, J., Coste, C.H., Nascimento, M.D., Siddiqui, R., Shaw, J.J., & Blackwell, J.M. (2001) Genetic epidemiology of visceral leishmaniasis in northeastern Brazil. *Genet Epidemiol*, **20**, 383–396.

Peacock, C.S., Sanjeevi, C.B., Shaw, M.A., Collins, A., Campbell, R.D., March, R., Silveira, F., Costa, J., Coste, C.H., Nascimento, M.D., Siddiqui, R., Shaw, J.J., & Blackwell, J.M. (2002) Genetic analysis of multicase families of visceral leishmaniasis in northeastern Brazil: no major role for class II or class III regions of HLA. *Genes Immun*, **3**, 350–358.

Perez, H., Arredondo, B., & Gonzalez, M. (1978) Comparative study of American cutaneous leishmaniasis and diffuse cutaneous leishmaniasis in two strains of inbred mice. *Infect Immun*, **22**, 301–307.

Perez, H., Labrador, F., & Torrealba, J.W. (1979) Variations in the response of five strains of mice to *Leishmania mexicana*. *Int J Parasitol*, **9**, 27–32.

Petzl-Erler, M.L., Belich, M.P., & Queiroz-Telles, F. (1991) Association of mucosal leishmaniasis with HLA. *Hum Immunol*, **32**, 254–260.

Reiner, S.L., Zheng, S., Wang, Z.E., Stowring, L., & Locksley, R.M. (1994) *Leishmania* promastigotes evade interleukin 12 (IL-12) induction by macrophages and stimulate a broad range of cytokines from CD4+ T cells during initiation of infection. *J Exp Med*, **179**, 447–456.

Roberts, L.J., Baldwin, T.M., Curtis, J.M., Handman, E., & Foote, S.J. (1997) Resistance to *Leishmania major* is linked to the H2 region on chromosome 17 and to chromosome 9. *J Exp Med*, **185**, 1705–1710.

Roberts, L.J., Baldwin, T.M., Speed, T.P., Handman, E., & Foote, S.J. (1999) Chromosomes X, 9, and the H2 locus interact epistatically to control *Leishmania major* infection. *Eur J Immunol*, **29**, 3047–3050.

Roberts, M., Alexander, J., & Blackwell, J.M. (1989) Influence of Lsh, H-2, and an H-11-linked gene on visceralization and metastasis associated with *Leishmania mexicana* infection in mice. *Infect Immun*, **57**, 875–881.

Roberts, M., Alexander, J., & Blackwell, J.M. (1990) Genetic analysis of *Leishmania mexicana* infection in mice: single gene (Scl-2) controlled predisposition to cutaneous lesion development. *J Immunogenet*, **17**, 89–100.

Roberts, M., Mock, B.A., & Blackwell, J.M. (1993) Mapping of genes controlling *Leishmania major* infection in CXS recombinant inbred mice. *Eur J Immunogenet*, **20**, 349–362.

Sadick, M.D., Locksley, R.M., Tubbs, C., & Raff, H.V. (1986) Murine cutaneous leishmaniasis: resistance correlates with the capacity to generate interferon-gamma in response to *Leishmania* antigens in vitro. *J Immunol*, **136**, 655–661.

Sadick, M.D., Heinzel, F.P., Holaday, B.J., Pu, R.T., Dawkins, R.S., & Locksley, R.M. (1990) Cure of murine leishmaniasis with anti-interleukin 4 monoclonal antibody. Evidence for a T cell-dependent, interferon gamma-independent mechanism. *J Exp Med*, **171**, 115–127.

Satoskar, A., Bluethmann, H., & Alexander, J. (1995) Disruption of the murine interleukin-4 gene inhibits disease progression during *Leishmania mexicana* infection but does not increase control of *Leishmania donovani* infection. *Infect Immun*, **63**, 4894–4899.

Satoskar, A.R., Elizondo, J., Monteforte, G.M., Stamm, L.M., Bluethmann, H., Katavolos, P., & Telford, S.R., 3rd (2000) Interleukin-4-deficient BALB/c mice develop an enhanced Th1-like response but control cardiac inflammation following *Borrelia burgdorferi* infection. *FEMS Microbiol Lett*, **183**, 319–325.

Scharton, T.M., & Scott, P. (1993) Natural killer cells are a source of interferon gamma that drives differentiation of CD4+ T cell subsets and induces early resistance to *Leishmania major* in mice. *J Exp Med*, **178**, 567–577.

Scharton-Kersten, T., Afonso, L.C., Wysocka, M., Trinchieri, G., & Scott, P. (1995) IL-12 is required for natural killer cell activation and subsequent T helper 1 cell development in experimental leishmaniasis. *J Immunol*, **154**, 5320–5330.

Schmitt, E., Hoehn, P., Huels, C., Goedert, S., Palm, N., Rude, E., & Germann, T. (1994) T helper type 1 development of naive CD4+ T cells requires the coordinate action of interleukin-12 and interferon-gamma and is inhibited by transforming growth factor-beta. *Eur J Immunol*, **24**, 793–798.

El-Safi, S.H., Bucheton, B., Kheir, M.M., Musa, H.A., M, E.L.-O., Hammad, A., & Dessein, A. (2002) Epidemiology of visceral leishmaniasis in Atbara River area, eastern Sudan: the outbreak of Barbar El Fugara village (1996–1997). *Microbes Infect*, **4**, 1439–1447.

Shaw, M.A., Davies, C.R., Llanos-Cuentas, E.A., & Collins, A. (1995) Human genetic susceptibility and infection with *Leishmania peruviana*. *Am J Hum Genet*, **57**, 1159–1168.

Singh, N., Sundar, S., Williams, F., Curran, M.D., Rastogi, A., Agrawal, S., & Middleton, D. (1997) Molecular typing of HLA class I and class II antigens in Indian kala-azar patients. *Trop Med Int Health*, **2**, 468–471.

Swihart, K., Fruth, U., Messmer, N., Hug, K., Behin, R., Huang, S., Del Giudice, G., Aguet, M., & Louis, J.A. (1995) Mice from a genetically resistant background lacking the interferon gamma receptor are susceptible to infection with *Leishmania major* but mount a polarized T helper cell 1-type CD4+ T cell response. *J Exp Med*, **181**, 961–971.

Sypek, J.P., Chung, C.L., Mayor, S.E., Subramanyam, J.M., Goldman, S.J., Sieburth, D.S., Wolf, S.F., & Schaub, R.G. (1993) Resolution of cutaneous leishmaniasis: interleukin 12 initiates a protective T helper type 1 immune response. *J Exp Med*, **177**, 1797–1802.

Titus, R.G., Muller, I., Kimsey, P., Cerny, A., Behin, R., Zinkernagel, R.M., & Louis, J.A. (1991) Exacerbation of experimental murine cutaneous leishmaniasis with CD4+ *Leishmania major*-specific T cell lines or clones which secrete interferon-gamma and mediate parasite-specific delayed-type hypersensitivity. *Eur J Immunol*, **21**, 559–567.

Tumang, M.C., Keogh, C., Moldawer, L.L., Helfgott, D.C., Teitelbaum, R., Hariprashad, J., & Murray, H.W. (1994) Role and effect of TNF-alpha in experimental visceral leishmaniasis. *J Immunol*, **153**, 768–775.

Turetz, M.L., Machado, P.R., Ko, A.I., Alves, F., Bittencourt, A., Almeida, R.P., Mobashery, N., Johnson, W.D., Jr., & Carvalho, E.M. (2002) Disseminated leishmaniasis: a new and emerging form of leishmaniasis observed in northeastern Brazil. *J Infect Dis*, **186**, 1829–1834.

Vidal, S., Tremblay, M.L., Govoni, G., Gauthier, S., Sebastiani, G., Malo, D., Skamene, E., Olivier, M., Jothy, S., & Gros, P. (1995) The Ity/Lsh/Bcg locus: natural resistance to infection with intracellular parasites is abrogated by disruption of the Nramp1 gene. *J Exp Med*, **182**, 655–666.

Vieth, M., Will, A., Schroppel, K., Rollinghoff, M., & Gessner, A. (1994) Interleukin-10 inhibits antimicrobial activity against *Leishmania major* in murine macrophages. *Scand J Immunol*, **40**, 403–409.

Vladimirov, V., Badalova, J., Svobodova, M., Havelkova, H., Hart, A.A., Blazkova, H., Demant, P., & Lipoldova, M. (2003) Different genetic control of cutaneous and visceral disease after *Leishmania major* infection in mice. *Infect Immun*, **71**, 2041–2046.

Wang, Z.E., Reiner, S.L., Zheng, S., Dalton, D.K., & Locksley, R.M. (1994) CD4+ effector cells default to the Th2 pathway in interferon gamma-deficient mice infected with *Leishmania major. J Exp Med,* **179**, 1367–1371.

Wilhelm, P., Ritter, U., Labbow, S., Donhauser, N., Rollinghoff, M., Bogdan, C., & Korner, H. (2001) Rapidly fatal leishmaniasis in resistant C57BL/6 mice lacking TNF. *J Immunol,* **166**, 4012–4019.

Wilson, M.E., Sandor, M., Blum, A.M., Young, B.M., Metwali, A., Elliott, D., Lynch, R.G., & Weinstock, J.V. (1996) Local suppression of IFN-gamma in hepatic granulomas correlates with tissue-specific replication of *Leishmania chagasi. J Immunol,* **156**, 2231–2239.

Wilson, M.E., Young, B.M., Davidson, B.L., Mente, K.A., & McGowan, S.E. (1998) The importance of TGF-beta in murine visceral leishmaniasis. *J Immunol,* **161**, 6148–6155.

Wyllie, S., Seu, P., & Goss, J.A. (2002) The natural resistance-associated macrophage protein 1 Slc11a1 (formerly Nramp1) and iron metabolism in macrophages. *Microbes Infect,* **4**, 351–359.

26

Schistosomiasis

Alain Dessein, Christophe Chevillard, & Nasr Eldin Elwali

Schistosomiasis is a disease caused by several species of 1- to 2-cm-long helminths—trematodes or flat worms—called schistosomes. Some 250 million people are believed to be infected, mainly in developing countries, and schistosomiasis causes 100,000–250,000 deaths annually.

The Parasite and Disease

Schistosoma Life Cycle

Schistosomes are disseminated by freshwater snails that release infective swimming larvae, the cercariae, in ponds, small rivers, and irrigation canals. Humans and animals are infected following exposure to the waters during agricultural activities such as irrigation and from bathing, washing, or drinking (animals). In the snails, the parasite undergoes asexual multiplication that increases the parasite population size by a thou-

sand times. In its vertebrate hosts, schistosomes undergo sexual reproduction, with female worms laying a few hundred eggs per day in the vessels of the host intestine and bladder. These eggs perforate the mucosa to enter the fecal or urinary stream, whereupon they shed into a river or pond and hatch and release a larva (miracidium) that infects the snails.

Species Specificity

Individual schistosome species have different geographical distributions, vectors, and tissue tropisms, and they cause different diseases. Four species cause important health problems in the tropics: S. *mansoni*, S. *japonicum*, and S. *mekongi* inhabit the mesenteric veins and the portal veins of their vertebrate host and cause intestinal and hepatosplenic disease; S. *haematobium* inhabits the vessels of the urinary system and causes disease of the urinary tract, including severe hydronephrosis. All schistosome infections can be lethal.

Diagnosis

Most clinical signs associated with infection by schistosomes are nonspecific. The diagnosis of schistosomal infection relies mostly on the detection by microscope examination of schistosome eggs in patient feces (S. mansoni, S. japonicum) or urine (S. haematobium). The shape of the eggs is characteristic of schistosome species. When necessary, the presence of eggs can be confirmed by rectal biopsy. Trained parasitologists can differentiate between live eggs and dead ones (from old or from treated infections). Serology cannot normally differentiate between active or past infection; however, it may be used to detect previous contact with schistosomes in cases of abnormal localization of the schistosome worms such as in neuroschistosomiasis. Evaluation of the most severe clinical form by ultrasonography can reveal periportal fibrosis (PPF), the presence of varices, or kidney and bladder alterations.

Pathology

Eggs trapped in tissues secrete proteolytic enzymes that are toxic for the surrounding cells. Damaged endothelial cells and activated platelets release inflammatory substances that attract inflammatory cells, including eosinophils, macrophages, T lymphocytes, and B lymphocytes (Warren, 1977). This periovular reaction persists for several weeks and becomes organized as a granuloma (von Lichtenberg, 1962, Warren et al., 1967). The early granuloma is inflammatory-necrotic and then becomes fibrotic. Fibrosis occurs with accumulation of extracellular matrix proteins (ECMPs), for example, laminin, collagen, and connectin produced by stellate cell (Ito cell)–derived myofibroblasts. These changes are regulated by a variety of cytokines and lipid-derived mediators (Gressner, 1995, Poli, 2000) produced by hepatocytes, endothelial cells, or Kupffer cells and by other inflammatory cells present in the granuloma. Thus, hepatic fibrosis in some subjects with S. mansoni or S. japonicum infection and also those with S. haematobium infections is due to an uncontrolled scarring process in the liver that grows into massive PPF. In addition to PPF, S. japonicum causes fibrosis of the hepatic parenchyma (parenchymal fibrosis [PaF]). PPF and possibly PaF cause portal hypertension, ascites, and varicose veins. Patients die of direct or indirect consequences of hematemesis (due to bleeding varices), heart failure, or superinfection with bacterial pathogens.

The anti-egg reaction also causes severe bladder and renal pathology, mostly in children and adolescents. Periovular inflammation and fibrosis cause thickening of the bladder and ureter walls that may ultimately contribute to hydronephrosis of variable severity. Finally, schistosomal infection is a major cause of bladder cancer and of hepatocarcinoma in adults.

Treatment

Parasitological cure can be achieved by a single treatment with praziquantel (all Schistosoma species) or oxamniquine (S. mansoni). Full cure may require two or three treatments at three-week intervals. The management of severe disease consists mostly of the classic treatment of portal hypertension; in patients with bleeding, varicose veins can be sclerified and the spleen can be removed. If the disease has not reached the stage of decompensation, these treatments allow long-term survival. Hepatic disease due to schistosomes is often aggravated by co-infection with hepatitis C virus.

Sterile Immunity Versus Clinical Immunity

Adult schistosomes are little affected by the immune response of their hosts. Young larvae, however, are targets of immunity when they invade the skin and when they migrate through the lungs. Eggs induce granulomatous reactions in intestinal and bladder tissues. The blood also carries large number of eggs to other locations, to the liver in particular, where they lodge in the sinusoidal veins. Here, the egg granuloma is essential to the host in preventing eggs from digesting hepatocytes, and the granuloma is progressively replaced by scar tissue. The scarring process may escape regulatory control and causes organ fibrosis.

Subjects living in endemic areas develop immunity that protects them against infection (sterile immunity). This immunity is directed toward schistosome larvae and reduces worm load. Most subjects living in endemic areas remain infected even after many years of exposure or become reinfected after parasitological cure with praziquantel. Thus, sterile immunity is almost never complete, even in the most resistant subjects. In contrast, clinical immunity, observed both in urinary and in intestinal schistosomiasis, can be very strong and provide full protection against clinical manifestations.

Genetic Effects

Control of Endemic Infection by Genes in a Major Chromosomal Region (5q31-q33)

In endemic populations with relatively uniformly high exposure, clustering of infection by family suggests that inherited factors partially determine the probability of infection (Dessein et al., 1992). This hypothesis was tested in a Brazilian population living in an area endemic for *S. mansoni*. Segregation analysis showed that the distribution of infection levels in families was best explained by a model that included age, gender, exposure and a major codominant gene effect (Abel et al., 1991). The gene effect accounted for half of the variance in infection levels. An estimated frequency of the deleterious allele at 0.22 meant that about 5% of the population were highly predisposed to infection, 60% were resistant, and 35% showed an intermediate level of resistance. This finding was replicated in Kenya (A. Dessein and K. Gachuhi, unpublished data).

This locus (*S. mansoni* 1, *SM1*) was mapped by linkage analysis in 142 Brazilian subjects from 11 informative families (Marquet et al., 1996). Only one region on chromosome 5 (5q31-q33) showed suggestive linkage: two adjacent markers provided maximum LOD scores of 3.18 and 3.06, respectively. Additional markers were analyzed in that region. The maximum two-point LOD score was observed for markers near a colony-stimulating factor receptor gene (*CSF1R*) and near the *IL4*, *IL13*, *IL5* cluster. Multipoint linkage analysis including five markers for this region indicated a maximum LOD score of 5.45 (Marquet et al., 1996, 1999). Muller-Myhsok et al (1997) tested this result in a newly emerged epidemic focus of intestinal schistosomiasis in Senegal, where the population had become heavily infected with *S. mansoni*. Complex segregation analysis initially failed to demonstrate the effect of a major gene; linkage analysis was then carried out by statistical methods that do not require defining a genetic model. Both the weighted pairwise correlation and the sib-pair methods confirmed the existence of a 5q31-q33 locus controlling infection by *S. mansoni*. The markers showing the strongest effect were the same as in the Brazilian study. Various reasons could explain why this second study failed to detect a major gene effect. Under- or overestimation of exposure in certain subjects was a likely explanation since the segregation analysis initially applied is very sensitive to errors in this factor. Selection against the major gene effect may have resulted from the shorter exposure to schistosomes among Senegalese, who had likely acquired infection within the past 10 years, compared with the Brazilian population. Nevertheless, of interest is that one or more genes in the 5q31-q33 region appeared to control *S. mansoni* infection in both endemic and epidemic situations, in Brazilian and Senegalese that are genetically different populations (table 26.1). The same genetic region also controls infection by another schistosome (*S. haematobium*) in the Dogons of Mali, who differ genetically from both the Senegalese and the Brazilians (Kouriba et al., 2005).

The strategy that combines complex segregation and linkage analysis cannot detect additional genetic effects. To search for involvement of additional loci in the control of intensity of infection by *S. mansoni*, a model-free analysis (weighted pairwise correlation) was applied to the data from the genome scan performed on the Brazilian pedigrees. The results showed significant linkage in the 5q31-q33 region, confirming the major effect of this locus (Zinn-Justin et al., 2001). Taking into account *SM1*, two additional regions, 1p21-q23 and 6p21-q21, showed statistically significant linkage. The effect of the 1p21-q23 region was independent of *SM1*, whereas the variation in the 6p21-q21 region was in interaction with *SM1*. The former region, which showed the higher multipoint linkage contains macrophage colony-stimulating factor 1 gene (*CSF1*), whose receptor gene, interestingly, is located in the 5q31-q33 region. Larger studies are required to confirm the existence of these minor loci of susceptibility to infection by *S. mansoni*.

Analysis of Candidate Genes in the 5q31-q33 Chromosomal Region

The 5q31-q33 region contains a cluster of genes encoding proteins that play a central role in the immune response, including in T-helper Th2/Th1 differentiation. These include loci for the granulocyte-macrophage colony-stimulating factor (*CSF2*), several interleukins (*IL3*, *IL4*, *IL5*, *IL9*, *IL12*, and *IL13*), interferon regulatory factor 1 (*IRF1*), and the colony-stimulating factor-1 receptor (*CSF1R*).

In vitro studies have shown that antibody-dependent cellular cytotoxicity involving eosinophils and macrophages is most efficient against schistosome larvae in the developmental stage most susceptible to immune attack. *In vivo* studies carried out to identify immunological

TABLE 26.1. Principal genetic regions, loci, and alleles linked or associated with susceptibility to schistosomal infection or to severe hepatic schistosomiasis.

Phenotype	Region (Gene)	Allele	Methods	Population	Reference
Infection levels (egg excretion): S. mansoni, S. haematobium	5q31-q33 SM1 (7911)	—	Segregation/linkage analysis	Brazil	(Marquet et al, 1996)
	5q31-q33	—	Nonparametric linkage analysis	Senegal	(Muller-Myhsok et al, 1997)
	5q31 IL13 (3596)	−1055C/T	Association test	Mali	(Kouriba et al, 2005)
Severe periportal fibrosis associated with portal hypertension: S. mansoni	6q22-q23 SM2 (53366)	—	Combined segregation / linkage	Sudan	(Dessein et al, 1999)
	12q24 IFNG (3458)	+2109 A/G +3810 G/A	Association test	Sudan	(Chevillard et al, 2003)
Mild to severe periportal fibrosis	6q23		Sib-pair linkage analysis	Egypt	(Blanton et al, 2005)
Periportal fibrosis, hepatosplenomegaly: S. mansoni	HLA[a]		Association tests	Egypt	(Abaza et al, 1985, Abdel-Salam et al, 1986, Cabello et al, 1991, Salam et al, 1979, Secor et al, 1996)
Fibrosis/hepatosplenomegaly: S. japonicum	HLA[a]		Association tests	China	(Hirayama, 2004, Hirayama et al, 1999, McManus et al, 2001, Waine et al, 1998)

[a]HLA alleles are not indicated because of their variability.

responses predictive of resistance to reinfection after praziquantel treatment have shown that IgE and IgG$_4$ are associated with resistance/susceptibility to reinfection (Hagan et al., 1991, Rihet et al., 1991). High IgE levels were associated with protection against reinfection, and elevated IgG$_4$ levels were associated with increased susceptibility to reinfection (Hagan et al., 1991, Rihet et al., 1991, 1992). The balancing effects of these isotypes were best demonstrated when analyzed simultaneously. IgG$_4$ was shown to compete with IgE for schistosomula antigens, suggesting that the balancing effect results from competition for antigen binding (Demeure et al., 1993). These results were confirmed later (Dunne et al., 1992). IgE and eosinophils are highly dependent on IL-4, IL-13, and IL-5. Protection against larvae is regulated by Th2 cytokines, the genes for which are located in 5q31-q33. In addition, larval-specific T-cell clones from resistant subjects are Th2 or Th0/2, whereas those from susceptible subjects are Th1 or TH0/1. Immunological studies have further demonstrated that the cluster of Th2 cytokine genes

(IL4, IL5, IL13) is the best candidate region for the control of infection in the 5q31-q33 region.

After this hypothesis was promulgated in the Brazilian cohort, it was tested in subjects recruited in a Dogon village in Mali who were highly exposed to S. haematobium. No association with levels of infection was found with polymorphisms in the promoters of IL4 and IL5; however, alleles of the IL13 promoter (−1055C and−591A) were associated with the highest frequency of infection (Kouriba et al., 2005). Previous studies had associated IL13−1055T/T with altered regulation of IL13 (van der Pouw Kraan et al., 1999), with elevated IgE levels (Liu et al., 2003), and with sensitization to food and outdoor allergens (Liu et al., 2004). IL-13 could increase immunity against invading larvae in several ways: First, IL-13 induces germline ε transcription and IgE switching (Oettgen, 2000) and stimulates IgE production (de Vries et al., 1993). Second, IL-13 induces the expression of the low-affinity FcεRII (CD23) (McKenzie et al., 1993, Punnonen et al., 1993), which should increase IgE—the helminthocide of monocytes and eosinophils (Capron and Capron, 1994, Capron and Goldman, 2001, Capron et al., 1995). IL-13 is unable to drive T-cell differentiation into Th2; however, it down-regulates IL-12 production and thus may contribute to the selection of the Th2 CD4[+] T lymphocytes observed in the resistant subjects. IL-13 also increases the recruitment and the longevity of eosinophils in tissues by altering vascular cellular adhesion molecule-1 expression on endothelial cells (Bochner et al., 1995), CD69 expression on eosinophils (Luttmann et al., 1996), and granulocyte-macrophage colony-stimulating factor production by various cell types, including epithelial cells (Bergmann et al., 2000).

Work on *IL13* and on IgE, eosinophils, and Th2 cytokines support the conclusion that polymorphisms in *IL13* determine susceptibility to schistosomal infection. In the Brazilians, one single nucleotide polymorphism (SNP) in *IL13* appeared to have a dramatic effect in a population where so many other factors operate (Kouriba et al., 2005). Figure 26.1 shows the effects of the *IL13*−1055T/T genotype on infection levels in females in populations living in conditions of high or low *S. haematobium* transmission. Multivariate analysis of that SNP as well as potential confounding factors such as age and gender showed statistically significant effects on level of infection in the population as a whole, in all age categories, in both sexes, and in subjects with high or low pathogen exposure. Infection levels in the subjects with C/C or C/T genotypes were not different, and data from these two groups were pooled. The protective effect of the T/T genotype was detected in both high- and low-transmission populations, but it is clearer in adolescents and in young adults than in children in the low-transmission village, probably because protective immunity develops slowly (i.e., at an older age) in these conditions. Other genes in the region probably contribute to the genetic control of infection; linkage studies that yield high and significant LOD scores in the Th2 cluster region and also in the region containing *CSF1R* support this view.

Control of Disease in Chronic Schistosome Infection by Genes in a Major Chromosomal Region (6q22-q23)

In regions endemic for *S. mansoni*, 5–30% of the residents are affected by advanced hepatic disease (PPF and hepatosplenomegaly, HSP) that may progress to complications (portal hypertension, ascites, and he-

matemesis). Risk factors for severe disease have been evaluated in endemic populations. In a study of a village in the irrigated region of Gezira in central Sudan (Mohamed-Ali et al., 1999), where agricultural activities depend heavily on water from irrigation channels, most inhabitants had been exposed to infection for more than 20 years. PPF was observed in 11.3% of the study subjects ($n = 792$) and 4.5 times more frequently in males than in females. About 20% of the population in every age category were free of PPF in spite of many years of exposure to infected waters. In contrast, advanced PPF was observed in 40–50% of the 20- to 30-year-old males. However, even in the older age groups, no more than 5–10% of males were affected by severe PPF; this difference indicates that not all subjects with advanced PPF progress to severe PPF.

The study in the Gezira population also pointed to a genetic predisposition. Severe PPF was frequent in certain families and absent in others, but analysis of living habits did not reveal sufficient heterogeneity to explain such family clustering and suggested inherited factors (Mohamed-Ali et al., 1999). Similar observations were made in populations infected by *S. japonicum* in China (Dessein et al., 2004, Ellis et al., 2006, Seto et al., 2005). Segregation analysis of 65 Sudanese families indicated that PPF segregated as a Mendelian trait. The analysis showed that codominant alleles of a gene (*SM2*) could account for the familial distribution of the phenotype. The frequency of the deleterious allele (A) was estimated as 0.16. The genetic model predicted 50% penetrance in AA males, AA females, and Aa males after 9, 14, and 19 years of residence in the area, respectively, whereas the penetrance remains lower than 0.02 for other subjects after 20 years of exposure. Nevertheless, all heterozygote males were likely to develop severe PPF if they had lived long enough in the village. Consequently, in this population, 30% (3% of homozygous and 27% of heterozygous) of untreated males could potentially develop severe schistosomiasis. The estimated penetrance of the *SM2* effect depended on gender; it accounted for the lower prevalence of fibrosis in females than in males.

In linkage studies of candidate regions to map the major locus, no linkage was found with the 5q31-q33 region, with the 6p21 region containing the human leukocyte antigen (HLA) and *TNF* genes, or with the 12q15 region including *IFNG* encoding interferon-γ (IFN-γ). Significant linkage was obtained in the 6q22-q23 region, with both the D6S310 microsatellite and the FA1 intragenic marker in the gene coding for the

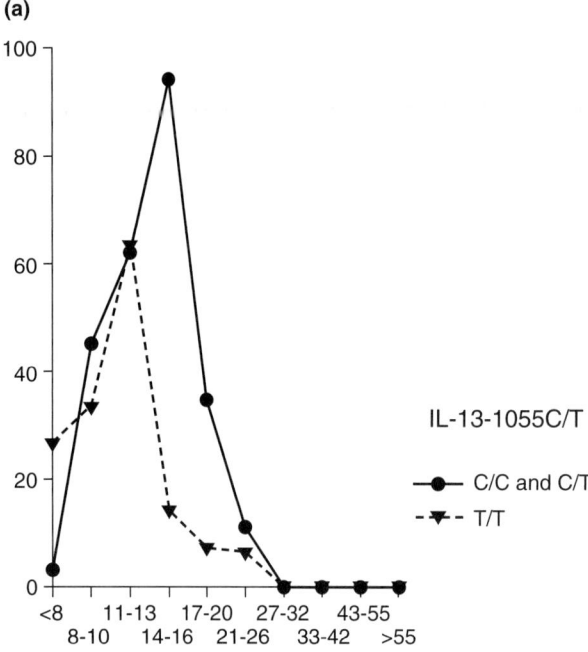

(a)

IL-13-1055C/T

— ●— C/C and C/T
--▼-- T/T

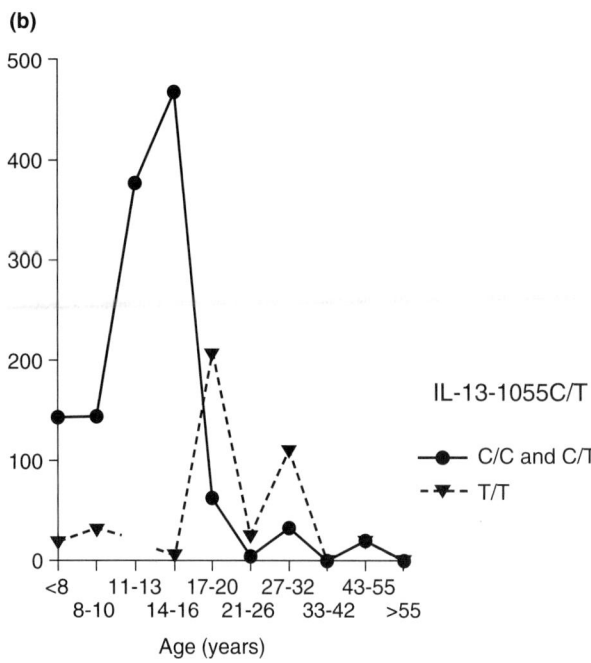

(b)

IL-13-1055C/T

— ●— C/C and C/T
--▼-- T/T

Age (years)

FIGURE 26.1. Infection levels in female carriers of IL13–1055 C/C or C/T versus T/T alleles in two Dogon villages. The data derive from one population that lives in an area of low schistosome transmission (a) and another that lives in an area of high transmission (b). The T/T genotype is protective in both conditions of transmission. The effect in the low transmission village is greater in older subjects who are more likely than younger subjects to have developed immunity. Immunity develops early in life in the high-transmission village.

α-chain of the IFN-γ receptor (*IFNGR1*) (Dessein et al., 1999). Combined segregation-linkage analysis with D6S310 in the 6q22-q23 region (table 26.1) yielded the maximum LOD score of 3.11 for a recombination fraction equal to 0. The penetrance of the disease allele (A) was almost complete in AA males and AA females after 12 and 17 years of exposure, respectively, whereas the penetrance in Aa males was 0.73 after 20 years of exposure. For others subjects, the *SM2* penetrance has remained <0.02 after 20 of residency in the area. Finally, multipoint analysis using four markers simultaneously provided a Z_{max} of 3.12 with D6S310 microsatellite and 2.5 with the FA1 marker. A genomewide scan performed on this population did not provide convincing evidence for involvement of additional loci in other chromosomal regions (N. el Wali and A.J. Dessein, unpublished observations).

More recently, Blanton et al. (2005), working in an Egyptian population, tested the linkage of advanced and severe PPF with several regions, including those containing *TGFB1*, *IL13*, and *IFNGR1*. This study employed a nonparametric sib-pair analysis that accommodes polygenic control better than segregation/ linkage analytic methods. The data confirmed the linkage to markers in the *IFNGR1* and suggested linkage to *IL13* and *TGFB1*.

These studies show, in genetically different populations, that a major locus on chromosome 6q23, distinct from the one on chromosome 5q31-q33, controls progression to advanced hepatic fibrosis. Thus, immunity against disease and immunity against infection are controlled by separate major genes.

Analysis of Candidate Genes in the 6q23 Chromosomal Region

Inflammation and fibrosis triggered by schistosome eggs in the liver are tightly dependent on cytokines such as IFN-γ, tumor necrosis factor (TNF), transforming growth factor-β (TGF-β), IL-13, IL-4, and IL-10. Stellate cells are activated by such substances as platelet-derived growth factor (PDGF), released by damaged hepatocytes, endothelial cells, and activated platelets. Myofibroblasts are regulated by a variety of cytokines, such as IFN-γ, which inhibits their multiplication and the production of ECMP (Duncan and Berman, 1985; Mallat et al., 1995). Conversely, IL-13, TGF-β, and IL-4 stimulate fibroblast division and ECMP production (Tiggelman et al., 1995). Tissue fibrosis results from the excessive production of ECMP and/or the insufficient

turnover of the fibrotic tissue. This process depends on the action of metalloprotease (MP)/metalloprotease inhibitors (MPI), the synthesis and activities of which are also regulated by the above-mentioned cytokines (i.e., IFN-γ stimulates the production of MP and inhibits the synthesis of MPI; Tamai et al., 1995).

Thus, IFN-γ is strong anti-fibrosing cytokine, whereas IL-13 and TGF-β are strongly pro-fibrogenic. IFN-γ was associated with protection and TNF with aggravation of PPF in endemic populations of Sudan and Uganda (Henri et al., 2002a). Recent studies suggest that T-regulatory cells may interfere with protective immunity to *Schistosoma*. Resolution of egg granulomatous lesions in experimental schistosomiasis requires the down-regulation of Th2 cytokines (IL-4, IL-13) and the up-regulation of IFN-γ (McKee and Pearce, 2004). Therefore, regulating the quality of the T-cell response is critical. Th cell deviation can be achieved by various mechanisms: inhibition by IFN-γ– producing Th1 cells, reduction of IL-4 producing T cells, or regulation by either constitutive (CD25[+] CD4[+]) or adaptive (Tr1 or Th3) T-regulatory cells (Cottrez and Groux, 2004).

There is evidence for the presence of IL-10 producing CD4[+] CD25[+] T cells at the chronic stage of *S. mansoni* infection in mice; T-regulatory cells were shown to control morbidity and mortality in a reconstituted recombination activating gene 2 (*Rag2–*) and *Il10*–deficient mice infected with *S. mansoni*. T-regulatory cells exert their suppressive effects via a number of molecules, among which are IL-10 and TGF-β (Hesse et al., 2004). Whether IL-10 or TGF-β production is increased or decreased in hepatic schistosomiasis is not known; excessive activity of T-regulatory cells in the liver of schistosome infected subjects could induce fibrosis by two extremely potent mechanisms (1) by inhibiting a most potent anti-fibrogenic cytokine (IFN-γ) and (2) by stimulating fibrosis by the strongly fibrogenic cytokine TGF-β.

Thus *IFNGR1*, which was associated with the highest LOD score in the linkage analysis, is also the best candidate gene in the 6q23 region for the control of fibrosis based on immunological studies. The studies described above also indicate that other chromosomal regions could also play a role in the control of fibrosis, including regions containing genes for PDGF, IFN-γ, TGF-β, TNF, and IL-13. So far, associations of PPF with only two polymorphisms in *IFNG* (Chevillard et al., 2002) have been reported (table 26.1). Both polymorphisms in *IFNG* affect the binding of nuclear transcription factors and possibly gene transcription (Chevillard et al., 2003). These results are consistent with all experimental work and studies in humans showing that IFN-γ protects against PPF.

It should be emphasized that the lack of linkage of PPF with the HLA-TNF region did not exclude contributions of polymorphisms in that region to disease. Reported associations between certain HLA class II alleles and biopsy-confirmed hepatic schistosomiasis in Brazil (Secor et al., 1996) indicate that alleles of class II genes may play a role (albeit less than the chromosome 6q23 region) in the control of disease (table 26.1). Serologically defined HLA class I alleles (A1 and B5) were associated with HSP in early studies in Egypt and Brazil (Salam et al., 1979, Abaza et al., 1985, Abdel-Salam et al., 1986, Cabello et al., 1991). However, HSP is not inevitably associated with lethal PPF, and most children with HSP do not exhibit PPF. Disease association studies in the era of serotyping for class I alleles are difficult to interpret without verification by molecular methods or biologic confirmation. Associations between fibrosis and certain HLA-DR-DQ alleles or haplotypes and HLA-DP alleles have also been reported in *S. japonicum* infections (Hirayama, 2002, 2004, Hirayama et al., 1999, McManus et al., 2001, Waine et al., 1998); there are, however, inconsistencies between studies and some weaknesses in clinical phenotype definition. Moreover, study groups are small, and not all associations are convincing after taking multiple comparisons into account. Finally, a study in the Sudanese population failed to detect an association between any of several functional *TNF* alleles and PPF (Moukoko et al., 2003), but more comprehensive study of *TNF* polymorphism is needed.

Conclusions

Studies on the genetics of schistosome infections in several distinct populations by different laboratories have shown that a few genes play a major role in the control of infection and hepatic disease. This contrasts with a more complex pattern of genetic control of leishmaniasis (see chapter 25). The difference may be due partly to the ease of evaluation of environmental risks factors in schistosome infections or to the biology of the parasites: *Leishmania* populations are heterogeneous, while pathogenicity and virulence of *Schistosoma* populations are more homogenous. Higher genomic plasticity may have permitted *Leishmania* to evolve more rapidly than

schistosomes, escape more readily from host defenses, and force their vertebrate host into a genetic race for resistance alleles that has resulted in more rapid accumulation of genetic variants in host and parasite.

Genetic studies of individuals resistant and susceptible to schistosome infections have demonstrated that the mechanisms of immune protection against infection and against severe hepatic disease are distinct. These observations on the distinct immunological pathways involved in protection can now inform the development of assays for protection that should be valuable in vaccine trials because they distinguish between the immune response to vaccines against infection and the response to vaccines against disease. Finally, susceptibility alleles can also be used to identify those individuals who are at higher risk of severe infection/disease and should be included in vaccination trials or protected with regular chemotherapy.

References

Abaza, H., Asser, L., el Sawy, M., Wasfy, S., Montaser, L., Hagras, M., & Shaltout, A. (1985) HLA antigens in schistosomal hepatic fibrosis patients with haematemesis. *Tissue Antigens*, **26**, 307–309.

Abdel-Salam, E., Abdel Khalik, A., Abdel-Meguid, A., Barakat, W., & Mahmoud, A.A. (1986) Association of HLA class I antigens (A1, B5, B8 and CW2) with disease manifestations and infection in human schistosomiasis mansoni in Egypt. *Tissue Antigens*, **27**, 142–146.

Abel, L., Demenais, F., Prata, A., Souza, A.E., & Dessein, A. (1991) Evidence for the segregation of a major gene in human susceptibility/resistance to infection by *Schistosoma mansoni*. Am J Hum Genet, **48**, 959–970.

Bergmann, M., Barnes, P.J., & Newton, R. (2000) Molecular regulation of granulocyte macrophage colony-stimulating factor in human lung epithelial cells by interleukin (IL)-1beta, IL-4, and IL-13 involves both transcriptional and post-transcriptional mechanisms. *Am J Respir Cell Mol Biol*, **22**, 582–589.

Blanton, R.E., Salam, E.A., Ehsan, A., King, C.H., & Goddard, K.A. (2005) Schistosomal hepatic fibrosis and the interferon gamma receptor: a linkage analysis using single-nucleotide polymorphic markers. *Eur J Hum Genet*, **13**, 660–668.

Bochner, B.S., Klunk, D.A., Sterbinsky, S.A., Coffman, R.L., & Schleimer, R.P. (1995) IL-13 selectively induces vascular cell adhesion molecule-1 expression in human endothelial cells. *J Immunol*, **154**, 799–803.

Cabello, P.H., Krieger, H., Lopes, J.D., & Sant'Ana, E.J. (1991) On the association between HLA-A1 and B5 and clinical forms of schistosomiasis mansoni. *Mem Inst Oswaldo Cruz*, **86**, 37–40.

Capron, M., & Capron, A. (1994) Immunoglobulin E and effector cells in schistosomiasis. *Science*, **264**, 1876–1877.

Capron, M., & Goldman, M. (2001) The eosinophil, a cell with multiple facets. *Therapie*, **56**, 371–375.

Capron, M., Soussi Gounni, A., Morita, M., Truong, M.J., Prin, L., Kinet, J.P., & Capron, A. (1995) Eosinophils: from low- to high-affinity immunoglobulin E receptors. *Allergy*, **50**, 20–23.

Chevillard, C., Henri, S., Stefani, F., Parzy, D., & Dessein, A. (2002) Two new polymorphisms in the human interferon gamma (IFN-gamma) promoter. *Eur J Immunogenet*, **29**, 53–56.

Chevillard, C., Moukoko, C.E., Elwali, N.E., Bream, J.H., Kouriba, B., Argiro, L., Rahoud, S., Mergani, A., Henri, S., Gaudart, J., Mohamed-Ali, Q., Young, H.A., & Dessein, A.J. (2003) IFN-gamma polymorphisms (IFN-gamma +2109 and IFN-gamma +3810) are associated with severe hepatic fibrosis in human hepatic schistosomiasis (*Schistosoma mansoni*). *J Immunol*, **171**, 5596–5601.

Cottrez, F., & Groux, H. (2004) Specialization in tolerance: innate CD(4+)CD(25+) versus acquired TR1 and TH3 regulatory T cells. *Transplantation*, **77**, S12–15.

Demeure, C.E., Rihet, P., Abel, L., Ouattara, M., Bourgois, A., & Dessein, A.J. (1993) Resistance to *Schistosoma mansoni* in humans: influence of the IgE/IgG4 balance and IgG2 in immunity to reinfection after chemotherapy. *J Infect Dis*, **168**, 1000–1008.

Dessein, A.J., Couissinier, P., Demeure, C., Rihet, P., Kohlstaedt, S., Carneiro-Carvalho, D., Ouattara, M., Goudot-Crozel, V., Dessein, H., Bourgois, A., & et al. (1992) Environmental, genetic and immunological factors in human resistance to *Schistosoma mansoni*. *Immunol Invest*, **21**, 423–453.

Dessein, A.J., Hillaire, D., Elwali, N.E., Marquet, S., Mohamed-Ali, Q., Mirghani, A., Henri, S., Abdelhameed, A.A., Saeed, O.K., Magzoub, M.M., & Abel, L. (1999) Severe hepatic fibrosis in *Schistosoma mansoni* infection is controlled by a major locus that is closely linked to the interferon-gamma receptor gene. *Am J Hum Genet*, **65**, 709–721.

Dessein, A., Kouriba, B., Eboumbou, C., Dessein, H., Argiro, L., Marquet, S., Elwali, N.E., Rodrigues, V., Li, Y., Doumbo, O., & Chevillard, C. (2004) Interleukin-13 in the skin and interferon-gamma in the liver are key players in immune protection in human schistosomiasis. *Immunol Rev*, **201**, 180–190.

de Vries, J.E., Punnonen, J., Cocks, B.G., de Waal Malefyt, R., & Aversa, G. (1993) Regulation of the human IgE response by IL4 and IL13. *Res Immunol*, **144**, 597–601.

Duncan, M.R., & Berman, B. (1985) Gamma interferon is the lymphokine and beta interferon the monokine responsible for inhibition of fibroblast collagen production and late but not early fibroblast proliferation. *J Exp Med*, **162**, 516–527.

Dunne, D.W., Butterworth, A.E., Fulford, A.J., Kariuki, H.C., Langley, J.G., Ouma, J.H., Capron, A., Pierce, R.J., & Sturrock, R.F. (1992) Immunity after treatment of human schistosomiasis: association between IgE antibodies to adult worm antigens and resistance to reinfection. *Eur J Immunol*, **22**, 1483–1494.

Ellis, M.K., Li, Y., Rong, Z., Chen, H., & McManus, D.P. (2006) Familial aggregation of human infection with *Schistosoma japonicum* in the Poyang Lake region, China. *Int J Parasitol*, **36**, 71–77.

Gressner, A.M. (1995) Cytokines and cellular crosstalk involved in the activation of fat-storing cells. *J Hepatol*, **22**, 28–36.

Hagan, P., Blumenthal, U.J., Dunn, D., Simpson, A.J., & Wilkins, H.A. (1991) Human IgE, IgG4 and resistance to reinfection with *Schistosoma haematobium*. *Nature*, **349**, 243–245.

Henri, S., Chevillard, C., Mergani, A., Paris, P., Gaudart, J., Camilla, C., Dessein, H., Montero, F., Elwali, N.E., Saeed, O.K., Magzoub, M., & Dessein, A.J. (2002) Cytokine regulation of periportal fibrosis in humans infected with *Schistosoma mansoni*: IFN-gamma is associated with protection against fibrosis and TNF-alpha with aggravation of disease. *J Immunol*, **169**, 929–936.

Hesse, M., Piccirillo, C.A., Belkaid, Y., Prufer, J., Mentink-Kane, M., Leusink, M., Cheever, A.W., Shevach, E.M., & Wynn, T.A. (2004) The pathogenesis of schistosomiasis is controlled by cooperating IL-10-producing innate effector and regulatory T cells. *J Immunol*, **172**, 3157–3166.

Hirayama, K. (2002) Genetic factors associated with development of cerebral malaria and fibrotic schistosomiasis. *Korean J Parasitol*, **40**, 165–172.

Hirayama, K. (2004) Immunogenetic analysis of postschistosomal liver fibrosis. *Parasitol Int*, **53**, 193–196.

Hirayama, K., Chen, H., Kikuchi, M., Yin, T., Gu, X., Liu, J., Zhang, S., & Yuan, H. (1999) HLA-DR-DQ alleles and HLA-DP alleles are independently associated with susceptibility to different stages of postschistosomal hepatic fibrosis in the Chinese population. *Tissue Antigens*, **53**, 269–274.

Kouriba, B., Chevillard, C., Bream, J.H., Argiro, L., Dessein, H., Arnaud, V., Sangare, L., Dabo, A., Beavogui, A.H., Arama, C., Traore, H.A., Doumbo, O., &

Dessein, A. (2005) Analysis of the 5q31-q33 locus shows an association between IL13−1055C/T IL-13−591A/G polymorphisms and *Schistosoma haematobium* infections. *J Immunol*, 174, 6274–6281.

Liu, X., Beaty, T.H., Deindl, P., Huang, S.K., Lau, S., Sommerfeld, C., Fallin, M.D., Kao, W.H., Wahn, U., & Nickel, R. (2003) Associations between total serum IgE levels and the 6 potentially functional variants within the genes IL4, IL13, and IL4RA in German children: the German Multicenter Atopy Study. *J Allergy Clin Immunol*, 112, 382–388.

Liu, X., Beaty, T.H., Deindl, P., Huang, S.K., Lau, S., Sommerfeld, C., Fallin, M.D., Kao, W.H., Wahn, U., & Nickel, R. (2004) Associations between specific serum IgE response and 6 variants within the genes IL4, IL13, and IL4RA in German children: the German Multicenter Atopy Study. *J Allergy Clin Immunol*, 113, 489–495.

Luttmann, W., Knoechel, B., Foerster, M., Matthys, H., Virchow, J.C., Jr., & Kroegel, C. (1996) Activation of human eosinophils by IL-13. Induction of CD69 surface antigen, its relationship to messenger RNA expression, and promotion of cellular viability. *J Immunol*, 157, 1678–1683.

Mallat, A., Preaux, A.M., Blazejewski, S., Rosenbaum, J., Dhumeaux, D., & Mavier, P. (1995) Interferon alfa and gamma inhibit proliferation and collagen synthesis of human Ito cells in culture. *Hepatology*, 21, 1003–1010.

Marquet, S., Abel, L., Hillaire, D., & Dessein, A. (1999) Full results of the genome-wide scan which localises a locus controlling the intensity of infection by *Schistosoma mansoni* on chromosome 5q31-q33. *Eur J Hum Genet*, 7, 88–97.

Marquet, S., Abel, L., Hillaire, D., Dessein, H., Kalil, J., Feingold, J., Weissenbach, J., & Dessein, A.J. (1996) Genetic localization of a locus controlling the intensity of infection by *Schistosoma mansoni* on chromosome 5q31-q33. *Nat Genet*, 14, 181–184.

McKee, A.S., & Pearce, E.J. (2004) CD25+CD4+ cells contribute to Th2 polarization during helminth infection by suppressing Th1 response development. *J Immunol*, 173, 1224–1231.

McKenzie, A.N., Culpepper, J.A., de Waal Malefyt, R., Briere, F., Punnonen, J., Aversa, G., Sato, A., Dang, W., Cocks, B.G., Menon, S., et al. (1993) Interleukin 13, a T-cell-derived cytokine that regulates human monocyte and B-cell function. *Proc Natl Acad Sci USA*, 90, 3735–3739.

McManus, D.P., Ross, A.G., Williams, G.M., Sleigh, A.C., Wiest, P., Erlich, H., Trachtenberg, E., Guanling, W., McGarvey, S.T., Li, Y.S., & Waine, G.J. (2001) HLA class II antigens positively and negatively associated with hepatosplenic schistoso-

miasis in a Chinese population. *Int J Parasitol*, 31, 674–680.

Mohamed-Ali, Q., Elwali, N.E., Abdelhameed, A.A., Mergani, A., Rahoud, S., Elagib, K.E., Saeed, O.K., Abel, L., Magzoub, M.M., & Dessein, A.J. (1999) Susceptibility to periportal (Symmers) fibrosis in human *Schistosoma mansoni* infections: evidence that intensity and duration of infection, gender, and inherited factors are critical in disease progression. *J Infect Dis*, 180, 1298–1306.

Moukoko, C.E., El Wali, N., Saeed, O.K., Mohamed-Ali, Q., Gaudart, J., Dessein, A.J., & Chevillard, C. (2003) No evidence for a major effect of tumor necrosis factor alpha gene polymorphisms in periportal fibrosis caused by *Schistosoma mansoni* infection. *Infect Immun*, 71, 5456–5460.

Muller-Myhsok, B., Stelma, F.F., Guisse-Sow, F., Muntau, B., Thye, T., Burchard, G.D., Gryseels, B., & Horstmann, R.D. (1997) Further evidence suggesting the presence of a locus, on human chromosome 5q31-q33, influencing the intensity of infection with *Schistosoma mansoni*. *Am J Hum Genet*, 61, 452–454.

Oettgen, H.C. (2000) Regulation of the IgE isotype switch: new insights on cytokine signals and the functions of epsilon germline transcripts. *Curr Opin Immunol*, 12, 618–623.

Poli, G. (2000) Pathogenesis of liver fibrosis: role of oxidative stress. *Mol Aspects Med*, 21, 49–98.

Punnonen, J., Aversa, G., Cocks, B.G., McKenzie, A.N., Menon, S., Zurawski, G., de Waal Malefyt, R., & de Vries, J.E. (1993) Interleukin 13 induces interleukin 4-independent IgG4 and IgE synthesis and CD23 expression by human B cells. *Proc Natl Acad Sci USA*, 90, 3730–3734.

Rihet, P., Demeure, C.E., Bourgois, A., Prata, A., & Dessein, A.J. (1991) Evidence for an association between human resistance to *Schistosoma mansoni* and high anti-larval IgE levels. *Eur J Immunol*, 21, 2679–2686.

Rihet, P., Demeure, C.E., Dessein, A.J., & Bourgeois, A. (1992) Strong serum inhibition of specific IgE correlated to competing IgG4 revealed by a new methodology in subjects from a *S. mansoni* endemic area. *Eur J Immunol*, 22, 2063–2070.

Salam, E.A., Ishaac, S., & Mahmoud, A.A. (1979) Histocompatibilty-linked susceptibility for hepatosplenomegaly in human schistosomiasis *mansoni*. *J Immunol*, 123, 1829–1831.

Secor, W.E., del Corral, H., dos Reis, M.G., Ramos, E.A., Zimon, A.E., Matos, E.P., Reis, E.A., do Carmo, T.M., Hirayama, K., David, R.A., David, J.R., & Harn, D.A., Jr. (1996) Association of hepatosplenic schistosomiasis with HLA-DQB1*0201. *J Infect Dis*, 174, 1131–1135.

Seto, E.Y., Zhong, B., Kouch, J., Hubbard, A., & Spear, R.C. (2005) Genetic and household risk factors for *Schistosoma japonicum* infection in the presence of larger scale environmental differences in the mountainous transmission areas of China. *Am J Trop Med Hyg*, **73**, 1145–1150.

Tamai, K., Ishikawa, H., Mauviel, A., & Uitto, J. (1995) Interferon-gamma coordinately upregulates matrix metalloprotease (MMP)-1 and MMP-3, but not tissue inhibitor of metalloproteases (TIMP), expression in cultured keratinocytes. *J Invest Dermatol*, **104**, 384–390.

Tiggelman, A.M., Boers, W., Linthorst, C., Sala, M., & Chamuleau, R.A. (1995) Collagen synthesis by human liver (myo)fibroblasts in culture: evidence for a regulatory role of IL-1 beta, IL-4, TGF beta and IFN gamma. *J Hepatol*, **23**, 307–317.

van der Pouw Kraan, T.C., van Veen, A., Boeije, L.C., van Tuyl, S.A., de Groot, E.R., Stapel, S.O., Bakker, A., Verweij, C.L., Aarden, L.A., & van der Zee, J.S. (1999) An IL-13 promoter polymorphism associated with increased risk of allergic asthma. *Genes Immun*, **1**, 61–65.

von Lichtenberg, F. (1962) Host response to eggs of S. mansoni. I. Granuloma formation in the unsensitized laboratory mouse. *Am J Pathol*, **41**, 711–731.

Waine, G.J., Ross, A.G., Williams, G.M., Sleigh, A.C., & McManus, D.P. (1998) HLA class II antigens are associated with resistance or susceptibility to hepatosplenic disease in a Chinese population infected with *Schistosoma japonicum*. *Int J Parasitol*, **28**, 537–542.

Warren, K.S. (1977) Modulation of immunopathology and disease in schistosomiasis. *Am J Trop Med Hyg*, **26**, 113–119.

Warren, K.S., Domingo, E.O., & Cowan, R.B. (1967) Granuloma formation around schistosome eggs as a manifestation of delayed hypersensitivity. *Am J Pathol*, **51**, 735–756.

Zinn-Justin, A., Marquet, S., Hillaire, D., Dessein, A., & Abel, L. (2001) Genome search for additional human loci controlling infection levels by *Schistosoma mansoni*. *Am J Trop Med Hyg*, **65**, 754–758.

27

Genetics and Immune Response to Vaccines

Gregory A. Poland, Inna G. Ovsyannikova, & Robert M. Jacobson

Much can be learned from reviewing relevant information concerning the relationship between vaccine-induced immune responses and the genes that influence and modify these responses. This chapter focuses on data regarding genes located in the human leukocyte antigen (HLA) gene cluster, because data support the importance of HLA genes in determining adaptive immune responses. In addition, this chapter focuses on the immune responses to specific vaccines for hepatitis B, measles, rubella, influenza, bacille Calmette-Guerin (BCG), and polio. Because the HLA–viral peptide complex is the vital structural unit for immune recognition (Racioppi et al., 1991), identifying HLA relationships with the most dramatic effects on adaptive immunity can elucidate HLA restriction—an important mechanism for understanding differential vaccine response. Further, defining HLA associations with specific vaccine antigens increases the knowledge base that could potentially lead to the development of the next generation of viral vaccines.

Genetic Influences on Disease Susceptibility

While this volume broadly addresses genetic susceptibility to infectious diseases, the specific focus in this chapter is on considering genetic influences upon vaccine response (Hill, 1998). In terms of heritable manifestations of infectious diseases, twin studies, HLA and non-HLA associations, and family studies all underscore the genetic interplay between infectious agent and host. First, twin studies have shown variable contributions of heredity and environment in infectious disease susceptibility (Gedda et al., 1984; Haverkorn et al., 1975). Among common pediatric infectious diseases studied, the immune response to measles infection has a particularly strong hereditary component (Gedda et al., 1984; Haverkorn et al., 1975). A twin study has also revealed variable genetic regulation of the degree of response to different antigens in the context of cell-mediated immunity (CMI) to tuberculosis (Jepson et al., 2001).

Second, HLA markers have been reported with elevated levels of antibodies against common infections such as influenza, measles, and rubella (Haverkorn et al., 1975; Galbraith et al., 1976), with both susceptibility and resistance to congenital rubella syndrome (Honeyman et al., 1975; Kato et al., 1980), and with paralytic polio (Lasch et al., 1979).

Third, severe complications of measles have been reported to cluster in families (Ito et al., 2000). Other studies report a familial association with a hyperimmune response to measles virus antigen in multiple sclerosis (Haghighi et al., 2000; Paty et al., 1976). Although multiple sclerosis is not a complication of measles, multiple sclerosis is associated with unusually elevated levels of various antibodies. Early studies of elevated measles antibody in multiple sclerosis have demonstrated HLA associations (Paty et al., 1976).

In addition, familial associations have been found with complications of hepatitis B (see chapter 21), suggesting a genetic influence on the immune response to the disease (Nasrallah et al., 1978; Eliakim et al., 1978; Munoz et al., 1989; Lynch et al., 1984). For example, HLA associations have been found with hepatitis B and membranous nephropathy (Bhimma et al., 2002). Similar associations have been found with the carrier state, chronic active hepatitis, and hepatocellular carcinoma following hepatitis B infection (Sampliner et al., 1981; Levo et al., 1982; Yang et al., 1989; Forzani et al., 1984; Scobie et al., 1983).

Although the data reported to date concentrate on relationships with HLA genes and the molecules that these genes encode, other genes are undoubtedly involved in the relationships with disease susceptibility and disease complications. In fact, non-HLA genes may play a larger role in the variability of CMI or other pathways in the immune response, as was particularly evident with tuberculosis (Jepson et al., 1997). Other relevant examples include recent reports of a 32-bp deletion in a chemokine receptor CCR5 gene that has been associated with a significant modulation in the immune response to HIV-1 (see chapter 19) and with decreased levels of circulating varicella zoster antibody but not other common herpesviruses (Wiencke et al., 2001).

Theoretical Constructs from Biology for a Genetic Role in Vaccine Response

The theoretical basis for genetic influences on vaccine response can be found in the extensive polymorphisms of the genetic machinery for the immune response. The normal spectrum for the repertoire of epitope response found in the HLA system provides the underlying rationale for hypothesizing that healthy individuals who vary in their HLA allele distribution across class I and class II HLA genes will, in turn, respond variably to vaccines and other antigens.

For a variety of reasons, vaccine response is frequently portrayed as binary, whereas the measures of immunity are in reality numerical and continuous. The artifice of a binary response dates back to the prevaccine era when it was recognized that many infectious diseases typically resulted in what appeared to be life-long immunity (e.g., measles, polio, rubella). Therefore, it was natural to consider an individual either "immune" if that individual had recovered from the disease or "susceptible" if the individual had succumbed. This dichotomization was further ratified in the context of public health, where receipt of a vaccine has often been equated with immunity. However, diseases such as measles have occurred in settings among individuals with decidedly positive responses to vaccine, and such experiences emphasize the quantitative spectrum of vaccine response (Chen et al., 1990). The landmark study by Chen et al. (1990) focused on the humoral response to measles vaccine even though many vaccines act and depend substantially upon cellular immunity. The relative difficulties of quantifying cellular immunity have often led to both denial and oversimplification of the variability in vaccine response. By ignoring the complexity of immune response, this convenient simplification has obfuscated the potential roles of environmental and genetic influences on the range of interindividual vaccine responses.

HLA and Vaccine Response

Various investigative groups have been particularly interested in examining the immunogenetic variables influencing humoral antibody, with the goal of understanding the influence of HLA genes on the continuous biologic spectrum of antibody level (Poland & Jacobson, 1998; Jacobson & Poland, 2004; Ovsyannikova et al., 2004a; Anders et al., 1996; Wang et al., 2004; Newport et al., 2004). The focus on humoral immunity is logical for several key reasons: (1) recognition that the measurement of antibody level following vaccination is the gold standard by which vaccines are standardized, licensed, and evaluated (Robbins et al., 1995); (2) a relative paucity of evidence across vaccines that any vaccine-induced entity other than serum antibody prevents disease, and concomitant evidence that passive immunization with pathogen-specific immunoglobulin confers protection, as in the case of measles infection (Robbins et al., 1995; Norrby, 1995); (3) evidence that passively transferred maternal humoral IgG antibody transiently protects newborns against specific viral diseases (e.g., measles for 12–15 months) (Norrby, 1995); (4) evidence that immuno-deficient children can be protected against viral disease when treated with immunoglobulin (Norrby, 1995); and (5) difficulty identifying a quantifiable and repro-ducible indicator of specific CMI that has been pro-spectively defined and validated in response to immu-nization. Even now, the methods available to measure CMI in response to immunization, to confirm their accuracy and meaning, and to relate them to long-term immunity remain promising but not fully validated.

Despite the ostensible predominance of humoral over cellular immunity, there is evidence that CMI is essential for recovery from certain diseases such as measles and that CMI provides for long-term immu-nity even in the absence of detectable circulating an-tibody (Bautista-López et al., 2000; Good & Zak, 1956; Ruckdeshel et al., 1975; Samb et al., 1995; Hickman et al., 1997; Mitus et al., 1965; Markowitz et al., 1988). The vital role of T-cell–mediated CMI is demonstrated by agammaglobulinemic children who recover from measles infection and develop protective immunity, while children with T-cell abnormalities suffer com-plications and die from infection (Burnet, 1968; Mar-kowitz et al., 1988; Nanan et al., 2000). Therefore, CMI may be as or more important than antibody for long-lasting immunity to viral infections such as mea-sles (Pabst et al., 1997).

As tools for evaluating CMI have become more informative, increasing effort has been made to un-derstand genetic regulation of vaccine-induced CMI responses (Ovsyannikova et al., 2003, 2004d; Doolan et al., 2000; Nanan et al., 1995). Studies of measures of cellular immune responses such as lymphoprolifera-tion, vaccine-specific T-helper 1 (Th1) and Th2 cyto-kine responses, and vaccine-specific $CD4^+$ and $CD8^+$ T-cell frequencies have been closely accompanied by the exploration of associations with genetic variability. Because response to foreign viral antigens is heavily determined by HLA polymorphisms, a leading hy-pothesis has been that HLA polymorphisms may ex-plain individual variability in cellular immune re-

sponses to viral vaccines (Poland & Jacobson, 1998; Poland, 1998, 1999; Berzofsky, 1988). T-cell activation results in T-cell proliferation and differentiation into $CD4^+$ or $CD8^+$ cells. $CD4^+$ cells further differentiate into Th1 or Th2 cells, each of which produces distinct profiles of cytokines that polarize the immune response toward a cell-mediated or antibody-mediated response, respectively. In this way, cellular immune responses (i.e., cytokine production and secretion) may be ge-netically regulated at a very early step in the immune response cascade—where the high degree of inherited variability represented by HLA alleles leads to selective presentation of antigens (Lanzavecchia & Sallusto, 2000). As discussed in chapters 4 and 5, HLA class I genes (A, B, and C genes) encode proteins that bind peptide for display to $CD8^+$ cytotoxic T lymphocytes (CTLs), leading to cellular immune responses. HLA class II genes (DRB, DQB, DQA, DPA, and DPB) play an important role in the humoral immune response to viral infections (Pamer, 1999), generally presenting peptides to $CD4^+$ Th cells, and certain alleles of those genes show associations with resistance or susceptibility to specific infections. Measles vaccine–induced im-mune responses have been used as one model for ex-amining genetic variation in CMI associated with live viral vaccines, with the understanding that this work can be conceptually extended to models of response to other similar vaccines (Poland & Jacobson, 1998; Poland, 1998, 1999). Studies in the measles model have con-centrated on dissecting those portions of the immune responses mediated by the HLA system (table 27.1).

Immunoglobulin Gm and Km Allotypes

Genes associated with human immunoglobulin allo-typic markers Gm (γ-chains) and Km (κ-type light chains) are located on chromosome 14 and chromo-some 2, respectively, (Pandey, 1990; Schanfield & Van Loghem, 1986). Gm groups are limited to IgG classes (IgG1–IgG4), and approximately 18 Gm specificities are currently determined. The Km allotypes are re-presented in all classes of immunoglobulins (IgG, IgA, IgM, IgD, and IgE) and are inherited through three alleles: Km*1, Km*1,2, and Km*3 (Pandey, 2000). Significant racial variation in Gm and Km allotypes and allelic associations with Gm and Km allotypes in the immune responses to some pathogens have been reported (Black et al., 1995; Pandey & Blaser, 1986; Biggar et al., 1994; Wachsmuth et al., 1987; Rodriguez-

TABLE 27.1. Associations between HLA polymorphisms and immune response to vaccines.

Vaccine	Gene	Variant	Effect	Selected References
Hepatitis B	HLA class I	B*8	Decreased antibody response (anti-HBsAg)	Kruskall et al, 1992; Desombere et al, 1998; Wang et al, 2004
	HLA class II	DRB1*03, DRB1*04, DRB1*07		
	HLA class I Chinese cohort	B*15, B*46	Decreased antibody response	Yap & Chan, 1996;
	HLA class II Japanese cohort	DRB1*08032, DPA1*0103, DPB1*0402, DQA1*0503	Decreased antibody response	Mineta et al, 1996
Measles (single dose)	HLA class I HLA class II	B*8, B*13, B*44 DRB1*03, DQA1*0201	Decreased antibody (IgG)	Poland et al, 2001; Jacobson et al, 2003
	HLA class I HLA class II	B*7 DRB1*08, DQA1*0104, DPA1*0202	Increased antibody (IgG)	Ovsyannikova et al, 2004c
Rubella	HLA class I	A*3, A*11, B*3503, Cw*1502	T-cell response (CTL, lymphocyte proliferation)	Ou et al, 1997, 1998;
	HLA class II	DRB1*0403, DRB1*0901 DRB1*03, DRB1*04, DRB1*0101, DRB1*1104, DQB1*0501, DPB1*0301	T-cell response (lymphocyte proliferation)	Nepom et al, 1997;
	HLA class II	DPB1*0301, DPB1*0401, DPB1*1301, DPB1*1501	Increased antibody (IgG)	Ovsyannikova et al, 2004b, 2005
Influenza	HLA class II	DRB1*07, DRB1*13, DQB1*0603-9/14, DQB1*0303	Decreased antibody response (hemagglutination-inhibition)	Gelder et al, 2002
Polio	HLA class I	A2, Aw*19, B*7, B*8, B*12, B*44	Increased antibody response	Lasch et al, 1979; Lindberg et al, 1979; Ermolovich et al, 2002

Abbreviations: HBsAg, surface polypeptide antigen of HBV; CTL, cytotoxic T lymphocytes; BCG, bacille Calmette-Guerin.

Barradas et al., 1996). Various studies have examined the role of Gm and Km allotype gene polymorphisms in humoral immune responses to vaccines and in the genetic predisposition to several infectious diseases (Pandey, 2000; Sarvas et al., 1990; Granoff et al., 1986, 1988; Goldblatt et al., 1994). In general, the lack of HLA, Gm, and Km polymorphisms was associated with elevated levels of infectious disease such as pneumonia (Black et al., 1995) and was specifically associated with lower antibody responses to pathogens and vaccine (influenza, measles, rubella) immunity (Goldblatt et al., 1994). The biologic function of Gm and Km allotype gene polymorphisms requires further understanding; however, some evidence suggests that certain of these polymorphisms are protective at the population level.

Immunoglobulin Gm and Km allotypes and immunity to *Haemophilus influenzae* type b (Hib) polysac-

charide vaccine has been investigated in studies of both children and adults. A significant negative association was found between the Km1 allotype and the immune response to one dose of Hib vaccine in white children but not in black children (Pandey et al., 1979). In addition, Km1-positive black children had an approximately 3-fold lower relative risk of developing Hib meningitis than did those who had the Km1-negative allotype (Pandey, 2000). The IgG1 antibody responses in children immunized with Hib polysaccharide were not affected by the Gm23 allotype; however, adults homozygous for Gm23 demonstrated higher IgG2 antibody levels following Hib vaccination (Granoff & Holmes, 1992; Granoff et al., 1988). Because the Gm23 allotype is known to influence the IgG2 subclass concentration (Pandey & French, 1996), Gm23-negative persons exhibit primarily IgG1 responses to Hib polysaccharide.

The role of IgG allotypes in the immune response to pneumococcal capsular polysaccharides (PPS) was studied in 72 unrelated Caucasian adults and 61 members of an extended Ashkenazic Jewish family (Musher et al., 1997). HLA type was not associated with the humoral response to PPS; however, an association between IgG level and Gm23 allotype was observed in unrelated Caucasians but not in Ashkenazic Jews. Another study demonstrated no relationship between Gm23 and Km1 allotypes and antibody responses to the type III group G streptococcal antigen (Pandey et al., 1984).

In an analysis of the relationship between immunoglobulin allotypes and immune responses to meningococcal A, B, and C polysaccharides, a heterozygous Gm phenotype was found to be significantly linked with low antibody responses to meningococcal polysaccharide A ($p < 0.01$) (Pandey et al., 1982). A second study found that the Km1 allotype was associated with the immune response to Hib and meningococcus C polysaccharides in Caucasian children (Pandey et al., 1979). The Km1-positive allotype and antibody responsiveness to meningococcal group B polysaccharide (MPS) has also been studied in 105 Caucasians (Pandey et al., 1981). No significant association was observed between Gm phenotypes and humoral immune response to MPS group B vaccine; however, a significant association was found between the Km1 allotype and antibody levels to this vaccine. Further, after immunization, bactericidal antibodies induced by MPS group B vaccine were significantly higher in Km-positive subjects than in Km-negative individuals (18.22 vs. 10.49 U/ml, $p = 0.03$) (Pandey et al., 1981). Again, Gm and Km allotype associations were studied in relation to other infectious pathogens and vaccine antigens, such as tetanus toxoid, BCG, *Pseudomonas aeruginosa* lipopolysaccharide, *Campylobacter jejuni*, and onchocerciasis, and revealed that these genetic markers may play an important role in susceptibility to disease, though the biologic role of the polymorphisms of Gm and Km remain uncertain (Schanfield et al., 1979; Matrakshin et al., 1993; Moss et al., 1987; Pandey & Blaser, 1986; Pandey et al., 1995). Together, this work suggests a potential role of Gm and Km polymorphisms in specific antibody responses to infectious pathogens and vaccines. It is important to elucidate the genes associated with immunoglobulin allotypic markers, because these markers may be involved in differential immunity to other lethal infectious pathogens.

The Heterozygote Advantage

In their explorations of HLA and the susceptibility to infectious disease, Black and Hedrick (Hedrick & Black, 1997; Black & Hedrick, 1997) developed a theory of the heterozygote advantage. This theory suggests that genetic, and specifically HLA, heterozygosity allows for *increased* responsiveness to foreign antigen(s), compared to homozygosity, which, by definition, leads to expression of a more restricted set of HLA antigen-presenting molecules (Hansen et al., 1993). In this manner, heterozygosity of class I and II HLA genes could confer a selective advantage to the host by increasing the diversity of peptides presented by antigen-presenting cells (Hughes & Nei, 1988). Of course, if certain HLA alleles mediate better specific responses, others might mediate worse responses. Further, homozygosity at an HLA gene locus might predispose to a more limited response and more likely a poorer one, and increasing homozygosity at more than one HLA locus might worsen this situation. Evidence for this concept derived from studies where individuals homozygous for a specific extended haplotype failed to make antibody in response to hepatitis B vaccine, suggesting that low antibody levels following immunization and HLA homozygosity are related (Kruskall, 1990; Deulofeut et al., 1993; Craven et al., 1986). McDermott et al. (1999) reported that individuals homozygous for the HLA-DRB1*0701, DQB1*0202 genotype failed to produce >100 IU/l of anti-HBs antibody regardless of the hepatitis B vaccine dose. HLA homozygosity has also been shown to be disadvantageous with regard to infectious diseases (Thio et al., 1999; Tang et al., 1999; Hohler et al., 1997; Pollicino et al., 1996; Carrington et al., 1999) and specifically for vaccine response, including hepatitis B (Kruskall et al., 1992) and measles vaccine (St. Sauver et al., 2002; Ovsyannikova et al., 2000; Poland et al., 1995, 1998 et al.,). In fact, some investigators have postulated that the deficiency of HLA homozygotes in a population may be caused by selection against homozygotes by infectious diseases (Hedrick, 1990; Black & Salzano, 1981). For example, Black et al. (1977) studied the pronounced susceptibility to rubella and measles among indigenous peoples and found an association with a high degree of homozygosity in HLA loci. This could, in turn, manifest as disease susceptibility, distinct vaccine response phenotypes, or perhaps even in susceptibility to specific vaccine-induced adverse events. On the other hand, others have questioned the concept of heterozygote advantage on a population level and suggested that further work is necessary before firm conclusions can be drawn (De Boer et al., 2004).

Associations of individual HLA alleles with negative and hyperpositive responses to measles vaccine and of homozygosity with a poor response to the vaccine have been documented, and these associations diminish in frequency and proportion with the receipt of a second dose of measles vaccine (St. Sauver et al., 2005). This implies that repeated antigen exposure can result in extinction of the disadvantage caused by a given HLA allele or homozygosity—at least in the case of measles.

Hepatitis B Vaccine

Variation in the immune response modulated by HLA genes is an important factor in the generation of protective immunity by hepatitis B virus (HBV) vaccines. Studies have shown relationships between HLA genes and nonresponse to the hepatitis B vaccine (Alper et al., 1989; Marescot et al., 1989; Pol et al., 1990; Kruskall et al., 1992; Li et al., 2002; Caillat-Zucman et al., 1998; Durupinar & Okten, 1996). In particular, the response to the surface polypeptide antigen of the HBV (HBsAg) has been shown to be HLA class II restricted (Alper et al., 1989). For example, in those of Caucasian and African ancestry, associations of low antibody responsiveness have been documented with haplotypes containing HLA-DR3, -DR4, or -DR7 (Desombere et al., 1998). In a population of Asian ancestry, an excess of certain class I alleles (HLA-B46 and -B15) were found among nonresponders to recombinant HBV vaccine (Yap & Chan, 1996). HLA-DR restricted cellular recognition of HBsAg, and midsequence HBsAg antigen peptide has also been reported (Deulofeut et al., 1993), suggesting that HLA-DR–linked genes control the human immune responses to hepatitis B (Desombere et al., 1998). A study of 339 healthy Japanese subjects immunized with recombinant HBV vaccine demonstrated an association between class I and class II HLA genes and HBV antibody nonresponse (Mineta et al., 1996). The contribution of the *HLA-DRB1* locus to antibody production was the greatest among the HLA loci studied. For instance, DRB1*08032 in the B46-DRB1*08032 haplotype, DPA1*0103 and DPB1*0402 in the B7-DRB1*0101–DPA1*0103–DPB1*0402 haplotype, and DQA1*0503 in the DRB1*1403–DQA1*0503 haplotype were demonstrated to be the primary positive contributors in those haplotypes to anti-HBsAg antibody production (Mineta et al., 1996).

The heritability of response to HBV vaccine also appears to be strong. Investigators studying twins to quantify the strength of the genetic effect on the immune response to HBsAg (Hohler et al., 2002) reported that the *DRB1* locus accounted for about 25% of the total heritability of the HBsAg vaccine response. Of the total contribution of genetic variability to the immune response to HBsAg, about 40% was ascribed to HLA and 60% to non-HLA genes. Recent work has corroborated high heritability (77%) for antibody responses to HBV vaccine in early life (Newport et al., 2004). Family studies of nonresponsiveness to HBV vaccine indicated that response to HBV vaccine in Caucasian adults is strongly associated with HLA-C4A3, DRB1*0701,DQB1*02 and HLA-C4AQ0,DRB1* 0301,DQB1*02 haplotypes (Desombere et al., 1998; McDermott et al., 1997), but also emphasized the importance of the *C4A* in the HLA class III region, and the C4AQ0 allele in particular (De Silvestri et al., 2001). Early studies demonstrated that out of nine HLA-B8,SC01,DR3-haplotype homozygous individuals, eight were low or nonresponders to the HBV vaccine (Kruskall et al., 1992).

It is well established that at least 5–7% of healthy HBV vaccinated individuals make poor or low antibody responses to the standard three-dose vaccine regimen (Kruskall et al., 1992; Lemon & Thomas, 1997; Desombere et al., 1998). Interestingly, many of the poor responders to HBV vaccine at birth carry up to four HLA-DQαβ heterodimers predisposing to insulin-dependent diabetes mellitus and celiac disease (Martinetti et al., 2000). Not surprisingly, patients with celiac disease, a condition strongly associated with HLA-DQ2 and the C4AQ0-containing haplotype, have a significant predisposition to HBV vaccine nonresponse (Noh et al., 2003). Recently, investigators examined associations between HLA class II alleles and Th1 and Th2 cytokine gene variants with differential responses to full-dose HBV vaccination in 164 HIV-infected North American adolescents (Wang et al., 2004). The HLA-DRB1*07 allele and HIV-1 infection were independently associated with antibody nonresponse to HBV vaccination. In addition, associations were found with cytokine single nucleotide polymorphisms in the interleukin-2 (IL-2) and IL-4 loci along with insertion/deletion variants at the IL-12B locus. These results indicate that HLA-DRB1*07 and immunoregulatory cytokine gene polymorphisms (*IL2*,

IL4, and *IL12B* variants) result in variable immune responses to recombinant HBV vaccines (Wang et al., 2004). In short, as predicted by family studies, evidence is now accumulating that the immune response to HBV vaccine is significantly influenced by more than just HLA polymorphisms.

Measles Vaccine

Investigation of the immune response to live measles virus vaccine has revealed familial clustering of antibody seronegativity following measles immunization and that genetic polymorphisms within the HLA genes significantly influence the immune responses to measles vaccine (Poland, 1999). After a single dose of measles vaccine, low antibody levels have been strongly associated with both class I (B8, B13, B44) and class II (DRB1*03 and DQA1*0201) alleles (Jacobson et al., 2003; Poland et al., 2001), as well as with homozygosity at both class I and class II loci (St. Sauver et al., 2002).

HLA alleles have also been associated with very high levels (or hyper-seroresponsiveness) of measles antibody (from the upper 10th percentile of IgG antibody titers of all subjects) after a single dose of measles vaccine. HLA-B7, DRB1*08, DQA1*0104, and DPA1*0202 alleles were overrepresented in hyperseropositive subjects (Ovsyannikova et al., 2004c). Thus, both measles vaccine antibody seronegativity and hyper-seropositivity appear to be influenced by HLA allelic variants. Further study is necessary to establish the definite role of these HLA molecules and differences in HLA-bound measles-derived peptides in the variation of vaccine response.

Rubella Vaccine

Rubella immunization induces long-lasting immunity with an efficacy greater than 90% (Banatvala & Brown, 2004). In an examination of the relationship between HLA alleles and rubella virus vaccine–induced humoral (serum antibody) and cell-mediated (lymphocyte proliferation) immune responses in children who had received two doses of rubella immunization, allelic variation at the *HLA-DPB1* locus was positively associated with variability in rubella antibody titers. Specifically, DPB1*0301, DPB1*0401, DPB1*1301, and DPB1*1501 alleles were significantly associated with high levels of rubella vaccine–induced antibodies (Ovsyannikova et al., 2005). Significant associations

were not seen with humoral immunity to rubella vaccine and any of the other class I or class II loci. This observation suggests that human *HLA-DPB1* molecules play an important role as restriction elements for the recognition of rubella virus epitopes by Th2 cells.

As for their role in CMI, several class I alleles (HLA-B*3503 and Cw*1502), and class II alleles (HLA-DPB1*0301, DQB1*0501, DRB1*0101, and DRB1*1104) were positively associated and several class II alleles (HLA-DPB1*1101, DQB1*0202, and DRB1*0701) were negatively associated with rubella virus–specific lymphoproliferation (Ovsyannikova et al., 2004b et al., 2005). These patterns of association may reflect strong linkage disequilibrium between alleles of the *DRB1* and *DQB1* loci. Others have also found evidence of HLA associations with rubella vaccine (Kato et al., 1982; Ou et al., 1994; Nepom et al., 1997; Chaye et al., 1992). One investigator has focused on restriction of T-cell responses to rubella antigens by HLA-DRB1*0403 and DRB1*0901 (Ou et al., 1998) and to rubella E1 envelope protein by HLA-DR3 and DR4 (Ou et al., 1994; Nepom et al., 1997) and in the class I CD8$^+$ CTL pathway by HLA-A*3 and A*11 (Ou et al., 1997). Besides their apparent role in modulating humoral and cellular responses, the distribution of several class II allele groups has been found to be distorted in individuals with arthropathy following rubella (Mitchell et al., 1998). Thus, both class I and class II HLA-mediated restricted antigen recognition appears to make important contributions to the physiologic and adverse responses to rubella vaccination.

Influenza Vaccine

Influenza vaccine nonresponsiveness is a serious concern due to the worldwide morbidity and mortality caused by the influenza virus. While early reports suggested possible class I alleles that would influence the early phase of the immune response to influenza A antigens, findings from these older studies have not been replicated or confirmed (Cunningham-Rundles et al., 1979; Mackenzie et al., 1977 et al., 1979; McMichael & Askonas, 1978; Spencer et al., 1976). An increased frequency of the two closely linked HLA-DRB1*07 and -DQB1*0303 alleles and a decreased frequency of HLA-DQB1*0603–9/14 and -DRB1*13 was found in nonresponders to the trivalent influenza vaccine when compared with matched responders to the same vaccine (Gelder et al., 2002). Further, following subunit vaccination individuals with HLA-DRB1*0701 were found to recognize identical CD4 T-cell epitopes from influenza A virus hemagglutinin (Gelder et al., 1998). Another group of investigators demonstrated that HLA serogroup DR3, DR4, or both are associated with lower immune responsiveness to influenza virus vaccine in patients with type 1 diabetes (Ruben et al., 1988). No associations were identified with HLA class III (tumor necrosis factor and lymphotoxin) genes (Gelder et al., 2002).

BCG Vaccine

The widely used BCG vaccine for the prevention of tuberculosis has shown highly variable protective efficacy (Brewer & Colditz, 1995; Fine, 1995). The reasons for this degree of variability are not fully understood (Fine & Vynnycky, 1998). Early studies reported that both HLA-DRB1 polymorphism and non-HLA genes play an important role in the human T-cell responsiveness to mycobacterial antigens; however, these relationships need confirmation (Ottenhoff et al., 1985; Hill, 1997). Recently, 207 Gambian infant twin pairs were reported to show 39–65% heritability in their response to some BCG vaccine antigens. Further work in this population demonstrated that interferon-γ (IFN-γ) responses to BCG antigens were predominantly influenced by *HLA-DRB1* alleles (Newport et al., 2004).

In India DRB1*1501 (DR2) and DQB1*0601 have been identified as high-risk susceptibility alleles for pulmonary tuberculosis (Ravikumar et al., 1999; Selvaraj et al., 1996). With the emergence of the Th1–Th2 paradigm, one group of investigators has focused on the role of non-HLA genes in tuberculosis pathogenesis in humans and in mouse models, with examination of IFN-γ, IL-4, and IL-10 cytokine expression in 71 adult pulmonary tuberculosis patients and 74 control individuals in south India (Dheenadhayalan et al., 2001). In particular, they documented increased IL-10 expression in association with HLA non-DRB1*02 status and *Mycobacterium bovis* BCG scar-negative status in adult pulmonary tuberculosis patients. Another report demonstrated that T-cell receptor Vβ usage in the context of class II DRB1*1501, DRB1*08, and DQB1*0601 alleles and *M. bovis* BCG scar status seem to play important roles in susceptibility and resistance to tuberculosis (Shanmugalakshmi et al., 2003). Geluk et al. (1998) reported that HLA-DR–restricted Th1 cells from transgenic DR3.Ab[0] mice and HLA-DR3[+]

humans recognize the same immunodominant determinants of *Mycobacterium tuberculosis*–derived proteins. The biologic function of these genetic polymorphisms remains tentative, but some evidence suggests that several mycobacterial antigens and peptides are promiscuous in their HLA-DR binding and could potentially be used to develop new subunit or recombinant vaccines against mycobacterial diseases (Mustafa et al., 1993; Mustafa, 2000).

Polio Vaccine

The Sabin oral polio vaccine (OPV) contains trivalent combination live attenuated poliovirus serotypes that protect against wild-virus–associated poliomyelitis by induction of humoral and cellular immunity. Since the elimination of wild-virus poliomyelitis in the Western Hemisphere in 1991 and rapid progress in global polio eradication, studies of the genetic factors in polio have been limited (Wattigney et al., 2001). Early papers reported that antibody response to vaccination with killed polio vaccine and tetanus toxoid was not higher in chronic active hepatitis patients carrying HLA-B8 and/or HLA-B12 alleles than in patients without these antigens (Lindberg et al., 1979). One report described an association between vaccine-associated paralytic poliomyelitis (VAPP) in children and the presence of HLA-A2 and -B44 alleles; however, the sample size was small (Ermolovich et al., 2002). Interestingly, 95% of serologically examined children with VAPP were found to have virus-neutralizing serum antibodies to poliovirus, suggesting the capacity of the immune system to respond to the administration of the vaccine virus, even in the face of the development of vaccine-associated disease. Additionally, in an early study of serologically defined alleles, HLA-Aw19 and -B7 were found more frequently in affected children during two outbreaks of paralytic poliomyelitis that occurred in a vaccine-protected infant population in the Gaza Strip in 1974 and 1976 (Lasch et al., 1979). A recent study explored the genetic regulation of immune responses to vaccines in early life and found high heritability (60%) for antibody responses to the first dose of Sabin OPV at birth (Newport et al., 2004). Characterization of poliovirus-specific CD4[+] T lymphocytes in the peripheral blood of Sabin OPV-immunized humans using synthetic peptides has mapped several epitopes to specific regions of poliovirus capsid protein VP1 (Simons et al., 1993). Importantly, monoclonal antibody–blocking experiments suggested that a peptide (residues 244–264) within this VP1 protein is presented by the HLA-DQ3 molecule.

Directed Vaccine Development

A primary reason for defining HLA associations with specific vaccine antigens in the context of specific genes is the notion that such data can guide development of new vaccines for use in heterogeneous outbred populations. For example, knowledge of defined class I and II associations with immune status following vaccination as well as the role of homozygosity upon vaccine failure potentially allows for identification of nonresponder or hyperresponder alleles and haplotypes. In addition, identifying such alleles may reveal important epitopes that could direct new vaccine design (Pougatcheva et al., 1999; Nepom et al., 1997). Similarly, it is theoretically plausible to isolate and immunize with only the most effective antigens to overcome the immaturity of the immune system or passively acquired neutralizing maternal antibody in infants. Alternatively, such studies might lead to the design of a cocktail of vaccine peptide components that bind to a wide spectrum of HLA molecules found in the population. Such a strategy could deliver multiple peptides immunogenic for virtually all members of a genetically diverse population (Poland & Jacobson, 1998). This strategy of designing population-specific vaccines based in part on profiles of HLA class I allele distribution is under active investigation among those developing HIV-1 vaccines (De Groot et al., 2003).

In addition, HLA molecules with binding grooves promiscuous enough to bind a common set of peptides have been grouped into HLA "supertypes." For example, the HLA-A2 supertype is composed of several distinct HLA-A alleles (A*0201–07, A*6802, and A*6901, and possibly alleles A*0208–14), all of which have sufficiently similar peptide binding grooves that a common set of peptides can be bound and presented (Sette & Sidney, 1998; Sidney et al., 2001). Alleles of the A2 supertype are present in approximately 50% of many populations (Ellis et al., 2000). From the relative frequency of HLA supertypes present in the population, it could theoretically be possible to select sets of viral peptides that would induce protective immune responses in that population (Sette & Sidney, 1998; Sidney et al., 1996). As an example, recently, Drexler et al. (2003) described an immunodominant HLA-

A*0201 restricted vaccinia virus-specific epitope that was recognized by murine and human CD8[+] T cells and conserved among *Orthpoxvirus* species, including the variola virus. In addition, a new naturally processed and A*0201-presented epitope derived from a peptide encoded by the vaccinia virus gene thymidylate kinase was identified using a mass spectrometry approach (Johnson et al., 2005). These two examples are relevant because A*0201 belongs to the most prevalent HLA-A2 supertype (Sette & Sidney, 1999; Ellis et al., 2000). The identification of such peptides within a class I *HLA-A* supertype may help design a highly promiscuous class I A peptide that is immunogenic in a sizable fraction of the population. Two additional viral epitopes from Epstein-Barr virus and cytomegalovirus that were recognized by CTLs in association with different alleles of the HLA-A24 supertype have also been defined (Burrows et al., 2003). These findings have important implications for the development of peptide-based immunotherapy and the monitoring of immune responses to viral vaccines (Sidney et al., 2001).

In summary, increasing attention is being paid to the important relationship between vaccine-induced immune responses and the genes that modify them. Early work focused on HLA genes and their mechanisms of action. In the future, understanding the genetically mediated mechanisms of vaccine success and failure should inform rational, directed design of new vaccines and might aid in predicting vaccine adverse events. A better understanding of the relationship between HLA genes and immune response could provide important generalizable principles for the directed development of viral vaccines by determining the basis for individual variation in immune response (Pougatcheva et al., 1999; Nepom et al., 1997). This approach may lead to clues about mechanisms of host defense, for applications in design strategies for new vaccines (e.g., for measles, rubella, smallpox, and HIV-1), for eradication of disease (e.g., HLA supertype vaccines), for use in specific nonresponder groups (Dawson et al., 2001). Finally, understanding possible genetically directed Th1- and Th2-type immune responses to vaccines offers further potential for favorable manipulation of the immune response to vaccine antigens.

References

Alper, C.A., Kruskall, M.S., Marcus-Bagley, D., Craven, D.E., Katz, A.J., Brink, S.J., Dienstag, J.L., Awdeh,

Z., & Yunis, E.J. (1989) Genetic prediction of non-response to hepatitis B vaccine. *New England Journal of Medicine*, 321, 708–712.

Anders, J.F., Jacobson, R.M., Poland, G.A., Jacobsen, S.J., & Wollan, P.C. (1996) Secondary failure rates of measles vaccines: A meta-analysis of published studies. *Pediatric Infectious Disease Journal*, 15, 62–66.

Banatvala, J.E., & Brown, D.W. (2004) Rubella. *Lancet*, 363, 1127–1137.

Bautista-López, N., Ward, B.J., Mills, E., McCormick, D., Martel, N., & Ratnam, S. (2000) Development and durability of measles antigen-specific lymphoproliferative response after MMR vaccination. *Vaccine*, 18, 1393–1401.

Berzofsky, J.A. (1988) Immunodominance in T lymphocyte recognition. *Immunology Letters*, 18, 83–92.

Bhimma, R., Hammond, M.G., Coovadia, H.M., Adhikari, M., & Connolly, C.A. (2002) HLA class I and II in black children with hepatitis B virus-associated membranous nephropathy. *Kidney International*, 61, 1510–1515.

Biggar, R.J., Pandey, J.P., Henle, W., Nkrumah, F.K., & Levine, P.H. (1994) Humoral immune response to Epstein-Barr virus antigens and immunoglobulin allotypes in African Burkitt lymphoma patients. *International Journal of Cancer*, 33, 577–580.

Black, F.L., & Hedrick, P.W. (1997) Strong balancing selection at HLA loci: Evidence from segregation in South Amerindian families. *Proceedings of the National Academy of Sciences of the United States of America*, 94, 12452–12456.

Black, F.L., Pinheiro, F.d., Hierholzer, W.J., & Lee, R.V. (1977) Epidemiology of infectious disease: The example of measles. In *Health and Disease in Tribal Societies* (ed. by Ciba Foundation), pp. 115–135. Elsevier, Amsterdam.

Black, F.L., & Salzano, F.M. (1981) Evidence for heterosis in HLA system. *American Journal of Human Genetics*, 33, 894–899.

Black, F.L., Schiffman, G., & Pandey, J.P. (1995) HLA, Gm, and Km polymorphisms and immunity to infectious diseases in South Amerinds. *Experimental and Clinical Immunogenetics*, 12, 206–216.

Brewer, T.F., & Colditz, G.A. (1995) Relationship between bacille calmette-guerin (BCG) strains and the efficacy of BCG vaccine in the prevention of tuberculosis. *Clinical Infectious Diseases*, 20, 126–135.

Burnet, F.M. (1968) Measles as an index of immunological function. *Lancet*, 2, 610–613.

Burrows, S.R., Elkington, R.A., Miles, J.J., Green, K.J., Walker, S., Haryana, S.M., Moss, D.J., Dunckley, H., Burrows, J.M., & Khanna, R. (2003) Promiscuous CTL recognition of viral epitopes on multiple human leukocyte antigens: Biological validation of the proposed HLA A24 supertype. *Journal of Immunology*, 171, 1407–1412.

Caillat-Zucman, S., Gimenez, J.-J., Wambergue, F., Albouze, G., Lebkiri, B., Naret, C., Moynot, A., Jungers, P., & Bach, J.-F. (1998) Distinct HLA class II alleles determine antibody response to vaccination with hepatitis B surface antigen. *Kidney International*, 53, 1626–1630.

Carrington, M., Nelson, G.W., Martin, M.P., Kissner, T., Vlahov, D., Goedert, J.J., Kaslow, R., Buchbinder, S., Hoots, K., & O'Brien, S.J. (1999) HLA and HIV-1: Heterozygote advantage and *B*35-Cw*04* disadvantage. *Science*, 283, 1748–1752.

Chaye, H.H., Mauracher, C.A., Tingle, A.J., & Gillam, S. (1992) Cellular and humoral immune responses to rubella virus structural proteins E1, E2, and C. *Journal of Clinical Microbiology*, 30(9), 2323–2329.

Chen, R.T., Markowitz, L.E., Albrecht, P., Stewart, J.A., Mofenson, L.M., Preblud, S.R., & Orenstein, W.A. (1990) Measles antibody: Reevaluation of protective titers. *Journal of Infectious Diseases*, 162, 1036–1042.

Craven, D.E., Awdeh, Z.L., Kunches, L.M., Yunis, E.J., Dienstag, J.L., Werner, B.G., Polk, B.F., Snydman, D.R., Platt, R., Crumpacker, C.S., Grady, G.F., & Alper, C.A. (1986) Nonresponsiveness to hepatitis B vaccine in health care workers. Results of revaccination and genetic typings. *Annals of Internal Medicine*, 105, 356–360.

Cunningham-Rundles, S., Brown, A., Gross, D., Braun, D., Hansen, J.A., Good, R.A., Armstrong, D., & Dupont, B. (1979) Association of HLA in immune response to influenza-A immunization. *Transplantation Proceedings*, 11, 1849–1852.

Dawson, D.V., Ozgur, M., Sari, K., Ghanayem, M., & Kostyu, D.D. (2001) Ramifications of HLA class I polymorphism and population genetics for vaccine development. *Genetic Epidemiology*, 20, 87–106.

De Boer, R.J., Borghans, J.A., van Boven, M., Kesmir, C., & Weissing, F.J. (2004) Heterozygote advantage fails to explain the high degree of polymorphism of the MHC. *Immunogenetics*, 55, 725–731.

De Groot, A.S., Jesdale, B., Martin, W., Saint Aubin, C., Sbai, H., Bosma, A., Lieberman, J., Skowron, G., Mansourati, F., & Mayer, K.H. (2003) Mapping cross-clade HIV-1 vaccine epitopes using a bioinformatics approach. *Vaccine*, 21, 4486–4504.

De Silvestri, A., Pasi, A., Martinetti, M., Belloni, C., Tinelli, C., Rondini, G., Salvaneschi, L., and Cuccia, M. (2001) Family study of non-responsiveness to hepatitis B vaccine confirms the importance of HLA class III C4A locus. *Genes and Immunity*, 2, 367–372.

Desombere, I., Willems, A., & Leroux-Roels, G. (1998) Response to hepatitis B vaccine: Multiple HLA genes are involved. *Tissue Antigens*, 51, 593–604.

Deulofeut, H., Iglesias, A., Mikael, N., Bing, D.H., Awdeh, Z., Yunis, J., Marcus-Bagley, D., Kruskall, M.S., Alper, C.A., & Yunis, E.J. (1993) Cellular recognition and HLA restriction of a midsequence HBsAg peptide in hepatitis B vaccinated individuals. *Molecular Immunology*, 30, 941–948.

Dheenadhayalan, V., Shanmugalakshmi, S., Vani, S., Muthuveeralakshmi, P., Arivarignan, G., Nageswari, A.D., & Pitchappan, R.M. (2001) Association of interleukin-10 cytokine expression status with HLA non-DRB1*02 and *Mycobacterium bovis* BCG scar-negative status in south Indian pulmonary tuberculosis patients. *Infection and Immunity*, 69, 5635–5642.

Doolan, D.L., Southwood, S., Chesnut, R., Appella, E., Gomez, E., Richards, A., Higashimoto, Y.I., Maewal, A., Sidney, J., Gramzinski, R.A., Mason, C., Koech, D., Hoffman, S.L., & Sette, A. (2000) HLA-DR promiscuous T cell epitopes from *Plasmodium falciparum* ore-erythrocytic-state antigens restricted by multiple HLA class II alleles. *Journal of Immunology*, 165, 1123–1137.

Drexler, I., Staib, C., Kastenmüller, W., Stevanovic, S., Schmidt, B., Lemonnier, F.A., Rammensee, H.-G., Busch, D.H., Bernhard, H., Erfle, V., & Sutter, G. (2003) Identification of vaccinia virus epitope-specific HLA-A*0201-restricted T cells and comparative analysis of smallpox vaccines. *Proceedings of the National Academy of Sciences of the United States of America*, 100, 217–222.

Durupinar, B., & Okten, G. (1996) HLA tissue types in nonresponders to hepatitis B vaccine. *Indian Journal of Pediatrics*, 63, 369–373.

Eliakim, M., Ligumski, M., Sandler, S.G., & Zlotnick, A. (1978) Familial clustering and immune response in family contacts of patients with HBsAg-positive liver cirrhosis. *American Journal of Digestive Diseases*, 23, 407–412.

Ellis, J.M., Henson, V., Slack, R., Ng, J., Hartzman, R.J., & Hurley, C.K. (2000) Frequencies of HLA-A2 alleles in five U.S. population groups. Predominance of A*02011 and identification of HLA-A*0231. *Human Immunology*, 61, 334–340.

Ermolovich, M.A., Fel'dman, E.V., Samoilovich, E.O., Kuzovkova, N.A., & Levin, V.I. (2002) Characterization of the immune status of patients with vaccine-associated poliomyelitis. *Zhurnal Mikrobiologii, Epidemiologii, i Immunobiologii*, 2, 42–50.

Fine, P.E. (1995) Variation in protection by BCG: Implications of and for heterologous immunity. *Lancet*, 346, 1339–1345.

Fine, P.E.M., & Vynnycky, E. (1998) The effect of heterologous immunity upon the apparent efficacy of (e.g. BCG) vaccines. *Vaccine*, 16, 1923–1928.

Forzani, B., Actis, G.C., Verme, G., Amoroso, A., Borelli, I., Curtoni, E.S., Rumi, M.G., Picciotto, A., Marinucci, G., & Freni, M.A. (1984) HLA-DR antigens in HBsAg-positive chronic active liver disease with and without associated delta infection. *Hepatology*, 4, 1107–1110.

Galbraith, R.M., Eddleston, A.L., Williams, R., Webster, A.D., Pattison, J., Doniach, D., Kennedy, L.A., & Batchelor, J.R. (1976) Enhanced antibody responses in active chronic hepatitis: Relation to HLA-B8 and HLA-B12 and porto-systemic shunting. *Lancet*, 1, 930–934.

Gedda, L., Rajani, G., Brenci, G., Lun, M.T., Talone, C., & Oddi, G. (1984) Heredity and infectious diseases: A twin study. *Acta Geneticae Medicae et Gemellologiae*, 33, 497–500.

Gelder, C., Davenport, M., Barnardo, M., Bourne, T., Lamb, J., Askonas, B., Hill, A., & Welsh, K. (1998) Six unrelated HLA-DR-matched adults recognize identical CD4$^+$ T cell epitopes from influenza A haemagglutinin that are not simply peptides with high HLA-DR binding affinities. *International Immunology*, 10, 211–222.

Gelder, C.M., Lambkin, R., Hart, K.W., Fleming, D., Williams, O.M., Bunce, M., Welsh, K.I., Marshall, S.E., & Oxford, J. (2002) Associations between human leukocyte antigens and nonresponsiveness to influenza vaccine. *Journal of Infectious Diseases*, 185, 114–117.

Geluk, A., Taneja, V., Van Meijgaarden, K.E., Zanelli, E., Abou-Zeid, C., Thole, J.E.R., De Vries, R.R.P., David, C.S., & Ottenhoff, T.H.M. (1998) Identification of HLA class II-restricted determinants of *Mycobacterium tuberculosis*-derived proteins by using HLA-transgenic, class II-deficient mice. *Proceedings of the National Academy of Sciences of the United States of America*, 95, 10797–10802.

Goldblatt, D., Scadding, G.K., Lund, V.J., Wade, A.M., Turner, M.W., & Pandey, J.P. (1994) Association of Gm allotypes with the antibody response to the outer membrane proteins of a common upper respiratory tract organism, *Moraxella catarrhalis*. *Journal of Immunology*, 153, 5316–5320.

Good, R.A., & Zak, S.J. (1956) Disturbances in gamma globulin synthesis as "experiments of nature." *Pediatrics*, 18, 109–149.

Granoff, D.M., & Holmes, S.J. (1992) G2m(23) immunoglobulin allotype and immunity to *Haemophilus influenzae* type b. *Journal of Infectious Diseases*, 165, S66–S69.

Granoff, D.M., Shackelford, P.G., Suarez, B.K., Nahm, M.H., Cates, K.L., Murphy, T.V., Karasic, R., Osterholm, M.T., Pandey, J.P., & Daum, R.S. (1986) *Hemophilus influenzae* type B disease in children vaccinated with type B polysaccharide vaccine. *New England Journal of Medicine*, 315, 1584–1590.

Granoff, D.M., Suarez, B.K., Pandey, J.P., & Shackelford, P.G. (1988) Genes associated with G2m(23) immunoglobulin allotype regulate the IgG subclass responses to *Haemophilus influenzae* type b polysaccharide vaccine. *Journal of Infectious Diseases*, 157, 1142–1149.

Haghighi, S., Andersen, O., Rosengren, L., Bergstrom, T., Wahlstrom, J., & Nilsson, S. (2000) Incidence of CSF abnormalities in siblings of multiple sclerosis patients and unrelated controls. *Journal of Neurology*, 247, 616–622.

Hansen, T.H., Carreno, B.M., & Sachs, D.H. (1993) The major histocompatibility complex. In *Fundamental Immunology* (ed. by W.E. Paul), pp. 577–628. Raven Press, New York.

Haverkorn, M.J., Hofman, B., Masurel, N., & Van Rood, J.J. (1975) HL-A linked genetic control of immune response in man. *Transplantation Reviews*, 22, 120–124.

Hedrick, P.W. (1990) Evolution at HLA: Possible explanations for the deficiency of homozygotes in two populations. *Human Heredity*, 40, 213–220.

Hedrick, P.W., & Black, F.L. (1997) Random mating and selection in families against homozygotes for HLA in south Amerindians. *Hereditas*, 127, 51–58.

Hickman, C.J., Khan, A.S., Rota, P.A., & Bellini, W.J. (1997) Use of synthetic peptides to identify measles nucleoprotein T-cell epitopes in vaccinated and naturally infected humans. *Virology*, 235, 386–397.

Hill, A.V. (1997) MHC polymorphism and susceptibility to intracellular infections in humans. In *Host Response to Intracellular Pathogens* (ed. by S.H.E. Kaufmann), pp. 47–59. R.G. Landes Company, Austin, TX.

Hill, A.V. (1998) The immunogenetics of human infectious diseases. *Annual Review of Immunology*, 16, 593–617.

Hohler, T., Gerken, G., Notghi, A., Knolle, P., Lubjuhn, R., Taheri, H., Schneider, P.M., Zumbuschenfelde, K.H.M., & Rittner, C. (1997) MHC class II genes influence the susceptibility to chronic active hepatitis C. *Journal of Hepatology*, 27, 259–264.

Hohler, T., Reuss, E., Evers, N., Dietrich, E., Rittner, C., Freitag, C.M., Vollmar, J., Schneider, P.M., & Fimmers, R. (2002) Differential genetic determination of immune responsiveness to hepatitis B surface antigen and to hepatitis A virus: A vaccination study in twins. *Lancet*, 360, 991–995.

Honeyman, M.C., Dorman, D.C., Menser, M.A., Forrest, M.J., Guinan, J.J., & Clark, P. (1975) HL-A antigens in congenital rubella and the role of antigens 1 and 8 in the epidemiology of natural rubella. *Tissue Antigens*, 5, 12–18.

Hughes, A.L., & Nei, M. (1988) Pattern of nucleotide substitution at major histocompatibility complex class I loci reveals overdominant selection. *Nature*, 335, 167–170.

Ito, I., Ishida, T., Hashimoto, T., Arita, M., Osawa, M., & Tsukayama, C. (2000) Familial cases of severe measles pneumonia. *Internal Medicine*, 39, 670–674.

Jacobson, R.M., & Poland, G.A. (2004) The genetic basis for measles vaccine failure. *Acta Paediatrica*, 445(suppl), 43–47.

Jacobson, R.M., Poland, G.A., Vierkant, R.A., Pankratz, V.S., Schaid, D.J., Jacobsen, S.J., St. Sauver, J.L., & Moore, S.B. (2003) The association of class I HLA alleles and antibody levels following a single dose of measles vaccine. *Human Immunology*, 64, 103–109.

Jepson, A., Banya, W., Sisay-Joof, F., Hassan-King, M., Nunes, C., Bennett, S., & Whittle, H. (1997) Quantification of the relative contribution of major histocompatibility complex (MHC) and non-MHC genes to human immune responses to foreign antigens. *Infection and Immunity*, 65, 872–876.

Jepson, A., Fowler, A., Banya, W., Singh, M., Bennett, S., Whittle, H., & Hill, A.V. (2001) Genetic regulation of acquired immune responses to antigens of Mycobacterium tuberculosis: A study of twins in West Africa. *Infection and Immunity*, 69, 3989–3994.

Johnson, K.L., Ovsyannikova, I.G., Madden, B.J., Poland, G.A., & Muddiman, D.C. (2005) Accurate mass precursor ion data and tandem mass spectrometry identify a class I Human Leukocyte Antigen A*0201-presented peptide originating from vaccinia virus. *Journal of American Society for Mass Spectrometry*, 16, 1812–1817.

Kato, S., Kimura, M., Takakura, I., Tsuji, K., & Ueda, K. (1980) HLA-linked genetic control in natural rubella infection. *Tissue Antigens*, 15, 86–89.

Kato, S., Muranaka, S., Takakura, I., Kimura, M., & Tsuji, K. (1982) HLA-DR antigens and the rubella-specific immune response in man. *Tissue Antigens*, 19, 140–145.

Kruskall, M.S. (1990) The major histocompatibility complex: The value of extended haplotypes in the analysis of associated immune diseases and disorders. *Yale Journal of Biology and Medicine*, 63, 477–486.

Kruskall, M.S., Alper, C.A., Awdeh, Z., Yunis, E.J., & Marcus-Bagley, D. (1992) The immune response to hepatitis B vaccine in humans: Inheritance patterns in families. *Journal of Experimental Medicine*, 175, 495–502.

Lanzavecchia, A., & Sallusto, F. (2000) Dynamics of T lymphocyte responses: Intermediates, effectors, and memory cells. *Science*, 290, 92–97.

Lasch, E.E., Joshua, H., Gazit, E., El Massri, M., Marcus, O., & Zamir, R. (1979) Study of the HLA antigen in

Arab children with paralytic poliomyelitis. *Israel Journal of Medical Sciences*, 15, 12–13.

Lemon, S.M., & Thomas, D.L. (1997) Vaccines to prevent viral hepatitis. *New England Journal of Medicine*, 336, 196–204.

Levo, Y., Tur-Kaspa, R., Shouval, D., Brautbar, C., & Eliakim, M. (1982) Histocompatibility antigens and cell-mediated immunity in carriers of hepatitis B virus; a study of a family. *Journal of Clinical and Laboratory Immunology*, 9, 105–107.

Li, M., Li, R., Huang, S., Gong, J., Zeng, X., Li, Y., Lu, M., & Li, H. (2002) The relationship between nonresponse to hepatitis B vaccine and HLA genotype/haplotype. *Zhonghua Yu Fang Yi Xue Za Zhi (Chinese Journal of Preventive Medicine)*, 36, 180–183.

Lindberg, J., Kaijser, B., Lindholm, A., Hermodsson, S., & Iwarson, S. (1979) Humoral immunoreactivity in chronic active hepatitis: Relation to HLA antigens. *International Archives of Allergy and Applied Immunology*, 58, 75–81.

Lynch, H.T., Srivatanskul, P., Phornthutkul, K., & Lynch, J.F. (1984) Familial hepatocellular carcinoma in an endemic area of Thailand. *Cancer Genetics and Cytogenetics*, 11, 11–18.

Mackenzie, J.S., Wetherall, J.D., Fimmel, P.J., Hawkins, B.R., & Dawkins, R.L. (1977) Host factors and susceptibility to influenza A infection: The effect of ABO blood groups and HL-A antigens. *Developments in Biological Standardization*, 39, 355–362.

Mackenzie, J.S., Wetherall, J.D., Flower, R.L., Fimmel, P.J., & Dawkins, R.L. (1979) HLA antigens and the response to influenza A virus. *Vox Sanguinis*, 37, 201–208.

Marescot, M.R., Budkowska, A., Pillot, J., & Debre, P. (1989) HLA linked immune response to S and pre-S2 gene products in hepatitis B vaccination. *Tissue Antigens*, 33, 495–500.

Markowitz, L.E., Chandler, F.W., Roldan, E.O., Saldana, M.J., Roach, K.C., Hutchins, S.S., Preblud, S.R., Mitchell, C.D., & Scott, G.B. (1988) Fatal measles pneumonia without rash in a child with AIDS. *Journal of Infectious Diseases*, 158, 480–483.

Martinetti, M., De Silvestri, A., Belloni, C., Pasi, A., Tinelli, C., Pistorio, A., Salvaneschi, L., Rondini, G., Avanzini, M.A., & Cuccia, M. (2000) Humoral response to recombinant hepatitis B virus vaccine at birth: Role of HLA and beyond. *Clinical Immunology*, 97, 234–240.

Matrakshin, A.G., Tsoi, K.N., Pospelov, L.E., Kapina, M.A., Kholod, O.N., & Pushkina, E.I. (1993) [A genotypic study of children ill with tuberculosis and of healthy BCG-revaccinated ones of Tuvinian nationality]. *Problemy Tuberkuleza*, 25–27.

McDermott, A.B., Cohen, S.B.A., Zuckerman, J.N., & Madrigal, J.A. (1999) Human leukocyte antigens influence the immune response to a pre-S/S hepatitis B vaccine. *Vaccine*, 17, 330–339.

McDermott, A.B., Zuckerman, J.N., Sabin, C.A., Marsh, S.G.E., & Madrigal, J.A. (1997) Contribution of human leukocyte antigens to the antibody response to hepatitis B vaccination. *Tissue Antigens*, 50, 8–14.

McMichael, A.J., & Askonas, B.A. (1978) Influenza virus-specific cytotoxic T cells in man; induction and properties of the cytotoxic cell. *European Journal of Immunology*, 8, 705–711.

Mineta, M., Tanimura, M., Tana, T., Yssel, H., Kashiwagi, S., & Sasazuki, T. (1996) Contribution of HLA class I and class II alleles to the regulation of antibody production to hepatitis B surface antigen in humans. *International Immunology*, 8, 525–531.

Mitchell, L.A., Tingle, A.J., MacWilliam, L., Horne, C., Keown, P., Gaur, L.K., & Nepom, G.T. (1998) HLA-DR class II associations with rubella vaccine-induced joint manifestations. *Journal of Infectious Diseases*, 177, 5–12.

Mitus, A., Holloway, A., Evans, A.E., & Enders, J.F. (1965) Attenuated measles vaccine in children with acute leukemia. *American Journal of Diseases of Children*, 103, 413–418.

Moss, R.B., Hsu, Y.P., Van Eede, P.H., Van Leeuwen, A.M., Lewiston, N.J., & De Lange, G. (1987) Altered antibody isotype in cystic fibrosis: Impaired natural antibody response to polysaccharide antigens. *Pediatric Research*, 22, 708–713.

Munoz, N., Lingao, A., Lao, J., Esteve, J., Viterbo, G., Domingo, E.O., & Lansang, M.A. (1989) Patterns of familial transmission of HBV and the risk of developing liver cancer: A case-control study in the Philippines. *International Journal of Cancer*, 44, 981–984.

Musher, D.M., Groover, J.E., Watson, D.A., Pandey, J.P., Rodriguez-Barradas, M.C., Baughn, R.E., Pollack, M.S., Graviss, E.A., de Andrade, M., & Amos, C.I. (1997) Genetic regulation of the capacity to make immunoglobulin G to pneumococcal capsular polysaccharides. *Journal of Investigative Medicine*, 45, 57–68.

Mustafa, A.S. (2000) HLA-restricted immune response to mycobacterial antigens: Relevance to vaccine design. *Human Immunology*, 61, 166–171.

Mustafa, A.S., Lundin, K.E., & Oftung, F. (1993) Human T cells recognize mycobacterial heat shock proteins in the context of multiple HLA-DR molecules: Studies with healthy subjects vaccinated with *Mycobacterium bovis* BCG and *Mycobacterium leprae*. *Infection and Immunity*, 61, 5294–5301.

Nanan, R., Carstens, C., & Kreth, H.W. (1995) Demonstration of virus-specific CD8[+] memory T cells in measles-seropositive individuals by *in vitro* peptide stimulation. *Clinical and Experimental Immunology*, 102, 40–45.

Nanan, R., Rauch, A., Kämpgen, E., Niewiesk, S., & Kreth, H.W. (2000) A novel sensitive approach for frequency analysis of measles virus-specific memory T-lymphocytes in healthy adults with a childhood history of natural measles. *Journal of General Virology*, 81, 1313–1319.

Nasrallah, S.M., Nassar, V.H., & Shammaa, M.H. (1978) Genetic and immunological aspects of familial chronic active hepatitis (type B). *Gastroenterology*, 75, 302–306.

Nepom, G.T., Domeier, M.E., Ou, D., Kovats, S., Mitchell, L.A., & Tingle, A.J. (1997) Recognition of contiguous allele-specific peptide elements in the rubella virus E1 envelope protein. *Vaccine*, 15, 648–652.

Newport, M.J., Goetghebuer, T., Weiss, H.A., Whittle, H., Siegrist, C.-A., & Marchant, A.; MRC Gambia Twin Study Group. (2004) Genetic regulation of immune responses to vaccines in early life. *Genes and Immunity*, 5, 122–129.

Noh, K.W., Poland, G.A., & Murray, J.A. (2003) Hepatitis B vaccine nonresponse and celiac disease. *American Journal of Gastroenterology*, 98, 2289–2292.

Norrby, E. (1995) The paradigms of measles vaccinology. *Current Topics in Microbiology and Immunology*, 191, 167–180.

Ottenhoff, T.H.M., Elferink, B.G., & De Vries, R.R.P. (1985) HLA class II restriction repertoire of antigen specific T cells 1. *Human Immunology*, 13, 105–116.

Ou, D., Mitchell, L.A., Décarie, D., Gillam, S., & Tingle, A.J. (1997) Characterization of an overlapping CD8+ and CD4+ T-cell epitope on rubella capsid protein. *Virology*, 235, 286–292.

Ou, D., Mitchell, L.A., Décarie, D., Tingle, A.J., & Nepom, G.T. (1998) Promiscuous T-cell recognition of a rubella capsid protein epitope restricted by DRB1*0403 and DRB1*0901 molecules sharing an HLA DR supertype. *Human Immunology*, 59, 149–157.

Ou, D., Mitchell, L.A., Ho, M., Décarie, D., Tingle, A.J., Nepom, G.T., LaCroix, M., & Zrein, M. (1994) Analysis of overlapping T- and B-cell antigenic sites on rubella virus E1 envelope protein. Influence of HLA-DR4 polymorphism on T-cell clonal recognition. *Human Immunology*, 39, 177–187.

Ovsyannikova, I.G., Dhiman, N., Jacobson, R.M., Vierkant, R.A., & Poland, G.A. (2003) Frequency of measles virus-specific CD4+ and CD8+ T cells in subjects seronegative or highly seropositive for measles vaccine. *Clinical and Diagnostic Laboratory Immunology*, 10, 411–416.

Ovsyannikova, I.G., Jacobson, R.M., & Poland, G.A. (2004a) Variation in vaccine response in normal populations. *Pharmacogenomics*, 5, 417–427.

Ovsyannikova, I.G., Jacobson, R.M., Vierkant, R.A., Jacobsen, S.J., Pankratz, V.S., & Poland, G.A. (2004b) The contribution of HLA class I antigens in immune status following two doses of rubella vaccination. *Human Immunology*, 65, 1506–1515.

Ovsyannikova, I.G., Jacobson, R.M., Vierkant, R.A., Jacobsen, S.J., Pankratz, V.S., & Poland, G.A. (2005) Human leukocyte antigen class II alleles and rubella-specific humoral and cell-mediated immunity following measles-mumps-rubella-II vaccination. *Journal of Infectious Diseases*, 191, 515–519.

Ovsyannikova, I.G., Jacobson, R.M., Vierkant, R.A., Pankratz, S.V., Jacobsen, S.J., & Poland, G.A. (2004c) Associations between human leukocyte antigen (HLA) alleles and very high levels of measles antibody following vaccination. *Vaccine*, 22, 1914–1920.

Ovsyannikova, I.G., Jacobson, R.M., Vierkant, R.A., Shitaye, H., Sohni, Y., Schaid, D.J., Pankratz, V.S., Jacobsen, S.J., & Poland, G.A. (2000) The role of class II HLA homozygosity in measles vaccine virus (MVV) antibody (Ab) nonresponse. (Abstract). In *Third Annual Conference on Vaccine Research*, National Foundation of Infectious Diseases, p. 58. Washington D.C.

Ovsyannikova, I.G., Poland, G.A., Easler, N.J., & Vierkant, R.A. (2004d) Influence of HLA-DRB1 alleles on lymphoproliferative responses to a naturally processed and presented measles virus phosphoprotein in measles immunized individuals. *Human Immunology*, 65, 209–217.

Pabst, H.F., Spady, D.W., Carson, M.M., Stelfox, H.T., Beeler, J.A., & Krezolek, M.P. (1997) Kinetics of immunologic responses after primary MMR vaccination. *Vaccine*, 15, 10–14.

Pamer, E.G. (1999) Antigen presentation in the immune response to infectious diseases. *Clinical Infectious Diseases*, 28, 714–716.

Pandey, J.P. (1990) Genetics of immunoglobulins. *Immunology Series*, 50, 107–121.

Pandey, J.P. (2000) Immunoglobulin GM and KM allotypes and vaccine immunity. *Vaccine*, 19, 613–617.

Pandey, J.P., Ambrosch, F., Fudenberg, H.H., Stanek, G., & Wiedermann, G. (1982) Immunoglobulin allotypes and immune response to meningococcal polysaccharides A and C. *Journal of Immunogenetics*, 9, 25–29.

Pandey, J.P., Baker, C.J., Kasper, D.L., & Fudenberg, H.H. (1984) Two unlinked genetic loci interact to control the human immune response to type III group B streptococcal antigen. *Journal of Immunogenetics*, 11, 159–163.

Pandey, J.P., & Blaser, M.J. (1986) Heterozygosity at the Km locus associated with humoral immunity to *Campylobacter jejuni. Experimental and Clinical Immunogenetics*, 3, 49–53.

Pandey, J.P., Elson, L.H., Sutherland, S.E., Guderian, R.H., Araujo, E., & Nutman, T.B. (1995) Immunoglobulin kappa chain allotypes (KM) in onchocerciasis. *Journal of Clinical Investigation*, 96, 2732–2734.

Pandey, J.P., & French, M.A.H. (1996) GM phenotypes influence the concentrations of the four subclasses of immunoglobulin G in normal human serum. *Human Immunology*, 51, 99–102.

Pandey, J.P., Fudenberg, H.H., Virella, G., Kyong, C.U., Loadholt, C.B., & Galbraith, R.M. (1979) Association between immunoglobulin allotypes and immune responses to *Haemophilus influenzae* and meningococcus polysaccharides. *Lancet*, 1, 190–192.

Pandey, J.P., Zollinger, W.D., Fudenberg, H.H., & Loadholt, C.B. (1981) Immunoglobulin allotypes and immune response to meningococcal group B polysaccharide. *Journal of Clinical Investigation*, 68, 1378–1380.

Paty, D.W., Furesz, J., Boucher, D.W., Rand, C.G., & Stiller, C.R. (1976) Measles antibodies as related to HL-A types in multiple sclerosis. *Neurology*, 26, 651–655.

Pol, S., Legendre, C., Mattlinger, B., Berthelot, P., & Kreis, H. (1990) Genetic basis of nonresponse to hepatitis B vaccine in hemodialyzed patients. *Journal of Hepatology*, 11, 385–387.

Poland, G.A. (1998) Variability in immune response to pathogens: Using measles vaccine to probe immunogenetic determinants of response. *American Journal of Human Genetics*, 62, 215–220.

Poland, G.A. (1999) Immunogenetic mechanisms of antibody response to measles vaccine: The role of the HLA genes. *Vaccine*, 17, 1719–1725.

Poland, G.A., Hayney, M.S., Schaid, D.J., Jacobson, R.M., & Lipsky, J.J. (1995) Class II HLA-DR homozygosity is associated with non-response to measles vaccine in U.S. children (Abstract). *FASEB Journal*, 9, A240.

Poland, G.A., & Jacobson, R.M. (1998) The genetic basis for variation in antibody response to vaccines. *Current Opinion in Pediatrics*, 10, 208–215.

Poland, G.A., Jacobson, R.M., Schaid, D.J., Moore, S.B., & Jacobsen, S.J. (1998) The association between HLA class I alleles and measles vaccine-induced antibody response: Evidence of a significant association. *Vaccine*, 16, 1869–1871.

Poland, G.A., Ovsyannikova, I.G., Jacobson, R.M., Vierkant, R.A., Jacobsen, S.J., Pankratz, V.S., & Schaid, D.J. (2001) Identification of an association between HLA class II alleles and low antibody levels after measles immunization. *Vaccine*, 20, 430–438.

Pollicino, T., Pernice, F., Campo, S., Mesiti, O., Misefari, V., Pernice, M., & Raimondo, G. (1996) Severe outcomes of hepatitis B virus (HBV) infection and lack of HBV e antigen-defective virus emergence in patients homozygous for HLA class I alleles. *Journal of General Virology*, 77, 1833–1836.

Pougatcheva, S.O., Abernathy, E.S., Vzorov, A.N., Compans, R.W., & Frey, T.K. (1999) Development of a rubella virus DNA vaccine. *Vaccine*, 17, 2104–2112.

Racioppi, L., Ronchese, F., Schwartz, R.H., & Germain, R.N. (1991) The molecular basis of class II MHC allelic control of T cell responses. *Journal of Immunology*, 147, 3718–3727.

Ravikumar, M., Dheenadhayalan, V., Rajaram, K., Lakshmi, S.S., Kumaran, P.P., Paramasivan, C.N., Balakrishnan, K., & Pitchappan, R.M. (1999) Associations of HLA-DRB1, DQB1 and DPB1 alleles with pulmonary tuberculosis in south India. *Tubercle and Lung Disease*, 79, 309–317.

Robbins, J.B., Schneerson, R., & Szu, S.C. (1995) Hypothesis: Serum IgG antibody is sufficient to confer protection against infectious diseases by inactivating the inoculum. *Journal of Infectious Diseases*, 171, 1387–1398.

Rodriguez-Barradas, M.C., Groover, J.E., Lacvke, C.E., Gump, D.W., Lahart, C.J., Pandey, J.P., & Musher, D.M. (1996) IgG antibody to pneumococcal capsular polysaccharide in human immunodeficiency virus-infected subjects: Persistence of antibody in responders, revaccination in nonresponders, and relationship of immunoglobulin allotype to response. *Journal of Infectious Diseases*, 173, 1347–1353.

Ruben, F.L., Fireman, P., LaPorte, R.E., Drash, A.L., Uhrin, M., & Vergona, R. (1988) Immune responses to killed influenza vaccine in patients with type 1 diabetes: Altered responses associated with HLA-DR 3 and DR4. *Journal of Laboratory and Clinical Medicine*, 112, 595–602.

Ruckdeshel, J.C., Graziano, K.D., & Mardiney, M.R. (1975) Additional evidence that the cell-associated immune system is the primary host defense against measles (rubeola). *Cellular Immunology*, 17, 11–18.

Samb, B., Aaby, P., Whittle, H.C., Coll Seck, A.M., Rahman, S., Bennett, J., Markowitz, L., & Simondon, F. (1995) Serologic status and measles attack rates among vaccinated and unvaccinated children in rural Senegal. *Pediatric Infectious Disease Journal*, 14, 203–209.

Sampliner, R.E., Bias, W.B., Carney, E., Hillis, A., & Hillis, W.D. (1981) HLA antigens and HBV infection: Evaluation in the chronic carrier state and in a large family. *Tissue Antigens*, 18, 247–251.

Sarvas, H., Rautonen, N., Kayhty, H., Kallio, M., & Makela, O. (1990) Effect of Gm allotypes on IgG2 antibody responses and IgG2 concentrations in children and adults. *International Immunology*, 2, 317–322.

Schanfield, M.S., & Van Loghem, E.V. (1986) Human immunoglobulin allotypes. In *Handbook of Experimental Immunology*, Blackwell, Oxford, UK.

Schanfield, M.S., Wells, J.V., & Fudenberg, H.H. (1979) Immunoglobulin allotypes and response to tetanus toxoid in Papua, New Guinea. *Journal of Immunogenetics*, 6, 311–315.

Scobie, B., Woodfield, D.G., & Fong, R. (1983) Familial hepatocellular carcinoma and hepatitis B antigenemia in a New Zealand Chinese family. *Australian and New Zealand Journal of Medicine*, 13, 236–239.

Selvaraj, P., Reetha, A.M., Uma, H., Xavier, T., Janardhanam, B., Prabhakar, R., & Narayanan, P.R. (1996) Influence of HLA-DR and -DQ phenotypes on tuberculin reactive status in pulmonary tuberculosis patients. *Tubercle and Lung Disease*, 77, 369–373.

Sette, A., & Sidney, J. (1998) HLA supertypes and supermotifs: A functional perspective on HLA polymorphism. *Current Opinion in Immunology*, 10, 478–482.

Sette, A., & Sidney, J. (1999) Nine major HLA class I supertypes account for the vast preponderance of HLA-A and -B polymorphism. *Immunogenetics*, 50, 201–212.

Shanmugalakshmi, S., Dheenadhayalan, V., Muthuveeralakshmi, P., Arivarignan, G., & Pitchappan, R.M. (2003) *Mycobacterium bovis* BCG scar status and HLA class II alleles influence purified protein derivative-specific T-cell receptor Vb expression in pulmonary tuberculosis patients from southern India. *Infection and Immunity*, 71, 4544–4553.

Sidney, J., Grey, H.M., Kubo, R.T., & Sette, A. (1996) Practical, biochemical and evolutionary implications of the discovery of HLA class I supermotifs. *Immunology Today*, 17, 261–266.

Sidney, J., Southwood, S., Mann, D.L., Fernandez-Vina, M.A., Newman, M.J., & Sette, A. (2001) Majority of peptides binding HLA-A*0201 with high affinity crossreact with other A2-supertype molecules. *Human Immunology*, 62, 1200–1216.

Simons, J., Kutubuddin, M., & Chow, M. (1993) Characterization of poliovirus-specific T lymphocytes in the peripheral blood of Sabin-vaccinated humans. *Journal of Virology*, 67, 1262–1268.

Spencer, M.J., Cherry, J.D., & Terasaki, P.I. (1976) HLA antigens and antibody response after influenza A vaccination. Decreased response associated with HLA type W16. *New England Journal of Medicine*, 294, 13–16.

St. Sauver, J.L., Dhiman, N., Ovsyannikova, I.G., Jacobson, R.M., Vierkant, R.A., Pankratz, S.V., Jacobsen, S.J., & Poland, G.A. (2005) Extinction of the human leukocyte antigen homozygosity effect after two doses of the measles-mumps-rubella vaccine. *Human Immunology*, 66, 788–798.

St. Sauver, J.L., Ovsyannikova, I.G., Jacobson, R.M., Jacobsen, S.J., Vierkant, R.A., Schaid, D.J., Pankratz, V.S., Green, E.M., & Poland, G.A. (2002) Associations between human leukocyte antigen homozygosity and antibody levels to measles vaccine. *Journal of Infectious Diseases*, 185, 1545–1549.

Tang, J.M., Costello, C., Keet, I.P.M., Rivers, C., LeBlanc, S., Karita, E., Allen, S., & Kaslow, R.A. (1999) HLA class I homozygosity accelerates disease progression in human immunodeficiency virus type I infection. *AIDS Research and Human Retroviruses*, 15, 317–324.

Thio, C.L., Carrington, M., Marti, D., O'Brien, S.J., Vlahov, D., Nelson, K.E., Astemborski, J., & Thomas, D.L. (1999) Class II HLA alleles and Hepatitis B virus persistence in African Americans. *Journal of Infectious Diseases*, 179, 1004–1006.

Wachsmuth, R.R., Pandey, J.P., Fedrick, J.A., Nishimura, Y., & Sasazuki, T. (1987) Interactive effect of Gm and Km allotypes on cellular immune responses to streptococcal cell wall antigen. *Experimental and Clinical Immunogenetics*, 4, 163–166.

Wang, C., Tang, J., Song, W., Lobashevsky, E., Wilson, C.M., & Kaslow, R.A. (2004) HLA and cytokine gene polymorphisms are independently associated with responses to hepatitis B vaccination. *Hepatology*, 39, 978–988.

Wattigney, W.A., Mootrey, G.T., Braun, M.M., & Chen, R.T. (2001) Surveillance for poliovirus vaccine adverse events, 1991 to 1998: Impact of a sequential vaccination schedule of inactivated poliovirus vaccine followed by oral poliovirus vaccine. *Pediatrics*, 107, E83.

Wiencke, J.K., Kelsey, K.T., Zuo, Z.F., Weinberg, A., & Wrensch, M.R. (2001) Genetic resistance factor for HIV-1 and immune response to varicella zoster virus. *Lancet*, 357, 360–361.

Yang, P.M., Sung, J.L., & Chen, D.S. (1989) HLA-A, B, C and DR antigens in chronic hepatitis B viral infection. *Hepatogastroenterology*, 36, 363–366.

Yap, I., & Chan, S.H. (1996) A new pre-S containing recombinant hepatitis B vaccine and its effect on non-responders: A preliminary observation. *Annals of the Academy of Medicine, Singapore*, 25, 120–122.

Appendix

Selected Useful Web Sites

There is an ever-growing number of online resources for work on human genetic variation. This appendix lists Web sites selected useful for their general information about methods and projects and for their more specific databases, including resequencing data for several hundred genes, many of which are relevant to infection and immunity. Some databases can be reached simultaneously using sites such as snpper.chip.org/bio/snpper-explain, while links to multiple databases can be found at key Web sites such as www.ncbi.nih.gov.

www.allelefrequencies.net	Commercial consortium for immune response gene information
www.bris.ac.uk/cellmolmed/services/GAI/cytokine4.htm	Disease associations of cytokine gene variants
snp.cshl.org/	The SNP Consortium, commercial consortium for genomewide SNP documentation)
www.ebi.ac.uk/imgt/hla	European Bioinformatics Institute's HLA database
www.ensembl.org	A gene browser
geneticassociationdb.nih.gov/cgi-bin/index.cgi	Database of genetic associations by disease
genome.perlegen.com/browser/index.html	Perlegen Genotype Browser
www.genome.utah.edu/genesnps/	Gene SNPs
www.genes.org.uk/	Online encyclopedia for genetic epidemiology studies
www.hapmap.org/	International HapMap Project
www.meb.ki.se/genestat/genestat.htm	Tutorials in statistical genetics methods
www.ncbi/nlm/entrez	A gene browser
www.ncbi.nih.gov/omim	Online Mendelian Inheritance of Man database
www.ncbi.nih.gov/SNP/	SNP database, also known as dbSNP
www.ornl.gov/sci/techresources/Human_Genome/home.shtml	Human Genome Project information, 1990–2003
pga.gs.washington.edu/finished_genes.html	SeattleSNPs, plus links to several other sites with SNP data from resequencing projects
123genomics.homestead.com/files/home.html	Genomics, proteomics, and bioinformatics knowledge bases

Glossary

allele An alternative form of a gene or **locus** marker due to changes at the DNA level. A locus can have many different alleles, which may differ from each other by as little as a single base or by the complete absence of a sequence. For example, at the ABO blood group locus, there are three alleles A, B, and O.

allotype A protein product of an **allele** that may be detected as an antigen in another member of the same species. For example, the products of HLA genes in one individual are histocompatibility antigens that are recognized as foreign by another individual.

centimorgan (cM) A measure of relative genetic distance equivalent to 1/100 of a morgan and encompassing 1% **recombination**. One cM covers roughly 1,000,000 bp of DNA (but this can vary by orders of magnitudes either way). This term is named for Thomas Hunt Morgan.

complex trait (disease) A trait (disease) that has a genetic component that does not show strictly **Mendelian inheritance**. Complex traits may involve the interaction of two or more genes to produce a phenotype or may involve gene–environment interactions.

diplotype Two parental haplotypes, each consisting of two or more neighboring alleles (SNPs or other variants) in allelic relation to each other. For example, **single nucleotide polymorphisms** at two nearby positions in the CCL5 promoter (−403G −28C/−403A −28C) form a diplotype.

dizygotic twins Two simultaneous births resulting from fertilization of two separate ova by two spermatozoa. Dizygotic (fraternal) twins share an average of 50% of their genes.

epigenetics Phenomena of change in gene expression due to alterations other than the gene sequence (e.g., DNA methylation or histone deacetylation).

epistasis An interaction between nonallelic genes, especially an interaction in which one gene suppresses another.

expressivity Clinically apparent variation in the expression of a genetically determined effect trait (disease).

genetic heterogeneity Similar phenotypic expression due to **polymorphism** in different genes in different individuals. It may confound **linkage** analysis or association studies by suggesting true genetic relationships or by producing more false-positive relationships than would be expected.

genomewide scan An approach to identifying genes and gene variants contributing to **complex traits (diseases)** through analysis of large numbers of polymorphisms distributed at relatively equal intervals throughout the genome. **Linkage** and association studies using this approach can establish the profile of genetic variation of an individual or locate a region or gene accounting for susceptibility.

haplotype A linear, ordered combination of alleles (two or more **single nucleotide polymorphisms** or genes) at closely linked loci, inherited as a unit on the same chromosome. Alleles of a stable haplotypes are in **linkage disequilibrium**. An "ancestral haplotype" refers to a stable one that has been preserved through evolution within or across species. An "extended haplotype" refers to one covering multiple genes.

Hardy-Weinberg equilibrium A condition in which, with random mating in the absence of immigration, mutation, and selection, the allele frequencies at a single **locus** in each population remain fixed at a particular value. Equilibrium allele frequencies may differ among populations. Various genetic, environmental, and social factors can contribute to the deviation from equilibrium.

heritability In the narrow sense, heritability is defined as the proportion of the total phenotypic variance in a trait (disease) that is due to the additive effects of genes, as opposed to dominance or environmental effects. In the broad sense, heritability is proportion of the total phenotypic variance of a trait that is due to all genetic effects, including additive and dominance effects.

433

heterozygote advantage Selection force favoring heterozygotes over homozygotes in protection against lethal or otherwise deleterious traits. The occurrence or degree of advantage is not predictable.

heterozygous The two paired alleles at a **locus** that differ from one another on a chromosome pair. An individual with blood type AB is heterozygous at the ABO blood group locus.

homolog A gene closely related to another by descent from common DNA sequence. Homologs may occur in the same species (see **paralog**) or in different species (see **ortholog**).

homozygous The two paired alleles at a **locus** that are identical to one another on a chromosome pair. An individual who has blood type O is homozygous for the O allele.

identity-by-descent (IBD) Two alleles determined with certainty to have been inherited from a common ancestor. For example, a mother with blood type O and father with blood type AB have two children, each with blood type A. Since the genotypes of the children are AO, the children share one allele IBD, the A allele. Whether the maternally inherited O allele is IBD in the children is unclear since the mother is **homozygous** for the O allele.

isoform A protein that has the same function as another protein but is encoded by a different gene. Isoforms may have small differences in their sequences.

linkage Inheritance of two or more genes physically located on the same chromosome as a single unit, with parallel inheritance of the functions of those genes. In general, the closer the two genes are to each other physically, the tighter the linkage.

linkage disequilibrium (LD) Nonrandom association of alleles at two or more loci, particularly neighboring loci. LD describes a situation in which some combinations of alleles or genetic markers occur more or less frequently in a population than would be expected from a random assortment of alleles based on their individual frequencies. "Disequilibrium" refers to deviation from the predicted **Hardy-Weinberg equilibrium**. LD is not the same as **linkage**).

locus Any genomic site (segment of DNA or position on a chromosome) that can be mapped through formal genetic analysis.

LOD score The base-10 logarithm of the likelihood of the odds ratio for **linkage**. Traditionally, LOD scores have been used to investigate genetic disorders where the mode of inheritance is well defined. LOD scores greater than or equal to 3.0 provide evidence in favor of linkage; LOD scores less than or equal to –2.0 provide evidence against linkage; LOD scores between –2.0 and 3.0 indicate that additional data are required before a definite conclusion can be reached. LOD scores may be reported in association with a theta, the **recombination fraction**.

Mendelian inheritance Referring to Gregor Mendel, the predictable manner in which he described individual genes and traits to be passed from parents to children. This may include autosomal dominant, autosomal recessive, and sex-linked genes and traits.

microsatellite A short block of DNA sequence (see **short tandem repeat**), often less than 150 bp long, that is repeated many times within the genome of an organism. Many repeats tend to be concentrated at the same **locus**. Microsatellites represent one type of **polymorphism** useful for population studies.

monozygotic twins Two simultaneous births resulting from the division of a single ovum fertilized by a single spermatozoon. Monozygotic (identical) twins share 100% of their genes. They represent subjects with maximum attainable heritability.

nonparametric analysis A type of **linkage** analysis that relies on some specification of components of the genetic model (in contrast to all components of the genetic model), but usually not the degree of dominance. For example, affected relative pair methods of linkage analysis require the specification of allele frequencies.

ortholog A gene closely related to another by mutation, occurring in a separate species but retaining the same function (see **homolog**). MHC class I and II genes are orthologous to each other in primates and humans.

overdominance A relationship in which the phenotypic expression of the heterozygote is greater than that of either homozygote; it may be an indication of heterozygote advantage.

paralog A gene closely related to another by duplication, occurring in the same species but with similar or new function (see **Homolog**). The 10 human Toll-like receptor genes are paralogous to each other.

parametric analysis A statistical test is considered to be parametric when it requires the specification of an underlying model. For example, the **LOD score** approach to **linkage** analysis is a parametric test since it requires the specification of all components of the genetic model.

penetrance The proportion of individuals with a specific genotype who display a specific phenotype associated with that genotype. Adjectives such as "incomplete," "complete," and "variable" are usually used as modifiers to reflect the influence of other genetic and environmental factors on the manifestation of the phenotype.

polymorphism The presence of alternative nucleotides at a specific site in genomic DNA of an organism—any mutation or variation (a single nucleotide change, a variable repeat motif, an insertion or deletion, or duplication of a chromosomal segment) detected at a reproducible frequency in a population (usually set as >1%). The frequency of a polymorphism may vary across populations and is therefore highly useful in studying population effects of genetic variation (see **single nucleotide polymorphism**, Segmental duplication).

population stratification (also ethnic stratification, population substructure, latent class effects) Differences in frequencies of alleles in affected and unaffected populations due to their different ethnic/geographic backgrounds. Population stratification may be more or less likely to confound disease association studies depending on the origins of the study populations.

proband The individual in a pedigree first identified by medical or research personnel.

quantitative trait A phenotype that can vary in a quantitative manner when measured among different individuals. The variation in expression can be due to combinations of genetic and environmental factors, as well as a chance. Quantitative traits are often controlled by the cumulative action of alleles at multiple loci. Such a region may be called a quantitative trait locus (QTL).

recombination Formation of new combinations and arrangements of genes during meiosis. Recombination is achieved by crossing over, independent assortment, and segregation.

recombination fraction (theta, θ) The frequency of crossing over between two loci. Estimates of the recombination fraction between two loci that are less than 0.50 are consistent with the loci being linked to one another;

estimates of the recombination fraction that are equal to 0.50 are consistent with the loci being unlinked to one another. Recombination fraction estimates > 0.50 for two loci may suggest an area of high recombination or data error. In **linkage** studies, when theta = 0, the marker and disease gene are at the same **locus**.

segmental duplication (also copy number variation, CNV, or copy number **polymorphism**) A specific type of polymorphism involving single genes or multiple linked genes (segments) that are duplicated, usually near each other, in numbers that may vary among populations.

short tandem repeat (STR) A series of repeated nucleotide sequences, with variable number of repeats and each repeat usually in a pattern of identical two to five nucleotides but occasionally longer. For example, TCCTCCTCC is a trinucleotide repeat element. STRs are found throughout the genome and have been used as polymorphic signature markers in population studies.

single nucleotide polymorphism (SNP) A site variation in a DNA sequence (see **polymorphism**).

stop codon One of three codons (UAA, UAG, UGA) that terminate polypeptide synthesis at the stage of translation.

variable number tandem repeat (VNTR) A **locus** or region of DNA with different numbers of tandemly repeated sequences (see **short tandem repeat**).

Index

Boldface entries denote in-depth coverage of a topic.